Comprehensive Evaluation & Treatment: Provides a step-wise approach to the evaluation and treatment of coma, seizures, shock, and other common complications of poisoning and to the proper use of gastric decontamination and dialysis procedures.

Emergency Treatment

Specific Poisons & Drugs: Diagnosis & Treatment: Alphabetical listing of specific drugs and poisons, including the pathophysiology, toxic dose and level, clinical presentation, diagnosis, and specific treatment associated with each substance.

Common Poisons & Drugs

Therapeutic Drugs & Antidotes: Descriptions of therapeutic drugs and antidotes discussed in the two preceding sections, including their pharmacology, indications, adverse effects, drug interactions, recommended dosage, and formulations.

Antidotes & Drug Therapy

Environmental & Occupational Toxicology: Approach to hazardous materials incidents; evaluation of occupational exposures; and the toxic effects, physical properties, and workplace exposure limits for over 500 common industrial chemicals.

Industrial Chemicals

Index: Includes generic drug and chemical names and numerous brand name drugs and commercial products.

Index

D1057690

third edition

POISONING
& DRUG
OVERDOSE

by the faculty, staff and associates of
the California Poison Control System

Edited by
Kent R. Olson, MD, FACEP
Medical Director
California Poison Control System, San Francisco Division
San Francisco General Hospital
Attending Emergency Physician
Eden Hospital Medical Center
Clinical Professor of Medicine, Pediatrics, and Pharmacy
University of California, San Francisco

Associate Editors

Ilene B. Anderson, PharmD
Senior Toxicology Management Specialist
California Poison Control System,
San Francisco Division
Associate Clinical Professor of Pharmacy
University of California, San Francisco

Neal L. Benowitz, MD
Associate Medical Director
California Poison Control System,
San Francisco Division
Professor of Medicine
Chief, Division of Clinical Pharmacology
& Toxicology
University of California, San Francisco

Paul D. Blanc, MD, MSPH
Assistant Medical Director
California Poison Control System,
San Francisco Division
Associate Professor of Medicine
Chief, Division of Occupational
& Environmental Medicine
University of California, San Francisco

Richard F. Clark, MD, FACEP
Medical Director
California Poison Control System,
San Diego Division
Associate Professor of Clinical Medicine
Director
Division of Medical Toxicology
University of California, San Diego

Thomas E. Kearney, PharmD, ABAT
Managing Director
California Poison Control System,
San Francisco Division
Clinical Professor of Pharmacy
University of California, San Francisco

John D. Osterloh, MD
Attending Toxicologist
California Poison Control System,
San Francisco Division
Associate Chief, Biochemistry/Toxicology
San Francisco General Hospital
Professor of Clinical Laboratory Medicine
University of California, San Francisco

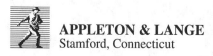
APPLETON & LANGE
Stamford, Connecticut

Copyright © 1999 by Appleton & Lange
A Simon & Schuster Company
Copyright © 1990, 1994 by Appleton & Lange

www.appletonlange.com

99 00 01 02 03 / 10 9 8 7 6 5 4 3 2 1

QV
39
S195p
1999

Prentice Hall International (UK) Limited, *London*
Prentice Hall of Australia Pty. Limited, *Sydney*
Prentice Hall Canada, Inc., *Toronto*
Prentice Hall Hispanoamericana, S.A., *Mexico*
Prentice Hall of India Private Limited, *New Delhi*
Prentice Hall of Japan, Inc., *Tokyo*
Simon & Schuster Asia Pte. Ltd., *Singapore*
Editor Prentice Hall do Brasil Ltda., *Rio de Janeiro*
Prentice Hall, Upper Saddle River, *New Jersey*

ISBN: 0-8385-0260-1
ISSN: 1048-8847

ISBN 0-8385-0260-1

Senior Acquisitions Editor: Shelley Reinhardt
Senior Development Editor: Cara Coffey
Production Editor: Jeanmarie Roche
Art Coordinator: Eve Siegel

PRINTED IN THE UNITED STATES OF AMERICA

Contents

Authors

Timothy E. Albertson, MD, PhD, FACEP, FACMT
Professor of Medicine and Medical Pharmacology/Toxicology, School of Medicine,
University of California, Davis, Davis Medical Center, Sacramento.
Internet: tealbertson@ucdavis.edu
Section II: Barbiturates; Dextromethorphan; Opiates and Opioids

Judith A. Alsop, PharmD, ABAT
Associate Clinical Professor, School of Pharmacy, University of California, San Francisco;
Associate Clinical Professor, School of Medicine, University of California, Davis.
Internet: jalsop@itsa.ucsf.edu
Section III: Metoclopramide; Ondansetron

Ilene B. Anderson, PharmD
Associate Clinical Professor of Pharmacy, University of California, San Francisco; Senior
Toxicology Management Specialist, California Poison Control System, San Francisco
Division.
Internet: iba@itsa.ucsf.edu
*Section II: Camphor and Other Essential Oils; Coumarin and Related Rodenticides;
Ethylene Glycol and Other Glycols; Lomotil and Other Antidiarrheals; Methanol; Nontoxic
or Minimally Toxic Household Products*

John R. Balmes, MD
Professor of Medicine, University of California, San Francisco; Chief, Division of
Occupational and Environmental Medicine, San Francisco General Hospital.
Section II: Asbestos; Formaldehyde; Gases, Irritant; Phosgene; Sulfur Dioxide

Neal L. Benowitz, MD
Professor of Medicine and Chief, Division of Clinical Pharmacology and Toxicology,
University of California, San Francisco; Associate Medical Director, California Poison
Control System, San Francisco Division.
Internet: nbeno@itsa. ucsf.edu
*Section II: Amphetamines; Anesthetics, Local; Antiarrhythmic Drugs; Antidepressants
(noncyclic); Beta-adrenergic Blockers; Calcium Antagonists; Cardiac Glycosides;
Chloroquine and Other Aminoquinolines; Cocaine; Colchicine; Ergot Derivatives; Lithium;
Marijuana; Monamine Oxidase Inhibitors; Nicotine; Nitrates and Nitrites;
Phenylpropanolamine and Related Decongestants; Quinidine and Other Type 1a
Antiarrhythmic Drugs; Quinine; Strychnine; Tricyclic Antidepressants; Vacor (PNU).
Section III: Dopamine; Epinephrine; Norepinephrine*

Paul D. Blanc, MD, MSPH
Associate Professor of Medicine and Chief, Division of Occupational and Environmental
Medicine, University of California, San Francisco; Assistant Medical Director, California
Poison Control System, San Francisco Division.
*Section II: Cyanide; Dioxins; Isocyanates; Manganese; Metal Fume Fever;
Methemoglobinemia.   Section IV: Evaluation of the Patient with Occupational Chemical
Exposure*

Christopher R. Brown, MD
Assistant Clinical Professor, University of California, San Francisco; Director, Intensive
Care Unit, California Pacific Medical Center, San Francisco.
Section II: Amantadine; Caffeine; Isoniazid

Randall G. Browning, MD, MPH
Tri-City Emergency Medical Group, Oceanside, California.
Internet: browning@tcemg.com
Section II: Carbon Tetrachloride; Chloroform

Alan Buchwald, MD, FACEP, ACMT
Staff Physician, Emergency Department, and Medical Director, Occupational Health Center, Dominican Santa Cruz Hospital, Santa Cruz, California.
Internet: albuchwald955@pol.net
Section II: Benzene

Richard F. Clark, MD, FACEP
Associate Professor of Clinical Medicine and Director, Division of Medical Toxicology, School of Medicine, University of California, San Diego; Medical Director, California Poison Control System, San Diego Division.
Internet: rfclark@ucsd.edu
Section II: Hymenoptera; Lionfish and Other Scorpaenidae; Scorpions; Snakebite; Spiders. Section III: Antivenin, Crotalidae (Rattlesnake); Antivenin, Latrodectus Mactans (Black Widow Spider); Antivenin, Micrurus Fulvius (Coral Snake)

Delia Dempsey, MD
Assistant Professor, Department of Pediatrics and Clinical Pharmacology, University of California, San Francisco.
Section I: Special Considerations in Pediatric Patients. Section II: Bromides; Lead; Methyl Bromide; Pentachlorophenol and Dinitrophenol

Jo Ellen Dyer, PharmD
Assistant Clinical Professor of Pharmacy, University of California, San Francisco; Senior Toxicology Management Specialist, California Poison Control System, San Francisco Division.
Section II: Azide, Sodium; GHB

Brent R. Ekins, PharmD, ABAT
Assistant Clinical Professor, School of Pharmacy, University of California, San Francisco; Adjunct Professor, School of Pharmacy, University of the Pacific, Stockton, California; Managing Director, California Poison Control System, Fresno Division.
Internet: bekins@valleychildrens.org
Section II: Chlorinated Hydrocarbon Pesticides; Pyrethrins and Pyrethroids. Section III: Atropine; Pralidoxime (2-PAM)

Thomas J. Ferguson, MD, PhD
Associate Clinical Professor of Internal Medicine, School of Medicine, University of California, Davis; Medical Director, Employee Health Services, University of California, Davis.
Internet: tjferguson@ucdavis.edu
Section II: Chromium; Thallium

Mark Galbo, MS
Environmental Toxicologist, California Poison Control System, San Francisco Division.
Internet: mjgalbo@itsa.ucsf.edu
Section II: Naphthalene and Paradichlorobenzene

Rick Geller, MD
Medical Director, California Poison Control System, Fresno Division.
Section II: Disulfiram; Paraquat and Diquat

Christine A. Haller, MD
Fellow in Clinical Pharmacology and Toxicology, University of California, San Francisco.
Section II: Table II–45.

Patricia H. Hiatt, BS
Administrative Operations Manager, California Poison Control System, San Francisco Division; University of California, San Francisco.
Internet: phiatt@itsa.ucsf.edu
Section IV: The Toxic Hazards of Industrial and Occupational Chemicals & Table IV–4

B. Zane Horowitz, MD
Associate Professor of Emergency Medicine and Clinical Toxicology, School of Medicine, University of California, Davis, and the Oregon Health Services University, Oregon Poison Center, Portland.
Internet: horowiza@ohsu.edu
Section II: Copper; Ethanol

Gerald Joe, PharmD
Assistant Clinical Professor of Pharmacy, University of California, San Francisco.
Internet: gerald@itsa.ucsf.edu
Section II: Fluoracetate; Jellyfish and Other Cnidaria; Metaldehyde; Vitamins

Thomas E. Kearney, PharmD, ABAT
Clinical Professor, School of Pharmacy, University of California, San Francisco; Managing Director, California Poison Control System, San Francisco Division.
Internet: pcctk@itsa.ucsf.edu
Section II: Valproic Acid. Section III: Introduction; Acetylcysteine (N-Acetylcysteine, NAC); Apomorphine; Benzodiazepines (Diazepam, Lorazepam, and Midazolam); Benztropine; Bicarbonate, Sodium; Botulin Antitoxin; Bretylium; Bromocriptine; Calcium; Charcoal-Activated; Cimetidine and H_2 Blockers; Dantrolene; Diazoxide; Digoxin-specific Antibodies; Diphenhydramine; Esmolol; Ethanol; Fromepizole (4-MP); Glucagon; Glucose; Haloperidol; Isoproterenol; Labetalol; Lidocaine; Methocarbamol; Morphine; Neuromuscular Blockers; Nicotinamide (niacinamide); Nifedipine; Nitroprusside; Octreotide; Oxygen; Penicillamine; Pentobarbital; Phenobarbital; Phentolamine; Physostigmine; Propranolol; Protamine; Pyridoxine (Vitamin B_6); Thiamine (Vitamin B_1); Vitamin K_1 (Phytonadione)

Kathryn H. Keller, PharmD
Associate Clinical Professor, Division of Clinical Pharmacy, University of California, San Francisco; Senior Toxicology Management Specialist, California Poison Control System, San Francisco Division.
Internet: kkeller@itsa.ucsf.edu
Section II: Bromates; Chlorates; Ipecac Syrup; Nonsteroidal Anti-inflammatory Drugs; Phenytoin.   Section III: Folic Acid; Hydroxocobalamin; Leucovorin Calcium; Methylene Blue; Nitrite, Sodium and Amyl; Phenytoin and Fosphenytoin

Susan Kim, PharmD
Associate Clinical Professor of Pharmacy, University of California, San Francisco; Senior Toxicology Management Specialist, California Poison Control System, San Francisco Division.
Internet: susank@itsa.ucsf.edu
Section II: Antidiabetic Agents; Antineoplastic Agents; Beta-2-Adrenergic Stimulants; Food Poisoning: Bacterial; Food Poisoning: Fish and Shellfish; Salicylates.   Section III: Thiosulfate; Sodium

Michael J. Kosnett, MD, MPH
Assistant Clinical Professor, Drew University of Medicine and Science, Los Angeles, and University of Colorado Health Sciences Center, Denver.
Internet: michael.kosnett@uchsc.edu
Section III: EDTA, Calcium

Diane Liu, MD, MPH
Assistant Clinical Professor of Medicine, University of California, San Francisco.
Section II: Polychlorinated Biphenyls (PCBs); Trichloroethane and Trichloroethylene

Anthony S. Manoguerra, PharmD, ABAT
Professor of Clinical Pharmacy, School of Pharmacy, University of California, San Francisco; Managing Director, California Poison Control System, San Diego Division.
Internet: amanoguerra@ucsd.edu
Section III: Amrinone; Deferoxamine; Ipecac Syrup

Timothy McCarthy, PharmD
Assistant Clinical Professor of Pharmacy, University of California, San Francisco.
Internet: tmccarthy@sfghpcc.ucsf.edu
Section II: Paraldehyde.

Kathryn Meier, PharmD
Assistant Clinical Professor of Pharmacy, University of California, San Francisco;
Toxicology Management Specialist, California Poison Control System, San Francisco
Division.
Section II: Dapsone; Fluoride; Magnesium

Walter Mullen, PharmD
Assistant Clinical Professor of Pharmacy, University of California, San Francisco;
Toxicology Management Specialist, California Poison Control System, San
Francisco Division.
Internet: w@wtnx.com
Section II: Caustic and Corrosive Agents; Iodine.   Section III: Flumazenil

Frank Mycroft, PhD, MPH
Toxicologist, California Environmental Protection Agency.
Internet: mycroft@pacbell.net
Section IV: Toxic Hazards of Industrial and Occupational Chemicals & Table IV–4

Kent R. Olson, MD, FACEP
Clinical Professor of Medicine, Pediatrics, & Pharmacy, University of California, San
Francisco; Attending Emergency Physician, Eden Hospital Medical Center, Castro Valley,
California; Medical Director, California Poison Control System, San Francisco Division.
Internet: olson@itsa.ucsf.edu
Section I: Emergency Evaluation & Treatment.   Section II: Acetaminophen; Cadmium;
Carbon Monoxide; Hydrogen Fluoride and Hydrofluoric Acid; Mushrooms; Nitrogen
Oxides; Nitrous Oxide; Oxalic Acid; PCP; Theophylline.   Section IV: Emergency Medical
Response to Hazmat

Michael O'Malley, MD, MPH
Associate Clinical Professor, School of Medicine, University of California, Davis.
Internet: maomalley@ucdavis.edu
Section II: Chlorophenoxy Herbicides

Gary Joseph Ordog, MD, FAACT, FACEP, FABFE, FABME
Medical Director, Department of Medical Toxicology, Henry Mayo Newhall Medical Center,
University of California, Los Angeles.
Section II: Detergents; Hydrocarbons

John D. Osterloh, MD
Professor of Clinical Laboratory Medicine, University of California, San Francisco;
Associate Chief, Biochemistry/Toxicology, San Francisco General Hospital; Attending
Toxicologist, California Poison Control System, San Francisco Division.
Section I: Toxicology Screening

Paul D. Pearigen, MD, FACEP
Residency Program Director, Department of Emergency Medicine, Naval Medical Center,
San Diego.
Internet: pearigen@snd10.med.navy.mil
Section II: Methylene Chloride; Sedative-Hypnotic Agents; Thyroid Hormone

Brett A. Roth, MD
Fellow in Clinical Pharmacology and Toxicology, University of California, San Francisco.
Section II: Hydrogen Sulfide; Isopropyl Alcohol; Vasodilators.   Section III: Nalaxone and
Nalmefene

Dennis J. Shusterman, MD, MPH
Associate Clinical Professor, Division of Occupational and Environmental Medicine,
University of California, San Francisco.
Internet; dennis@itsa.ucsf.edu
Section II: Freons and Halons

Karl A. Sporer, MD
Assistant Clinical Professor of Surgery, University of California, San Francisco; Attending
Emergency Physician, San Francisco General Hospital.
Section II: Benzodiazepines; LSD and Other Hallucinogens; Phenothiazines and Other
Antipsychotic Drugs; Skeletal Muscle Relaxants; Tetanus

S. Alan Tani, PharmD
Assistant Clinical Professor of Pharmacy, University of California, San Francisco;
Toxicology Management Specialist, California Poison Control System, San Francisco
Division.
Internet: atani@itsa.ucsf.edu
Section II: Anticholinergics; Antihistamines

R. Steven Tharratt, MD
Associate Professor of Medicine, School of Medicine, University of California, Davis;
Associate Regional Medical Director, California Poison Control System, Davis Division.
Internet: rstharratt@ucdavis.edu
Section II: Ammonia; Chlorine.   Section IV: Emergency Medical Response to Hazmat

Peter Wald, MD, MPH
Associate Clinical Professor of Occupational Medicine, School of Medicine, University of
Southern California, Los Angeles; Corporate Medical Director, ARCO, Los Angeles.
Internet: pwald@mail.arco.com
Section II: Antimony and Stibine; Arsine; Phosphine and Phosphides; Phosphorus

Jonathan Wasserberger, MD
Professor of Emergency Medicine, Charles R. Drew University of Medicine, King Drew Med-
ical Center, Los Angeles, and School of Medicine, University of California, Los Angeles.
Section II: Detergents; Hydrocarbons

Janet S. Weiss, MD
Adjunct Assistant Clinical Professor of Medicine, Department of Occupational Medicine,
University of California, San Francisco.
Internet: jweiss@pacbell.net
Section II: Ethylene Dibromide; Selenium; Toluene and Xylene

Saralyn R. Williams, MD
Assistant Clinical Professor of Medicine, School of Medicine, University of California, San
Diego; Assistant Medical Director, California Poison Control System, San Diego Division.
Internet: srwilliams@ucsd.edu
Section II: Arsenic; Mercury. Section III: BAL (Dimercaprol); DMSA (Succimer)

Olga F. Woo, PharmD
Associate Clinical Professor of Pharmacy, University of California, San Francisco.
Internet: ow4849@itsa.ucsf.edu
*Section II: Ace Inhibitors; Antibiotics; Antiseptics and Disinfectants; Barium; Boric Acid
and Boron; Botulism; Carbamazepine; Clonidine and Related Drugs; Iron;
Organophosphates and Carbamates; Phenol and Related Compounds; Plants and Herbal
Medicines*

Evan Wythe, MD
Associate Director, Eden Emergency Medical Group, Inc., Castro Valley, California
Internet: wythe@aol.com
Section II: Radiation (Ionizing)

Shoshana Zevin, MD
Department of Internal Medicine, Shaare Zedek Medical Center, Jerusalem, Israel.
Internet: szevia@md2.huji.ac.il
Section II: Diuretics; Mushrooms

Preface

Poisoning & Drug Overdose provides practical advice for the diagnosis and management of poisoning and drug overdose and concise information about common industrial chemicals. The manual is divided into four sections and an index, each identified by a black tab in the right margin. **Section I** leads the reader through initial emergency management, including treatment of coma, hypotension, and other common complications; physical and laboratory diagnosis; and methods of decontamination and enhanced elimination of poisons. **Section II** provides detailed information for about 150 common drugs and poisons. **Section III** describes the use and side effects of about 60 antidotes and therapeutic drugs. **Section IV** describes the medical management of chemical spills and occupational chemical exposures and includes a table of over 500 chemicals. The **Index** is comprehensive and extensively cross-referenced.

The manual is designed to allow the reader to move quickly from section to section, obtaining the needed information from each. For example, in managing a patient with isoniazid intoxication, the reader will find specific information about isoniazid toxicity in **Section II,** practical advice for gut decontamination and management of complications such as seizures in **Section I,** and detailed information about dosing and side effects for the antidote pyridoxine in **Section III.**

ACKNOWLEDGMENTS

The success of the first and second editions of this manual would not have been possible without the combined efforts of the staff, faculty, and fellows of the San Francisco Bay Area Regional Poison Control Center, to whom I am deeply indebted. From its inception, this book has been a project by and for our poison center; as a result, all royalties from its sale have gone to our center's operating fund and not to any individual editor or author.

In January 1997, four independent poison control centers joined their talents and vision to become the California Poison Control System, administered by the University of California, San Francisco. With this change, the manual becomes a project of our statewide system, bringing in new authors and editors.

On behalf of the authors and editors of the third edition, my sincere thanks go to all those who contributed to the first and second editions:

Ilene Brewer Anderson, PharmD (1st & 2nd ed.)
Margaret Atterbury, MD (1st ed.)
Georgeanne M. Backman (1st ed.)
John Balmes, MD (2nd ed.)
Charles E. Becker, MD (1st & 2nd ed.)
Neal L. Benowitz, MD (1st & 2nd ed.)
Bruce Bernard, MD (1st ed.)
Paul D. Blanc, MD, MSPH (1st & 2nd ed.)
James F. Buchanan, PharmD (1st ed.)
Delia Dempsey, MD (2nd ed.)
Chris Dutra, MD (1st ed.)
Jo Ellen Dyer, PharmD (2nd ed.)
Donna E. Foliart, MD, MPH (1st ed.)
Mark J. Galbo, MS (2nd ed.)
Gail M. Gullickson, MD (1st ed.)
Patricia H. Hiatt, BS (1st & 2nd ed.)
Gerald Joe, PharmD (2nd ed.)

Jeffrey R. Jones, MPH, CIH (1st ed.)
Belle L. Lee, PharmD (1st ed.)
Diane Liu, MD, MPH (2nd ed.)
Thomas E. Kearney, PharmD, ABAT (2nd ed.)
Kathryn H. Keller, PharmD (1st & 2nd ed.)
Michael T. Kelley, MD (1st ed.)
Susan Y. Kim, PharmD (1st & 2nd ed.)
Michael Kosnett, MD (2nd ed.)
Timothy D. McCarthy, PharmD (1st & 2nd ed.)
Howard E. McKinney, PharmD (1st ed.)
Kathryn H. Meier, PharmD (2nd ed.)
Frank J. Mycroft, PhD, MPH (1st & 2nd ed.)
Kent R. Olson, MD (1st & 2nd ed.)
John D. Osterloh, MD (1st & 2nd ed.)
Gary Pasternak, MD (1st ed.)
Karl A. Sporer, MD (2nd ed.)

S. Alan Tani, PharmD (2nd ed.)   Olga F. Woo, PharmD (1st & 2nd ed.)
Mary Tweig, MD (1st ed.)   Evan T. Wythe, MD (1st & 2nd ed.)
Peter H. Wald, MD, MPH (1st ed.)   Peter Yip, MD (1st ed.)

We are also grateful for the numerous comments and suggestions received from colleagues, students, and the editorial staff at Appleton & Lange, which helped us to improve the manual with each edition.

Finally, a special thanks to Donna, Brad, Marlene, and Greg, for their patience, love, and support.

Kent R. Olson, MD, FACEP

San Francisco, California
September 1998

SECTION I. Comprehensive Evaluation and Treatment

▶ EMERGENCY EVALUATION AND TREATMENT

Kent R. Olson, MD

Even though they may not appear acutely ill, all poisoned patients should be treated as if they have a potentially life-threatening intoxication. Below is a checklist (Figure I–1) of emergency evaluation and treatment procedures. More detailed information on diagnosis and treatment for each emergency step is referenced by page and presented immediately after the checklist.

When you are treating suspected poisoning cases, **quickly review the checklist** to determine the scope of appropriate interventions and **begin needed life-saving treatment.** If further information is required for any step, turn to the cited pages for detailed discussion of each topic. Although the checklist is presented in a **sequential format,** many steps may be performed **simultaneously** (eg, airway management, naloxone and dextrose administration, and gastric lavage).

AIRWAY

I. **Assessment.** The most common factor contributing to death from drug overdose or poisoning is loss of airway-protective reflexes with subsequent airway obstruction caused by the flaccid tongue, pulmonary aspiration of gastric contents, or respiratory arrest. All poisoning patients should be suspected of having a potentially compromised airway.

A. **Patients who are awake** and talking are likely to have intact airway reflexes, but should be monitored closely because worsening intoxication can result in rapid loss of airway control.

B. **In lethargic or obtunded patients,** the gag or cough reflex may be an indirect indication of the patient's ability to protect the airway. If there is any doubt, it is best to perform endotracheal intubation (see below).

II. **Treatment.** Optimize the airway position and perform endotracheal intubation if necessary. Early use of naloxone (see pp 19 and 384) or flumazenil (see pp 19 and 369) may awaken a patient intoxicated with opiates or benzodiazepines, respectively, and obviate the need for endotracheal intubation.

A. **Position the patient and clear the airway** (see Figure I–2).

1. **Optimize the airway position** to force the flaccid tongue forward and to maximize the airway opening. The following techniques are useful. *Caution:* Do *not* perform neck manipulation if you suspect a neck injury.

a. Place the neck and head in the **"sniffing" position,** with the neck flexed forward and the head extended (Figure I–2b).

b. Apply the **"jaw thrust"** to create forward movement of the tongue without flexing or extending the neck. Pull the jaw forward by placing the fingers of each hand on the angle of the mandible just below the ears (Figure I–2c). (This motion also provides a painful stimulus to the angle of the jaw, the response to which indicates the patient's depth of coma.)

c. Place the patient in a **head-down, left-sided position** that allows the tongue to fall forward and secretions or vomitus to drain out of the mouth (Figure I–2d).

2. If the airway is still not patent, examine the oropharynx and **remove any obstruction or secretions** by suction, by a sweep with the finger, or with Magill forceps.

3. The airway can also be maintained with **artificial oropharyngeal or nasopharyngeal airway devices.** These are placed in the mouth or nose to lift the tongue and push it forward. They are only temporary measures. A

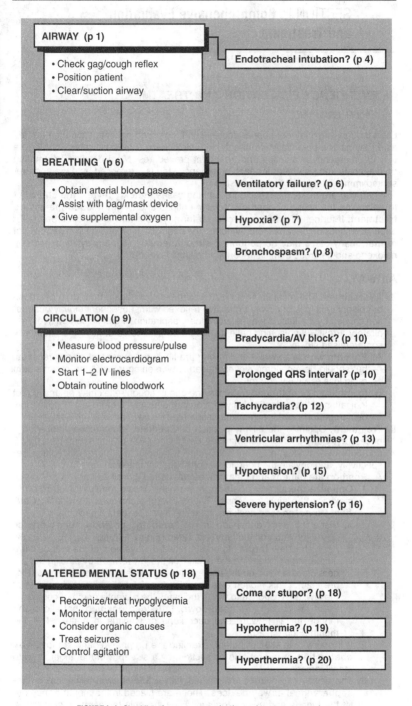

FIGURE I–1. Checklist of emergency evaluation and treatment procedures.

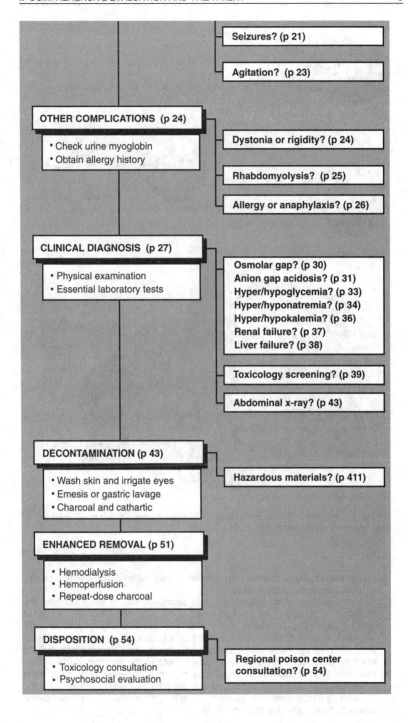

Seizures? (p 21)

Agitation? (p 23)

OTHER COMPLICATIONS (p 24)

• Check urine myoglobin
• Obtain allergy history

Dystonia or rigidity? (p 24)

Rhabdomyolysis? (p 25)

Allergy or anaphylaxis? (p 26)

CLINICAL DIAGNOSIS (p 27)

• Physical examination
• Essential laboratory tests

Osmolar gap? (p 30)
Anion gap acidosis? (p 31)
Hyper/hypoglycemia? (p 33)
Hyper/hyponatremia? (p 34)
Hyper/hypokalemia? (p 36)
Renal failure? (p 37)
Liver failure? (p 38)

Toxicology screening? (p 39)

Abdominal x-ray? (p 43)

DECONTAMINATION (p 43)

• Wash skin and irrigate eyes
• Emesis or gastric lavage
• Charcoal and cathartic

Hazardous materials? (p 411)

ENHANCED REMOVAL (p 51)

• Hemodialysis
• Hemoperfusion
• Repeat-dose charcoal

DISPOSITION (p 54)

• Toxicology consultation
• Psychosocial evaluation

Regional poison center
consultation? (p 54)

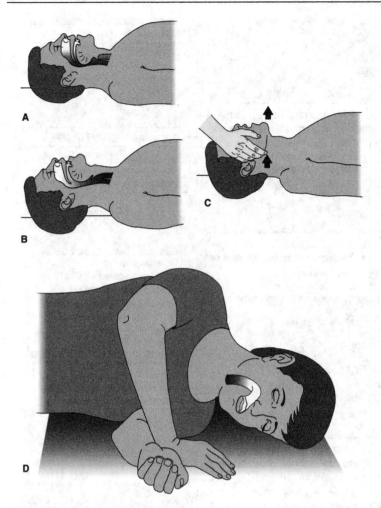

FIGURE I–2. Airway positioning. A: Normal position. B: "Sniffing" position. C: "Jaw thrust" maneuver. D: Left-side, head-down position, showing nasal and oral airway.

patient who can tolerate an artificial airway without complaint probably needs an endotracheal tube.

B. Perform endotracheal intubation if personnel trained in the procedure are available. Intubation of the trachea provides the most reliable protection of the airway, preventing aspiration and obstruction and allowing for mechanically assisted ventilation. However, it is not a simple procedure and *should be attempted only by those with training and experience*. Complications include vomiting with pulmonary aspiration; local trauma to the oropharynx, nasopharynx, and larynx; inadvertent intubation of the esophagus or a main stem bronchus; and failure to intubate the patient after respiratory arrest has been induced by a neuromuscular blocker. There are two routes for endotracheal intubation: nasotracheal and orotracheal.

1. Nasotracheal intubation. In nasotracheal intubation, a soft flexible tube is passed through the nose and into the trachea, by using a "blind" technique (Figure I–3a).

  a. Technique

    (1) Instill local anesthetic and insert a vasoconstrictor into the patient's nose before the procedure to limit pain and bleeding. Use phenylephrine spray and 2% lidocaine jelly or 3–4 mL of a 5% cocaine solution.

    (2) Pass the nasotracheal tube gently through the nose and into the nasopharynx. As the patient inspires, gently but firmly push the tube into the trachea. Success is usually marked by abrupt coughing.

    (3) Check breathing sounds to rule out accidental esophageal intubation or intubation of the right main-stem bronchus.

    (4) Secure the tube and fill the cuff balloon. (Tubes used for children do not have inflatable cuffs.)

    (5) Obtain a chest x-ray to confirm appropriate tube placement.

  b. Advantages

    (1) May be performed in a conscious patient without requiring neuromuscular paralysis.

    (2) Once placed, it is better tolerated than an orotracheal tube.

  c. Disadvantages

    (1) Perforation of the nasal mucosa with epistaxis.

    (2) Stimulation of vomiting in an obtunded patient.

    (3) Patient must be breathing spontaneously.

    (4) Anatomically more difficult in infants because of their anterior epiglottis.

2. Orotracheal intubation. In orotracheal intubation, the tube is passed through the patient's mouth into the trachea under direct vision (Figure I–3b).

  a. Technique

    (1) If the patient is not fully relaxed (eg, if the jaw is not flaccid or neck mobility is restricted), induce neuromuscular paralysis with succinylcholine (1–1.5 mg/kg intravenously [IV]), vecuronium or pancuronium (0.1 mg/kg IV), or another neuromuscular blocking agent (see p 386). *Caution:* In children, succinylcholine may induce excessive vagal tone, resulting in bradycardia or asystole. Patients with digitalis intoxication (see p 128) may have a similar response to succinylcholine. Pretreat with atropine (0.01 mg/kg IV), or use vecuronium or pancuronium for paralysis.

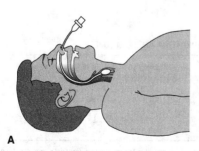
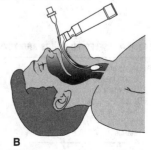

A   **B**

FIGURE I–3. Two routes for endotracheal intubation. A: Nasotracheal intubation. B: Orotracheal intubation.

    (2) Ventilate the patient manually with 100% oxygen while awaiting full paralysis (1–2 minutes for succinylcholine or vecuronium, 3–5 minutes for pancuronium).

    (3) Using a lighted laryngoscope, visualize the larynx and pass the endotracheal tube into the trachea under direct vision. Have an assistant apply firm pressure over the cricoid cartilage to prevent passive reflux of gastric contents into the oropharynx.

    (4) Check breathing sounds to rule out accidental esophageal intubation or intubation of the right main-stem bronchus.

    (5) Secure the tube and inflate the cuff balloon. (Tubes used for children do not have inflatable cuffs.)

    (6) Obtain a chest x-ray to confirm the appropriate tube position.

  b. Advantages

    (1) Performed under direct vision, making accidental esophageal intubation unlikely.

    (2) Insignificant risk of bleeding.

    (3) Patient need not be breathing spontaneously.

    (4) Higher success rate than that achieved via the nasotracheal route.

  c. Disadvantages

    (1) Frequently requires neuromuscular paralysis, creating a risk of fatal respiratory arrest if intubation is unsuccessful.

    (2) Requires neck manipulation, which may cause spinal cord injury if the patient has also had neck trauma.

BREATHING

Along with airway problems, breathing difficulties are the major cause of morbidity and death in patients with poisoning or drug overdose. Patients may have one or more of the following complications: ventilatory failure, hypoxia, or bronchospasm.

I. Ventilatory failure.

  A. Assessment. Ventilatory failure has multiple causes, including failure of the ventilatory muscles, central depression of respiratory drive, and severe pneumonia or pulmonary edema. Examples of drugs and toxins that cause ventilatory failure and the causative mechanisms are listed in Table I–1.

  B. Complications. Ventilatory failure is the most common cause of death in poisoned patients.

    1. Hypoxia may result in brain damage, cardiac arrhythmias, and cardiac arrest.

    2. Hypercarbia results in acidosis, which may contribute to arrhythmias, especially in patients with tricyclic antidepressant overdose.

  C. Differential diagnosis. Rule out the following:

    1. Bacterial or viral pneumonia.

    2. Viral encephalitis or myelitis (eg, polio).

    3. Traumatic or ischemic spinal cord or central nervous system injury.

    4. Tetanus, causing chest wall muscle rigidity.

TABLE I–1. SELECTED DRUGS AND TOXINS CAUSING VENTILATORY FAILURE[a]

Paralysis of ventilatory muscles	Depression of central respiratory drive
Botulin toxin	Barbiturates
Neuromuscular blockers	Clonidine and other sympatholytic agents
Organophosphates and carbamates	Ethanol and alcohols
Snakebite	Opiates
Strychnine	Sedative-hypnotics
Tetanus	Tricyclic antidepressants

[a]Adapted, with permission, from Olson KR, Pentel PR, Kelly MT: Physical assessment and differential diagnosis of the poisoned patient. *Med Toxicol* 1987;2:52.

D. Treatment. Obtain measurements of arterial blood gases. Quickly estimate the adequacy of ventilation from the pCO_2 level; obtundation with an elevated or rising pCO_2 (eg, > 60 mm Hg) indicates a need for assisted ventilation. Do *not* wait until the patient is apneic or until the pCO_2 is above 60 mm to begin assisted ventilation.

1. **Assist breathing manually** with a bag-valve-mask device or bag-valve-endotracheal-tube device until the mechanical ventilator is ready for use.
2. If not already accomplished, **perform endotracheal intubation.**
3. **Program the ventilator** for tidal volume (usually 15 mL/kg), rate (usually 12–15 breaths/min), and oxygen concentration (usually 30–35% to start). Monitor the patient's response to ventilator settings frequently by obtaining arterial blood gas values.
   a. If the patient has some spontaneous ventilation, the machine can be set to allow the patient to breathe spontaneously with only intermittent mandatory ventilation (usually 10–12 breaths/min).
   b. If the endotracheal tube has been placed only for airway protection, the patient can be left to breathe entirely spontaneously with blow-by oxygen mist (T-piece).

II. **Hypoxia.**
   A. **Assessment.** Examples of drugs or toxins causing hypoxia are listed in Table I–2. Hypoxia can be caused by the following conditions:
   1. **Insufficient oxygen** in ambient air (eg, displacement of oxygen by inert gases).
   2. **Disruption of oxygen absorption** by the lung (eg, resulting from pneumonia or pulmonary edema).
      a. **Pneumonia.** The most common cause of pneumonia in overdosed patients is pulmonary aspiration of gastric contents. Pneumonia may also be caused by intravenous injection of foreign material or bacteria, aspiration of petroleum distillates, or inhalation of irritant gases.
      b. **Pulmonary edema.** All agents that can cause chemical pneumonia (eg, irritant gases and hydrocarbons) can also cause pulmonary edema. This usually involves an alteration of permeability in pulmonary capillaries, resulting in **noncardiogenic** pulmonary edema (adult respiratory-distress syndrome [ARDS]). In noncardiogenic pulmonary edema, the pulmonary capillary wedge pressure (reflecting filling pressure in the left ventricle) is usually normal or low. In contrast, **cardiogenic** pulmonary edema caused by cardiac-depressant drugs is characterized by low cardiac output with elevated pulmonary wedge pressure.

TABLE I–2. SELECTED CAUSES OF HYPOXIA[a]

Inert gases	**Pneumonia or noncardiogenic pulmonary edema**
Carbon dioxide	Aspiration of gastric contents
Methane and propane	Aspiration of hydrocarbons
Nitrogen	Chlorine and other irritant gases
Cardiogenic pulmonary edema	Cocaine
Beta blockers	Ethchlorvynol (IV and oral)
Quinidine, procainamide,	Ethylene glycol
and disopyramide	Mercury vapor
Tricyclic antidepressants	Metal fumes ("metal fumes fever")
Verapamil	Nitrogen dioxide
Cellular hypoxia	Opiates
Carbon monoxide	Paraquat
Cyanide	Phosgene
Hydrogen sulfide	Salicylates
Methemoglobinemia	Sedative-hypnotic drugs
Sulfhemoglobinemia	Smoke inhalation

[a]See also Table I–1.

3. **Cellular hypoxia,** which may be present despite a normal arterial blood gas value.

   a. **Carbon monoxide** poisoning (see p 124) and **methemoglobinemia** (p 220) may severely limit oxygen binding to hemoglobin (and, therefore, the oxygen-carrying capacity of blood) without altering the pO_2, because routine blood gas determination measures dissolved oxygen in the plasma but does not measure actual oxygen content. In such cases, only the direct measurement of oxygen saturation (not its calculation from the pO_2) will reveal decreased oxyhemoglobin saturation. *Note:* Pulse oximetry gives falsely normal or nearly normal results and is not reliable.

   b. **Cyanide** (p 150) and **hydrogen sulfide** poisoning (p 188) interfere with cellular oxygen utilization, resulting in decreased oxygen uptake by the tissues, and may cause abnormally high venous oxygen saturation.

B. **Complications.** Significant or sustained hypoxia may result in brain damage and cardiac arrhythmias.

C. **Differential diagnosis.** Rule out the following:

  1. Erroneous sampling (eg, inadvertently measuring venous blood gases rather than arterial blood gases).

  2. Bacterial or viral pneumonia.

  3. Pulmonary contusion caused by trauma.

  4. Acute myocardial infarction with pump failure.

D. **Treatments**

  1. **Correct hypoxia.** Administer supplemental oxygen as indicated based on arterial pO_2. Intubation and assisted ventilation may be required.

    a. If carbon monoxide poisoning is suspected, give 100% oxygen (see p 125).

    b. See also treatment guides for cyanide (p 150), hydrogen sulfide (p 188), and methemoglobinemia (p 220).

  2. **Treat pneumonia.** Obtain frequent sputum samples and initiate appropriate antibiotic therapy when there is evidence of infection.

    a. There is no basis for prophylactic antibiotic treatment of aspiration- or chemical-induced pneumonia.

    b. Although some physicians recommend corticosteroids for chemical-induced pneumonia, there is little evidence of their benefit.

  3. **Treat pulmonary edema.**

    a. Avoid excessive fluid administration. Pulmonary artery cannulation and wedge pressure measurements may be necessary to guide fluid therapy.

    b. Administer supplemental oxygen to maintain a pO_2 of at least 60–70 mm Hg. Endotracheal intubation and use of positive end-expiratory pressure (PEEP) ventilation may be necessary to maintain adequate oxygenation.

III. **Bronchospasm.**

A. **Assessment.** Examples of drugs and toxins that cause bronchospasm are listed in Table I–3. Bronchospasm may result from the following:

  1. **Direct irritant injury** from inhaled gases or pulmonary aspiration of petroleum distillates or stomach contents.

  2. **Pharmacologic effects** of toxins, eg, organophosphate or carbamate insecticides or beta-adrenergic blockers.

  3. **Hypersensitivity** or allergic reactions.

TABLE I–3. SELECTED DRUGS AND TOXINS CAUSING BRONCHOSPASM

Beta blockers	Organophosphates and other anticholinesterases
Chlorine and other irritant gases	Smoke inhalation
Hydrocarbon aspiration	Sulfites (eg, in foods)
Isocyanates	

B. Complications. Severe bronchospasm may result in hypoxia and ventilatory failure.
C. Differential diagnosis. Rule out the following:
 1. Asthma or other preexisting bronchospastic disorders.
 2. Stridor caused by upper-airway injury and edema (progressive airway edema may result in acute airway obstruction).
D. Treatment
 1. Administer supplemental oxygen. Assist ventilation and perform endotracheal intubation if needed.
 2. Remove the patient from the source of exposure to any irritant gas or other offending agent.
 3. Immediately discontinue any beta-blocker treatment.
 4. Administer bronchodilators:
   a. Aerosolized beta-2 stimulant (eg, albuterol [2.5–5 mg] in nebulizer).
   b. If this is not effective, and particularly for beta-blocker-induced wheezing, give aminophylline (6 mg/kg IV over 30 minutes).
 5. For patients with bronchospasm and bronchorrhea caused by organophosphate or other anticholinesterase poisoning, give atropine (see p 340).

CIRCULATION

I. General assessment and initial treatment.
A. Check blood pressure and pulse rate and rhythm. Perform cardiopulmonary resuscitation (CPR) if there is no pulse and perform advanced cardiac life support (ACLS) for arrhythmias and shock. Note that some ACLS drugs may be ineffective or dangerous in patients with drug- or poison-induced cardiac disorders. For example, procainamide is contraindicated in patients with tricyclic antidepressant overdose, and atropine and isoproterenol are ineffective in patients with beta blocker poisoning.
B. Begin continuous electrocardiographic (ECG) monitoring. Arrhythmias may complicate a variety of drug overdoses, and all patients with potentially cardiotoxic drug poisoning should be monitored in the emergency department or an intensive care unit for at least 6 hours after the ingestion.
C. Secure venous access. Antecubital or forearm veins are usually easy to cannulate. Alternative sites include femoral, subclavian, internal jugular, or other central veins. Access to central veins is technically more difficult but allows measurement of central venous pressure and placement of a pacemaker or pulmonary artery lines.
D. Draw blood for routine studies (see p 30).
E. Begin intravenous infusion of normal saline (NS), 5% dextrose in NS (D5-NS), D5 in 0.5 NS, or 5% dextrose in water (D5W) at a keep-open rate; for children, use 5% dextrose in 0.25 NS. If the patient is hypotensive (see p 15), normal saline or another isotonic crystalloid solution is preferred.

TABLE I–4. SELECTED DRUGS AND TOXINS CAUSING BRADYCARDIA OR ATRIOVENTRICULAR BLOCK[a]

Cholinergic or vagotonic agents	Symphatholytic agents
Carbamate insecticides	Beta blockers
Digitalis glycosides	Clonidine
Organophosphates	Opiates
Physostigmine	**Other**
Membrane-depressant drugs	Calcium antagonists
Beta blockers	Lithium
Encainide and flecainide	Phenylpropanolamine and other alpha-adrenergic
Quinidine, procainamide, and disopyramide	agonists
Tricyclic antidepressants	Propoxyphene

[a]Adapted, with permission, from Olson KR et al. *Med Toxicol* 1987;2:71.

F. In seriously ill patients (eg, those who are hypotensive, obtunded, convulsing, or comatose), **place a Foley catheter** in the bladder, obtain urine for routine and toxicologic testing, and measure hourly urine output.

II. Bradycardia and atrioventricular (AV) block.

    A. Assessment. Examples of drugs and toxins causing bradycardia or AV block and their mechanisms are listed in Table I–4.

        1. Bradycardia and AV block are common features of intoxication with calcium antagonists (see p 119) and drugs that depress sympathetic tone or increase parasympathetic tone. These conditions may also result from severe intoxication with membrane-depressant drugs (eg, tricyclic antidepressants, quinidine, or other type Ia and Ic antiarrhythmic agents).

        2. Bradycardia or AV block may also be a reflex response (baroreceptor reflex) to hypertension induced by alpha-adrenergic agents such as phenylpropanolamine.

        3. In children, bradycardia is commonly caused by respiratory compromise and usually responds to ventilation and oxygenation.

    B. Complications. Bradycardia and AV block frequently cause hypotension, which may progress to asystolic cardiac arrest.

    C. Differential diagnosis. Rule out the following:

        1. Hypothermia.

        2. Myocardial ischemia or infarction.

        3. Electrolyte abnormality (eg, hyperkalemia).

        4. Metabolic disturbance (eg, hypothyroidism).

        5. Physiologic origin, due to an intrinsically slow pulse rate (common in athletes) or an acute vaso-vagal reaction.

        6. Cushing reflex (caused by severe intracranial hypertension).

    D. Treatment. Do *not* treat bradycardia or AV block unless the patient is symptomatic (eg, exhibits signs of syncope or hypotension). *Note:* Bradycardia or even AV block may be a protective reflex to lower the blood pressure in a patient with life-threatening hypertension (see item VII, below).

        1. Maintain an open airway and assist ventilation (see pp 1–7) if necessary. Administer supplemental oxygen.

        2. Rewarm hypothermic patients. A sinus bradycardia of 40–50/min is normal when the body temperature is 32–35 °C (90–95 °F).

        3. Administer atropine, 0.01–0.03 mg/kg IV (p 340). If this is not successful, use isoproterenol 1–10 µg/min IV (p 376), titrated to the desired rate, or use an emergency transcutaneous or transvenous pacemaker.

        4. Use the following specific antidotes if appropriate:

            a. For beta-blocker overdose, give glucagon (p 371).

            b. For digitalis intoxication, use Fab fragments (p 357).

            c. For tricyclic antidepressant or membrane-depressant drug overdose, administer sodium bicarbonate (p 345).

            d. For calcium antagonist overdose, give calcium (p 350).

III. QRS interval prolongation.

    A. Assessment. Examples of drugs and toxins causing QRS interval prolongation are listed in Table I–5.

        1. QRS interval prolongation of greater than 0.12 seconds in the limb leads (Figure I–4) strongly indicates serious poisoning by tricyclic antidepressants (see p 310) or other membrane-depressant drugs (eg, quinidine [p 277], flecainide [p 72], chloroquine [p 138], and propranolol [p 107]).

        2. QRS interval prolongation may also result from a ventricular escape rhythm in a patient with complete heart block (eg, from digitalis, calcium antagonist poisoning, or intrinsic cardiac disease).

    B. Complications. QRS interval prolongation in patients with tricyclic antidepressant or similar drug poisonings is often accompanied by hypotension, AV block, and seizures.

    C. Differential diagnosis. Rule out the following:

TABLE I–5. SELECTED DRUGS AND TOXINS CAUSING QRS INTERVAL PROLONGATION[a]

Beta blockers (propranolol)	Hyperkalemia
Chloroquine and related agents	Phenothiazines (thioridazine)
Digitalis glycosides (complete heart block)	Propoxyphene
Diphenhydramine	Quinidine, procainamide, and disopyramide
Encainide and flecainide	Tricyclic antidepressants

[a]Adapted, in part, with permission, from Olson KR et al. *Med Toxicol* 1987;2:71.

1. Intrinsic conduction system disease (bundle branch block or complete heart block) caused by coronary artery disease. Check an old ECG if available.
2. Hyperkalemia with critical cardiac toxicity may appear as a "sine wave" pattern with markedly wide QRS complexes. These are usually preceded by peaked T waves (Figure I–5).
3. Hypothermia with a core temperature of less than 32 °C (90 °F) often causes an extra terminal QRS deflection (J wave or Osborne wave), resulting in a widened QRS appearance (Figure I–6).

D. Treatment

1. Maintain the airway and assist ventilation if necessary (see pp 1–7). Administer supplemental oxygen.
2. Treat hyperkalemia (see p 36) and hypothermia (p 19) if they occur.
3. Treat AV block with atropine (p 340), isoproterenol (p 376), and a pacemaker if necessary.

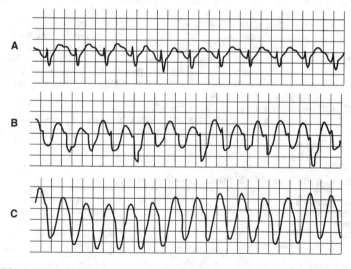

FIGURE I–4. Widened QRS interval caused by tricyclic antidepressant overdose. A: Delayed intraventricular conduction results in prolonged QRS interval (0.18 s). B and C: Supraventricular tachycardia with progressive widening of QRS complexes mimics ventricular tachycardia. (Modified and reproduced, with permission, from Benowitz NL, Goldschlager N. Cardiac disturbances in the toxicologic patient. (Page 71 in *Clinical Management of Poisoning and Drug Overdose*. Haddad LM, Winchester JF [editors]. Saunders, 1983.)

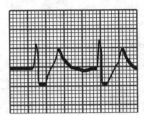 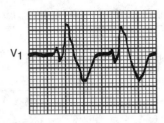

FIGURE I–5. Electrocardiogram of patient with hyperkalemia. (Modified and reproduced, with permission, from Goldschlager N, Goldman MJ: Effect of drugs and electrolytes on the electrocardiogram, p 199. In: *Electrocardiography: Essentials of Interpretation.* Goldschlager N, Goldman MJ [editors]. Lange, 1984.)

4. For tricyclic antidepressant or other sodium channel blocking drug over-dose, give sodium bicarbonate, 1–2 mEq/kg IV bolus (p 345); repeat as needed.
5. Give other antidotes if appropriate:
   a. Digoxin-specific Fab antibodies for complete heart block induced by digitalis (p 357).
   b. Glucagon for beta-blocker intoxication (p 371).
   c. Calcium for calcium antagonist poisoning (p 350).

IV. **Tachycardia.**
   A. **Assessment.** Examples of drugs and toxins causing tachycardia and their mechanisms are shown in Table I–6.
      1. Sinus tachycardia and supraventricular tachycardia are often caused by excessive sympathetic system stimulation or inhibition of parasympathetic tone. Sinus tachycardia may also be a reflex response to hypotension or hypoxia.
      2. Sinus tachycardia and supraventricular tachycardia accompanied by QRS interval prolongation (eg, with tricyclic antidepressant poisoning) may have the appearance of ventricular tachycardia (Figure I–4, p 11).
   B. **Complications.** Simple sinus tachycardia (heart rate < 140/min) is rarely of hemodynamic consequence; children and healthy adults easily tolerate rates up to 160–180/min. However, sustained rapid rates may result in hypotension, chest pain, or syncope.
   C. **Differential diagnosis.** Rule out the following:
      1. Occult blood loss (eg, from gastrointestinal bleeding, or trauma).
      2. Fluid loss (eg, from gastritis or gastroenteritis).
      3. Hypoxia.

TABLE I–6. SELECTED DRUGS AND TOXINS CAUSING TACHYCARDIA[a]

Sympathomimetic agents	**Anticholinergic agents**
Amphetamines and derivatives	*Amanita muscaria* mushrooms
Caffeine	Antihistamines
Cocaine	Atropine and other anticholinergics
Ephedrine and pseudoephedrine	Phenothiazines
Phencyclidine (PCP)	Plants (many)
Theophylline	Tricyclic antidepressants
Agents causing cellular hypoxia	**Other**
Carbon monoxide	Ethanol or sedative-hypnotic drug
Cyanide	withdrawal
Hydrogen sulfide	Hydralazine and other vasodilators
Oxidizing agents (methemoglobinemia)	Thyroid hormone

[a]Adapted, with permission, from Olson KR et al. *Med Toxicol* 1987;2:71.

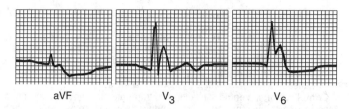

aVF   V₃   V₆

FIGURE I–6. Electrocardiogram of patient with hypothermia, showing prominent J waves. (Modified and reproduced, with permission, from Goldschlager N, Goldman MJ: Miscellaneous abnormal electrocardiogram patterns, p 227. In: *Electrocardiography: Essentials of Interpretation.* Goldschlager N, Goldman MJ (ed.). Lange, 1984.)

   4. Fever and infection.
   5. Myocardial infarction.
   6. Anxiety.
   7. Intrinsic conduction system disease (eg, Wolff-Parkinson-White syndrome).
   D. Treatment. If tachycardia is not associated with hypotension or chest pain, observation and sedation (especially for stimulant intoxication) are usually adequate.
   1. For sympathomimetic-induced tachycardia, give propranolol, 0.01–0.03 mg/kg IV (p 405); or esmolol, 25–100 µg/kg/min IV (p 366).
   2. For anticholinergic-induced tachycardia, give physostigmine, 0.01–0.03 mg/kg IV (p 402); or neostigmine, 0.01–0.03 mg/kg IV. *Caution:* Do **not** use these drugs in patients with tricyclic antidepressant overdose, because additive depression of conduction may result in asystole.
V. Ventricular arrhythmias.
   A. Assessment. Examples of drugs and toxins causing ventricular arrhythmias are listed in Table I–7.
   1. Ventricular irritability is commonly associated with excessive sympathetic stimulation (eg, from cocaine or amphetamines). Patients intoxicated by chlorinated, fluorinated, or aromatic hydrocarbons may have heightened myocardial sensitivity to the arrhythmogenic effects of catecholamines.
   2. Ventricular tachycardia may also be a manifestation of intoxication by a tricyclic antidepressant or other sodium blocking drug, although with these drugs true ventricular tachycardia may be difficult to distinguish from sinus

TABLE I–7. SELECTED DRUGS AND TOXINS CAUSING VENTRICULAR ARRHYTHMIAS[a]

Ventricular tachycardia or fibrillation	QT prolongation or torsades de pointes[b]
Amphetamines and other sympathomimetic agents	Amiodarone
Aromatic hydrocarbon solvents	Arsenic
Caffeine	Astemizole and terfenadine
Chloral hydrate	Chloroquine, quinine, and related agents
Chlorinated or fluorinated hydrocarbon solvents	Citrate
Cocaine	Fluoride
Digitalis glycosides	Organophosphate insecticides
Fluoride	Quinidine, procainamide, and disopyramide
Phenothiazines	Thallium
Theophylline	Thioridazine
Tricyclic antidepressants	Tricyclic antidepressants

[a]Adapted, in part, with permission, from Olson KR et al. *Med Toxicol* 1987;2:71.
[b]These agents can also cause ventricular tachycardia or fibrillation.

or supraventricular tachycardia accompanied by QRS interval prolongation (Figure I–4, p 11).

3. Agents that cause QT interval prolongation (QTc > 0.42 seconds) may produce "atypical" ventricular tachycardia (Torsades de pointes). Torsades is characterized by polymorphous ventricular tachycardia that appears to rotate its axis continuously (Figure I–7). Torsades may also be caused by hypocalcemia or hypomagnesemia.

B. **Complications.** Ventricular tachycardia in patients with a pulse may be associated with hypotension or may deteriorate into pulseless ventricular tachycardia or ventricular fibrillation.

C. **Differential diagnosis.** Rule out the following possible causes of ventricular premature beats, ventricular tachycardia, or ventricular fibrillation:
   1. Hypoxemia.
   2. Hypokalemia.
   3. Metabolic acidosis.
   4. Myocardial ischemia or infarction.
   5. Electrolyte disturbances (eg, hypocalcemia or hypomagnesemia) or congenital disorders that may cause QT prolongation and Torsades.

D. **Treatment.** Perform CPR if necessary, and follow advanced cardiac life support (ACLS) guidelines for management of arrhythmias, with the exception that procainamide and bretylium should **not** be used, especially if tricyclic antidepressant or sodium channel blocking drug overdose is suspected.
   1. Maintain an open airway and assist ventilation if necessary (see pp 1–7). Administer supplemental oxygen.
   2. Correct acid-base and electrolyte disturbances.
   3. **For ventricular fibrillation,** immediately apply direct-current countershock at 3–5 J/kg. Repeat once if needed. Continue CPR if the patient is still without a pulse, and administer epinephrine, repeated countershocks, and lidocaine as recommended in ACLS guidelines.
   4. **For ventricular tachycardia in patients without a pulse,** immediately give a precordial thump or apply synchronized direct-current countershock at 1–3 J/kg. If this is not successful, begin CPR and apply countershock at 3–5 J/kg; administer lidocaine and repeated countershocks as recommended in ACLS guidelines.
   5. **For ventricular tachycardia in patients with a pulse,** use lidocaine, 1–3 mg/kg IV (p 379). Do **not** use procainamide (Pronestyl) or other type Ia antiarrhythmic agents. For suspected myocardial sensitivity caused by chloral hydrate or halogenated or aromatic hydrocarbons, use esmolol, 25–100 µg/kg/min IV (see p 366), or propranolol, 0.5-3 mg IV (see p 405).

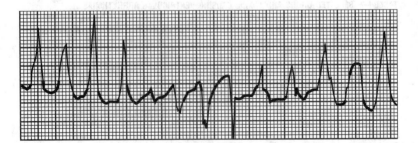

FIGURE I–7. Polymorphic ventricular tachycardia (Torsades de pointes). (Modified and reproduced, with permission, from Goldschlager N, Goldman MJ: Effect of drugs and electrolytes on the electrocardiogram, p 197. In: *Electrocardiography: Essentials of Interpretation.* Goldschlager N, Goldman MJ (ed.). Lange, 1984.)

6. **For tricyclic antidepressant or other sodium channel blocking drug overdose,** administer sodium bicarbonate, 1–2 mEq/kg IV (p 345), in repeated boluses until the QRS interval narrows or the serum pH exceeds 7.7.

7. **For "atypical" or polymorphic ventricular tachycardia (Torsades),** do the following:

    a. Use overdrive pacing or isoproterenol, 1–10 μg/min IV (p 376), to increase the heart rate (this makes repolarization more homogeneous and abolishes the arrhythmia).

    b. Alternately, administer magnesium sulfate, 1–2 g in adults, followed by infusion at 3–20 mg/min.

VI. Hypotension.

  A. Assessment. Examples of drugs and toxins causing hypotension and their mechanisms are listed in Table I–8.

    1. Physiologic derangements resulting in hypotension include volume loss because of vomiting, diarrhea, or bleeding; apparent volume depletion caused by venodilation; arteriolar dilation; depression of cardiac contractility; arrhythmias that interfere with cardiac output; and hypothermia.

    2. Volume loss, venodilation, and arteriolar dilation are likely to result in hypotension with reflex tachycardia. In contrast, hypotension accompanied by bradycardia should suggest intoxication by sympatholytic agents, membrane-depressant drugs, calcium channel blockers, or cardiac glycosides or the presence of hypothermia.

  B. Complications. Severe or prolonged hypotension can cause acute renal tubular necrosis, brain damage, and cardiac ischemia. Metabolic acidosis is a common finding.

  C. Differential diagnosis. Rule out the following:

    1. Hypothermia, which results in a decreased metabolic rate and lowered blood pressure demands.

    2. Hyperthermia, which causes arteriolar dilation and venodilation and direct myocardial depression.

    3. Fluid loss caused by gastroenteritis.

TABLE I–8. SELECTED DRUGS AND TOXINS CAUSING HYPOTENSION[a]

HYPOTENSION WITH RELATIVE BRADYCARDIA	HYPOTENSION WITH TACHYCARDIA
Sympatholytic agents	**Fluid loss or third spacing**
Beta blockers	Amatoxin-containing mushrooms
Bretylium	Arsenic
Clonidine and methyldopa	Colchicine
Hypothermia	Copper sulfate
Opiates	Hyperthermia
Reserpine	Iron
Tetrahydrozoline and oxymetazoline	Rattlesnake envenomation
	Sedative-hypnotic agents
Membrane-depressant drugs	
Beta blockers (mainly propranolol)	**Peripheral venous or arteriolar dilation**
Encainide and flecainide	β_2-stimulants (eg, metaproterenol, terbutaline)
Quinidine, procainamide, and disopyramide	Caffeine
Propoxyphene	Hydralazine
Tricyclic antidepressants	Hyperthermia
	Nitrites
Others	Prazosin
Barbiturates	Sodium nitroprusside
Calcium antagonists	Phenothiazines
Fluoride	Theophylline
Organophosphates and carbamates	Tricyclic antidepressants
Sedative-hypnotic agents	

[a]Adapted, in part, with permission, from Olson KR et al. *Med Toxicol* 1987;2:57.

4. Blood loss (eg, from trauma or gastrointestinal bleeding).
5. Myocardial infarction.
6. Sepsis.
7. Spinal cord injury.
D. **Treatment.** Fortunately, hypotension usually responds readily to empirical therapy with intravenous fluids and low doses of pressor drugs (eg, dopamine). When hypotension does not resolve after simple measures, a systematic approach should be followed to determine the cause of hypotension and to select the appropriate treatment.
   1. Maintain an open airway and assist ventilation if necessary (see pp 1–7). Administer supplemental oxygen.
   2. Treat cardiac arrhythmias that may contribute to hypotension (heart rate < 40–50/min or > 180–200/min [pp 10–14]).
   3. Hypotension associated with hypothermia often will not improve with routine fluid therapy but will rapidly normalize upon rewarming of the patient. A systolic blood pressure of 80–90 mm Hg is expected when the body temperature is 32 °C (90 °F).
   4. Give a fluid challenge using normal saline, 10–20 mL/kg, or another crystalloid solution.
   5. Administer dopamine, 5–15 µg/kg/min (p 362). Note that dopamine may be ineffective in some patients with depleted neuronal stores of catecholamines (eg, from disulfiram [p 158], reserpine, or tricyclic antidepressant [p 310] overdose). In such cases norepinephrine, 0.1 µg/kg/min IV (p 393), may be more effective.
   6. Consider specific antidotes:
      a. Sodium bicarbonate (p 345) for tricyclic antidepressant or other sodium channel blocking drug overdose.
      b. Glucagon (p 371) for beta-blocker overdose.
      c. Calcium (p 350) for calcium antagonist overdose.
      d. Propranolol (p 405) or esmolol (p 366) for theophylline, caffeine, or metaproterenol or other beta-agonist overdose.
   7. If the above measures are unsuccessful, insert a central venous pressure (CVP) monitor or pulmonary artery catheter to determine whether further fluids are needed and to measure the cardiac output (CO) and calculate the systemic vascular resistance (SVR) as follows:

$$SVR = 80(MAP - CVP)/CO$$

   where MAP is the mean arterial pressure, CVP is the central venous pressure, CO is the cardiac output, and normal SVR = 770–1500.
   Select further therapy based on the following results:
      a. If the central venous pressure or pulmonary artery wedge pressure remains low, give more intravenous fluids.
      b. If the cardiac output is low, give more dopamine (p 362) or dobutamine.
      c. If the systemic vascular resistance is low, administer norepinephrine, 4–8 µg/min (p 393).
VII. **Hypertension.**
   A. **Assessment.** Hypertension is frequently overlooked in drug-intoxicated patients and often goes untreated. Many young persons have normal blood pressures in the range of 90/60 mm Hg to 100/70 mm Hg; in such a person an abrupt elevation to 170/100 is much more significant (and potentially catastrophic) than the same blood pressure elevation in an older person with chronic hypertension. Examples of drugs and toxins causing hypertension are listed in Table I–9. Hypertension may be caused by a variety of mechanisms:
      1. Amphetamines and other related drugs cause hypertension and tachycardia through generalized sympathetic stimulation.

TABLE I–9. SELECTED DRUGS AND TOXINS CAUSING HYPERTENSION[a]

HYPERTENSION WITH TACHYCARDIA

Generalized sympathomimetic agents	**Anticholinergic agents**[b]
Amphetamines and derivatives	Antihistamines
Cocaine	Atropine and other anticholinergics
Ephedrine and pseudoephedrine	Tricyclic antidepressants
Epinephrine	**Other**
Levodopa	Ethanol and sedative-hypnotic drug withdrawal
LSD (lysergic acid diethylamide)	Nicotine (early stage)
Marihuana	Organophosphates (early stage)
Monoamine oxidase inhibitors	

HYPERTENSION WITH BRADYCARDIA OR ATRIOVENTRICULAR BLOCK

Clonidine, tetrahydrozoline, and oxymetazoline[c]	Norepinephrine
Ergot derivatives	Phenylephrine
Methoxamine	Phenylpropanolamine

[a]Adapted, in part, with permission, from Olson KR et al. *Med Toxicol* 1987;2:56.
[b]Hypertension usually mild and associated with therapeutic or slightly supratherapeutic levels. Overdose may cause hypotension, especially with tricyclics.
[c]Hypertension often transient and followed by hypotension.

2. Selective alpha-adrenergic agents cause hypertension with reflex (baroreceptor-mediated) bradycardia or even AV block.
3. Anticholinergic agents cause mild hypertension with tachycardia.
4. Substances that stimulate nicotinic cholinergic receptors (eg, organophosphates) may initially cause tachycardia and hypertension, followed later by bradycardia and hypotension.

B. **Complications.** Severe hypertension can result in intracranial hemorrhage, aortic dissection, myocardial infarction, and congestive heart failure.

C. **Differential diagnosis.** Rule out the following:
1. Idiopathic hypertension (which is common in the general population). However, without a prior history of hypertension, it should not be initially assumed to be the cause of the elevated blood pressure.
2. Increased intracranial pressure caused by spontaneous hemorrhage, trauma, or other causes. This may result in hypertension with reflex bradycardia (Cushing reflex).

D. **Treatment.** Rapid lowering of the blood pressure is desirable as long as it does not result in hypotension, which can potentially cause an ischemic cerebral infarction in older patients with cerebrovascular disease. For a patient with chronic hypertension, lowering the diastolic pressure to 100 mm Hg is acceptable. On the other hand, for a young person whose normal diastolic blood pressure is 60 mm Hg, the diastolic pressure should be lowered to 80 mm Hg.
1. **For hypertension with little or no tachycardia,** use phentolamine, 0.02–0.1 mg/kg IV (see p 400); or nitroprusside, 2–10 μg/kg/min IV (p 392).
2. **For hypertension with tachycardia,** add to the treatment in item 1 above propranolol, 0.02–0.1 mg/kg IV (p 405); or esmolol, 25–100 μg/kg/min IV (p 366); or labetalol, 0.2–0.3 mg/kg IV (p 377). *Caution:* Do *not* use propranolol or esmolol alone to treat hypertensive crisis; beta blockers may paradoxically worsen hypertension if it is caused primarily by alpha-adrenergic stimulation.
3. **If hypertension is accompanied by a focally abnormal neurologic examination** (eg, hemiparesis), perform a computed tomography (CT) scan as quickly as possible. In a patient with a cerebrovascular accident, hypertension should generally not be treated unless specific complications of the elevated pressure (eg, heart failure or cardiac ischemia) are present. Consult a neurologist.

ALTERED MENTAL STATUS
I. Coma and stupor.
A. Assessment. A decreased level of consciousness is the most common serious complication of drug overdose or poisoning. Examples of drugs and toxins causing coma are listed in Table I–10.
1. Coma is most often a result of global depression of the brain's reticular activating system, caused by anticholinergic agents, sympatholytic drugs, generalized central nervous system depressants, or toxins that result in cellular hypoxia.
2. Coma sometimes represents a post-ictal phenomenon after a drug- or toxin-induced seizure.
3. Coma may also be caused by brain injury associated with infarction or intracranial bleeding. Brain injury is suggested by the presence of focal neurologic deficits and is confirmed by a CT scan.

B. Complications. Coma is frequently accompanied by respiratory depression, which is a major cause of death. Other conditions that may accompany or complicate coma include hypotension (see p 15), hypothermia (p 19), hyperthermia (p 20), and rhabdomyolysis (p 25).

C. Differential diagnosis. Rule out the following:
1. Head trauma or other causes of intracranial bleeding.
2. Abnormal levels of blood glucose, sodium, or other electrolytes.
3. Hypoxia.
4. Hypothyroidism.
5. Liver or renal failure.
6. Environmental hyperthermia or hypothermia.
7. Serious infections such as encephalitis or meningitis.

D. Treatment
1. Maintain the airway and assist ventilation if necessary (see pp 1–7). Administer supplemental oxygen.
2. Give dextrose, thiamine, and naloxone.
   a. **Dextrose.** All patients with depressed consciousness should receive concentrated dextrose unless hypoglycemia is ruled out with an immediate bedside glucose determination. Use a secure vein and avoid extravasation; concentrated dextrose is highly irritating to tissues. Initial doses include the following:
   (1) Adults: 50% dextrose, 50 mL (25 g) IV.
   (2) Children: 25% dextrose, 2 mL/kg IV.

TABLE I–10. SELECTED DRUGS AND TOXINS CAUSING COMA OR STUPOR[a]

General CNS depressants	Cellular hypoxia
Anticholinergics	Carbon monoxide
Antihistamines	Cyanide
Barbiturates	Hydrogen sulfide
Benzodiazepines	Methemoglobinemia
Carbamazepine	Sodium azide
Ethanol and other alcohols	**Other or unknown mechanisms**
GHB (gamma hydroxybutyrate)	Bromide
Phenothiazines	Diquat
Sedative-hypnotic agents	Disulfiram
Tricyclic antidepressants	Hypoglycemic agents
Valproic acid	Lithium
Sympatholytic agents	Phencyclidine
Clonidine, tetrahydrozoline, and oxymetazoline	Phenylbutazone and enolic acid derivatives
Methyldopa	Salicylates
Opiates	

[a]Adapted, in part, with permission, from Olson KR et al. *Med Toxicol* 1987;2:61.

b. **Thiamine.** Thiamine is given to prevent abrupt precipitation of Wernicke's syndrome resulting from thiamine deficiency in alcoholic patients and others with suspected vitamin deficiencies. It is **not** given routinely to children. Give thiamine, 100 mg, in the IV bottle or intramuscularly (p 408).

c. **Naloxone.** All patients with respiratory depression should receive naloxone (p 384); if a patient is already intubated and being artificially ventilated, then naloxone is not immediately necessary and can be considered a diagnostic rather than therapeutic drug. **Caution:** Although naloxone has no depressant activity of its own and can normally be given safely in large doses, it may precipitate abrupt opiate withdrawal. If amphetamines or cocaine has been injected along with heroin, reversal of the opiate-induced sedation may unmask stimulant-mediated hypertension, tachycardia, or psychosis. In addition, acute pulmonary edema is sometimes temporally associated with abrupt naloxone reversal of opiate intoxication.

(1) Give naloxone, 0.4 mg IV (may also be given intramuscularly [IM]).
(2) If there is no response within 1–2 minutes, give naloxone, 2 mg IV.
(3) If there is still no response and opiate overdose is highly suspected by history or clinical presentation (pinpoint pupils, apnea, or hypotension), give naloxone, 10–20 mg IV.

d. Consider **flumazenil** (Romazicon) if benzodiazepines are the suspected cause of coma and there are no contraindications (see p 369).

3. Normalize the body temperature (see hypothermia, p 19, or hyperthermia, p 20).
4. If there is any possibility of central nervous system trauma or cerebrovascular accident, perform a CT scan.
5. If meningitis or encephalitis is suspected, perform a lumbar puncture and treat with appropriate antibiotics.

II. Hypothermia.

A. **Assessment.** Hypothermia may mimic or complicate drug overdose and should be suspected in every comatose patient. Examples of drugs and toxins causing hypothermia are listed in Table I–11.

1. Hypothermia is usually caused by exposure to low ambient temperatures in a patient with blunted thermoregulatory-response mechanisms. Drugs and toxins may induce hypothermia by causing vasodilation, inhibiting the shivering response, decreasing metabolic activity, or causing loss of consciousness in a cold environment.
2. A patient whose temperature is lower than 32 °C (90 °F) may appear to be dead, with a barely detectable pulse or blood pressure and without reflexes. The ECG may reveal an abnormal terminal deflection (J wave or Osborne wave, Figure I–6, p 13).

B. **Complications.** Because there is a generalized reduction of metabolic activity and less demand for blood flow, hypothermia is commonly accompanied by hypotension and bradycardia.

1. Mild hypotension (systolic blood pressure of 70–90 mm Hg) in a patient with hypothermia should **not** be aggressively treated; excessive intravenous fluids may cause fluid overload and further lowering of the temperature.

TABLE I–11. SELECTED DRUGS AND TOXINS ASSOCIATED WITH HYPOTHERMIA[a]

Barbiturates	Phenothiazines
Ethanol and other alcohols	Sedative-hypnotic agents
Hypoglycemic agents	Tricyclic antidepressants
Opiates	Vasodilators

[a]Adapted, in part, with permission, from Olson KR et al. *Med Toxicol* 1987;2:60.

    2. Severe hypothermia (temperature < 28–30 °C) may cause intractable ventricular fibrillation and cardiac arrest. This may occur abruptly, such as when the patient is moved or rewarmed too quickly or when CPR is performed.

C. Differential diagnosis. Rule out the following:
    1. Sepsis.
    2. Hypoglycemia.
    3. Hypothyroidism.
    4. Environmental hypothermia, caused by exposure to a cold environment.

D. Treatment
    1. Maintain the airway and assist ventilation if necessary (see pp 1–7). Administer supplemental oxygen.
    2. Because the pulse rate may be profoundly slow (10/min) and weak, perform careful cardiac evaluation before assuming that the patient is in cardiac arrest. Do *not* treat bradycardia; it will resolve with rewarming.
    3. Unless the patient is in cardiac arrest (asystole or ventricular fibrillation), rewarm slowly (using blankets, warm intravenous fluids, and warmed-mist inhalation) to prevent rewarming arrhythmias.
    4. For patients in cardiac arrest, usual antiarrhythmic agents and direct current countershock are frequently ineffective until the core temperature is above 32–35 °C (90–95 °F). Provide gastric or peritoneal lavage with warmed fluids and perform CPR. For ventricular fibrillation, bretylium, 5–10 mg/kg IV (see p 347), may be effective.
    5. Open cardiac massage, with direct warm irrigation of the ventricle, or a partial cardiopulmonary bypass may be necessary in hypothermic patients in cardiac arrest who are unresponsive to the above treatment.

III. Hyperthermia.
  A. Assessment. Hyperthermia (temperature > 40 °C or 104 °F) may be a catastrophic complication of intoxication by a variety of drugs and toxins (Table I–12). It may be caused by excessive heat generation because of sustained seizures, rigidity, or other muscular hyperactivity; an increased metabolic rate; impaired dissipation of heat secondary to impaired sweating (eg, anticholinergic agents); or hypothalamic disorders.
    1. Neuroleptic malignant syndrome (NMS) is a hyperthermic disorder seen in some patients who use antipsychotic agents and is characterized by hyperthermia, muscle rigidity (often so severe as to be called "lead-pipe" rigidity), metabolic acidosis, and confusion.

TABLE I–12. SELECTED DRUGS AND TOXINS ASSOCIATED WITH HYPERTHERMIA[a]

Excessive muscular hyperactivity, rigidity, or seizures	Impaired heat dissipation or disrupted thermoregulation
Amoxapine	Amoxapine
Amphetamines and derivatives	Anticholinergic agents
Cocaine	Antihistamines
Lithium	Phenothiazines and other antipsychotic agents
LSD (lysergic acid diethylamide)	Tricyclic antidepressants
Maprotiline	**Other**
Monoamine oxidase inhibitors	Exertional heatstroke
Phencyclidine	Malignant hyperthermia
Tricyclic antidepressants	Metal fume fever
Increased metabolic rate	Neuroleptic malignant syndrome (NMS)
Dinitrophenol and pentachlorophenol	Serotonin syndrome
Salicylates	Withdrawal from ethanol or sedative-hypnotic
Thyroid hormone	drugs

[a]Adapted, with permission, from Olson KR et al. *Med Toxicol* 1987;2:59.

2. **Malignant hyperthermia** is an inherited disorder that causes severe hyperthermia, metabolic acidosis, and rigidity after certain anesthetic agents (most commonly halothane and succinylcholine) are used.

3. **Serotonin syndrome** occurs primarily in patients taking monoamine oxidase (MAO) inhibitors (see p 225) who also take serotonin-enhancing drugs, such as meperidine (Demerol), fluoxetine (Prozac), or other serotonin reuptake inhibitors (SSRIs; see Noncyclic and Other Newer Antidepressants, p 79), and is characterized by irritability, rigidity, myoclonus, diaphoresis, autonomic instability, and hyperthermia. It may also occur in people taking combinations of SSRIs even without concurrent use of MAO inhibitors.

B. Complications. Untreated, severe hyperthermia is likely to result in hypotension, rhabdomyolysis, coagulopathy, cardiac and renal failure, brain injury, and death. Survivors often have permanent neurologic sequelae.

C. Differential diagnosis. Rule out the following:
1. Sedative–hypnotic-drug or ethanol withdrawal (delirium tremens).
2. Exertional or environmental heat stroke.
3. Thyrotoxicosis.
4. Meningitis or encephalitis.
5. Other serious infections.

D. Treatment. Immediate rapid cooling is essential to prevent death or serious brain damage.
1. Maintain the airway and assist ventilation if necessary (see pp 1–7). Administer supplemental oxygen.
2. Administer glucose-containing intravenous fluids, and give concentrated glucose bolus (pp 18 and 372) if the patient is hypoglycemic.
3. Rapidly gain control of seizures (p 21), agitation (p 23), or muscular rigidity (p 24).
4. Begin external cooling with tepid (lukewarm) sponging and fanning. This evaporative method is the most efficient method of cooling. Other methods include iced gastric or colonic lavage or even ice-water immersion.
5. Shivering often occurs with rapid external cooling, and shivering may generate yet more heat. Some physicians recommend chlorpromazine to abolish shivering, but this agent can lower the seizure threshold, inhibit sweating, and cause hypotension. It is preferable to use diazepam, 0.1–0.2 mg/kg IV; lorazepam, 0.05–0.1 mg/kg IV; or midazolam, 0.05–0.1 mg/kg IV or IM (p 342); or use neuromuscular paralysis (see below).
6. The most rapidly effective and reliable means of lowering the temperature is by neuromuscular paralysis. Administer pancuronium, 0.1 mg/kg IV (p 386); or vecuronium, 0.1 mg/kg IV. *Caution:* The patient will stop breathing; be prepared to ventilate and intubate endotracheally.
7. **Malignant hyperthermia.** If muscle rigidity persists despite administration of neuromuscular blockers, a defect at the muscle cell level (ie, malignant hyperthermia) should be suspected. Give dantrolene, 1–10 mg/kg IV (p 354).
8. **Neuroleptic malignant syndrome.** Consider bromocriptine (see p 348).
9. **Serotonin syndrome.** Anecdotal case reports suggest benefit with cyproheptadine (Periactin), 4 mg orally (PO) every hour for 3–4 doses; or methysergide, 2 mg PO every 6 hours for 3–4 doses.

IV. Seizures.
A. Assessment. Seizures are a major cause of morbidity and mortality from drug overdose or poisoning. Seizures may be single and brief or multiple and sustained and may result from a variety of mechanisms (Table I–13).
1. Generalized seizures usually result in loss of consciousness, often accompanied by tongue biting and fecal and urinary incontinence.
2. Other causes of muscular hyperactivity or rigidity (see p 24) may be mistaken for seizures, especially if the patient is also unconscious.

B. Complications
1. Any seizure can cause airway compromise, resulting in apnea or pulmonary aspiration.

TABLE I–13. SELECTED DRUGS AND TOXINS CAUSING SEIZURES[a]

Adrenergic-sympathomimetic agents	Antidepressants and antipsychotics
Amphetamines and derivatives	Amoxapine
Caffeine	Haloperidol and butyrophenones
Cocaine	Loxapine, clozapine, and olanzapine
Phencyclidine	Phenothiazines
Phenylpropanolamine	Tricyclic antidepressants
Theophylline	Venlafaxine, other newer serotonin reuptake
	inhibitors (SSRI's)

Others	
Antihistamines (diphenhydramine, hydroxyzine)	GHB (gamma hydroxybutyrate)
Beta blockers (primarily propranolol; not reported for atenolol, metoprolol, pindolol, or practolol)	Isoniazid (INH)
	Lead and other heavy metals
	Lidocaine and other local anesthetics
Boric acid	Lithium
Camphor	Mefenamic acid
Carbamazepine	Meperidine (normeperidine metabolite)
Cellular hypoxia (eg, carbon monoxide, cyanide, hydrogen sulfide)	Metaldehyde
	Methanol
Chlorinated hydrocarbons	Methyl bromide
Cholinergic agents (carbamates, nicotine, organophosphates)	Phenols
	Phenylbutazone
Cicutoxin and other plant toxins	Piroxicam
Citrate	Salicylates
DEET (diethyltoluamide)	Strychnine (opisthotonus and rigidity)
Ethylene glycol	Withdrawal from ethanol or sedative-hypnotic
Fluoride	drugs

[a]Adapted, in part, with permission, from Olson KR et al. *Med Toxicol* 1987;2:63.

    2. Multiple or prolonged seizures may cause severe metabolic acidosis, hyperthermia, rhabdomyolysis, and brain damage.

C. Differential diagnosis. Rule out the following:

    1. Any serious metabolic disturbance (eg, hypoglycemia, hyponatremia, hypocalcemia, or hypoxia).

    2. Head trauma with intracranial injury.

    3. Idiopathic epilepsy.

    4. Withdrawal from alcohol or a sedative-hypnotic drug.

    5. Exertional or environmental hyperthermia.

    6. Central nervous system infection such as meningitis or encephalitis.

D. Treatment

    1. Maintain an open airway and assist ventilation if necessary (see pp 1–7). Administer supplemental oxygen.

    2. Administer naloxone (pp 19 and 384) if seizures are thought to be caused by hypoxia resulting from narcotic-associated respiratory depression.

    3. Check for hypoglycemia and administer dextrose and thiamine as for coma (p 18).

    4. Use one or more of the following anticonvulsants. *Caution:* Anticonvulsants can cause hypotension, cardiac arrest, or respiratory arrest if administered too rapidly.

        a. Diazepam, 0.1–0.2 mg/kg IV (p 342).

        b. Lorazepam, 0.05–0.1 mg/kg IV (p 342).

        c. Midazolam, 0.1–0.2 mg/kg IM (useful when intravenous access is difficult) or 0.05–0.1 mg/kg IV (p 342).

        d. Phenobarbital, 10–15 mg/kg IV; slow infusion over 15–20 minutes (p 399).

        e. Phenytoin, 15–20 mg/kg IV; slow infusion over 25–30 minutes (p 401). *Note:* Phenytoin is ineffective for convulsions caused by theophylline and is considered the anticonvulsant of last choice for most drug-induced seizures.

f. Pentobarbital, 5–6 mg/kg IV; slow infusion over 8–10 minutes, then continuous infusion at 0.5–3 mg/kg/h titrated to effect (p 398).

5. Immediately check the rectal or tympanic temperature and cool the patient rapidly (p 20) if the temperature is above 40 °C (104 °F). The most rapid and reliably effective method of temperature control is neuromuscular paralysis with pancuronium, 0.1 mg/kg IV (p 386). ***Caution:*** If paralysis is used, the patient must be intubated and ventilated; in addition, monitor the electroencephalogram (EEG) for continued brain seizure activity because peripheral muscular hyperactivity is no longer visible.

6. Use the following specific antidotes if available:
   a. Pyridoxine (p 407) for isoniazid (INH; p 195).
   b. Pralidoxime (2–PAM, p 403) or atropine (p 340), or both, for organophosphate or carbamate insecticides (p 244).

V. Agitation, delirium, or psychosis.
   A. Assessment. Agitation, delirium, or psychosis may be caused by a variety of drugs and toxins (Table I–14). In addition, such symptoms may result from a functional thought disorder or metabolic encephalopathy caused by medical illness.
      1. Functional psychosis or stimulant-induced agitation and psychosis are usually associated with an intact sensorium, and hallucinations are predominantly auditory.
      2. With metabolic encephalopathy or drug-induced delirium, there is usually alteration of the sensorium (manifested by confusion or disorientation). Hallucinations, when they occur, are predominantly visual.
   B. Complications. Agitation, especially if accompanied by hyperkinetic behavior and struggling, may result in hyperthermia (see p 20) and rhabdomyolysis (see p 25).
   C. Differential diagnosis. Rule out the following:
      1. Serious metabolic disturbance (hypoxia, hypoglycemia, or hyponatremia).
      2. Alcohol or sedative–hypnotic drug withdrawal.
      3. Thyrotoxicosis.
      4. Central nervous system infection such as meningitis or encephalitis.
      5. Exertion-induced or environmental hyperthermia.
   D. Treatment. Sometimes the patient can be calmed with reassuring words and reduction of noise, light, and physical stimulation. If this is not quickly effec-

TABLE I–14. SELECTED DRUGS AND TOXINS CAUSING AGITATION, DELIRIUM, OR CONFUSION[a]

Predominant confusion or delirium	Predominant agitation or psychosis
Amantadine	Amphetamines and derivatives
Anticholinergic agents	Caffeine
Antihistamines	Cocaine
Bromide	Cycloserine
Carbon monoxide	LSD (lysergic acid diethylamide)
Cimetidine and other H-2 blockers	Marihuana
Disulfiram	Mercury
Lead and other heavy metals	Phencyclidine (PCP)
Levodopa	Phenylpropanolamine
Lidocaine and other local anesthetics	Procaine
Lithium	Serotonin reuptake inhibitors (SSRIs)
Salicylates	Steroids (eg, prednisone)
Withdrawal from ethanol or sedative-hypnotic drugs	Theophylline

[a]Adapted, in part, with permission, from Olson KR et al. *Med Toxicol* 1987;2:62.

tive, rapidly gain control of the patient to determine the rectal or tympanic temperature and begin rapid cooling and other treatment if needed.

1. Maintain an open airway and assist ventilation if necessary (see pp 1–7). Administer supplemental oxygen.
2. Treat hypoglycemia (p 33), hypoxia (p 7), or other metabolic disturbances.
3. Administer one of the following sedatives:
   a. Midazolam, 0.05–0.1 mg/kg IV over 1 minute, or 0.1–0.2 mg/kg IM (p 342).
   b. Lorazepam, 0.05–0.1 mg/kg IV over 1 minute (p 342).
   c. Diazepam, 0.1–0.2 mg/kg IV over 1 minute (p 342).
   d. Droperidol, 2.5–5 mg IV; or haloperidol, 0.1–0.2 mg/kg IM or IV over 1 minute (p 373). *Note:* Do not give haloperidol decanoate salt intravenously.
4. If hyperthermia occurs as a result of excessive muscular hyperactivity, then skeletal-muscle paralysis is indicated. Use pancuronium, 0.1 mg/kg IV (see p 386). *Caution:* Be prepared to ventilate and endotracheally intubate the patient after muscle paralysis.

OTHER COMPLICATIONS

I. **Dystonia, dyskinesia, and rigidity.**
   A. **Assessment.** Examples of drugs and toxins causing abnormal movements or rigidity are listed in Table I–15.
      1. **Dystonic reactions** are common with therapeutic or toxic doses of many antipsychotic agents and with some antiemetics. The mechanism triggering these reactions is thought to be related to central dopamine blockade. Dystonias usually consist of forced, involuntary, and often painful neck rotation (torticollis), tongue protrusion, jaw extension, or trismus. Other extrapyramidal or parkinsonian movement disorders (eg, pill rolling, bradykinesia, or masked facies) may also be seen with these agents.
      2. In contrast, **dyskinesias** are usually rapid, repetitive body movements that may involve small localized muscle groups (eg, tongue darting, focal myoclonus) or may consist of generalized hyperkinetic activity. The cause is not dopamine blockade but, more commonly, increased dopamine effects or blockade of central cholinergic effects.
      3. **Rigidity** may also be seen with a number of toxins and may be caused by central nervous system effects or spinal cord stimulation. Neuroleptic malignant syndrome and serotonin syndrome (see p 20) are characterized by rigidity, hyperthermia, metabolic acidosis, and an altered mental status.

TABLE I–15. SELECTED DRUGS AND TOXINS CAUSING DYSTONIAS, DYSKINESIAS, AND RIGIDITY[a]

Dystonia	Dyskinesias
Haloperidol and butyrophenones	Amphetamines
Metoclopramide	Anticholinergic agents
Phenothiazines (prochlorperazine)	Antihistamines
Rigidity	Caffeine
Black widow spider bite	Carbamazepine
Lithium	Carisoprodol
Malignant hyperthermia	Cocaine
Methaqualone	GHB (gamma hydroxybutyrate)
Monoamine oxidase inhibitors	Ketamine
Neuroleptic malignant syndrome	Levodopa
Phencyclidine (PCP)	Lithium
Strychnine	Phencyclidine (PCP)
	Serotonin reuptake inhibitors (SSRIs)
	Tricyclic antidepressants

[a]Adapted, in part, with permission, from Olson KR et al. *Med Toxicol* 1987;2:64.

Rigidity seen with malignant hyperthermia (see p 21) is caused by a defect at the muscle cell level and may not reverse with neuromuscular blockade.

B. Complications. Sustained muscular rigidity or hyperactivity may result in rhabdomyolysis (see p 25), hyperthermia (p 20), ventilatory failure (p 6), or metabolic acidosis (p 31).

C. Differential diagnosis. Rule out the following:

1. Catatonic rigidity caused by functional thought disorder.
2. Tetanus.
3. Cerebrovascular accident.
4. Postanoxic encephalopathy.
5. Idiopathic parkinsonism.

D. Treatment

1. Maintain the airway and assist ventilation if necessary (see pp 1–7). Administer supplemental oxygen.
2. Check the rectal or tympanic temperature, and treat hyperthermia (p 20) rapidly if the temperature is above 39 °C (102.2 °F).
3. **Dystonia.** Administer an anticholinergic agent such as diphenhydramine (Benadryl, p 359), 0.5–1 mg/kg IM or IV; or benztropine (Cogentin, p 344), 1–4 mg IM in adults. Follow this treatment with oral therapy for 2–3 days.
4. **Dyskinesia.** Do *not* treat with anticholinergic agents. Instead, administer a sedative such as diazepam, 0.1–0.2 mg/kg IV (p 342); lorazepam, 0.05–0.1 mg IV or IM, or midazolam, 0.05–0.1 mg/kg IV or 0.1–0.2 mg/kg IM (p 342).
5. **Rigidity.** Do *not* treat with anticholinergic agents. Instead, administer a sedative (see item **4,** directly above) or provide specific pharmacologic therapy as follows:
   a. Intravenous calcium (p 350) for a black widow spider bite (p 296).
   b. Dantrolene (p 354) for malignant hyperthermia (p 21).
   c. Bromocriptine (p 348) for neuroleptic malignant syndrome (p 20).

II. Rhabdomyolysis.

A. Assessment. Muscle cell necrosis is a common complication of poisoning. Examples of drugs and toxins causing rhabdomyolysis are listed in Table I–16.

1. Causes of rhabdomyolysis include prolonged immobilization on a hard surface, excessive seizures or muscular hyperactivity, hyperthermia, or direct cytotoxic effects of the drug or toxin (eg, carbon monoxide, colchicine, *Amanita phalloides* mushrooms, and some snake venoms).
2. The diagnosis is made by finding hematest-positive urine with few or no intact red blood cells or an elevated serum creatinine phosphokinase (CPK) level.

TABLE I–16. SELECTED DRUGS AND TOXINS ASSOCIATED WITH RHABDOMYOLYSIS

Excessive muscular hyperactivity, rigidity, or seizures	Direct cellular toxicity
Amphetamines and derivatives	Amatoxin-containing mushrooms
Clozapine and olanzapine	Carbon monoxide
Cocaine	Colchicine
Lithium	Ethylene glycol
Monoamine oxidase inhibitors	
Phencyclidine (PCP)	**Other or unknown mechanisms**
Seizures caused by a variety of agents	Barbiturates (prolonged immobility)
Strychnine	Chlorophenoxy herbicides
Tetanus	Clofibrate
Tricyclic antidepressants	Ethanol
	Hemlock
	Hyperthermia caused by a variety of agents
	Sedative-hypnotic agents (prolonged immobility)
	Trauma

B. Complications. Myoglobin released by damaged muscle cells may precipitate in the kidneys, causing acute tubular necrosis and renal failure. This is more likely when the serum CPK level exceeds several thousand IU/L and if the patient is dehydrated. With severe rhabdomyolysis, hyperkalemia, hyperphosphatemia, hyperuricemia, and hypocalcemia may also occur.

C. Differential diagnosis. Hemolysis with hemoglobinuria may also produce hematest-positive urine.

D. Treatment

1. Aggressively restore volume in dehydrated patients. Then establish a steady urine flow rate (3–5 mL/kg/h) with intravenous fluids. For massive rhabdomyolysis accompanied by oliguria, also consider a bolus of mannitol, 0.5 g/kg IV.
2. Alkalinize the urine by adding 100 mEq of sodium bicarbonate to each L of 5% dextrose. (Acidic urine promotes deposition of myoglobin in the tubules.)
3. Provide intensive supportive care, including hemodialysis if needed, for acute renal failure. Kidney function is usually regained in 2–3 weeks.

III. Anaphylactic and anaphylactoid reactions.

A. Assessment. Examples of drugs and toxins causing anaphylactic or anaphylactoid reactions are listed in Table I–17. These reactions are characterized by bronchospasm and increased vascular permeability that may lead to laryngeal edema, skin rash, and hypotension.

1. **Anaphylaxis** occurs when a patient with antigen-specific immunoglobulin E (IgE) bound to the surface of mast cells and basophils is exposed to the antigen, triggering the release of histamine and various other vasoactive compounds.
2. **Anaphylactoid reactions** are also caused by release of active compounds from mast cells but do not involve prior sensitization or mediation through IgE.

B. Complications. Severe anaphylactic or anaphylactoid reactions can result in laryngeal obstruction, respiratory arrest, hypotension, and death.

C. Differential diagnosis. Rule out the following:

1. Anxiety, with vasodepressor syncope or hyperventilation.
2. Pharmacologic effects of the drug or toxin (eg, procaine reaction with procaine penicillin).
3. Bronchospasm or laryngeal edema from irritant gas exposure.

D. Treatment

1. Maintain the airway and assist ventilation if necessary (see pp 1–7). Endotracheal intubation may be needed if laryngeal swelling is severe. Administer supplemental oxygen.
2. Treat hypotension with intravenous crystalloid fluids (eg, normal saline) and place the patient in a supine position.
3. Administer epinephrine (p 365) as follows:

TABLE I-17. EXAMPLES OF DRUGS AND TOXINS CAUSING ANAPHYLACTIC OR ANAPHYLACTOID REACTIONS

Anaphylactic reactions (IgE-mediated)	Anaphylactoid reactions (not IgE-mediated)
Antisera (antivenins)	Acetylcysteine
Foods (nuts, fish, shellfish)	Blood products
Hymenoptera and other insect stings	Iodinated contrast media
Immunotherapy allergen extracts	Opiates
Penicillins and other antibiotics	Scombroid
Vaccines	Tubocurarine

Other or unclassified
Exercise
Sulfites
Tartrazine dye

      a. For mild to moderate reactions, administer 0.3–0.5 mg subcutaneously (SC) (children, 0.01 mg/kg; maximum 0.5 mg).

      b. For severe reactions, administer 0.05–0.1 mg IV bolus every 5 minutes, or give an infusion starting at a rate of 1–4 µg/min and titrating upward as needed.

   4. Administer diphenhydramine (Benadryl, p 359), 0.5–1 mg/kg IV over 1 minute. Follow with oral therapy for 2–3 days. Cimetidine (Tagamet, see p 353), 300 mg IV every 8 hours, is also helpful.

   5. Administer a corticosteroid such as hydrocortisone, 200–300 mg IV; or methylprednisolone, 40–80 mg IV.

DIAGNOSIS OF POISONING

Diagnosis and treatment of poisoning often must proceed rapidly without the results of extensive toxicologic screening. Fortunately, in most cases the correct diagnosis can be made by using carefully collected data from the history, a directed physical examination, and commonly available laboratory tests.

  I. History. Although frequently unreliable or incomplete, the history of ingestion may be very useful if carefully obtained.

    A. Ask the patient about all drugs taken, including nonprescription drugs, herbal medicines, and vitamins.

    B. Ask family members, friends, and paramedical personnel about any prescriptions or over-the-counter medications known to be used by the patient or others in the house.

    C. Obtain any available drugs or drug paraphernalia for later testing, but handle them very carefully to avoid poisoning by skin contact or an inadvertent needle stick with potential for hepatitis B or HIV transmission.

    D. Check with the pharmacy on the label of any medications found with the patient to determine whether other prescription drugs have been obtained there.

  II. Physical examination.

    A. General findings. Perform a carefully directed examination emphasizing key physical findings that may uncover one of the common **autonomic syndromes**. Important variables in the autonomic physical examination include blood pressure, pulse rate, pupil size, sweating, and peristaltic activity. The autonomic syndromes are summarized in Table I–18.

TABLE I–18. AUTONOMIC SYNDROMES[a,b]

	Blood Pressure	Pulse Rate	Pupil Size	Sweating	Peristalsis
Alpha-adrenergic	+	−	+	+	−
Beta-adrenergic	±	+	±	±	±
Mixed adrenergic	+	+	+	+	−
Sympatholytic	−	−	- -	−	−
Nicotinic	+	+	±	+	+
Muscarinic	−	- -	- -	+	+
Mixed cholinergic	±	±	- -	+	+
Anticholinergic	±	+	+	- -	- -

[a]Key to symbols: + = increased; ++ = markedly increased; − = decreased; - - = markedly decreased; ± = mixed effect, no effect, or unpredictable.
[b]Adapted, with permission, from Olson KR et al. *Med Toxicol* 1987;2:54.

1. **Alpha-adrenergic syndrome.** Hypertension with reflex bradycardia is characteristic of alpha-adrenergic syndrome. The pupils are usually dilated. (Examples: phenylpropanolamine, phenylephrine, and methoxamine.)
2. **Beta-adrenergic syndrome.** Beta-2-mediated vasodilation may cause hypotension. Tachycardia is common. (Examples: albuterol, metaproterenol, theophylline, and caffeine.)
3. **Mixed alpha- and beta-adrenergic syndrome.** Hypertension is accompanied by tachycardia. The pupils are dilated. The skin is sweaty, although mucous membranes are dry. (Examples: cocaine and amphetamines.)
4. **Sympatholytic syndrome.** Blood pressure and pulse rate are both decreased (peripheral alpha blockers such as hydralazine may cause hypotension with reflex tachycardia). The pupils are small, often of pinpoint size. Peristalsis is often decreased. (Examples: centrally acting alpha-2 agonists [clonidine and methyldopa], opiates, and phenothiazines.)
5. **Nicotinic cholinergic syndrome.** Stimulation of nicotinic receptors at autonomic ganglia activates both parasympathetic and sympathetic systems, with unpredictable results. Excessive stimulation frequently causes depolarization blockage. Thus, initial tachycardia may be followed by bradycardia, and muscle fasciculations may be followed by paralysis. (Examples: nicotine; in addition, the depolarizing neuromuscular blocker succinylcholine, which acts on nicotinic receptors in skeletal muscle.)
6. **Muscarinic cholinergic syndrome.** Muscarinic receptors are located at effector organs of the parasympathetic system. Stimulation causes bradycardia, miosis, sweating, hyperperistalsis, bronchorrhea, wheezing, excessive salivation, and urinary incontinence. (Examples: None. There are no pure muscarinic drugs.)
7. **Mixed cholinergic syndrome.** Because both nicotinic and muscarinic receptors are stimulated, mixed effects may be seen. The pupils are usually miotic (of pinpoint size). The skin is sweaty, and peristaltic activity is increased. Fasciculations are a manifestation of nicotinic stimulation and may progress to muscle weakness or paralysis. (Examples: organophosphate and carbamate insecticides and physostigmine.)
8. **Anticholinergic syndrome.** Tachycardia with mild hypertension is common. The pupils are widely dilated. The skin is flushed, hot, and dry. Peristalsis is decreased, and urinary retention is common. Patients may have myoclonic jerking or choreoathetoid movements. Agitated delirium is common, and hyperthermia may occur. (Examples: atropine, scopolamine, benztropine, antihistamines, and antidepressants; all of these drugs are primarily antimuscarinic.)

B. **Eye findings**
   1. **Pupil size** is affected by a number of drugs acting on the autonomic nervous system. Table I–19 lists common causes of miosis and mydriasis.
   2. **Horizontal-gaze nystagmus** is common with a variety of drugs and toxins, including barbiturates, ethanol, carbamazepine, phenytoin, and scorpion envenomation. Phencyclidine (PCP) may cause horizontal, vertical, and even rotatory nystagmus.

C. **Neuropathy.** A variety of drugs and poisons can cause sensory or motor neuropathy, usually after chronic repeated exposure (see Table I–20). Some agents (eg, arsenic and thallium) can cause neuropathy after a single large exposure.

D. **Abdominal findings.** Peristaltic activity is commonly affected by drugs and toxins (see Table I–18 on autonomic syndromes).
   1. Ileus may also be caused by **mechanical factors** such as injury to the gastrointestinal tract with perforation and peritonitis or mechanical obstruction by a swallowed foreign body.
   2. Abdominal distension and ileus may also be a manifestation of acute **bowel infarction,** a rare but catastrophic complication that results from prolonged hypotension or mesenteric artery vasospasm (caused, for ex-

TABLE I–19. SELECTED CAUSES OF PUPIL SIZE CHANGES[a]

CONSTRICTED PUPILS (MIOSIS)	DILATED PUPILS (MYDRIASIS)
Sympatholytic agents	**Sympathomimetic agents**
Clonidine	Amphetamines and derivatives
Opiates	Cocaine
Phenothiazines	Dopamine
Tetrahydrozoline and oxymetazoline	LSD (lysergic acid diethylamide)
Valproic acid	Monoamine oxidase inhibitors
Cholinergic agents	Nicotine[b]
Carbamate insecticides	**Anticholinergic agents**
Nicotine[b]	Antihistamines
Organophosphates	Atropine and other anticholinergics
Physostigmine	Glutethimide
Pilocarpine	Tricyclic antidepressants
Others	
Heatstroke	
Pontine infarct	
Subarachnoid hemorrhage	

[a]Adapted, in part, with permission, from Olson KR et al. *Med Toxicol* 1987;2:66.
[b]Nicotine can cause pupils to be dilated (rare) or constricted (common).

ample, by ergot or amphetamines). Radiographs or CT scans may reveal air in the intestinal wall, biliary tree, or hepatic vein. The serum phosphorus and alkaline phosphatase levels are often elevated.

    3. Vomiting, especially with hematemesis, may indicate the ingestion of a corrosive substance.

E. Skin findings

    1. Sweating or absence of sweating may provide a clue to one of the autonomic syndromes (Table I–18).

    2. Flushed red skin may be caused by carbon monoxide poisoning, boric acid intoxication, chemical burns from corrosives or hydrocarbons, or anticholinergic agents. It may also result from vasodilation (eg, phenothiazines or disulfiram-ethanol interaction).

TABLE I–20. SELECTED CAUSES OF NEUROPATHY

Cause	Comments
Acrylamide	Sensory and motor distal axonal neuropathy
Antineoplastic agents	Vincristine most strongly associated (see p 88)
Antiretroviral agents	Nucleoside reverse transcriptase inhibitors
Arsenic	Sensory predominant mixed axonal neuropathy (see p 95)
Buckthorn (*K humboltiana*)	Livestock and human demyelinating neuropathy
Carbon disulfide	Sensory and motor distal axonal neuropathy
Dimethylaminoproprionitrile	Urogenital and distal sensory neuropathy
Disulfiram	Sensory and motor distal axonal neuropathy
Ethanol	Sensory and motor distal axonal neuropathy (see p 162)
n-Hexane	Sensory and motor distal axonal neuropathy
Isoniazid (INH)	Preventable with co-administration of pyridoxine (see p 195)
Lead	Motor predominant mixed axonal neuropathy (see p 199)
Mercury	Organic mercury compounds (see p 213)
Methyl *n*-butyl ketone	Acts like *n*-hexane, via 2,5-hexanedione metabolite
Nitrofurantoin	Sensory and motor distal axonal neuropathy
Nitrous oxide	Sensory axonal neuropathy with loss of proprioception (see p 236)
Organophosphate insecticides	Specific agents only (eg, triorthocresylphosphate)
Pyridoxine (Vitamin B_6)	Sensory neuropathy with chronic excessive dosing
Thallium	Sensory and motor distal axonal neuropathy (see p 302)
Tick paralysis	Ascending flaccid paralysis after bites by several tick species

      3. Pale coloration with diaphoresis is frequently caused by sympath-omimetic agents. Severe localized pallor should suggest possible arterial vasospasm, such as that caused by ergot (see p 160) or some ampheta-mines (p 68).

      4. Cyanosis may indicate hypoxia, sulfhemoglobinemia, or methemoglobine-mia (p 220).

    F. Odors. A number of toxins may have characteristic odors (Table I–21). How-ever, the odor may be subtle and may be obscured by the smell of emesis or by other ambient odors. In addition, the ability to smell an odor may vary; for example, only about 50% of the general population can smell the "bitter-al-mond" odor of cyanide. Thus, the absence of an odor does not guarantee the absence of the toxin.

III. Essential clinical laboratory tests. Simple, readily available clinical laboratory tests may provide important clues to the diagnosis of poisoning and may guide the investigation toward specific toxicology testing.

    A. Routine tests. The following tests are recommended for routine screening of the overdose patient:

      1. Serum osmolality and osmolar gap.

      2. Electrolytes for determination of sodium, potassium, and anion gap.

      3. Serum glucose.

      4. Blood urea nitrogen (BUN) and creatinine for evaluation of renal function.

      5. Hepatic transaminases and hepatic function tests.

      6. Urinalysis to check for crystalluria, hemoglobinuria, or myoglobinuria.

      7. Electrocardiogram (ECG).

      8. Stat serum acetaminophen level and serum ethanol level.

      9. Pregnancy test (females of childbearing age).

    B. Serum osmolality and osmolar gap. Serum osmolality may be measured in the laboratory with the freezing-point-depression osmometer or the heat-of-vaporization osmometer. Under normal circumstances the measured serum osmolality is approximately 290 mOsm/L and can be calculated from the results of the sodium, glucose, and BUN tests. The difference between the calculated osmolality and the osmolality measured in the laboratory is the osmolal gap, more commonly referred to as the osmolar gap (Table I–22).

      1. Causes of an elevated osmolar gap (Table I–22)

        a. The osmolar gap may be increased in the presence of low-molecular-weight substances such as ethanol, other alcohols, and glycols, any of which can contribute to the measured but not the calculated osmolality. Table I–23 describes how to estimate alcohol and glycol levels based on the osmolar gap.

        b. An osmolar gap accompanied by anion gap acidosis should immedi-ately suggest poisoning by methanol or ethylene glycol. *Note:* A falsely

TABLE I–21. SOME COMMON ODORS CAUSED BY TOXINS AND DRUGS[a]

Odor	Drug or Toxin
Acetone	Acetone, isopropyl alcohol
Acrid or pearlike	Chloral hydrate, paraldehyde
Bitter almonds	Cyanide
Carrots	Cicutoxin (water hemlock)
Garlic	Arsenic, organophosphates, selenium, thallium
Mothballs	Naphthalene, paradichlorobenzene
Pungent aromatic	Ethchlorvynol
Rotten eggs	Hydrogen sulfide, stibine, mercaptans, old sulfa drugs
Wintergreen	Methyl salicylate

[a]Adapted, in part, with permission, from Olson KR et al. *Med Toxicol* 1987;2:67.

TABLE I–22. CAUSES OF ELEVATED OSMOLAR GAP[a]

Acetone	Mannitol
Dimethyl sulfoxide (DMSO)	Metaldehyde
Ethanol	Methanol
Ethyl Ether	Osmotic contrast dyes
Ethylene glycol and other low-molecular-weight glycols	Propylene glycol
Isopropyl alcohol	Renal failure without dialysis
Magnesium	Severe alcoholic ketoacidosis, diabetic ketoacidosis, or lactic acidosis

[a]Osmolar gap = measured – calculated osmolality. Normal = 0 ± 5.

Calculated osmolality = $2[Na] = \dfrac{[glucose]}{18} + \dfrac{[BUN]}{2.8} = 290$ mOsm/l

Na (serum sodium) in meq/L; glucose and BUN (urea nitrogen) in mg/dL.

Note: The osmolality may be measured as falsely normal if a vaporization point osmometer is used instead of the freezing point device, because volatile alcohols will be boiled off.

normal osmolar gap despite the presence of alcohols may result from using a heat-of-vaporization method to measure osmolality, because the alcohols will boil off before the serum boiling point is reached.
2. **Differential diagnosis**
   a. Combined osmolar- and anion-gap elevation may also be seen with severe alcoholic ketoacidosis or diabetic ketoacidosis, due to accumulation of beta hydroxybutyrate.
   b. Patients with chronic renal failure who are not undergoing hemodialysis may have an elevated osmolar gap owing to accumulation of low-molecular-weight solutes.
   c. False elevation of the osmolar gap may be caused by the use of an inappropriate sample tube (lavender top, EDTA; gray top, fluoride-oxalate; blue top, citrate); see Table I–33, p 41.
   d. A falsely elevated gap may occur in patients with severe hyperlipidemia.
3. **Treatment** depends on the cause. If ethylene glycol (p 166) or methanol (p 218) poisoning is suspected, based upon an elevated osmolar gap not accounted for by ethanol or other alcohols and on the presence of metabolic acidosis, then ethanol infusion therapy and hemodialysis may be indicated.
C. **Anion-gap metabolic acidosis.** The normal anion gap of 8–12 mEq/L accounts for unmeasured anions (eg, phosphate, sulfate, and anionic proteins) in the plasma. Metabolic acidosis is usually associated with an elevated anion gap.

TABLE I–23. ESTIMATION OF ALCOHOL AND GLYCOL LEVELS FROM THE OSMOLAR GAP[a]

Alcohol or Glycol	Molecular Weight (mg/mmol)	Conversion Factor[b]
Acetone	58	5.8
Ethanol	46	4.6
Ethylene glycol	62	6.2
Isopropyl alcohol	60	6
Methanol	32	3.2
Propylene glycol	72	7.2

[a]Adapted, with permission, from *Current Emergency Diagnosis & Treatment,* 3rd ed. Ho MT, Saunders CE (editors). Appleton & Lange, 1990.
[b]To obtain estimated serum level (in mg/dL), multiply osmolar gap by conversion factor.

1. **Causes of elevated anion gap** (Table I–24)
   a. An elevated anion-gap acidosis is usually caused by an accumulation of lactic acid but may also be caused by other unmeasured acid anions such as formate (eg, methanol poisoning) or oxalate (eg, ethylene glycol poisoning).
   b. In any patient with an elevated anion gap, also check the osmolar gap; a combination of elevated anion and osmolar gaps suggests poisoning by methanol or ethylene glycol. *Note:* Combined osmolar- and anion-gap elevation may also be seen with severe alcoholic ketoacidosis and diabetic ketoacidosis.
   c. A narrow anion gap may occur with an overdose by lithium, bromide, or nitrate, all of which can increase the serum chloride level measured by some laboratory instruments.
2. **Differential diagnosis.** Rule out the following:
   a. Common causes of lactic acidosis such as hypoxia or ischemia.
   b. False depression of the serum bicarbonate and pCO_2 measurements, which can occur from incomplete filling of the red-topped Vacutainer blood collection tube.
   c. False depression of the pCO_2 and calculated bicarbonate measurements, which can result from excess heparin when obtaining arterial blood gases (0.25 mL heparin in 2 mL blood falsely lowers pCO_2 by about 8 mm and bicarbonate by about 5 mEq/L).
3. **Treatment**
   a. Treat the underlying cause of the acidosis.
      (1) Treat seizures (see p 21) with anticonvulsants or neuromuscular paralysis.
      (2) Treat hypoxia (p 7) and hypotension (p 15) if they occur.
      (3) Treat methanol (p 218) or ethylene glycol (p 166) poisoning with fomepizole or ethanol and hemodialysis.
      (4) Treat salicylate intoxication (p 284) with alkaline diuresis and hemodialysis.
   b. Treatment of the acidemia itself is not generally necessary, unless the pH is less than 7–7.1. In fact, mild acidosis may be beneficial by promoting oxygen release to tissues. However, acidemia may be harmful in poisoning by salicylates or tricyclic antidepressants.
      (1) In salicylate intoxication (p 277), acidemia enhances salicylate entry into the brain and must be prevented. Alkalinization of the urine promotes salicylate elimination.

TABLE I–24. SELECTED DRUGS AND TOXINS CAUSING ELEVATED ANION GAP ACIDOSIS[a,b]

Lactic acidosis	Other
Acetaminophen (levels >600 mg/L)	Alcoholic ketoacidosis
Beta-adrenergic drugs	Benzyl alcohol
Caffeine	Diabetic ketoacidosis
Carbon monoxide	Ethylene glycol
Cyanide	Exogenous organic and mineral acids
Hydrogen sulfide	Formaldehyde
Iron	Ibuprofen (propionic acid)
Isoniazid (INH)	Metaldehyde
Phenformin (common) and metformin (rare)	Methanol
Salicylates	Salicylates (salicylic acid)
Seizures, shock, or hypoxia	Valproic acid
Sodium azide	
Theophylline	

[a]Anion gap = [Na] − [Cl] − [HCO_3] = 8 –12 meq/L.
[b]Adapted, in part, with permission, from Olson KR et al. *Med Toxicol* 1987;2:73.

    (2) In a tricyclic antidepressant overdose (p 310), acidemia enhances cardiotoxicity. Maintain the serum pH at 7.45–7.5 with boluses of sodium bicarbonate.

D. Hyperglycemia and hypoglycemia. A variety of drugs and disease states can cause alterations in the serum glucose level (Table I–25). A patient's blood glucose level can be altered by nutritional state, endogenous insulin levels, and endocrine and liver functions and by the presence of various drugs or toxins.

  1. Hyperglycemia, especially if severe (> 500 mg/dL) or sustained, may result in dehydration and electrolyte imbalance caused by the osmotic effect of excess glucose in the urine; the shifting of water from the brain into plasma may result in hyperosmolar coma. More commonly, hyperglycemia in poisoning or drug overdose cases is mild and transient. Significant or sustained hyperglycemia should be treated if it is not resolving spontaneously or if the patient is symptomatic.

    a. If the patient has an altered mental status, maintain an open airway, assist ventilation if necessary, and administer supplemental oxygen (see pp 1–7).

    b. Replace fluid deficits with intravenous normal saline or another isotonic crystalloid solution. Monitor serum potassium levels, which may fall sharply as blood glucose is corrected, and give supplemental potassium as needed.

    c. Correct acid-base and electrolyte disturbances.

    d. Administer regular insulin, 5–10 U IV initially, followed by infusion of 5–10 U/h, while monitoring the effects on serum glucose level (children: administer 0.1 U/kg initially and 0.1 U/kg/h).

  2. Hypoglycemia, if severe (serum glucose < 40 mg/dL) and sustained, can rapidly cause permanent brain injury. For this reason, whenever hypoglycemia is suspected as a cause of seizures, coma, or altered mental status, immediate empirical treatment with dextrose is indicated.

    a. If the patient has an altered mental status, maintain an open airway, assist ventilation if necessary, and administer supplemental oxygen (see pp 1–7).

    b. If available, perform rapid bedside blood glucose testing (now possible in most emergency departments).

    c. If the blood glucose is low (< 70 mg/dL) or if bedside testing is not available, administer concentrated 50% dextrose, 50 mL IV (25 g). In children, give 25% dextrose, 2 mL/kg (see p 372).

    d. In malnourished or alcoholic patients, also give thiamine, 100 mg IM or IV, to prevent acute Wernicke's syndrome.

TABLE I–25. SELECTED CAUSES OF ALTERATIONS IN SERUM GLUCOSE

Hyperglycemia	Hypoglycemia
β_2-adrenergic drugs	Akee fruit
Caffeine intoxication	Endocrine disorders (hypopituitarism, Addison's
Corticosteroids	disease, myxedema)
Dextrose administration	Ethanol intoxication (especially pediatric)
Diabetes mellitus	Fasting
Diazoxide	Hepatic failure
Excessive circulating epinephrine	Insulin
Glucagon	Oral sulfonylurea hypoglycemic agents
Theophylline intoxication	Propranolol intoxication
Thiazide diuretics	Renal failure
Vacor	Salicylate intoxication
	Valproic acid intoxication

e. For hypoglycemia caused by oral sulfonylurea drug overdose (p 81), consider antidotal therapy with diazoxide (p 356) or octreotide (p 394).

E. Hypernatremia and hyponatremia. Sodium disorders occur infrequently in poisoned patients (see Table I–26). More commonly they are associated with underlying disease states. Antidiuretic hormone (ADH) is responsible for concentrating the urine and preventing excess water loss.

1. **Hypernatremia** (serum sodium > 145 mEq/L) may be caused by excessive sodium intake, excessive free-water loss, or impaired renal concentrating ability.

   a. Dehydration with normal kidney function. Excessive sweating, hyperventilation, diarrhea, or osmotic diuresis (eg, hyperglycemia or mannitol administration) may cause disproportional water loss. The urine osmolality is usually greater than 400 mOsm/kg, and the ADH function is normal.

   b. Impaired renal concentrating ability. Excess free water is lost in the urine, and urine osmolality is usually less than 250 mOsm/L. This may be caused by hypothalamic dysfunction with reduced ADH production **(diabetes insipidus [DI])** or impaired kidney response to ADH **(nephrogenic DI).** Nephrogenic DI has been associated with chronic lithium therapy.

2. **Treatment of hypernatremia.** Treatment depends on the cause, but in most cases, the patient is hypovolemic and needs fluids. *Caution:* Do **not** reduce the serum sodium level too quickly, because osmotic imbalance may cause excessive fluid shift into brain cells, resulting in cerebral edema. The correction should take place over 24–36 hours; the serum sodium should be lowered about 1 mEq/L/h.

   a. Hypovolemia. Administer normal saline (0.9% saline) to restore fluid balance, then half-normal saline in dextrose (D5W-0.45NS saline).

   b. Volume overload. Treat with a combination of sodium-free or low-sodium fluid (eg, 5% dextrose or D5W-0.25NS) and a loop diuretic such as furosemide (Lasix), 0.5–1 mg/kg.

   c. Lithium-induced nephrogenic DI. Administer fluids (see **a**, above). Discontinue lithium therapy. Partial improvement may be seen with oral administration of indomethacin, 50 mg 3 times a day, and hydrochlorothiazide, 50–100 mg/d.

3. **Hyponatremia** (serum sodium < 130 mEq/L) is a common electrolyte abnormality and may result from a variety of mechanisms. Severe hyponatremia (serum sodium < 110–120 mEq/L) can result in seizures and altered mental status.

   a. Pseudohyponatremia may result from a shift of water from the extracellular space (eg, hyperglycemia). Plasma sodium falls by about 1.6 mEq/L for each 100-mg/dL rise in glucose. Reduced relative blood water volume (eg, hyperlipidemia or hyperproteinemia) may produce

TABLE I–26. SELECTED DRUGS AND TOXINS ASSOCIATED WITH ALTERED SERUM SODIUM

Hypernatremia	Hyponatremia
Cathartic abuse	Beer potomania
Lactulose therapy	Diuretics
Lithium therapy	Iatrogenic (IV fluid therapy)
Mannitol	Psychogenic polydipsia
Severe gastroenteritis (many poisons)	Syndrome of inappropriate ADH (SIADH):
Sodium overdose	Amitriptyline
Valproic acid (divalproex sodium)	Chlorpropamide
	Clofibrate
	Oxytocin
	Phenothiazines

pseudohyponatremia if older (flame emission) devices are used, but this is unlikely with current direct-measurement electrodes.

b. **Hyponatremia with hypovolemia** may be caused by excessive volume loss (sodium and water) that is partially replaced by free water. To maintain intravascular volume, the body secretes ADH, which causes water retention. A urine sodium level of less than 10 mEq/L suggests that the kidney is appropriately attempting to compensate for volume losses. An elevated urine sodium level (> 20 mEq/L) implies renal salt wasting, which can be caused by diuretics, adrenal insufficiency, or nephropathy.

c. **Hyponatremia with volume overload** occurs in conditions such as congestive heart failure and cirrhosis. Although the total body sodium is increased, baroreceptors sense an inadequate circulating volume and stimulate release of ADH. The urine sodium level is normally less than 10 mEq/L, unless the patient has been on diuretics.

d. **Hyponatremia with normal volume** occurs in a variety of situations. Measurement of the serum and urine osmolalities may help determine the diagnosis.

  (1) Syndrome of inappropriate ADH secretion (SIADH). In patients with SIADH, ADH is secreted independently of volume or osmolality. Causes include malignancies, pulmonary disease, and some drugs (see Table I–26). The serum osmolality is low, but the urine osmolality is inappropriately increased (> 300 mOsm/L). The serum blood urea nitrogen (BUN) is usually low (< 10 mg/dL).

  (2) Psychogenic polydipsia, or compulsive water drinking (generally > 10 L/d), causes reduced serum sodium because of the excessive free-water intake and because the kidney excretes sodium to maintain euvolemia. The urine sodium level may be elevated, but urine osmolality is appropriately low because the kidney is attempting to excrete the excess water and ADH secretion is suppressed.

  (3) Beer potomania may result from chronic daily excessive beer drinking (> 4 L/d). It usually occurs in patients with cirrhosis who already have elevated ADH levels.

  (4) Other causes of euvolemic hyponatremia include hypothyroidism, postoperative state, and idiosyncratic reactions to diuretics (generally thiazides).

4. **Treatment of hyponatremia.** Treatment depends on the cause, the patient's volume status, and most important, the patient's clinical condition. *Caution:* Avoid overly rapid correction of the sodium, because brain damage (central pontine myelinolysis) may occur if the sodium is increased by more than 25 mEq/L in the first 24 hours. Obtain frequent measurements of serum and urine sodium levels and adjust the rate of infusion as needed to increase the serum sodium by no more than 1–1.5 mEq/h. Arrange consultation with a nephrologist as soon as possible. **For patients with profound hyponatremia** (serum sodium < 110 mEq/L) accompanied by coma or seizures, administer hypertonic (3%) saline, 100–200 mL.

  a. **Hyponatremia with hypovolemia.** Replace lost volume with normal saline (0.9NS). If adrenal insufficiency is suspected, give hydrocortisone, 100 mg every 6–8 hours. Hypertonic saline (3% saline) is rarely indicated.

  b. **Hyponatremia with volume overload.** Restrict water (0.5–1 L/d) and treat the underlying condition (eg, congestive heart failure). If diuretics are given, do *not* allow excessive free-water intake. Hypertonic saline is dangerous in these patients; if it is used, also administer furosemide, 0.5–1 mg/kg. Consider hemodialysis to reduce volume and restore the sodium level.

  c. **Hyponatremia with normal volume.** Asymptomatic patients may be treated conservatively with water restriction (0.5–1 L/d). Psychogenic compulsive water drinkers may have to be restrained or separated from all sources of water, including washbasins and toilets. Demeclocycline (a tetracycline antibiotic that can produce nephrogenic DI), 300–600 mg twice a day, is used to treat mild SIADH. The onset of action may require a week. For patients with coma or seizures, give hypertonic (3%) saline, 100–200 mL, along with furosemide, 0.5–1 mg/kg.

F. **Hyperkalemia and hypokalemia.** A variety of drugs and toxins can cause serious alterations in the serum potassium level (Table I–27). Potassium levels are dependent on potassium intake and release (eg, from muscles), diuretic use, proper functioning of the ATPase pump, serum pH, and beta-adrenergic activity. Changes in serum potassium levels do not always reflect overall body gain or loss but may be caused by intracellular shifts (eg, acidosis drives potassium out of cells, but beta-adrenergic stimulation drives it into cells).

1. **Hyperkalemia** (serum potassium > 5 mEq/L) produces muscle weakness and interferes with normal cardiac conduction. Peaked T waves and prolonged PR intervals are the earliest signs of cardiotoxicity. Critical hyperkalemia produces widened QRS intervals, AV block, ventricular fibrillation, and cardiac arrest (see Figure I–5, p 12).
   a. Hyperkalemia caused by **fluoride intoxication** (see p 170) is usually accompanied by hypocalcemia.
   b. **Digitalis intoxication** associated with hyperkalemia is an indication for administration of digoxin-specific Fab antibodies (p 357).
2. **Treatment of hyperkalemia.** A potassium level higher than 6 mEq/L is a medical emergency; a level greater than 7 mEq/L is critical.
   a. Monitor the ECG. QRS prolongation indicates critical cardiac poisoning.
   b. Administer calcium chloride, 10–20 mg/kg IV (p 350), if there are signs of critical cardiac toxicity. *Caution:* Do **not** use calcium in patients with digitalis glycoside poisoning; intractable ventricular fibrillation may result.
   c. Sodium bicarbonate, 1–2 mEq/kg IV (p 345), rapidly drives potassium into cells and lowers the serum level.
   d. Glucose plus insulin also promotes intracellular movement of potassium. Give 50% dextrose, 50 mL (25% dextrose, 2 mL/kg in children), plus regular insulin, 0.1 U/kg IV.
   e. Inhaled beta-2 adrenergic agonists such as albuterol also enhance potassium entry into cells and can provide a rapid supplemental method of lowering serum potassium levels.
   f. Kayexalate (sodium polystyrene sulfonate), 0.3–0.6 g/kg PO in 2 mL/kg 70% sorbitol, is effective but takes several hours.
   g. Hemodialysis rapidly lowers serum potassium levels.

TABLE I–27. SELECTED DRUGS AND TOXINS AND OTHER CAUSES OF ALTERED SERUM POTASSIUM[a]

Hyperkalemia	Hypokalemia
Alpha-adrenergic agents	Barium
Angiotensin converting enzyme (ACE) inhibitors	Beta-adrenergic drugs
Beta blockers	Caffeine
Digitalis glycosides	Diuretics (chronic)
Fluoride	Epinephrine
Lithium	Theophylline
Potassium	Toluene (chronic)
Renal failure	
Rhabdomyolysis	

[a]Adapted, with permission, from Olson KR et al. *Med Toxicol* 1987;2:73.

3. **Hypokalemia** (serum potassium < 3.5 mEq/L) may cause muscle weakness, hyporeflexia, and ileus. Rhabdomyolysis may occur. The ECG shows flattened T waves and prominent U waves. In severe hypokalemia, AV block, ventricular arrhythmias, and cardiac arrest may occur.

   a. **With theophylline, caffeine, or beta-2 agonist intoxication,** an intracellular shift of potassium may produce a very low serum potassium level with normal total body stores. Patients usually do not have serious symptoms or ECG signs of hypokalemia, and aggressive potassium therapy is not required.

   b. **With barium poisoning** (p 103), profound hypokalemia may lead to respiratory muscle weakness and cardiac and respiratory arrest, and therefore intensive potassium therapy is necessary. Up to 420 mEq has been given in 24 hours.

   c. **Hypokalemia resulting from diuretic therapy** may contribute to ventricular arrhythmias, especially those associated with chronic digitalis glycoside poisoning.

4. **Treatment of hypokalemia.** Mild hypokalemia (potassium 3–3.5 mEq/L) is usually not associated with serious symptoms.

   a. Administer potassium chloride orally or intravenously. Do **not** give more than 10–15 mEq/h IV (0.25–0.5 mEq/kg/h in children).

   b. Monitor serum potassium and the ECG for signs of hyperkalemia from excessive potassium therapy.

   c. If hypokalemia is caused by diuretic therapy or gastrointestinal fluid losses, measure and replace other ions such as magnesium, sodium, and chloride.

G. **Renal failure.** Examples of drugs and toxins causing renal failure are listed in Table I–28. Renal failure may be caused by a direct nephrotoxic action of the poison or acute massive tubular precipitation of myoglobin (rhabdomyolysis), hemoglobin (hemolysis), or calcium oxalate crystals (ethylene glycol); or it may be secondary to shock caused by blood or fluid loss or cardiovascular collapse.

1. **Assessment.** Renal failure is characterized by a progressive rise in the serum creatinine and blood urea nitrogen (BUN) levels, usually accompanied by oliguria or anuria.

   a. The serum creatinine level usually rises about 1 mg/dL/d after total anuric renal failure.

   b. A more abrupt rise should suggest rapid muscle breakdown (rhabdomyolysis), which increases the creatine load and also results in elevated creatinine phosphokinase (CPK) levels that may interfere with determination of the serum creatinine level.

TABLE I–28. EXAMPLES OF DRUGS AND TOXINS AND OTHER CAUSES OF ACUTE RENAL FAILURE

Direct nephrotoxic effect	Hemolysis
Acetaminophen	Arsine
Amanita phalloides mushrooms	Naphthalene
Analgesics (eg, ibuprofen, phenacetin)	Oxidizing agents (esp. with G6PD deficiency)
Antibiotics (eg, aminoglycosides)	
Bromates	**Rhabdomyolysis (see also Table I–16)**
Chlorates	Amphetamines and cocaine
Chlorinated hydrocarbons	Coma with prolonged immobility
Cortinarius sp. mushrooms	Hyperthermia
Cyclosporin	Phencyclidine (PCP)
Ethylene glycol (oxalate)	Status epilepticus
Heavy metals (eg, mercury)	Strychnine

      c. Oliguria may be seen before renal failure occurs, especially with hypovolemia. In this case, the BUN level is usually elevated out of proportion to the serum creatinine level.

  2. Complications. The earliest complication of acute renal failure is hyperkalemia (see p 36); this may be more pronounced if the cause of the renal failure is rhabdomyolysis or hemolysis, both of which release large amounts of intracellular potassium into the circulation. Later complications include metabolic acidosis, delirium, and coma.

  3. Treatment

      a. Prevent renal failure, if possible, by administering specific treatment (eg, acetylcysteine for acetaminophen overdose, BAL [dimercaprol] chelation for mercury poisoning, and intravenous fluids for rhabdomyolysis or shock).

      b. Monitor the serum potassium level frequently and treat hyperkalemia (see p 36) if it occurs.

      c. Do *not* give supplemental potassium, and avoid cathartics or other medications containing magnesium, phosphate, or sodium.

      d. Perform hemodialysis as needed.

H. Hepatic failure. A variety of drugs and toxins may cause hepatic failure (Table I–29). Mechanisms of toxicity include direct hepatocellular damage (eg, *Amanita phalloides* mushrooms [p 228]), metabolic creation of a hepatotoxic intermediate (eg, acetaminophen [p 62] or carbon tetrachloride [p 127]), or hepatic vein thrombosis (eg, pyrrolizidine alkaloids).

  1. Assessment. Laboratory and clinical evidence of hepatitis usually does not become apparent until at least 24–36 hours after exposure to the poison. Then transaminase levels rise sharply and may fall to normal over the next 3–5 days. If hepatic damage is severe, measures of hepatic function (eg, bilirubin and prothrombin time) will continue to worsen after 2–3 days, even as transaminase levels are returning to normal. Metabolic acidosis and hypoglycemia usually indicate a poor prognosis.

  2. Complications

      a. Abnormal hepatic function may result in excessive bleeding owing to insufficient production of vitamin K-dependent coagulation factors.

      b. Hepatic encephalopathy may lead to coma and death, usually within 5–7 days of massive hepatic failure.

  3. Treatment

      a. Prevent hepatic injury if possible by administering specific treatment (eg, acetylcysteine for acetaminophen overdose).

      b. Obtain baseline and daily transaminase, bilirubin, and glucose levels and prothrombin time.

      c. Provide intensive supportive care for hepatic failure and encephalopathy (eg, glucose for hypoglycemia, fresh frozen plasma for coagulopathy, or lactulose for encephalopathy).

      d. Liver transplant may be the only effective treatment once massive hepatic necrosis has resulted in severe encephalopathy.

TABLE I–29. EXAMPLES OF DRUGS AND TOXINS CAUSING HEPATIC DAMAGE

Acetaminophen	Nitrosamine
Amanita phalloides and similar mushrooms	Pennyroyal oil
Arsenic	Phenol
Carbon tetrachloride and other chlorinated hydrocarbons	Phosphorus
Copper	Polychlorinated biphenyls (PCBs)
Dimethylformamide	Pyrrolizidine alkaloids
Ethanol	Thallium
Halothane	2-Nitropropane
Iron	Valproic acid

IV. Toxicology screening.* To maximize the utility of the toxicology laboratory, it is necessary to understand what the laboratory can and cannot do and how knowledge of the results will affect the patient. Comprehensive blood and urine screening is of little practical value in the initial care of the poisoned patient. On the other hand, specific toxicologic analyses and quantitative levels of certain drugs may be extremely helpful. Before ordering any tests, always ask these two questions: (i) How will the result of the test alter the approach to treatment, and (ii) can the result of the test be returned in time to affect therapy positively?

    A. Limitations of toxicology screens. Owing to long turnaround time, lack of availability, reliability factors, and the low risk of serious morbidity with supportive clinical management, toxicology screening is estimated to affect management in less than 15% of all cases of poisoning or drug overdose.

        1. Comprehensive toxicology screens or panels may look specifically for only 40–50 drugs out of more than 10,000 possible drugs or toxins (or 6 million chemicals). However, these 40–50 drugs (Tables I–30 and I–31) account for more than 80% of overdoses.

        2. To detect many different drugs, comprehensive screens usually include methods with broad specificity, and sensitivity may be poor for some drugs

---

*By John D. Osterloh, MD.

TABLE I-30. DRUGS COMMONLY INCLUDED IN A COMPREHENSIVE URINE SCREEN[a]

Alcohols
  Acetone
  Ethanol
  Isopropyl alcohol
  Methanol

Analgesics
  Acetaminophen
  Salicylates

Anticonvulsants
  Carbamazepine
  Phenobarbital
  Phenytoin
  Primidone

Antihistamines
  Benztropine
  Chlorpheniramine
  Diphenhydramine
  Pyrilamine
  Trihexylphenidyl

Opiates
  Codeine
  Dextromethorphan
  Hydrocodone
  Meperidine
  Methadone
  Morphine
  Oxycodone
  Pentazocine
  Propoxyphene

Phenothiazines
  Chlorpromazine
  Prochlorperazine

Promethazine
Thioridazine
Trifluoperazine

Sedative-hypnotic drugs
  Barbiturates
  Benzodiazepines
  Carisoprodol
  Chloral hydrate
  Ethchlorvynol
  Glutethimide
  Meprobamate
  Methaqualone

Stimulants
  Amphetamines
  Caffeine
  Cocaine and benzoylecgonine
  Phencyclidine (PCP)
  Strychnine

Tricyclic antidepressants
  Amitriptyline
  Desipramine
  Doxepin
  Imipramine
  Nortriptyline
  Protriptyline

Other drugs
  Diltiazem
  Lidocaine
  Procainamide
  Propranolol
  Quinidine and quinine
  Verapamil

---

[a]Newer drugs in any category may not be included in screening.

TABLE I–31. DRUGS COMMONLY INCLUDED IN A COMPREHENSIVE BLOOD SCREEN

Alcohols	**Sedative-hypnotic drugs**
Acetone	Barbiturates
Ethanol	Carisoprodol
Isopropyl alcohol	Chlordiazepoxide
Methanol	Diazepam
Analgesics	Ethchlorvynol
Acetaminophen	Glutethimide
Salicylates	Meprobamate
Anticonvulsants	Methaqualone
Ethosuximide	
Carbamazepine	
Phenobarbital	
Phenytoin	

(resulting in analytic false-negative results). On the other hand, some drugs present in therapeutic amounts may be detected on the screen even though they are causing no clinical symptoms (clinical false-positives).

3. Because many agents are neither sought nor detected during a toxicology screening (Table I–32), a negative result does not always rule out poisoning; the negative predictive value of the screen is only about 70%. In contrast, a positive result has a predictive value of about 90%.

4. The specificity of toxicologic tests is dependent on the method and the laboratory. The presence of other drugs, drug metabolites, disease states, or incorrect sampling may cause erroneous results (Table I–33).

B. Uses for toxicology screens

1. Comprehensive screening of urine and blood should be carried out whenever the diagnosis of brain death is being considered, to rule out the presence of common depressant drugs that might result in temporary loss of brain activity and mimic brain death.

2. Toxicology screens may be used to confirm clinical impressions during hospitalization and can be inserted in the permanent medicolegal record. This may be important if homicide, assault, or child abuse is suspected.

TABLE I–32. DRUGS AND TOXINS *NOT* COMMONLY INCLUDED IN TOXICOLOGIC SCREENING PANELS[a]

Anesthetic gases	Fentanyl and other opiate derivatives
Antiarrhythmic agents	Fluoride
Antibiotics	Formate
Antidepressants (newer)	Hypoglycemic agents
Antihypertensives	Isoniazid (INH)
Antipsychotic agents (newer)	Lithium
Benzodiazepines (newer)	LSD (lysergic acid diethylamide)
Beta blockers other than propranolol	MAO inhibitors
Borate	Marihuana
Bromide	Noxious gases
Calcium antagonists (newer)	Plant, fungal, and microbiologic toxins
Colchicine	Pressors (eg, dopamine)
Cyanide	Solvents and hydrocarbons
Digitalis glycosides	Theophylline
Diuretics	Valproic acid
Ergot alkaloids	Vasodilators
Ethylene glycol	

[a]Many of these are available as separate specific tests.

TABLE I–33. INTERFERENCES IN TOXICOLOGIC BLOOD TESTS

Drug or Toxin	Method[a]	Causes of Falsely Increased Blood Level
Acetaminophen	SC[b]	Salicylate, salicylamide, methyl salicylate (each will increase acetaminophen level by 10% of their level in mg/L); bilirubin; phenols; renal failure (each 1 mg/dL increase in creatinine = 30 mg/L acetaminophen).
	GC, IA	Phenacetin.
	HPLC[b]	Cephalosporins; sulfonamides.
Amitriptyline	HPLC, GC	Cyclobenzaprine.
Amphetamines (urine)	GC[c]	Other volatile stimulant amines (misidentified). GC mass spectrometry poorly distinguishes d-methamphetamine from l-methamphetamine (found in Vicks inhaler).
	IA[c], TLC[c]	Phenylpropanolamine, ephedrine, phentermine, phenmetrazine, labetalol; many phenylethylamine and amphetamine derivatives.
Chloride	SC	Bromide (0.8 meq Cl = 1 meq Br).
Creatinine	SC	Ketoacidosis (may increase Cr up to 2–3 mg/dL in non-rate methods); cephalosporins; creatine (eg, with rhabdomyolysis).
	EZ	Creatinine, lidocaine metabolite, 5-fluorouracil
Digoxin	IA	Endogenous digoxinlike natriuretic substances in newborns and in patients with renal failure (up to 1 ng/mL); bufotoxins; Chan Su; oleander ingestion (other cardiac glycosides identified as digoxin); after digoxin antibody (Fab) administration.
Ethanol	SC[b]	Other alcohols, ketones (by oxidation methods); isopropyl alcohol (by enzymatic methods).
	EZ	Isopropyl alcohol; patient with elevated lactate and LDH
Ethylene glycol	EZ	Other glycols; elevated triglycerides.
	SC, GC	Propylene glycol.
Glucose	EC	Acetaminophen; ascorbate (Medisense device).
Iron	SC	Deferoxamine causes 15% lowering of total iron-binding capacity (TIBC). Lavender-top Vacutainer tube contains EDTA, which lowers total iron.
Isopropanol	GC	Skin disinfectant containing isopropyl alcohol used before venipuncture (highly variable, usually trivial, but up to 40 mg/dL).
Ketones	SC	Acetylcysteine; valproic acid; captopril; levodopa.
Lithium	FE	Green-top Vacutainer specimen tube (contains lithium heparin) may cause marked elevation (up to 6–8 meq/L).
	SC	Procainamide, quinidine can produce 5–15% elevation.
Methemoglobin	SC	Sulfhemoglobin (cross-positive ~10% by co-oximeter); methylene blue (2 mg/kg dose gives transient false-positive 15% methemoglobin level); hyperlipidemia (triglyceride level of 6000 mg/dL may give false methemoglobin of 28.6%).
		Falsely decreased level with in vitro spontaneous reduction to hemoglobin in Vacutainer tube (~10%/h). Analyze within 1 hour.

(*continued*)

TABLE I–33. INTERFERENCES IN TOXICOLOGIC BLOOD TESTS (CONTINUED)

Drug or Toxin	Method[a]	Causes of Falsely Increased Blood Level
Morphine/codeine (urine)	TLC[c]	Hydromorphone; hydrocodone; oxycodone (misidentification)
	IA[c]	Cross-reactants: hydrocodone; hydromorphone; oxycodone; monoacetylmorphine; morphine from poppy-seed ingestion. Also rifampin and ofloxacin in different IAs.
Osmolality	Osm	Lavender-top (EDTA) Vacutainer specimen tube (15 mosm/L); gray-top (fluoride-oxalate) tube (150 mosm/L); blue-top (citrate) tube (10 mosm/L); green-top (lithium heparin) tube (theoretically, up to 6–8 mosm/L).
		Falsely normal if vapor pressure method used (alcohols are volatilized).
Phencyclidine (urine)	IA[c]	Diphenhydramine; methadone; dextromethorphan; chlorpromazine.
Salicylate	SC	Phenothiazines; diflunisal; ketosis[c]; salicylamide; accumulated salicylate metabolites in patients with renal failure (~10% increase).
	IA	Diflunisal.
	SC	**Decreased or altered salicylate level:** bilirubin; phenylketones.
	GC[b]	Methyl salicylate; eucalyptol; theophylline.
	HPLC[b]	Theophylline; antibiotics.
Theophylline	HPLC[b]	Acetazolamide; cephalosporins; endogenous xanthines and accumulated theophylline metabolites in renal failure (minor effect).
	IA	Caffeine overdose; accumulated theophylline metabolites in renal failure.

[a]GC = gas chromatography (interferences primarily with older methods); HPLC = high-pressure liquid chromatography; IA = immunoassay; SC = spectrochemical; TLC = thin-layer chromatography; EC = electrochemical; EZ = enzymatic; FE = flame emission.
[b]Uncommon methodology.
[c]More common with urine test. Confirmation by a second test is required.

    3. Selective screens (eg, for "drugs of abuse") with rapid turnaround times are often used to confirm clinical impressions and may aid in disposition of the patient. Positive results should be subjected to confirmatory testing with a second method.

  C. Approach to toxicology testing

    1. Communicate clinical suspicions to the laboratory.

    2. Obtain blood and urine specimens on admission and have the laboratory store them temporarily. If the patient rapidly recovers, they can be discarded.

    3. Urine and gastric specimens are the best samples for broad qualitative screening. Blood samples should be saved for possible quantitative testing, but blood is not a good specimen for screening for many common drugs, including psychotropic agents, opiates, and stimulants.

    4. Decide if a specific quantitative blood level may assist in management decisions (eg, use of an antidote or dialysis; Table I–34). Quantitative levels are helpful only if there is a predictable correlation between the serum level and toxic effects.

    5. A regional poison control center (see Table I–42) or toxicology consultant may provide assistance in considering certain drug etiologies and in selecting specific tests.

V. Abdominal x-rays. Abdominal x-rays may reveal radiopaque tablets, drug-filled condoms, or other toxic material.

TABLE I–34. SPECIFIC QUANTITATIVE LEVELS AND POTENTIAL INTERVENTIONS[a]

Drug or Toxin	Potential Intervention
Acetaminophen	Acetylcysteine
Carbamazepine	Repeat-dose charcoal, hemoperfusion
Carboxyhemoglobin	100% oxygen
Digoxin	Digoxin-specific antibodies
Ethanol	Low level indicates search for other toxins
Ethylene glycol	Ethanol or fomepizole therapy, hemodialysis
Iron	Deferoxamine chelation
Lithium	Hemodialysis
Methanol	Ethanol or fomepizole therapy, hemodialysis
Methemoglobin	Methylene blue
Salicylate	Alkalinization, hemodialysis
Theophylline	Repeat-dose charcoal, hemoperfusion
Valproic acid	Hemodialysis, repeat-dose charcoal

A. The radiograph is useful only if positive; recent studies suggest that few types of tablets are predictably visible (Table I–35).
B. Do *not* attempt to determine the radiopacity of a tablet by placing it directly on the x-ray plate. This often produces a false-positive result because of an air contrast effect.

DECONTAMINATION

I. Surface decontamination
A. Skin. Corrosive agents rapidly injure the skin and must be removed immediately. In addition, many toxins are readily absorbed through the skin, and systemic absorption can be prevented only by rapid action. Table II–17 (p 130)

TABLE I–35. RADIOPAQUE DRUGS AND POISONS[a]

Usually visible
  Bismuth subsalicylate (Pepto-Bismol)
  Calcium carbonate (Tums)
  Iron tablets
  Lead and lead-containing paint
  Metallic foreign bodies
  Potassium tablets
Sometimes/weakly visible
  Acetazolamide
  Arsenic
  Brompheniramine and dexbrompheniramine
  Busulfan
  Chloral hydrate
  Enteric-coated or sustained-release preparations (highly variable)
  Meclizine
  Perphenazine with amitriptyline
  Phosphorus
  Prochlorperazine
  Sodium chloride
  Thiamine
  Tranylcypromine
  Trifluoperazine
  Trimeprazine
  Zinc sulfate

[a]Reference: Savitt DL, Hawkins HH, Roberts JR: The radiopacity of ingested medications. *Ann Emerg Med* 1987; 16:331.

lists several corrosive chemical agents that can have systemic toxicity, and many of them are readily absorbed through the skin.

1. Be careful not to expose yourself or other care providers to potentially contaminating substances. Wear protective gear (gloves, gown, and goggles) and wash exposed areas promptly. Contact a regional poison center for information about the hazards of the chemicals involved; in the majority of cases, health care providers are not at significant personal risk for secondary contamination, and simple measures such as emergency department gowns and plain latex gloves are sufficient protection. For radiation and other hazardous materials incidents, see also Section IV (p 411).

2. Remove contaminated clothing and flush exposed areas with copious quantities of tepid (lukewarm) water or saline. Wash carefully behind ears, under nails, and in skin folds. Use soap and shampoo for oily substances.

3. There is rarely a need for chemical neutralization of a substance spilled on the skin. In fact, the heat generated by chemical neutralization can potentially create worse injury. Some of the few exceptions to this rule are listed in Table I–36.

B. **Eyes.** The cornea is especially sensitive to corrosive agents and hydrocarbon solvents that may rapidly damage the corneal surface and lead to permanent scarring.

1. Act quickly to prevent serious damage. Flush exposed eyes with copious quantities of tepid tap water or saline. If available, instill local anesthetic drops in the eye first to facilitate irrigation. Remove the victim's contact lenses if they are being worn.

2. Place the victim in a supine position under a tap or use intravenous tubing to direct a stream of water across the nasal bridge into the medial aspect of the eye (Figure I–8). Use at least 1 L to irrigate each eye.

3. If the offending substance is an acid or a base, check the pH of the victim's tears after irrigation and continue irrigation if the pH remains abnormal.

4. Do *not* instill any neutralizing solution; there is no evidence that such treatment works, and it may further damage the eye.

5. After irrigation is complete, check the conjunctival and corneal surfaces carefully for evidence of full-thickness injury. Perform a fluorescein examination of the eye by using fluorescein dye and a Wood's lamp to reveal corneal injury.

6. Patients with serious conjunctival or corneal injury should be referred to an ophthalmologist immediately.

C. **Inhalation.** Agents that injure the pulmonary system may be acutely irritating gases or fumes and may have good or poor warning properties (see p 181).

1. Be careful not to expose yourself or other care providers to toxic gases or fumes without adequate respiratory protection (see pp 415 and 416).

2. Remove the victim from exposure and give supplemental humidified oxygen, if available. Assist ventilation if necessary (see pp 1–7).

3. Observe closely for evidence of upper respiratory tract edema, which is heralded by a hoarse voice and stridor and may progress rapidly to com-

TABLE I–36. SOME TOPICAL AGENTS FOR CHEMICAL EXPOSURES TO THE SKIN[a]

Chemical Corrosive Agent	Topical Treatment
Hydrofluoric acid	Calcium soaks
Oxalic acid	Calcium soaks
Phenol	Mineral oil or other oil; isopropyl alcohol
Phosphorus (white)	Copper sulfate 1% (colors embedded granules blue, facilitates removal)

[a]Reference: Edelman PA; Chemical and electrical burns. Pages 183–202 in: *Management of the Burned Patient.* Achauer BM (editor). Appleton & Lange, 1987.

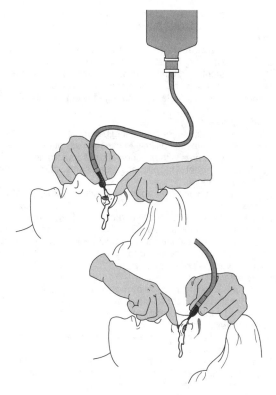

FIGURE I–8. Irrigation of the eyes after chemical injury, showing technique for irrigating both upper and lower eyelids.

plete airway obstruction. Endotracheally intubate patients who show evidence of progressive airway compromise.

4. Also observe for late-onset noncardiogenic pulmonary edema resulting from slower-acting toxins, which may take several hours to appear. Early signs and symptoms include dyspnea, hypoxemia, and tachypnea (see p 181).

II. **Gastrointestinal decontamination.** There is still considerable controversy about the roles of emesis, gastric lavage, activated charcoal, and cathartics to decontaminate the gastrointestinal tract. There is little support in the medical literature for gut emptying procedures, and it is now well established that after a delay of 60 minutes or more, very little of the ingested dose is removed by emesis or gastric lavage. Moreover, recent studies suggest that, in the average overdosed patient, simple oral administration of activated charcoal without prior gut emptying is probably just as effective as the traditional sequence of gut emptying followed by charcoal.

A. **Emesis.** Syrup of ipecac-induced emesis is often used for prehospital treatment of some ingestions (eg, in the home, a factory clinic, or private office) and may be of value *if the ipecac can be given within a few minutes of the ingestion.* It is rarely used in emergency departments because of the ready availability of activated charcoal. After syrup of ipecac administration, vomiting usually occurs within 20–30 minutes. If the ingestion occurred more than 30–60 minutes before ipecac administration, emesis is not very effective.

Moreover, persistent vomiting after ipecac use is likely to delay the administration of activated charcoal (see **C**, below).

1. **Indications**
   a. Early prehospital management of selected potentially serious oral poisonings, particularly in the home immediately after ingestion.
   b. Possibly useful to remove ingested agents not adsorbed by activated charcoal (eg, iron, lithium, potassium; see Table I–37). However, many of these cases are preferably managed with whole-bowel irrigation (see below).
2. **Contraindications**
   a. Obtunded, comatose, or convulsing patient.
   b. Ingestion of a substance likely to cause onset of central nervous system depression seizures within a short clinical time frame (eg, opioids, sedative-hypnotic agents, tricyclic antidepressants, camphor, cocaine, isoniazid, or strychnine).
   c. Ingestion of a corrosive agent (eg, acids, alkali, or strong oxidizing agents).
   d. Ingestion of a simple aliphatic hydrocarbon (see p 183). These are likely to cause pneumonitis if aspirated, but usually do not cause systemic poisoning once they enter the stomach. For those hydrocarbons that do carry a potential for systemic toxicity, activated charcoal with or without gastric lavage is preferable.
3. **Adverse effects**
   a. Persistent vomiting may delay administration of activated charcoal or oral antidotes (eg, acetylcysteine).
   b. Protracted forceful vomiting may result in hemorrhagic gastritis or a Mallory-Weiss tear.
   c. Vomiting may promote passage of toxic material into the small intestine, enhancing absorption.
   d. Drowsiness occurs in about 20% and diarrhea in 25% of children.
   e. Repeated daily use (eg, by bulimic patients) may result in cardiac arrhythmias and cardiomyopathy owing to accumulation of cardiotoxic alkaloids.
4. **Technique.** Use only syrup of ipecac, *not* the fluid extract (which contains much higher concentrations of emetic and cardiotoxic alkaloids).
   a. Administer 30 mL of syrup of ipecac orally (15 mL for children under age 5 years; 10 mL for children under age 1 year; not recommended for children under age 6 months). After 10–15 minutes, give 2–3 glasses of water (there is no consensus on the quantity of water or the timing of administration).
   b. If emesis has not occurred after 20 minutes, a second dose of ipecac may be given. Repeat the fluid administration. Have the patient sit up or move around, because this sometimes stimulates vomiting.

TABLE I–37. DRUGS AND TOXINS POORLY ADSORBED BY ACTIVATED CHARCOAL[a]

Alkali	Inorganic salts
Cyanide[b]	Iron
Ethanol and other alcohols	Lithium
Ethylene glycol	Mineral acids
Fluoride	Potassium

[a]Few studies have been performed to determine in vivo adsorption of these and other toxins to activated charcoal. Adsorption may also depend on the specific type and concentration of charcoal.
[b]Charcoal should still be given because usual doses of charcoal (60–100g) will adsorb usual lethal ingested doses of cyanide (200–300 mg).

    c. If the second dose of ipecac does not induce vomiting, use an alternative method of gut decontamination (eg, activated charcoal). It is not necessary to empty the stomach just to remove the ipecac.

    d. A soapy-water solution may be used as an alternate emetic. Use only standard dishwashing liquid or lotion soap, two tablespoons in a glass of water. Do **not** use powdered laundry or dishwasher detergent or liquid dishwashing concentrate; these products are corrosive. There is no other acceptable alternative to syrup of ipecac. Manual digital stimulation, copper sulfate, salt water, mustard water, apomorphine, and other emetics are unsafe and should not be used.

B. Gastric lavage. Gastric lavage is a more invasive procedure than ipecac-induced emesis, but it is commonly used in hospital emergency departments and is safe if carefully performed. Although there is little evidence to support its use, gastric lavage is probably slightly more effective than ipecac, especially for recently ingested liquid substances. However, it does not reliably remove undissolved pills or pill fragments (especially sustained-release or enteric-coated products). In addition, the procedure may delay administration of activated charcoal and may push poisons into the small intestine, especially if the patient is supine or in the right decubitus position. Gastric lavage is not necessary for small to moderate ingestions of most substances if activated charcoal can be given promptly.

  1. Indications

    a. To remove ingested liquid and solid drugs and poisons when the patient has taken a massive overdose or a particularly toxic substance. Lavage is more likely to be effective if initiated within 30–60 minutes of the ingestion, although it may still be useful several hours after ingestion of agents that slow gastric emptying (eg, salicylates or anticholinergic drugs).

    b. To administer activated charcoal and whole-bowel irrigation to patients unwilling or unable to swallow them.

    c. To dilute and remove corrosive liquids from the stomach and to empty the stomach in preparation for endoscopy.

  2. Contraindications

    a. Obtunded, comatose, or convulsing patients. Because it may disturb the normal physiology of the esophagus and airway protective mechanisms, gastric lavage must be used with caution in obtunded patients whose airway reflexes are dulled. In such cases, endotracheal intubation with a cuffed endotracheal tube should be performed first to protect the airway.

    b. Ingestion of sustained-release or enteric-coated tablets. Lavage is unlikely to return intact tablets, even through a 40F orogastric hose. In such cases, whole-bowel irrigation (see p 50) is preferable.

    c. Ingestion of a corrosive substance is *not* a contraindication; in fact, many gastroenterologists recommend that lavage be performed after liquid caustic ingestion to remove corrosive material from the stomach and to prepare for endoscopy.

  3. Adverse effects

    a. Perforation of the esophagus or stomach.

    b. Nosebleed from nasal trauma during passage of the tube.

    c. Inadvertent tracheal intubation.

    d. Vomiting resulting in pulmonary aspiration of gastric contents in an obtunded patient without airway protection.

  4. Technique (see Figure I–9)

    a. If the patient is deeply obtunded, protect the airway by intubating the trachea with a cuffed endotracheal tube.

    b. Place the patient in the left lateral decubitus position. This helps prevent ingested material from being pushed into the duodenum during lavage.

    c. Insert a large gastric tube through the mouth or nose and into the stomach (36–40F [catheter size] in adults; a smaller tube will suffice for liquid

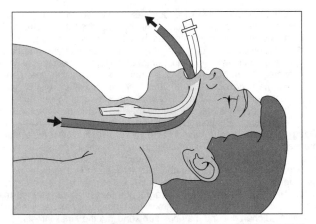

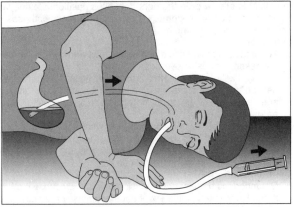

FIGURE I–9. Gastric lavage.

poisons or if simple administration of charcoal is all that is intended).
Check tube position with air insufflation while listening with a stetho-
scope positioned on the patient's stomach.

    d. Withdraw as much of the stomach contents as possible. If the ingested
poison is a toxic chemical that may contaminate hospital personnel (eg,
cyanide, organophosphate insecticide, etc), take steps to immediately
isolate it (eg, use a self-contained wall suction unit).

    e. Administer activated charcoal, 60–100 g (1 g/kg; see **C,** below), down
the tube before starting lavage to begin adsorption of material that may
enter the intestine during the lavage procedure.

    f. Instill tepid (lukewarm) water or saline, 200- to 300-mL aliquots, and re-
move by gravity or active suction. Use repeated aliquots for a total of 2 L
or until the return is free of pills or toxic material. ***Caution:*** Use of excessive volumes of lavage fluid or plain tap water can result in hypothermia
or electrolyte imbalance in infants and small children.

C. Activated charcoal. Activated charcoal is a highly adsorbent powdered material made from a distillation of wood pulp. Owing to its very large surface area,
it is highly effective in adsorbing most toxins. Only a few toxins are poorly adsorbed to charcoal (Table I–37). Recent studies suggest that activated char-

coal given alone without prior gastric emptying is as effective or even more effective than emesis and lavage procedures (see **A** and **B,** above).

1. **Indications**
   a. Used after virtually any toxic ingestion to limit drug absorption from the gastrointestinal tract.
   b. Charcoal is usually given even if the offending substance is not known to be well adsorbed to charcoal, in case other substances have been co-ingested.
   c. Repeated oral doses of activated charcoal may enhance elimination of some drugs from the bloodstream (see p 54).
2. **Contraindications.** Ileus without distension is not a contraindication for a single dose of charcoal.
3. **Adverse effects**
   a. Constipation or intestinal impaction or bezoar is a potential complication, especially if multiple doses of charcoal are given.
   b. Distension of the stomach with a potential risk of pulmonary aspiration.
   c. Many commercially available charcoal products contain charcoal and the cathartic sorbitol in a premixed suspension. Even single doses of sorbitol often cause stomach cramps and vomiting, and repeated doses may cause serious fluid shifts to the intestine, diarrhea, dehydration, and hypernatremia, especially in young children and elderly persons.
   d. May bind coadministered ipecac or acetylcysteine (not clinically significant).
4. **Technique**
   a. Give activated charcoal, 60–100 g (1 g/kg) PO or by gastric tube. If the quantity of an ingested substance is known, give at least 10 times the ingested dose of toxin by weight to prevent desorption of the toxin in the lower gastrointestinal tract.
   b. One or two additional doses of activated charcoal may be given at 1- or 2-hour intervals to ensure adequate gut decontamination, particularly after large ingestions. In rare cases, as many as 8 or 10 repeated doses may be needed to achieve a 10:1 ratio of charcoal to poison (eg, after an ingestion of 200 aspirin tablets); in such circumstances, the doses should be given over a period of several hours.

D. **Cathartics.** Controversy remains over the use of cathartics to hasten elimination of toxins from the gastrointestinal tract. Many toxicologists use cathartics, even though little data exist to support their efficacy.

1. **Indications**
   a. To enhance gastrointestinal transit of the charcoal-toxin complex, decreasing the likelihood of desorption of toxin or development of a charcoal bezoar.
   b. To hasten passage of iron tablets and other ingestions not adsorbed by charcoal.
2. **Contraindications**
   a. Ileus or intestinal obstruction.
   b. Sodium- and magnesium-containing cathartics should not be used in patients with fluid overload or renal insufficiency, respectively.
   c. There is no role for oil-based cathartics (previously recommended for hydrocarbon poisoning).
3. **Adverse effects**
   a. Severe fluid loss, hypernatremia, and hyperosmolarity may result from overuse or repeated doses of cathartics.
   b. Hypermagnesemia may occur in patients with renal insufficiency who are given magnesium-based cathartics.
   c. Abdominal cramping and vomiting may occur, especially with sorbitol.
4. **Technique**
   a. Administer the cathartic of choice (10% magnesium citrate, 3–4 mL/kg; or 70% sorbitol, 1–2 mL/kg) along with activated charcoal or mixed together as a slurry.

   b. Repeat with one-half the original dose if there is no charcoal stool after 6–8 hours.
E. Whole bowel irrigation. Whole bowel irrigation has become an accepted method for elimination of some drugs and poisons from the gut. The technique makes use of a surgical bowel-cleansing solution containing a nonabsorbable polyethylene glycol in a balanced electrolyte solution, formulated to pass through the intestinal tract without being absorbed. This solution is given at high flow rates to force intestinal contents out by sheer volume.

   1. Indications
      a. Large ingestions of iron, lithium, or other drugs poorly adsorbed to activated charcoal.
      b. Large ingestions of sustained-release or enteric-coated tablets (eg, Theo-Dur, Ecotrin, Calan SR, Cardizem CD, etc), or ingestion of foreign bodies or drug-filled packets or condoms.

   2. Contraindications
      a. Ileus or intestinal obstruction.
      b. Obtunded, comatose, or convulsing patient unless the airway is protected.

   3. Adverse effects
      a. Nausea and bloating.
      b. Regurgitation and pulmonary aspiration.
      c. Activated charcoal may not be as effective when given with whole-bowel irrigation.

   4. Technique
      a. Administer bowel preparation solution (eg, CoLyte or GoLYTELY), 2 L/h by gastric tube (children, 500 mL/h or 35 mL/kg/h), until rectal effluent is clear.
      b. Be prepared for large-volume stool within 1–2 hours. Pass a rectal tube or, preferably, have the patient sit on a commode.
      c. Stop administration after 4 L (children, 100 mL/kg) if no rectal effluent has appeared.

F. Other oral binding agents. Other binding agents may be given in certain circumstances to trap toxins in the gut, although activated charcoal is the most widely used effective adsorbent. Table I–38 lists some alternative binding agents and the toxin(s) for which they may be useful.

G. Surgical removal. Occasionally, drug-filled packets or condoms, intact tablets, or tablet concretions persist despite aggressive gastric lavage or whole-gut lavage, and surgical removal may be necessary. Consult a regional poison control center (Table I–42, p 55) or a medical toxicologist for advice.

TABLE I–38. SELECTED ORAL BINDING AGENTS

Drug or Toxin	Binding Agent(s)
Calcium	Cellulose sodium phosphate
Chlorinated hydrocarbons	Cholestyramine resin
Digitoxin[a]	Cholestyramine resin
Heavy metals (arsenic, mercury)	Demulcents (egg white, milk)
Iron	Sodium bicarbonate
Lithium	Sodium polystyrene sulfonate (Kayexalate)
Paraquat[a]	Fuller's earth, Bentonite
Potassium	Sodium polystyrene sulfonate (Kayexalate)
Thallium	Prussian blue

[a]Activated charcoal is also very effective.

ENHANCED ELIMINATION

Measures to enhance elimination of drugs and toxins have been overemphasized in the past. Although a desirable goal, rapid elimination of most drugs and toxins is frequently not practical and may be unsafe. A logical understanding of pharmacokinetics as they apply to toxicology (toxicokinetics) is necessary for the appropriate use of enhanced removal procedures.

I. **Assessment.** Three critical questions must be answered.
   A. **Does the patient need enhanced removal?** Ask the following questions. How is the patient doing? Will supportive care enable the patient to recover fully? Is there an antidote or other specific drug that might be used? Important indications for enhanced drug removal include the following:
      1. Obviously severe or critical intoxication with a deteriorating condition despite maximal supportive care (eg, phenobarbital overdose with intractable hypotension).
      2. The normal or usual route of elimination is impaired (eg, lithium overdose in a patient with renal failure).
      3. The patient has ingested a known lethal dose or has a lethal blood level (eg, theophylline or methanol).
      4. The patient has underlying medical problems that could increase the hazards of prolonged coma or other complications (eg, severe chronic obstructive pulmonary disease or congestive heart failure).
   B. **Is the drug or toxin accessible to the removal procedure?** For a drug to be accessible to removal by extracorporeal procedures, it should be located primarily within the bloodstream or in the extracellular fluid. If it is extensively distributed to tissues, it is not likely to be easily removed.
      1. **The volume of distribution (Vd)** is a numerical concept that provides an indication of the accessibility of the drug:

      $$Vd = \text{Apparent volume into which the drug is distributed}$$
      $$= \text{(Amount of drug in the body)/(plasma concentration)}$$
      $$= \text{(mg/kg)/(mg/L)} = \text{L/kg}$$

      A drug with a very large Vd has a very low plasma concentration. In contrast, a drug with a small Vd is potentially quite accessible by extracorporeal removal procedures. Table I–39 lists some common volumes of distribution.
      2. **Protein binding** may affect accessibility; highly protein-bound drugs have low free-drug concentrations and are difficult to remove by dialysis.
   C. **Will the method work?** Does the removal procedure efficiently extract the toxin from the blood?
      1. **The clearance (Cl)** is the rate at which a given volume of fluid can be "cleared" of the substance.
         a. The Cl may be calculated from the extraction ratio across the dialysis machine or hemoperfusion column, multiplied by the blood flow rate through the following system:

         $$Cl = \text{extraction ratio} \times \text{blood flow rate}$$

TABLE I–39. VOLUME OF DISTRIBUTION (Vd) OF SOME DRUGS AND TOXINS

Large Vd (>5–10 L/kg)	Small Vd (<1 L/kg)
Antidepressants	Alcohols
Digoxin	Carbamazepine
Lindane	Lithium
Opiates	Phenobarbital
Phencyclidine (PCP)	Salicylate
Phenothiazines	Theophylline

b. A crude urinary Cl measurement may be useful for estimating the effectiveness of fluid therapy for enhancing renal elimination of substances not secreted or absorbed by the renal tubule (eg, lithium):

$$\text{Renal Cl} = \frac{\text{urine level} \times \text{urine flow rate}}{\text{serum level}}$$

Note: The units of clearance are milliliters per minute. Clearance is not the same as elimination rate (milligrams per minute). If the blood concentration is small, the actual amount of drug removed is also small.

2. Total clearance is the sum of all sources of clearance (eg, renal excretion plus hepatic metabolism plus respiratory and skin excretion plus dialysis). If the contribution of dialysis is small compared with the total clearance rate, then the procedure will contribute little to overall elimination rate (Table I–40).

3. The **half-life** ($T_{1/2}$) depends on the volume of distribution and the clearance:

$$t_{1/2} = \frac{0.693 \times \text{Vd}}{\text{Cl}}$$

where the unit of measurement of Vd is L (liters) and of Cl is L/min.

II. Methods available for enhanced elimination.

A. Urinary manipulation. These methods require that the renal route be a significant contributor to total clearance.

  1. Forced diuresis may increase glomerular filtration rate, and ion trapping by urinary pH manipulation may enhance elimination of polar drugs.

  2. Alkalinization is commonly used for salicylate overdose, but "forced" diuresis (producing urine volumes of up to 1 L/h) is generally not used because of the risk of fluid overload.

B. Hemodialysis. Blood is taken from a large vein (usually a femoral vein) with a double-lumen catheter and is pumped through the hemodialysis system. The patient must be anticoagulated to prevent clotting of blood in the dialyzer. Drugs and toxins flow passively across the semipermeable membrane down a concentration gradient into a dialysate (electrolyte and buffer) solution. Fluid and electrolyte abnormalities can be corrected concurrently.

  1. Flow rates of up to 300–500 mL/min can be achieved, and clearance rates may reach 200–300 mL/min.

  2. Characteristics of the drug or toxin that enhance its extractability include small size (molecular weight < 500 daltons), water solubility, and low protein binding.

  3. *Note:* Smaller, portable dialysis units that utilize a resin column or filter to recycle a smaller volume dialysate ("mini-dialysis") do not efficiently remove drugs or poisons and should not be used.

C. Hemoperfusion. Using equipment and vascular access similar to that for hemodialysis, the blood is pumped directly through a column containing an adsorbent material (either charcoal or Amberlite resin). Systemic anticoagulation is required, often in higher doses than for hemodialysis, and thrombocytopenia is a common complication.

  1. Because the drug or toxin is in direct contact with the adsorbent material, drug size, water solubility, and protein binding are less important limiting factors.

  2. For most drugs, hemoperfusion can achieve greater clearance rates than hemodialysis. For example, the hemodialysis clearance for phenobarbital is 60–80 mL/min, whereas the hemoperfusion clearance is 200–300 mL/min.

D. Peritoneal dialysis. Dialysate fluid is infused into the peritoneal cavity through a transcutaneous catheter and drained off, and the procedure is repeated with fresh dialysate. The gut wall and peritoneal lining serve as the semipermeable membrane.

  1. Peritoneal dialysis is easier to perform than hemodialysis or hemoperfusion and does not require anticoagulation, but it is only about 10–15% as effec-

TABLE I-40. ELIMINATION OF SELECTED DRUGS AND TOXINS[a]

Drug or Toxin	Volume of Distribution (L/kg)	Usual Body Clearance (mL/min)	Reported Clearance by:	
			Dialysis (mL/min)	Hemoperfusion[b] (mL/min)
Acetaminophen	0.8–1	400	120–150	125–300
Amitriptyline	6–10	500–800	NHD[c]	240[d]
Bromide	0.7	5	100	NA[c]
Carbamazepine	1.2	60–90	NHD	80–130
Digitoxin	0.6	4	10–26	NA
Digoxin	5–7	150–200	NHD	90–140
Ethanol	0.7	100–300	100–200	NHP[c]
Ethchlorvynol	2–4	120–140	20–80	150–300[d]
Ethylene glycol	0.6–0.8	200	100–200	NHP
Glutethimide	2.7	200	70	300[d]
Isopropyl alcohol	0.7	30	100–200	NHP
Lithium	0.6–1	25–30	50–150	NHP
Meprobamate	0.75	60	60	85–150
Methanol	0.7	40–60	100–200	NHP
Methaqualone	5.8	130–175	23	150–270
Methotrexate	0.5–1	50–100	NA	54
Nadolol	2	135	46–102	NA
Nortriptyline	20–40	500–1000	24–34	216[d]
Paraquat	2.8	30–200	10	50–155
Pentobarbital	0.8–1	27–36	23–55	200–300
Phenobarbital	0.8	2–15	60–75	100–300
Phenytoin	0.6	15–30	NHD	76–189
Procainamide	1.9	650	70	75
N-acetylprocainamide (NAPA)	1.4	220	48	75
Salicylate	0.15	30	35–80	57–116
Theophylline	0.3–0.6	80–120	30–50	60–225
Trichloroethanol (chloral hydrate)	0.6–1.6	25	68–162	119–200
Valproic acid	0.15–0.4	10	23	55

[a]Adapted in part from Pond SM: Diuresis, dialysis, and hemoperfusion: Indications and benefits. *Emerg Med Clin North Am* 1984;2:29, and Cutler RE et al: Extracorporeal removal of drugs and poisons by hemodialysis and hemoperfusion. *Ann Rev Pharmacol Toxicol* 1987;27:169.
[b]Hemoperfusion data are mainly for charcoal hemoperfusion.
[c]Abbreviations: NHD = not hemodialyzable; NA = not available; NHP = not hemoperfusable.
[d]Data are for XAD-4 resin hemoperfusion.

tive owing to poor extraction ratios and slower flow rates (clearance rates, 10–15 mL/min).

2. However, peritoneal dialysis can be performed continuously, 24 hours a day; a 24-hour peritoneal dialysis with dialysate exchange every 1–2 hours is approximately equal to 4 hours of hemodialysis.

E. **Hemofiltration.** Continuous arteriovenous or venovenous hemodiafiltration (CAVHD or CVVHD, respectively) has been suggested as an alternative to conventional hemodialysis when the need for rapid removal of the drug is less urgent. Like peritoneal dialysis, these procedures are associated with lower clearance rates but have the advantage of being minimally invasive, with no significant impact on hemodynamics, and can be carried out "continuously" for many hours. However, their role in management of acute poisoning remains uncertain.

F. **Repeat-dose activated charcoal.** Repeated doses of activated charcoal (20–30 g or 0.5–1 g/kg every 2–3 hours) are given orally or via gastric tube. The presence of a slurry of activated charcoal throughout several meters of the intestinal lumen reduces blood concentrations by interrupting enterohepatic or enteroenteric recirculation of the drug or toxin, a mode of action quite distinct from simple adsorption of ingested but unabsorbed tablets. This technique is easy and noninvasive and has been shown to shorten the half-life of phenobarbital, theophylline, and several other drugs (Table I–41). However, it has not been shown in clinical trials to alter patient outcome. *Caution:* Repeat-dose charcoal may cause serious fluid and electrolyte disturbance secondary to large-volume diarrhea, especially if premixed charcoal-sorbitol suspensions are used. Also, it should not be used in patients with ileus or obstruction.

DISPOSITION OF THE PATIENT

I. **Emergency department discharge or intensive care unit admission?**
  A. All patients with potentially serious overdose should be observed for at least 6 hours before discharge or transfer to a nonmedical (eg, psychiatric) facility. If signs or symptoms of intoxication develop during this time, admission for further observation and treatment is required. *Caution:* Beware of delayed complications from slow absorption of medications (eg, from a tablet concretion or bezoar, or sustained-release or enteric-coated preparations). If specific drug levels are determined, obtain repeated serum levels to be certain that they are decreasing as expected.
  B. Most patients admitted for poisoning or drug overdose will need observation in an intensive care unit, although this depends on the potential for serious cardiorespiratory complications. Any patient with suicidal intent must be kept under close observation.

II. **Regional poison control center consultation.** Consult with a regional poison control center to determine the need for further observation or admission, administration of antidotes or therapeutic drugs, selection of appropriate laboratory tests, or decisions about extracorporeal removal. An experienced clinical toxicologist is usually available for immediate consultation. See Table I–42 for a list of regional poison control centers.

III. **Psychosocial evaluation.**
  A. **Psychiatric consultation for suicide risk.** All patients with intentional poisoning or drug overdose should have psychiatric evaluation for suicidal intent.
    1. It is not appropriate to discharge a potentially suicidal patient from the emergency department without a careful psychiatric evaluation. Most states have provisions for the physician to place an emergency psychiatric hold, forcing involuntary patients to remain under psychiatric observation for up to 72 hours.

TABLE I–41. SOME DRUGS REMOVED BY REPEAT-DOSE ACTIVATED CHARCOAL

Carbamazepine	Phenobarbital
Chlordecone	Phenylbutazone
Dapsone	Phenytoin
Digitoxin	Salicylate
Nadolol	Theophylline

TABLE I-42. REGIONAL POISON CONTROL CENTERS IN THE USA[a]

State	Poison Center	Phone Number
Alabama	Alabama Poison Center, Tuscaloosa	(800) 462-0800 (AL only) (205) 345-0600
	Children's Hospital of Alabama, Birmingham	(800) 292-6678 (AL only) (205) 939-9201
Arizona	Arizona Poison and Drug Information Center, Tucson	(800) 362-0101 (AZ only) (602) 626-6016
	Samaritan Regional Poison Center, Phoenix	(800) 362-0101 (AZ only) (602) 253-3334
California	California Poison Control System	(800) 876-4766 (CA only) (415) 502-8600 (Admin)
Colorado	Rocky Mountain Poison Center, Denver	(800) 332-3073 (CO only) (303) 629-1123
Connecticut	Connecticut Regional Poison Center	(800) 343-2722 (CT only)
District of Columbia	National Capitol Poison Center, Washington, DC	(202) 625-3333
Florida	Florida Poison Information Center (Network)	(800) 282-3171 (FL only)
Georgia	Georgia Poison Center, Atlanta	(800) 282-5846 (GA only) (404) 616-9000
Indiana	Indiana Poison Center, Indianapolis	(800) 382-9097 (IN only) (317) 929-2323
Kentucky	Kentucky Regional Poison Center, Louisville	(502) 589-8222
Louisiana	Louisiana Drug and Poison Information Center, Monroe	(800) 256-9822 (LA only)
Maryland	Maryland Poison Center, Baltimore	(800) 492-2414 (MD only) (410) 528-7701
Massachusetts	Massachusetts Poison Control System, Boston	(800) 682-9211 (MA only) (617) 232-2120
Michigan	Blodgett Regional Poison Center, Grand Rapids	(800) 764-7661 (MI only)
	Poison Control Center, Children's Hospital, Detroit	(800) 764-7661 (MI only) (313) 745-5711
Minnesota	Hennepin Regional Poison Center, Minneapolis	(612) 347-3141
	Minnesota Regional Poison Center	(800) 222-1222 (MN only) (612) 221-2113
Missouri	Cardinal Glennon Children's Hospital Regional Poison Center, St. Louis	(314) 772-5200
Montana	Rocky Mountain Poison Center, Denver, CO	(800) 525-5042 (MT only)
Nebraska	Mid-Plains Poison Center, Omaha	(800) 955-9119 (NE only)
New Jersey	New Jersey Poison Information and Education System	(800) 764-7661 (NJ only)
New Mexico	New Mexico Poison and Drug Information Center, Albuquerque	(800) 432-6866 (NM only) (505) 843-2551
New York	Central New York Poison Center, Syracuse	(800) 252-5665 (315) 476-4766
	Finger Lakes Regional Poison Center	(800) 333-0542 (NY only) (716) 275-3252
	Hudson Valley Poison Center, Nyack	(800) 336-6997 (NY only) (914) 353-1000
	Long Island Regional Poison Control Center	(516) 542-2323
	New York City Poison Center, New York City	(212) 340-4494 (212) 764-7667

TABLE I–42. REGIONAL POISON CONTROL CENTERS IN THE USA[a] *(Continued)*

State	Poison Center	Phone Number
North Carolina	Carolinas Poison Center, Charlotte	(800 848–6946 (NC only) (704) 355–4000
Ohio	Central Ohio Poison Center, Columbus	(800) 682–7625 (OH only) (614) 228–1323
	Cincinnati Drug and Poison Information Center, Cincinnati	(800) 872–5111 (513) 558–5111
Oregon	Oregon Poison Center, Portland	(800) 452–7165 (OR only) (503) 494–8968
Pennsylvania	Central Pennsylvania Poison Center, Hershey	(800) 521–6110
	Pittsburgh Poison Center, Pittsburgh	(412) 681–6669
	The Poison Center, Philadelphia	(800) 722–7112 (PA only) (215) 386–2100
Rhode Island	Life Span Poison Center, Providence	(401) 444–5727
Tennessee	Middle Tennessee Poison Center, Nashville	(800) 288–9999 (TN only) (615) 936–2034
Texas	Texas Poison Center Network	(800) 764–7661 (TX only)
Utah	Utah Poison Center, Salt Lake City	(800) 456–7707 (UT only) (801) 581–2151
Virginia	Blue Ridge Poison Center, Charlottesville	(800) 451–1428 (VA only) (804) 924–5543
West Virginia	West Virginia Poison Center, Charleston	(800) 642–3625 (WV only) (304) 348–4211
Wyoming	Mid-Plains Poison Center, Omaha, NE	(800) 955–9119 (WY only)

[a]AAPCC (American Association of Poison Control Centers) Regional Certification Committee, September, 1997.

2. Patients calling from home after an intentional ingestion should always be referred to an emergency department for medical and psychiatric evaluation.
B. **Child abuse** (see also p 58) or sexual abuse
   1. Children should be evaluated for the possibility that the ingestion was not accidental. Sometimes parents or other adults intentionally give children sedatives or tranquilizers to control their behavior.
   2. Accidental poisonings may also warrant social services referral. Occasionally children get into stimulants or other abused drugs that are left around the home. Repeated ingestions suggest overly casual or negligent parental behavior.
   3. Intentional overdose in a child or adolescent should raise the possibility of physical or sexual abuse. Teenage girls may have overdosed because of unwanted pregnancy.
IV. **Overdose in the pregnant patient.**
   A. In general, it is prudent to check for pregnancy in any young woman with drug overdose or poisoning. Unwanted pregnancy may be a cause for intentional overdose, or special concerns may be raised about treatment of the pregnant patient.
   B. Inducing emesis with syrup of ipecac is probably safe in early pregnancy, but protracted vomiting is unwelcome, especially in the third trimester. Gastric lavage or oral activated charcoal is preferable in all trimesters.
   C. Some toxins are known to be teratogenic or mutagenic (Table I–43). However, adverse effects on the fetus are generally associated with chronic, repeated use as opposed to acute, single exposure.

TABLE I-43. HUMAN TERATOGENS[a]

Alcohol (ethanol)
Alkylating agents (busulfan, chlorambucil, cyclophosphamide, mustine/mechlorethamine)
Antimetabolic agents (aminopterine, azauridine, cytarabine, fluorouracil, 6-mercaptopurine, methotrexate)
Carbon monoxide
Coumadins
Diethylstibestrol (DES)
Disulfiram
Heparin
Lithium carbonate
Mercuric sulfide
Methyl mercury
Phenytoin
Polychlorinated biphenyls (PCBs)
Tetracycline
Thalidomide
Tretinoin (retinoic acid)
Trimethadione
Valproic acid

[a]Reference: Bologa-Campeanu M et al: Prenatal adverse effects of various drugs and chemicals: A review of substances of frequent concern to mothers in the community. *Med Toxicol Adverse Drug Exp* 1988;3:307.

► SPECIAL CONSIDERATIONS IN PEDIATRIC PATIENTS

Delia A. Dempsey, MD, MS

The majority of calls to poison control centers involve children under 5 years of age. Fortunately, children account for a minority of serious poisonings requiring emergency hospital treatment. Most common childhood ingestions involve nontoxic substances or nontoxic doses of potentially toxic drugs or products (see p 239). The leading causes of serious or fatal childhood poisoning include iron supplements (see p 192); tricyclic antidepressants (see p 310); cardiovascular medications such as digitalis (see p 128), beta blockers (p 107) or calcium antagonists (p 119); methyl salicylate (p 284); and hydrocarbons (p 183). See Table I-44.

I. **High-risk populations.** Two age groups are commonly involved in pediatric poisonings: children between 1 and 5 years old and adolescents.

A. **Ingestions in toddlers and young children** usually result from oral exploration. Unintentional ingestion in children under 6 months of age or between the ages of 5 and adolescence is rare. In young infants, consider the possibility of intentional administration by an older child or adult. In school-age children, suspect abuse or neglect as a reason for the ingestion, and in adolescents, suspect a suicide attempt.

B. **In adolescents and young adults,** overdoses are usually suicidal but may also result from drug abuse or experimentation. Common underlying reasons for adolescents' suicide attempts include pregnancy; sexual, physical, or mental abuse; school failure; conflict with peers; conflict with homosexual or lesbian orientation; a sudden or severe loss; and alcoholism or illicit drug use. Any adolescent who makes a suicide attempt or gesture needs psychiatric evaluation and follow-up.

II. **Poisoning prevention.** Young children with an unintentional ingestion are at higher risk for a second ingestion than the general pediatric population. After an incident, prevention strategies need to be reviewed. If the family does not understand the instructions or it is the second poisoning incident, consider a home evaluation for childproofing by a public health nurse or other health care professional.

A. **Childproof** the home, day-care setting, and households the child commonly visits (eg, grandparents and other relatives). Store medicines, chemicals, and

TABLE I–44. EXAMPLES OF POTENT PEDIATRIC POISONS

Drug or Poison	Potentially Fatal Dose in a 10–kg Toddler	No. of Pediatric Deaths Reported to AAPCC 1983–1990
Benzocaine	2 mL of a 10% gel	
Camphor	5 mL of 20% oil	
Chloroquine	One 500-mg tablet	2
Chlorpromazine	One or two 200-mg tablets	1
Codeine	Three 60-mg tablets	
Desipramine	Two 75-mg tablets	4
Diphenoxylate/Atropine (Lomotil)	Five 2.5-mg tablets	2
Hydrocarbons (eg, kerosene)	One swallow (if aspirated)	12
Hypoglycemic sulfonylureas	Two 5-mg glyburide tablets	
Imipramine	One 150-mg tablet	3
Iron	Ten adult-strength tablets	16
Lindane	Two teaspoons (10 mL)	
Methyl salicylate	Less than 5 mL of oil of wintergreen	4
Quinidine	Two 300-mg tablets	1
Selenious acid (gun bluing)	One swallow	4
Theophylline	One 500-mg tablet	
Thioridazine	One 200-mg tablet	
Verapamil	One or two 240-mg tablets	3

References: Koren G: Medications which can kill a toddler with one teaspoon or tablet. *Clin Toxicol* 1993;31(3):407; Osterhoudt K: Toxtalk 1997;8(7); Litovitz T and Manoguerra A: Comparison of pediatric poisoning hazards: An analysis of 3.8 million exposure incidents. *Pediatrics* 1992;89(6):999.

cleaning products out of the reach of children or in locked cabinets. Do not store chemicals in food containers, and do not store chemicals in the same cabinets as food. Common places children find medications include visitors' purses or backpacks and bedside tables.

B. **Use child-resistant containers** to store prescription and nonprescription medications. However, child-resistant containers are not childproof; they only slow down the time it takes a determined child to get into the container.

C. **Dispense syrup of ipecac** (see p 375) to the home and day-care setting for possible use after an ingestion. (A poison control center or medical provider should be consulted before administration of the ipecac.)

III. **Child abuse.** Consider the possibility that the child was intentionally given the drug or toxin. Most states require that all health care professionals report suspected cases of child abuse or neglect, which means that it is not a discretionary decision but a *legal obligation to report any suspicious incident.* The parents or guardians should be informed in a straightforward, nonjudgmental manner that a report is being made under this legal obligation. In serious cases, the suspected abuse report should be made before the child is released, and the local child-protective services should decide whether it is safe to release the child to the parents or guardians. In unclear situations, the child can be admitted for "observation" to allow time for social services to make an expeditious evaluation. The following should alert medical personnel to the possibility of abuse or neglect:

A. The story does not make sense or does not ring true, or it changes over time, or different people give different stories.

    B. The child is nonambulatory (eg, child under 6 months of age). Carefully review how the child gained access to the drug or toxin.

    C. The child is over 4–5 years old. Accidental ingestions are rare in older children, and ingestion may be a signal of abuse or neglect.

    D. The drug ingested was a tranquilizer (eg, haloperidol or chlorpromazine), a drug of abuse (eg, cocaine or heroin), a sedative (eg, diazepam), or ethanol, or the parents are intoxicated.

    E. There is a long interval between the time of ingestion and the time the child is taken for medical evaluation.

    F. There are signs of physical or sexual abuse or neglect: multiple or unusual bruises; a broken bone or burns; a very dirty, unkempt child; a child with a flat affect or indifferent or inappropriate behavior.

    G. A history of repeated episodes of possible or documented poisonings or a history of prior abuse.

    H. Munchausen syndrome by proxy: drugs or toxins are given to the child to simulate illness. Most perpetrators are mothers, often with some medical background. This is a rare diagnosis.

IV. Clinical evaluation. The physical and laboratory evaluation is essentially the same as for adults. However, normal vital signs vary with age (see Table I–45).

    A. Heart rate. Newborns may have normal heart rates as high as 190/min, and 2-year-olds up to 120/min. Abnormal tachycardia or bradycardia suggests the possibility of hypoxemia, in addition to the numerous drugs and poisons that affect heart rate and rhythm (see Tables I–4 through I–7).

    B. Blood pressure is a very important vital sign in a poisoned child. The blood pressure cuff must be of the proper size; cuffs that are too small can falsely elevate the pressure. The blood pressures of infants are difficult to obtain by auscultation but are easily obtained by Doppler.

        1. Many children normally have a lower blood pressure than adults. However, low blood pressure in the context of a poisoning should be regarded as normal only if the child is alert, active, appropriate, and has normal peripheral perfusion.

        2. Idiopathic or essential hypertension is rare in children. Elevated blood pressure should be assumed to indicate an acute condition, although the systolic blood pressure can be transiently elevated if the child is vigorously

TABLE I–45. PEDIATRIC VITAL SIGNS[a]

Age	Respiratory Rate (/min)	Heart Rate (/min)	Blood Pressure (mm Hg)			
			Lower Limit	Average	Upper Limit	Severe
Newborn	30–80	110–190	52/25	50–55[b]	95/72	110/85
1 month	30–50	100–170	64/30	85/50	105/68	120/85
6 months	30–50	100–170	60/40	90/55	110/72	125/85
1 year	20–40	100–160	66/40	90/55	110/72	125/88
2 years	20–30	100–160	74/40	90/55	110/72	125/88
4 years	20–25	80–130	79/45	95/55	112/75	128/88
8 years	15–25	70–110	85/48	100/60	118/75	135/92
12 years	15–20	60–100	95/50	108/65	125/84	142/95

[a]References: Dieckmann RA, Coulter K: Pediatric emergencies. Page 811 in *Current Emergency Diagnosis and Treatment,* 4th ed. Saunders CE, Ho MT (editors). Appleton & Lange, 1992; Gundy JH: The pediatric physical exam. Page 68 in: *Primary Pediatric Care.* Hoekelman RA et al (editors). Mosby, 1987; Hoffman JIE: Systemic arterial hypertension. Page 1438 in *Rudolph's Pediatrics.* 19th ed. Rudolph AM et al (editors). Appleton & Lange 1991; Liebman J, Freed MD: Cardiovascular system. Page 447 in: *Nelson's Essentials of Pediatrics.* Behrman RE, Kleigman R (editors). Saunders, 1990; Lum GM: Kidney and urinary tract. Page 624 in *Current Pediatric Diagnosis and Treatment,* 10th ed. Hathaway WE et al (editors). Appleton & Lange, 1991.
[b]Mean arterial pressure range on the first day of life.

crying or screaming. Unless a child's baseline blood pressure is known, values at the upper limit of normal should be assumed to be "elevated." The decision to treat elevated blood pressure must be made on an individual basis, based on the clinical scenario and the toxin involved.

V. **Neonates** present specific problems, including unique pharmacokinetics and potentially severe withdrawal from prenatal drug exposure.

A. **Neonatal pharmacokinetics.** The newborn (birth to 1 month) and infants (1–12 months) are unique from a toxicologic and pharmacologic perspective. Drug absorption, distribution, and elimination are different from those of older children and adults. Incorrect dosing, transplacental passage proximate to the time of birth, breast-feeding, dermal absorption, and intentional poisoning are potential routes of toxic exposure. Of particular importance are enhanced skin absorption and reduced drug elimination, which may lead to toxicity after relatively mild exposure.

1. **Skin absorption.** Neonates have a very high surface area to body weight, which predisposes them to poisoning via percutaneous absorption (eg, hexachlorophene, boric acid, or alcohols).

2. **Elimination** of many drugs (eg, acetaminophen, many antibiotics, caffeine, lidocaine, morphine, phenytoin, and theophylline) is prolonged in neonates. For example, the half-life of caffeine is approximately 3 hours in adults but may be greater than 100 hours in newborns.

B. **Neonatal drug withdrawal** may occur in infants with chronic prenatal exposure to illicit or therapeutic drugs. The onset is usually within 72 hours of birth, but a postnatal onset as late as 14 days has been reported. Signs usually commence in the nursery, and infants are not discharged until clinically stable. However, with early discharge from nurseries becoming the norm, an infant in withdrawal may first present to an emergency department or acute-care clinic. The presentation may be as mild as colic or severe as withdrawal seizures or profound diarrhea.

1. **Opioids** (especially methadone and heroin; also pentazocine and propoxyphene) are the most common cause of serious neonatal drug withdrawal symptoms. **Other drugs** for which a withdrawal syndrome has been reported include phencyclidine (PCP), cocaine, amphetamines, tricyclic antidepressants, phenothiazines, benzodiazepines, barbiturates, ethanol, clonidine, diphenhydramine, lithium, meprobamate, and theophylline. A careful drug history from the mother should include illicit drugs, alcohol, and prescription and over-the-counter medications, and whether she is breast-feeding.

2. **The manifestations of neonatal opioid withdrawal** include inability to sleep, irritability, tremulousness, inconsolability, high-pitched incessant cry, hypertonia, hyperreflexia, sneezing and yawning, lacrimation, disorganized suck, poor feeding, vomiting, diarrhea, tachypnea or respiratory distress, tachycardia, autonomic dysfunction, sweating, fevers, and seizures. Morbidity and mortality from untreated opioid withdrawal can be significant and commonly result from weight loss, metabolic acidosis, respiratory alkalosis, dehydration, electrolyte imbalance, and seizures. Withdrawal is a diagnosis of exclusion; immediately rule out sepsis, hypoglycemia, hypocalcemia, and hypoxia, and consider hyperbilirubinemia, hypomagnesemia, hyperthyroidism, and intracranial hemorrhage. Seizures do not usually occur as the only clinical manifestation of opioid withdrawal.

3. **Treatment of neonatal opioid withdrawal** is mainly supportive and includes swaddling, rocking, a subdued room, frequent small feedings with high-caloric formula, and IV fluids if necessary. A variety of drugs have been used, including morphine, paregoric, tincture of opium, diazepam, lorazepam, chlorpromazine, and phenobarbital. Numerous abstinence-scoring systems exist to objectively evaluate and treat opioid withdrawal. *The scoring and treatment of a neonate in withdrawal should be supervised by a neonatologist or a pediatrician experienced with neonatal withdrawal.*

GENERAL TEXTBOOKS AND OTHER REFERENCES IN CLINICAL TOXICOLOGY

Bryson PD: *Comprehensive Review in Toxicology for Emergency Clinicians*, 3rd ed. Taylor & Francis, 1996.

Doull J, Klaassen C, Amdur M (editors): *Casarett and Doull's Toxicology: The Basic Science of Poisons*, 3rd ed. MacMillan, 1990.

Ellenhorn M: *Ellenhorn's Medical Toxicology*, 2nd ed. Elsevier, 1997.

Goldfrank LR et al (editors): *Goldfrank's Toxicologic Emergencies*, 6th ed. Appleton & Lange, 1998.

Haddad LM, Winchester JF, Shannon M (editors): *Clinical Management of Poisoning and Drug Overdose*, 3rd ed. Saunders, 1998.

Rumack BH (editor): *Poisindex* [computerized poison information system]. Micromedex [updated quarterly]. Medical Economics, Inc.

SECTION II. Specific Poisons and Drugs: Diagnosis and Treatment

▶ ACE INHIBITORS

Olga F. Woo, PharmD

The angiotensin-converting enzyme (ACE) inhibitors are widely used for the treatment of renovascular and idiopathic hypertension. Captopril (Capoten) was introduced in 1981, and eight more related ACE inhibitors have been marketed in the United States since then. The small number of acute overdoses reported with these drugs suggests that toxicity is mild.

I. **Mechanism of toxicity.** These agents inhibit vasoconstriction by inhibiting the enzyme peptidyldipeptide carboxyhydrolase, which converts angiotensin I to angiotensin II. All of the agents except captopril and lisinopril must be metabolized to their active moieties (eg, enalapril is converted to enalaprilat).

   Pharmacokinetics: The volume of distribution (Vd) of these drugs is fairly small (eg, 0.7 L/kg for captopril). The parent drugs are rapidly converted to their active metabolites, with half-lives of 0.75–1.5 hours. The active metabolites have elimination half-lives of 5.9–35 hours. (See also Table II–55.)

II. **Toxic dose.** Only mild toxicity has resulted from most reported overdoses of up to 7.5 g of captopril, 440 mg of enalapril (serum level 2.8 mg/L at 15 hours), and 420 mg of lisinopril. A 75-year-old man was found dead after ingesting approximately 1,125 mg of captopril, and he had a postmortem serum level of 60.4 mg/L. A 33 year old survived a level of 5.98 mg/L.

III. **Clinical presentation.** Mild hypotension, usually responsive to fluid therapy, has been the only toxic effect seen with acute overdose. Bradycardia may also occur. Hyperkalemia has been reported with therapeutic use, especially in patients with renal insufficiency and those taking nonsteroidal anti-inflammatory drugs. Persistent coughing, and acute angioedema (sometimes severe and life-threatening) have also been reported with therapeutic use.

IV. **Diagnosis** is based on a history of exposure.
   A. **Specific levels.** Blood levels are not readily available and do not correlate with clinical effects.
   B. **Other useful laboratory studies** include electrolytes, glucose, blood urea nitrogen (BUN), and creatinine.

V. **Treatment.**
   A. **Emergency and supportive measures.** If hypotension occurs, treat it with supine positioning and intravenous fluids (see p 15). Vasopressors are rarely necessary.
   B. **Specific drugs and antidotes.** No specific antidote is available.
   C. **Decontamination** (see p 43)
      1. **Prehospital.** Administer activated charcoal if available. Ipecac-induced vomiting may be useful for initial treatment at the scene (eg, children at home) if it can be given within a few minutes of exposure.
      2. **Hospital.** Administer activated charcoal. Gastric emptying is not necessary if activated charcoal can be given promptly.
   D. **Enhanced elimination.** Hemodialysis may effectively remove these drugs but is not likely to be indicated clinically.

▶ ACETAMINOPHEN

Kent R. Olson, MD

Acetaminophen (Anacin-3, Liquiprin, Panadol, Paracetamol, Tempra, Tylenol, many others) is a widely used drug found in many over-the-counter and prescription analgesics and cold remedies. When it is combined with another drug such as codeine or propoxyphene, the more dramatic acute symptoms caused by the other toxin may mask the mild and nonspecific symptoms of early acetaminophen toxicity, resulting in missed diagnosis or delayed antidotal treatment. Common combination products containing acetaminophen include Comtrex, Darvocet, Excedrin ES, Nyquil, Percocet, Unisom Dual Relief Formula, Sominex 2, Tylenol with codeine, Tylox, Vicks Formula 44-D, and Vicodin.

I. **Mechanism of toxicity.**

A. **Hepatic injury.** One of the minor products of normal metabolism of acetaminophen by the cytochrome P-450 mixed-function oxidase system is highly toxic; normally this reactive metabolite is rapidly detoxified by glutathione in liver cells. However, in an overdose, production of the toxic metabolite exceeds glutathione capacity and the metabolite reacts directly with hepatic macromolecules, causing liver injury.

B. **Renal damage** may occur by the same mechanism, owing to renal metabolism.

C. Overdose during **pregnancy** has been associated with fetal death and spontaneous abortion.

D. **Pharmacokinetics.** Rapidly absorbed, with peak levels usually reached within 30–120 min (***Note:*** absorption may be delayed after ingestion of sustained-release products or with co-ingestion of opioids or anticholinergics). Volume of distribution (Vd) = 0.8–1 L/kg. Eliminated by liver congugation (90%) to glucuronides or sulfates; cytochrome P-450 mixed-function oxidase accounts for only about 3–8% but produces a toxic intermediate (see A, above). The elimination half-life is 1–3 hours after therapeutic dose and may be greater than 12 hours after overdose. (See also Table II–55, p 319)

II. **Toxic dose.**

A. **Acute ingestion** of more than 150–200 mg/kg in children or 6–7 g in adults is potentially hepatotoxic.

1. Children younger than 10–12 years of age appear to be less susceptible to hepatotoxicity because of the smaller contribution of cytochrome P-450 to acetaminophen metabolism.

2. On the other hand, the margin of safety is lower in patients with induced cytochrome P-450 microsomal enzymes, because more of the toxic metabolite may be produced. **High-risk patients** include alcoholics and patients taking anticonvulsant medications or isoniazid. Fasting and malnutrition also increase the risk of hepatotoxicity, presumably by lowering cellular glutathione stores.

B. **Chronic toxicity** has been reported after daily consumption of high therapeutic doses (4–6 g/day) by alcoholic patients. Children have developed toxicity after receiving as little as 60–150 mg/kg/day for 2–8 days.

III. **Clinical presentation.** Clinical manifestations depend on the time after ingestion.

A. **Early** after acute acetaminophen overdose, there are usually no symptoms other than anorexia, nausea, or vomiting. Rarely, a massive overdose may cause altered mental status and metabolic acidosis.

B. **After 24–48 hours,** when transaminase levels (AST and ALT) rise, hepatic necrosis becomes evident. If acute fulminant hepatic failure occurs, encephalopathy and death may ensue. Encephalopathy, metabolic acidosis, and a continuing rise in the prothrombin time (PT) indicate a poor prognosis. Acute renal failure occasionally occurs, with or without concomitant liver failure.

IV. **Diagnosis.** Prompt diagnosis is possible only if the ingestion is suspected and a serum acetaminophen level is obtained. However, patients may fail to provide the history of acetaminophen ingestion, because they are unable (eg, comatose from another ingestion), unwilling, or unaware of its importance. Therefore, many clinicians routinely order acetaminophen levels in all overdose patients, regardless of the history of substances ingested.

A. **Specific levels.**

1. After an **acute overdose,** obtain a 4-hour-postingestion acetaminophen level and use the nomogram (Figure II–1) to predict the likelihood of toxic-

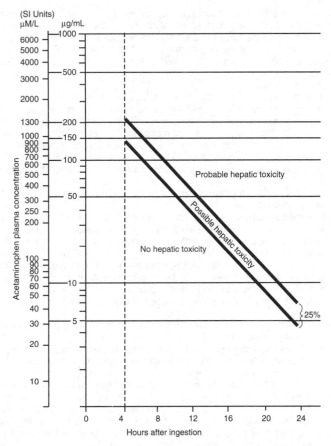

Figure II-1. Nomogram for prediction of acetaminophen hepatotoxicity after acute overdose. The upper line defines serum acetaminophen concentrations likely to be associated with hepatotoxicity; the lower line defines serum levels 25% below those expected to cause hepatotoxicity. (Courtesy of McNeil Consumer Products, Inc.).

ity. Do not attempt to interpret a level drawn before 4 hours, unless it is "nondetectable."

2. The nomogram should not be used to assess chronic or repeated ingestions.

3. Falsely elevated acetaminophen levels may occur in the presence of high levels of salicylate and other interferents by certain methods (see Table I–33, p 41).

B. **Other useful laboratory studies** include electrolytes, glucose, BUN, creatinine, liver transaminases, and prothrombin time.

V. **Treatment.**

A. **Emergency and supportive measures**

1. **Spontaneous vomiting** may delay the administration of antidote and charcoal (see below) and should be treated with metoclopramide (see p 382) or ondansetron (p 395).

2. Provide general supportive care for hepatic or renal failure if it occurs. Emergency **liver transplant** may be necessary for fulminant hepatic fail-

ure. Encephalopathy, metabolic acidosis, hypoglycemia, and progressive rise in the prothrombin time are indications of severe liver injury.

B. **Specific drugs and antidotes.** If the serum level falls above the upper ("probable toxicity") line on the nomogram or if stat serum levels are not immediately available, initiate antidotal therapy with **N-acetylcysteine** (NAC, Mucomyst, p 334), with a loading dose of 140 mg/kg orally. The effectiveness of NAC depends on **early treatment,** before the metabolite accumulates; it is of maximal benefit if started within 8–10 hours and of diminishing value after 12–16 hours (however, treatment should not be withheld, even if the delay is 24 hours or more). If vomiting interferes with oral acetylcysteine administration, give it by gastric tube and use high-dose metoclopramide (1–2 mg/kg intravenously (IV); see p 382) or ondansetron (p 395), or give the NAC intravenously (see p 334) if necessary.

1. If the serum level falls between the two nomogram lines, consider giving NAC if the patient is at increased risk for toxicity, eg, the patient is alcoholic, malnourished or fasting, or taking drugs that induce P-450 activity (eg, anticonvulsants, INH); multiple or subacute overdoses; or time of ingestion is uncertain or unreliable.

2. If the serum level falls below the lower nomogram line, treatment is not indicated unless the time of ingestion is uncertain or the patient is considered to be at particularly high risk.

3. *Note:* after ingestion of **Tylenol Extended Relief** tablets, which are designed for prolonged absorption, there may be a delay before the peak acetaminophen level is reached. This can also occur after co-ingestion of drugs that delay gastric emptying, such as opioids or anticholinergics. In such circumstances, repeat the serum acetaminophen level at 8 hours and possibly 12 hours.

4. **Duration of NAC treatment.** The current widely-used U.S. protocol for treatment of acetaminophen poisoning calls for 17 doses of oral NAC given over approximately 72 hours. However, successful protocols in Canada, the United Kingdom, and Europe utilize intravenous NAC for only 20 hours. We give NAC orally until 36 hours have passed since the time of ingestion. Then, if the serum acetaminophen level is below the limits of detection and liver transaminase levels are normal, NAC can be stopped. If there is evidence of hepatic toxicity, then NAC should be continued until liver function tests are improving.

5. **Chronic** acetaminophen ingestions: patients may give a history of several doses taken over 24 hours or more, in which case the nomogram cannot accurately estimate the risk of hepatotoxicity. In such cases, we advise NAC treatment if the amount ingested was more than 150–200 mg/kg or 6–7 g within a 24-hour period, or if liver enzymes are elevated, or if the patient falls within a high-risk group (see above). Treatment may be stopped 36 hours after the last dose of acetaminophen if the liver enzymes are normal.

C. **Decontamination** (see p 43)

1. **Prehospital.** Administer activated charcoal, if available. Ipecac-induced vomiting may be useful for initial treatment of children at home if it can be given within 30 minutes of exposure.

2. **Hospital.** Administer activated charcoal. Although activated charcoal adsorbs some of the orally administered antidote N-acetylcysteine, this effect is not considered clinically important. Gastric emptying is not necessary if charcoal can be given promptly. Do not administer charcoal if more than 3–4 hours have passed since ingestion, unless delayed absorption is suspected (eg, as with Tylenol Extended Relief or co-ingestants containing opioids or anticholinergic agents).

D. **Enhanced elimination.** Hemoperfusion effectively removes acetaminophen from the blood but is not generally indicated because antidotal therapy is so effective.

▶ AMANTADINE

Christopher R. Brown, MD

Amantadine (Symmetrel) is an antiviral agent that is also effective in the treatment of Parkinson's disease and for prophylaxis against the parkinsonian side effects of neuroleptic agents. It has also been advocated for use in therapy of cocaine addiction. Although there is limited information about its effects in acute overdose, it has been associated with seizures, arrhythmias, neuroleptic malignant syndrome, and death.

I. **Mechanism of toxicity.** Amantadine is thought to both enhance the release of dopamine and prevent dopamine reuptake in the peripheral and central nervous systems. In addition, it has anticholinergic properties, especially in overdose.

   Pharmacokinetics. Peak absorption = 1–4 hours; Volume of distribution (Vd) = 4–8 L/kg. Eliminated renally with a half-life of 7–37 hours (see also Table II–55).

II. **Toxic dose.** The toxic dose has not been determined. Because the elimination of amantadine depends entirely on kidney function, elderly patients with renal insufficiency may develop intoxication with therapeutic doses.

III. **Clinical presentation.**

   A. **Amantadine intoxication** causes agitation, visual hallucinations, nightmares, disorientation, delirium, slurred speech, ataxia, myoclonus, tremor, and sometimes seizures. Anticholinergic manifestations include dry mouth, urinary retention, and mydriasis. Rarely, ventricular arrhythmias including torsades de pointes (see p 13) and multifocal premature ventricular contractions may occur. Amantadine has also been reported to cause heart failure.

   B. **Amantadine withdrawal,** either after standard therapeutic use or in the days following an acute overdose, may result in hyperthermia and rigidity (possibly a form of neuroleptic malignant syndrome; see p 20).

IV. **Diagnosis** is based on a history of acute ingestion or is made by noting the above-mentioned constellation of symptoms and signs in a patient taking amantadine.

   A. **Specific levels** are not readily available. Serum levels above 1.5 mg/L have been associated with toxicity.

   B. **Other useful laboratory studies** include electrolytes, BUN, creatinine, and ECG.

V. **Treatment.**

   A. **Emergency and supportive measures**

   1. Maintain an open airway and assist ventilation if necessary (see pp 1–7).

   2. Treat coma (p 18), seizures (p 21), arrhythmias (p 13), and hyperthermia (p 20) if they occur.

   3. Monitor the asymptomatic patient for at least 8–12 hours after acute ingestion.

   B. **Specific drugs and antidotes.** There is no known antidote. Although some of the manifestations of toxicity are caused by the anticholinergic effects of amantadine, physostigmine should not be used.

   1. Treat **tachyarrhythmias** with beta blockers such as propranolol (see p 405) or esmolol (p 366).

   2. **Hyperthermia** requires urgent cooling measures (p 20) and may respond to specific pharmacologic therapy with dantrolene (p 354). When hyperthermia occurs in the setting of amantadine withdrawal, some have advocated using amantadine as therapy.

   C. **Decontamination** (see p 43)

   1. **Prehospital.** Administer activated charcoal, if available.

   2. **Hospital.** Administer activated charcoal. Gastric emptying is not necessary if activated charcoal can be given promptly.

   D. **Enhanced elimination.** Amantadine is not effectively removed by dialysis, because the volume of distribution is very large (5 L/kg). The serum elimination half-life ranges from 12 hours to 34 days, depending on renal function. In a patient with no renal function, dialysis or hemoperfusion may be necessary.

▶ AMMONIA

R. Steven Tharratt, MD

Ammonia is widely used as a refrigerant, a fertilizer, and a household and commercial cleaning agent. Anhydrous ammonia (NH_3) is a highly irritating gas that is very water-soluble. Aqueous solutions of ammonia may be strongly alkaline, depending on the concentration. Solutions for household use are usually 5–10% ammonia, but commercial solutions may be 25–30% or more. The addition of ammonia to chlorine or hypochlorite solutions will produce chloramine gas, an irritant with properties similar to those of chlorine (see p 134).

I. **Mechanism of toxicity.** Ammonia gas is highly water-soluble and rapidly produces an alkaline corrosive effect on contact with moist tissues such as the eyes and upper respiratory tract. Exposure to aqueous solutions causes corrosive alkaline injury to the eyes, skin, or gastrointestinal tract (see Caustic and Corrosive Agents, p 129).

II. **Toxic dose.**
   A. **Ammonia gas.** The odor of ammonia is detectable at 3–5 ppm, and persons without protective gear will experience respiratory irritation at 50 ppm and will usually self-evacuate the area. Eye irritation is common at 100 ppm. The workplace recommended exposure limit (ACGIH TLV-TWA) for anhydrous ammonia gas is 25 ppm as an 8-hour time-weighted average. The level considered immediately dangerous to life or health (IDLH) is 300 ppm.
   B. **Aqueous solutions.** Diluted aqueous solutions of ammonia (eg, < 5%) rarely cause serious burns but are moderately irritating. More concentrated industrial cleaners (eg, 25–30% ammonia) are much more likely to cause serious corrosive injury.

III. **Clinical presentation.** Clinical manifestations depend on physical state and route of exposure.
   A. **Inhalation of ammonia gas.** Symptoms are rapid in onset owing to the high water-solubility of ammonia and include immediate burning of the eyes, nose, and throat, accompanied by coughing. With serious exposure, upper-airway swelling may rapidly cause airway obstruction, preceded by croupy cough, hoarseness, and stridor. Bronchospasm with wheezing may occur. Massive inhalational exposure may cause noncardiogenic pulmonary edema.
   B. **Ingestion of aqueous solutions.** Immediate burning in the mouth and throat is common. With more concentrated solutions, serious esophageal and gastric burns are possible, and victims may have dysphagia, drooling, and severe throat, chest, and abdominal pain. Hematemesis and perforation of the esophagus or stomach may occur. The absence of oral burns does not rule out significant esophageal or gastric injury.
   C. **Skin or eye contact with gas or solution.** Serious alkaline corrosive burns may occur.

IV. **Diagnosis** is based on a history of exposure and description of the typical ammonia smell, accompanied by typical irritative or corrosive effects on the eyes, skin, and upper respiratory or gastrointestinal tract.
   A. **Specific levels.** Blood ammonia levels may be elevated (normal 8–33 μmol/L) but are not predictive of toxicity.
   B. **Other useful laboratory studies** include electrolytes, arterial blood gases or pulse oximetry, chest x-ray, and pH paper test strips.

V. **Treatment.**
   A. **Emergency and supportive measures.** Treatment depends on the physical state of the ammonia and the route of exposure.
      1. **Inhalation of ammonia gas**
         a. Observe carefully for signs of progressive upper-airway obstruction, and intubate early if necessary (see p 4).
         b. Administer humidified supplemental oxygen and bronchodilators for wheezing (p 8). Treat noncardiogenic pulmonary edema (p 7) if it occurs.

    c. Asymptomatic or mildly symptomatic patients may be sent home after a brief (1–2 hour) observation.
  2. Ingestion of aqueous solution. If a solution of 10% or greater has been ingested or if there are any symptoms of corrosive injury (dysphagia, drooling, or pain), perform flexible endoscopy to evaluate for serious esophageal or gastric injury. Obtain a chest x-ray to look for mediastinal air, which suggests esophageal perforation.
  3. Eye exposure. After eye irrigation, perform fluorescein examination and refer the patient to an ophthalmologist if there is evidence of corneal injury.
B. Specific drugs and antidotes. There is no specific antidote for these or other common caustic burns. The use of corticosteroids in alkaline corrosive ingestions has been proved ineffective and may be harmful in patients with perforation or serious infection.
C. Decontamination
  1. Inhalation. Remove immediately from exposure, and give supplemental oxygen if available.
  2. Ingestion (see p 45)
    a. Prehospital. Immediately give water by mouth to dilute the ammonia. Do *not* induce vomiting, as this may aggravate corrosive effects.
    b. Hospital. Gastric lavage is recommended in order to remove any liquid caustic in the stomach and to prepare for endoscopy; use a small, flexible tube and pass gently to avoid injury to damaged mucosa.
    c. Do *not* use activated charcoal; it does not adsorb ammonia, and it may obscure the endoscopist's view.
  3. Skin and eyes. Remove contaminated clothing and wash exposed skin with water. Irrigate exposed eyes with copious amounts of tepid water or saline (see p 43).
D. Enhanced elimination. There is no role for dialysis or other enhanced elimination procedures.

▶ AMPHETAMINES

Neal L. Benowitz, MD

Dextroamphetamine (Dexedrine) and methylphenidate (Ritalin) are used for the treatment of narcolepsy and for attention-deficit disorders in children. Several amphetaminelike drugs (benzphetamine, diethylpropion, phendimetrazine, phenmetrazine, and phentermine) are marketed as prescription anorectic medications for use in weight reduction (Table II–1). Fenfluramine and dexfenfluramine were marketed as anorectic medications but were withdrawn from the market in 1997 because of concerns about cardiopulmonary toxicity with long-term use. Methamphetamine (crank, speed), 3,4-methylenedioxymethamphetamine (MDMA, ecstasy), and several other amphetamine derivatives (see Lysergic Acid Diethylamide [LSD] and Other Hallucinogens, p 207), as well as a number of prescription drugs, are used orally and intravenously as illicit stimulants. "Ice" is a smokable form of methamphetamine. Phenylpropanolamine, ephedrine, and other over-the-counter decongestants are discussed on p 259.
I. Mechanism of toxicity. Amphetaminelike drugs act primarily by activating the sympathetic nervous system via central nervous system (CNS) stimulation, peripheral release of catecholamines, inhibition of neuronal reuptake of catecholamines, or inhibition of monoamine oxidase. Fenfluramine and dexfenfluramine cause serotonin release and block neuronal serotonin uptake. The various drugs have different profiles of action resulting from different levels of CNS and peripheral stimulation.
  Pharmacokinetics. All these drugs are well absorbed orally and have large volumes of distribution (Vd = 3–33 L/kg, except pemoline, with Vd = 0.2–0.6 L/kg), and they are generally extensively metabolized by the liver. Excretion of

TABLE II–1. COMMON AMPHETAMINELIKE DRUGS[a]

Drugs	Clinical Indications	Typical Adult Dose (mg)	Half Life (hours)[b]
Benzphetamine	Anorectant	25–50	6–12
Dexfenfluramine[c]	Anorectant	15	17–20
Dextroamphetamine	Narcolepsy, hyperactivity (children)	5–15	10–12
Diethylpropion	Anorectant	25, 75 (SR)	2.5–6
Fenfluramine[c]	Anorectant	20–40	10–30
Mazindol	Anorectant	1–2	10
Methamphetamine	Narcolepsy, hyperactivity (children)	5–15	4–5
Methylphenidate	Hyperactivity (children)	5–20	2–7
Pemoline	Narcolepsy, hyperactivity (children)	18.7–75	9–14
Phendimetrazine	Anorectant	35, 105 (SR)	5–12.5
Phenmetrazine	Anorectant	25,75 (SR)	
Phentermine	Anorectant	8, 30 (SR)	7–24

[a]See also Table II–28, p 208 (LSD and other hallucinogens).
[b]Half-life variable, dependent on urine pH
[c]Withdrawn from the U.S. market September 1997.

most amphetamines is highly dependent on urine pH, with amphetamines being more rapidly eliminated in an acidic urine (see also Table II–55, p 319).

II. **Toxic dose.** These drugs have a low therapeutic index, with toxicity at levels only slightly above usual doses. However, a high degree of tolerance can develop after repeated use. Acute ingestion of more than 1 mg/kg of dextroamphetamine (or an equivalent dose of other drugs; see Table II–1) should be considered potentially life-threatening.

III. **Clinical presentation.**

A. **Acute CNS effects** of intoxication include euphoria, talkativeness, anxiety, restlessness, agitation, seizures, and coma. Intracranial hemorrhage may occur owing to hypertension or cerebral vasculitis.

B. **Acute peripheral manifestations** include sweating, tremor, muscle fasciculations and rigidity, tachycardia, hypertension, acute myocardial ischemia, and infarction (even with normal coronary arteries). Inadvertent intra-arterial injection may cause vasospasm resulting in gangrene; this has also occurred with oral use of DOB (2,5-dimethoxy-4-bromoamphetamine; see Lysergic Acid Diethylamide [LSD] and Other Hallucinogens, p 207).

C. **Death** may be caused by ventricular arrhythmia, status epilepticus, intracranial hemorrhage, or hyperthermia. **Hyperthermia** frequently results from seizures and muscular hyperactivity and may cause brain damage, rhabdomyolysis, and myoglobinuric renal failure (see p 20).

D. **Chronic effects** of amphetamine abuse include weight loss, cardiomyopathy, stereotypic behavior (such as picking at the skin), paranoia, and paranoid psychosis. Psychiatric disturbances may persist for days or weeks. After cessation of habitual use, patients may suffer fatigue, hypersomnia, hyperphagia, and depression lasting several days.

E. Prolonged use (usually 3 months or longer) of fenfluramine or dexfenfluramine in combination with phentermine ("fen-phen") has been associated with an increased risk of pulmonary hypertension and of fibrotic valvular heart disease (primarily aortic, mitral, and tricuspid regurgitation). The pathology of the valvular disease is identical to that seen with carcinoid syndrome.

IV. Diagnosis is usually based on a history of amphetamine use and clinical features of sympathomimetic drug intoxication.
  A. Specific levels. Amphetamines and many related drugs can be detected in urine and gastric samples, providing confirmation of exposure. However, quantitative serum levels do not correlate well with severity of clinical effects and are not generally available. Amphetamine derivatives and adrenergic amines may cross-react in immunoassays (see Table I–33, p 41), and distinguishing the specific drug requires confirmatory testing (eg, with thin-layer chromatography, gas chromatography, or mass-spectrometry).
  B. Other useful laboratory studies include electrolytes, glucose, BUN and creatinine, CPK, urinalysis, urine dipstick test for occult hemoglobin (positive in patients with rhabdomyolysis with myoglobinuria), ECG and ECG monitoring, and CT scan of the head (if hemorrhage is suspected). Echocardiogram and right heart catheterization may be useful for detecting valvular disease or pulmonary hypertension.
V. Treatment.
  A. Emergency and supportive measures
    1. Maintain an open airway and assist ventilation if necessary (see pp 1–7).
    2. Treat agitation (p 23), seizures (p 21), coma (p 18), and hyperthermia (p 20) if they occur.
    3. Continuously monitor the temperature, other vital signs, and the ECG for a minimum of 6 hours.
  B. Specific drugs and antidotes. There is no specific antidote.
    1. Hypertension (see p 15) is best treated with a parenteral vasodilator such as phentolamine (p 400) or nitroprusside (p 392).
    2. Treat **tachyarrhythmias** (p 12) with propranolol (see p 405) or esmolol (p 366).
    3. Treat **arterial vasospasm** as described for ergots (p 160).
  C. Decontamination (see p 43)
    1. Prehospital. Administer activated charcoal, if available. Do *not* induce vomiting because of the risk of abrupt onset of seizures.
    2. Hospital. Administer activated charcoal. Gastric emptying is not necessary if activated charcoal can be given promptly.
  D. Enhanced elimination. Dialysis and hemoperfusion are not effective. Repeat-dose charcoal has not been studied. Renal elimination of dextroamphetamine may be enhanced by acidification of the urine, but this is not recommended because of the risk of aggravating the nephrotoxicity of myoglobinuria.

► **ANESTHETICS, LOCAL**

Neal L. Benowitz, MD

Local anesthetics are widely used to provide anesthesia via local subcutaneous injection; topical application to skin and mucous membranes; and epidural, spinal, and regional nerve blocks. In addition, lidocaine (see p 70) is used intravenously as an antiarrhythmic agent and cocaine (see p 142) is a popular drug of abuse. Commonly used agents are divided into two chemical groups: ester-linked and amide-linked (Table II–2).
  Toxicity from local anesthetics (other than cocaine) is usually caused by therapeutic overdosage (ie, excessive doses for local nerve blocks), inadvertent acceleration of intravenous infusions (lidocaine), or accidental injection of products meant for dilution (eg, 20% lidocaine) instead of those formulated for direct administration (2% solution). Acute injection of lidocaine has also been used as a method of homicide.
  I. Mechanism of toxicity. Local anesthetics bind to sodium channels in nerve fibers, blocking the sodium current responsible for nerve conduction and thereby increasing the threshold for conduction and reversibly slowing or blocking impulse generation. In therapeutic concentrations, this results in local anesthesia.

TABLE II–2. COMMON LOCAL ANESTHETICS

Anesthetic	Usual Half-Life	Maximum Adult Single Dose[a] (mg)
Ester-linked		
Benzocaine[b]		N/A
Benzonatate[c]		200
Butacaine[b]		N/A
Butamben[b]		N/A
Chlorprocaine	1.5–6 min	800
Cocaine[b]	1–2.5 h	N/A
Cyclomethylcaine[b]		N/A
Hexylcaine[b]		N/A
Procaine	7–8 min	600
Proparacaine[b]		N/A
Propoxycaine		75
Tetracaine	5–10 min	15
Amide-linked		
Bupivacaine	2–5 h	400
Dibucaine		10
Etidocaine	1.5 h	400
Lidocaine	1.2 h	300
Lidocaine with epinephrine	2 h	500
Mepivacaine		400
Prilocaine		600
Other (neither ester- nor amide-linked)		
Dyclonine[b]		N/A
Pramoxine[b]		N/A

[a]Maximum single dose for subcutaneous infiltration. N/A, Not applicable.
[b]Used only for topical anesthesia.
[c]Given orally as an antitussive.

In high concentrations, such actions may result in CNS and cardiovascular toxicity. In addition, some local anesthetics (eg, benzocaine) have been reported to cause methemoglobinemia (see p 220).

Pharmacokinetics. With local subcutaneous injection, peak blood levels are reached in 10–60 minutes, depending on the vascularity of the tissue and whether a vasoconstrictor such as epinephrine has been added. **Ester-type** drugs are rapidly hydrolyzed by plasma cholinesterase and have short half-lives. **Amide-type** drugs are metabolized by the liver, have a longer duration of effect, and may accumulate after repeated doses in patients with hepatic insufficiency. For other kinetic vaues, see Table II–55, p 319.

II. **Toxic dose.** Systemic toxicity occurs when brain levels exceed a certain threshold. Toxic levels can be achieved with a single large subcutaneous injection, with rapid intravenous injection of a smaller dose, or by accumulation of drug with repeated doses. The recommended maximum single subcutaneous doses of the common agents are listed in Table II–2.

III. Clinical presentation.
- **A.** Toxicity owing to **local anesthetic effects** includes prolonged anesthesia and, rarely, permanent sensory or motor deficits. Spinal anesthesia may block nerves to the muscles of respiration, causing respiratory arrest, or may cause sympathetic blockade, resulting in hypotension.
- **B.** Toxicity resulting from **systemic absorption** of local anesthetics affects primarily the CNS, with headache, confusion, perioral paresthesias, slurred speech, muscle twitching, convulsions, coma, and respiratory arrest. Cardiotoxic effects include sinus arrest, atrioventricular block, asystole, and hypotension.
- **C.** **Methemoglobinemia** (see also p 220) may occur after exposure to benzocaine.
- **D.** **Allergic reactions** (bronchospasm, hives, and shock) are uncommon and occur almost exclusively with ester-linked local anesthetics. Methylparaben, used as a preservative in some multidose vials, may be the cause of some reported hypersensitivity reactions.
- **E.** Features of toxicity caused by **cocaine** are discussed on p 142.

IV. Diagnosis is based on a history of local anesthetic use and typical clinical features. Abrupt onset of confusion, slurred speech, or convulsions in a patient receiving lidocaine infusion for arrhythmias should suggest lidocaine toxicity.
- **A. Specific levels.** Serum levels of some local anesthetics may confirm their role in producing suspected toxic effects, but these must be obtained promptly because the levels rapidly fall.
  - **1.** Serum concentrations of lidocaine greater than 6–10 mg/L are considered toxic.
  - **2.** Lidocaine is often detected in comprehensive urine toxicology screening as a result of use either as a local anesthetic (eg, for minor procedures in the emergency department) or as a cutting agent for drugs of abuse.
- **B. Other useful laboratory studies** include electrolytes, glucose, BUN and creatinine, ECG monitoring, arterial blood gases or pulse oximetry, and methemoglobin level (benzocaine).

V. Treatment.
- **A. Emergency and supportive measures**
  - **1.** Maintain an open airway and assist ventilation if necessary (see pp 1–7).
  - **2.** Treat coma (p 18), seizures (p 21), hypotension (p 15), arrhythmias (p 13), and anaphylaxis (p 26) if they occur. Extracorporeal circulatory assistance (eg, balloon pump or partial cardiopulmonary bypass) has been used for short-term support for patients with acute massive overdose with 20% lidocaine solution.
  - **3.** Monitor vital signs and ECG for at least 6 hours.
- **B. Specific drugs and antidotes.** There is no specific antidote.
- **C. Decontamination**
  - **1. Parenteral exposure.** Decontamination is not feasible.
  - **2. Ingestion** (see p 45)
    - **a. Prehospital.** Administer activated charcoal if available. Do **not** induce vomiting because of the risk of abrupt onset of seizures.
    - **b. Hospital.** Administer activated charcoal. Consider gastric lavage only for large recent ingestion.
- **D. Enhanced elimination.** Because lidocaine has a moderate volume of distribution, hemoperfusion is potentially beneficial, particularly after a massive overdose or when metabolic elimination is impaired because of circulatory collapse or severe liver disease.

▶ ANTIARRHYTHMIC DRUGS

Neal L. Benowitz, MD

Because of their actions on the heart, antiarrhythmic drugs are extremely toxic and overdoses are often life-threatening. Several classes of antiarrhythmic drugs are discussed elsewhere in Section II: type Ia drugs (quinidine, disopyramide, and procainamide; p 277); type II drugs (beta blockers, p 107); type IV drugs (calcium antagonists, p 119); and the older type Ib drugs (lidocaine, p 70; and phenytoin, p 261). This section describes toxicity caused by newer antiarrhythmic drugs: type Ib (tocainide and mexiletine); type Ic (flecainide, encainide, propafenone, and moricizine); and type III (bretylium and amiodarone). Sotalol, which also has type III antiarrhythmic actions, is discussed in the chapter on beta-adrenergic blockers (see p 107).

I. **Mechanism of toxicity.**
A. **Type I drugs** in general act by inhibiting the fast sodium channel responsible for initial cardiac cell depolarization and impulse conduction. Type Ia and type Ic drugs (which also block potassium channels) slow depolarization and conduction in normal cardiac tissue, and even at normal therapeutic doses the QT (types Ia and Ic) and QRS intervals (type Ic) are prolonged. Type Ib drugs slow depolarization primarily in ischemic tissue and have little effect on normal tissue or on the ECG. In overdose, all type I drugs have the potential to markedly depress myocardial automaticity, conduction, and contractility.
B. **Type II and type IV drugs** act by blocking beta-adrenergic receptors (type II) or calcium channels (type IV). Their actions are discussed elsewhere (type II, p 107; type IV, p 119).
C. **Type III drugs** act primarily by blocking potassium channels to prolong the duration of the action potential and the effective refractory period, resulting in QT interval prolongation at therapeutic doses.
  1. Intravenous administration of **bretylium** initially causes release of catecholamines from nerve endings, followed by inhibition of catecholamine release.
  2. **Amiodarone** is also a noncompetitive beta-adrenergic blocker and has calcium channel blocking effects, which may explain its tendency to cause bradyarrhythmias. Amiodarone may also release iodine, and chronic use has resulted in altered thyroid function (both hyper- and hypothyroidism).
D. **Relevant pharmacokinetics.** All drugs discussed in this section are widely distributed to body tissues. Most are extensively metabolized, but significant fractions of tocainide (40%), flecainide (30%), and bretylium (> 90%) are excreted unchanged by the kidneys. (See also Table II–55, p 319.)

II. **Toxic dose.** In general, these drugs have a narrow therapeutic index, and severe toxicity may occur slightly above or sometimes even within the therapeutic range, especially if combinations of antiarrhythmic drugs are taken together.
A. Ingestion of **twice the daily therapeutic dose** should be considered potentially life-threatening (usual therapeutic doses are given in Table II–3).
B. An exception to this rule of thumb is amiodarone, which is so extensively distributed to tissues that even massive single overdoses produce little or no toxicity (toxicity usually occurs only after accumulation during chronic amiodarone dosing).

III. **Clinical presentation.**
A. **Tocainide and mexiletine**
  1. **Side effects** with therapeutic use may include dizziness, paresthesias, tremor, ataxia, and gastrointestinal disturbance.
  2. **Overdose** may cause sedation, confusion, coma, seizures, respiratory arrest, and cardiac toxicity (sinus arrest, atrioventricular [AV] block, asystole, and hypotension). As with lidocaine, the QRS and QT intervals are usually normal, although they may be prolonged after massive overdose.
B. **Flecainide, encainide, propafenone, and moricizine**
  1. **Side effects** with therapeutic use include dizziness, blurred vision, headache, and gastrointestinal upset. Ventricular arrhythmias (monomorphic or polymorphic ventricular tachycardia; see p 13) may occur at therapeutic levels, especially in persons receiving high doses and those with reduced ventricular function.
  2. **Overdose** causes hypotension, bradycardia, AV block, and asystole. The QRS and QT intervals are prolonged, and ventricular arrhythmias may occur.

TABLE II–3. ANTIARRHYTHMIC DRUGS

Class	Drug	Usual Half-Life (hrs)	Therapeutic Daily Dose (mg)	Therapeutic Serum Levels (mg/L)	Major Toxicity[a]
Ia	Quinidine and related (p 277)				
Ib	Tocainide	11–15	1200–2400	5–12	S,B,H
	Mexiletine	10–12	300–1200	0.8–2	S,B,H
	Lidocaine (p 70)				
	Phenytoin (p 261)				
Ic	Flecainide	14–15	200–600	0.2–1	B,V,H
	Encainide[b, d]	2–11	75–300	[b]	S,B,V,H
	Propafenone[b]	2–10[c]	450–900	0.5–1	S,B,V,H
	Moricizine	1.5–3.5	600–900		B,V,H
II	Beta Blockers (p 107)				
III	Amiodarone	50 days	200–600	0.5–3	B,V,H
	Bretylium	5–14	5–10 mg/kg (IV loading dose)	0.7–1.5	H
	Sotalol (p 108)				
IV	Calcium Antagonists (p 119)				

[a]Major toxicity: S = Seizures   H = Hypotension
                    B = Bradyarrhythmias   V = Ventricular arrhythmias
[b]Active metabolite may contribute to toxicity; level not established.
[c]Genetically slow metabolizers may have half-lives of 10–32 hours. Also, metabolism is nonlinear, so half-lives may be longer in patients with overdose.
[d]Encainide no longer sold in the United States.

    C. Bretylium
        1. The major toxic **side effect** of bretylium is hypotension caused by inhibition of catecholamine release. Orthostatic hypotension may persist for several hours.
        2. After **rapid intravenous injection**, transient hypertension, nausea, and vomiting may occur.
    D. Amiodarone
        1. Acute overdose in a person not already on amiodarone is not expected to cause toxicity.
        2. With **chronic use**, amiodarone may cause ventricular arrhythmias (monomorphic or polymorphic ventricular tachycardia; see p 13) or bradyarrhythmias (sinus arrest, AV block). Amiodarone may cause pneumonitis or pulmonary fibrosis, hepatitis, photosensitivity dermatitis, corneal deposits, hypothyroidism or hyperthyroidism, tremor, ataxia, and peripheral neuropathy.
IV. Diagnosis is usually based on a history of antiarrhythmic drug use and typical cardiac and electrocardiographic findings. Syncope in any patient taking these drugs should suggest possible drug-induced arrhythmia.
    A. Specific levels. Serum levels are available for most type Ia and type Ib drugs (Table II–3); however, because toxicity is immediately life-threatening, measurement of drug levels is used primarily for therapeutic drug monitoring or to confirm the diagnosis rather than to determine emergency treatment. The following drugs are likely to be detected in comprehensive urine toxicology screening: diltiazem, lidocaine, metoprolol, phenytoin, propranolol, quinidine, and verapamil.

    B. **Other useful laboratory studies** include electrolytes, glucose, BUN and creatinine, liver enzymes, thyroid panel (chronic amiodarone), and ECG and ECG monitoring.

V. Treatment.

    A. **Emergency and supportive measures**

        1. Maintain an open airway and assist ventilation if necessary (see pp 1–7).

        2. Treat coma (p 18), seizures (p 21), hypotension (p 15), and arrhythmias (pp 10–14) if they occur. *Note:* Type Ia antiarrhythmic agents should not be used to treat cardiotoxicity caused by type Ia, type Ic, or type III drugs.

        3. Continuously monitor vital signs and ECG for a minimum of 6 hours after exposure, and admit the patient for 24 hours of intensive monitoring if there is evidence of toxicity.

    B. **Specific drugs and antidotes.** In patients with intoxication by type Ia or type Ic drugs, QRS prolongation, bradyarrhythmias, and hypotension may respond to **sodium bicarbonate**, 1–2 mEq/kg IV (see p 345). The sodium bicarbonate reverses cardiac-depressant effects caused by inhibition of the fast sodium channel.

    C. **Decontamination** (see p 43)

        1. **Prehospital.** Administer activated charcoal, if available.

        2. **Hospital.** Administer activated charcoal. Consider gastric lavage for large ingestions.

    D. **Enhanced elimination.** Owing to extensive tissue binding with resulting large volumes of distribution, dialysis and hemoperfusion are not likely to be effective for most of these agents. Hemodialysis may be of benefit for tocainide or flecainide overdose in patients with renal failure, but prolonged and repeated dialysis would be necessary. No data are available on the effectiveness of repeat-dose charcoal.

▶ ANTIBIOTICS

Olga F. Woo, PharmD

The antibiotic class of drugs has proliferated immensely since the first clinical use of sulfonamide in 1936 and the mass production of penicillin in 1941. In general, harmful effects have resulted from allergic reactions or inadvertent intravenous overdose. Serious toxicity from a single acute ingestion is rare. Table II–4 lists common antibiotics and their toxicities.

    I. **Mechanism of toxicity.** The precise mechanisms underlying toxic effects vary depending on the agent and are not well understood. In some cases, toxicity is caused by an extension of pharmacologic effects, while in other cases allergic or idiosyncratic reactions are responsible.

    II. **Toxic dose.** The toxic dose is highly variable, depending on the agent. Life-threatening allergic reactions may occur after subtherapeutic doses in hypersensitive individuals.

    III. **Clinical presentation.** After acute oral overdose, most agents cause only nausea, vomiting, and diarrhea. Specific features of toxicity are described in Table II–4.

    IV. **Diagnosis** is usually based on the history of exposure.

    A. **Specific levels.** Serum levels for most commonly used antibiotics are usually available. Levels are particularly useful for predicting toxic effects of **aminoglycosides, chloramphenicol,** and **vancomycin.**

    B. **Other useful laboratory studies** include complete blood count (CBC), electrolytes, glucose, BUN and creatinine, liver function tests, urinalysis, and methemoglobin level (for patients with dapsone overdose).

    V. **Treatment.**

    A. **Emergency and supportive measures**

TABLE II-4. COMMON ANTIBIOTICS AND THEIR TOXICITIES

Drug	Half-Life*	Toxic Dose or Serum Level	Toxicity
Acyclovir		Chronic	High-dose chronic therapy has caused crystalluria and renal failure. Acute overdose not likely to cause symptoms.
Aminoglycosides			
Amikacin	2–3 h	> 35 mg/L	Ototoxicity to vestibular and cochlear cells; neph-
Gentamicin	2 h	> 12 mg/L	rotoxicity causing proximal tubular damage and
Kanamycin	2–3 h	> 30 mg/L	acute tubular necrosis; competitive neuromuscu-
Neomycin		0.5–1 g/d	lar blockade if given rapidly intravenously with
Streptomycin	2.5 h	> 40–50 mg/L	other neuromuscular blocking drugs.
Tobramycin	2–2.5 h	> 10 mg/L	
Bacitracin		Unknown	Ototoxicity and nephrotoxicity.
Cephalosporins			
Cefazolin	90–120 min	Unknown	Convulsions reported in patients with renal insuffi-
Cephalothin			ciency; coagulopathy associated with cefazolin.
Cephaloridine		6 g/d	Proximal tubular necrosis.
Cefaclor	0.6–0.9 h		Neutropenia
Cefoperazone	102–156 min	3-4 mg/L	One case of symptomatic hepatitis. All of these
Cefamandole	30–60 min		antibiotics have the N-methyltetrazolethiol side
Cefotetan	3–4.6 h		chain which may inhibit aldehyde dehydrogenase
Moxalactam	114–150 min		to cause a disulfiramlike interaction with ethanol
Cefmetazole	72 min		(see p 158) and coagulopathy (inhibition of vitamin K_1 production).
Ceftriaxone	4.3–4.6 h Extensive excretion in bile	Intravenous bolus over < 3–5 min	Pseudolithiasis ("gall-bladder sludge"). Should be administered IV over 30 min
Chloramphenicol	4 h	> 50 mg/L	Leukopenia, reticulocytopenia; circulatory collapse (gray baby syndrome).
Dapsone	10–50 h	As little as 100 mg in an 18-month-old	Methemoglobinemia, sulfhemoglobinemia, hemolysis; metabolic acidosis; hallucinations, confusion; hepatitis.
Erythromycin	1.4 h	Unknown	Abdominal pain; idiosyncratic hepatotoxicity with estolate salt. Interaction with terfenadine or astemizole can induce QT prolongation and torsades de pointes.
Gramicidin		Unknown	Hemolysis.
Isoniazid (INH)	0.5–4 h	1–2g orally	Convulsions, metabolic acidosis (see p 195); hepatotoxicity with chronic use.
Lincomycin, clindamycin	4.4–6.4 h 2.4–3 h	Unknown	Hypotension and cardiopulmonary arrest after rapid intravenous administration.
Metronidazole	8.5 h	5 g/d	Convulsions; at therapeutic doses may cause disulfiramlike interaction with ethanol (see p 158).
Nalidixic acid	1.1–2.5 h	50 mg/kg/d	Seizures, hallucinations, confusion; visual disturbances; metabolic acidosis; intracranial hypertension.
Nitrofurantoin	20 min	Unknown	Hemolysis in G6PD-deficient patients.
Penicillins			
Penicillin	30 min	10 million units/d IV, or CSF > 5 mg/L	Seizures with single high dose or chronic excessive doses in patients with renal dysfunction.
Methicillin	30 min	Unknown	Interstitial nephritis, leukopenia.

TABLE II–4. COMMON ANTIBIOTICS AND THEIR TOXICITIES (CONTINUED)

Drug	Half-Life*	Toxic Dose or Serum Level	Toxicity
Nafcillin	1.0 h	Unknown	Neutropenia.
Ampicillin, amoxicillin	1.5 h 1.3 h	Unknown	Acute renal failure caused by crystal deposition.
Penicillins, anti-pseudomonal			
Carbenicillin	1.0–1.5	> 300 mg/kg/d	Bleeding disorders due to impaired platelet function;
Mezlocillin	0.8–1.1	> 300 mg/kg/d	hypokalemia. Risk of toxicity higher in patients with
Piperacillin	0.6–1.2	> 300 mg/kg/d	renal insufficiency.
Ticarcillin	1.0–1.2	> 275 mg/kg/d	
Polymyxins Polymyxin B	4.3–6 h	30,000 units/kg/d	Nephrotoxicity and noncompetitive neuromuscular blockade.
Polymyxin E		250 mg IM in a 10-month-old	
Rifampin	1.7 h	100 mg/kg/d	Facial edema, pruritus; headache, vomiting, diarrhea; red urine and tears.
Spectinomycin	1.2–2.8 h		Acute toxicity not reported.
Tetracyclines	6–12 h	> 1g/d in infants	Benign intracranial hypertension.
		> 4 g/d in pregnancy or > 15 mg/L	Acute fatty liver.
Demeclocycline	10–17 h	Chronic	Nephrogenic diabetes insipidus.
Minocycline	11–26 h	Chronic	Vestibular symptoms.
Sulfonamides		Unknown	Acute renal failure caused by crystal deposition.
Trimethoprim	8–11 h	Unknown	Bone marrow depression; methemoglobinemia; hyperkalemia
Vancomycin	4–6 h	> 80 mg/L	Ototoxic and nephrotoxic. Hypertension, skin rash/flushing ("red-man syndrome") associated with IV administration.
Zidovudine (AZT)	1.0 h	Unknown	Seizures (36 g overdose), bone marrow supression (20 g overdose).

*Normal renal function

1. Maintain an open airway and assist ventilation if necessary (see pp 1–7).
2. Treat coma (p 18), seizures (p 21), hypotension (p 15), anaphylaxis (p 26), and hemolysis (See Rhabdomyolysis, p 25) if they occur.
3. Replace fluid losses resulting from gastroenteritis with intravenous crystalloids.
4. Maintain steady urine flow with fluids to alleviate crystalluria from overdoses of sulfonamides, ampicillin and amoxicillin.

B. **Specific drugs and antidotes**
   1. **Trimethoprim** poisoning: administer **leucovorin** (folinic acid; see p 378). Folic acid is not effective.
   2. **Dapsone** overdose: administer **methylene blue** (see p 381) for symptomatic methemoglobinemia.
C. **Decontamination** (see p 43)
   1. **Prehospital.** Administer activated charcoal, if available.
   2. **Hospital.** Administer activated charcoal. Gastric emptying is not necessary if activated charcoal can be given promptly.

D. Enhanced elimination. Most antibiotics are excreted unchanged in the urine, so maintenance of adequate urine flow is important. The role of forced diuresis is unclear. Hemodialysis is not usually indicated, except perhaps in patients with renal dysfunction and a high level of a toxic agent.

1. Charcoal hemoperfusion effectively removes **chloramphenicol** and is indicated after a severe overdose with a high serum level and metabolic acidosis.
2. **Dapsone** undergoes enterohepatic recirculation and is more rapidly eliminated with repeat-dose activated charcoal (see p 54).

▶ ANTICHOLINERGICS

S. Alan Tani, PharmD

Anticholinergic intoxication can occur with a wide variety of prescription and over-the-counter medications and numerous plants and mushrooms. Common drugs that possess anticholinergic activity include antihistamines (see p 84), antipsychotics (see p 257), antispasmodics, skeletal muscle relaxants (see p 291), and tricyclic antidepressants (see p 310). *Common combination products containing anticholinergic drugs* include Atrohist, Donnagel, Donnatal, Hyland's Teething Tablets, Lomotil, Motofen, Ru-Tuss, Urised, and Urispas. Common anticholinergic medications are described in Table II–5. Plants and mushrooms containing anticholinergic alkaloids include jimsonweed (*Datura stramonium*), deadly nightshade (*Atropa belladonna*), and the fly agaric (*Amanita muscaria*).

I. Mechanism of toxicity. Anticholinergic agents competitively antagonize the effects of acetylcholine at peripheral muscarinic and central receptors. Exocrine glands, such as those responsible for sweating and salivation, and smooth muscle are mostly affected. The inhibition of muscarinic activity in the heart leads to rapid heart beat. Tertiary amines such as atropine are well absorbed centrally, whereas quaternary amines such as glycopyrrolate have a less central effect.

TABLE II–5. COMMON ANTICHOLINERGIC DRUGS[a]

Tertiary Amines	Usual Adult Single Dose (mg)	Quarternary Amines	Usual Adult Single Dose (mg)
Atropine	0.4–1	Anisotropine	50
Benztropine	1–6	Clidinium	2.5–5
Biperiden	2–5	Glycopyrrolate	1
Dicyclomine	10–20	Hexocyclium	25
Flavoxate	100–200	Ipratropium bromide	N/A[b]
L-Hyoscyamine	0.15–0.3	Isopropamide	5
Oxybutynin	5	Mepenzolate	25
Oxyphencyclimine	10	Methantheline	50–100
Procyclidine	5	Methscopolamine	2.5
Scopolamine	0.4–1	Propantheline	7.5–15
Trihexyphenidyl	6–10	Tridihexethyl	25–50

[a]These drugs act mainly at muscarinic cholinergic receptors, and are sometimes more correctly referred to as antimuscarinic drugs
[b]Not used orally; available as metered-dose inhaler and 0.02% inhalation solution and 0.03% nasal spray.

Pharmacokinetics. Absorption may be delayed because of the pharmacologic effects of these drugs on gastrointestinal motility. The duration of toxic effects can be quite prolonged (eg, benztropine intoxication may persist for 2–3 days). (See also Table II–55, p 319)

II. **Toxic dose.** The range of toxicity is highly variable and unpredictable. Fatal atropine poisoning has occurred after as little as 1–2 mg was instilled in the eye of a young child. Intramuscular injection of 32 mg of atropine was fatal in an adult.

III. **Clinical presentation.** The anticholinergic syndrome is characterized by warm, dry, flushed skin; dry mouth; mydriasis; delirium; tachycardia; ileus; and urinary retention. Jerky myoclonic movements and choreoathetosis are common. Hyperthermia, coma, and respiratory arrest may occur. Seizures are rare with pure antimuscarinic agents, although they may result from other pharmacologic properties of the drug (eg, tricyclic antidepressants and antihistamines).

IV. **Diagnosis** is based on a history of exposure and the presence of typical features such as dilated pupils and flushed skin. A trial dose of physostigmine (see below) can be used to confirm the presence of anticholinergic toxicity; rapid reversal of signs and symptoms is consistent with the diagnosis.
   A. **Specific levels.** Concentrations in body fluids are not generally available. Common over-the-counter agents are usually detectable on general urine toxicology screening.
   B. **Other useful laboratory studies** include electrolytes, glucose, arterial blood gases or pulse oximetry, and ECG monitoring.

V. **Treatment.**
   A. **Emergency and supportive measures**
      1. Maintain an open airway and assist ventilation if needed (see pp 1–7).
      2. Treat hyperthermia (p 20), coma (p 18), and seizures (p 21) if they occur.
   B. **Specific drugs and antidotes.** If a pure anticholinergic poisoning is suspected, a small dose of **physostigmine** (see p 402), 0.5–1 mg IV in an adult, can be given to patients with severe toxicity (eg, hyperthermia, severe delirium, or tachycardia). *Caution:* physostigmine is capable of causing atrioventricular block, asystole, and seizures, especially in patients with tricyclic antidepressant overdoses.
   C. **Decontamination** (see p 43)
      1. **Prehospital.** Administer activated charcoal if available.
      2. **Hospital.** Administer activated charcoal. Gastric emptying is not necessary if activated charcoal can be given promptly.
   D. **Enhanced elimination.** Hemodialysis, hemoperfusion, peritoneal dialysis, and repeat-dose charcoal are not effective in removing anticholinergic agents.

▶ ANTIDEPRESSANTS (NONCYCLIC)

Neal L. Benowitz, MD

Many noncyclic antidepressants are now available, including trazodone (Desyrel), nefazodone (Serzone), fluoxetine (Prozac), sertraline (Zoloft), paroxetine (Paxil), fluvoxamine (Luvox), venlafaxine (Effexor), and bupropion (Wellbutrin). Bupropion is also marketed under the brand name Zyban for smoking cessation. Mirtazapine (Remeron), a tetracyclic antidepressant, has recently become available. In general, these drugs are much less toxic than the tricyclic antidepressants (see p 310) and the monoamine oxidase (MAO) inhibitors (see p 225), although serious effects such as seizures and hypotension occasionally occur. Noncyclic and other antidepressants are described in Table II–6.

I. **Mechanism of toxicity.**
   A. Most agents cause CNS depression. Bupropion is a stimulant that can also cause seizures, presumably related to inhibition of reuptake of dopamine and norepinephrine.

TABLE II–6. NONCYCLIC AND OTHER NEWER ANTIDEPRESSANTS

Drug	Action[a]	Usual Adult Daily Dose (mg)	Typical Elimination Half-life (h)[b]
Bupropion	D	200–450	16
Fluoxetine	S	20–80	70
Fluvoxamine	S	50–300	15
Mirtazapine	A	15–45	20–40
Nefazodone	S,A	100–600	3
Paroxetine	S	20–50	21
Sertraline	S	50–200	28
Trazodone	S,A	50–400	3–9
Venlafaxine	S,N	30–600	5

[a]A = alpha-adrenergic blocker; D = dopamine uptake blocker; S = serotonin uptake blocker; N = norepinephrine uptake blocker
[b]Most have active metabolites, many with longer half-lives than the parent drug.

    B. Trazodone and mirtazapine produce peripheral alpha-adrenergic blockade, which can result in hypotension and priapism.

    C. Serotonin uptake inhibitors (often called selective serotonin reuptake inhibitors or SSRIs) such as fluoxetine, sertraline, paroxetine, fluvoxamine, venlafaxine, and trazodone may interact with each other or with chronic use of an MAO inhibitor (see p 225) to produce the **"serotonin syndrome"** (see below and p 21).

    D. None of the drugs in this group has significant anticholinergic effects.

    E. Pharmacokinetics. These drugs have large volumes of distribution (Vd = 12–88 L/kg, except trazodone [Vd = 1.3 L/kg]). Most are eliminated via hepatic metabolism (paroxetine is 65% renal). (See also Table II–55, p 319)

II. Toxic dose. The noncyclic antidepressants generally have a wide therapeutic index, with doses in excess of 10 times the usual therapeutic dose tolerated without serious toxicity. Bupropion can cause seizures in some patients with moderate overdose or even in therapeutic doses.

III. Clinical presentation.

    A. Central nervous system. The usual presentation after overdose includes ataxia, sedation, and coma. Respiratory depression may occur, especially with co-ingestion of alcohol or other drugs. These agents, particularly bupropion, can cause restlessness, anxiety, and agitation. Tremor and seizures are common with bupropion but occur occasionally after overdose with an SSRI.

    B. Cardiovascular effects are usually minimal, although trazodone can cause hypotension and orthostatic hypotension, bupropion can cause sinus tachycardia, and fluoxetine may cause minor ST-T wave changes.

    C. Serotonin syndrome (see p 21) is characterized by confusion, hypomania, restlessness, myoclonus, hyperreflexia, diaphoresis, shivering, tremor, incoordination, and hyperthermia. This reaction may be seen when a patient taking an MAO inhibitor (see p 225) ingests a serotonin uptake blocker. Because of the long duration of effects of MAO inhibitors and most of the serotonin uptake blockers, this reaction can occur up to several days to weeks after either treatment regimen has been discontinued. The syndrome has also been described in patients taking combinations of various SSRIs without concomitant MAO inhibitor use.

IV. Diagnosis. A noncyclic-antidepressant overdose should be suspected in patients with a history of depression who develop lethargy, coma, or seizures. These agents do not generally affect cardiac conduction, and QRS interval prolongation should suggest a tricyclic antidepressant overdose (see p 310).

A. **Specific levels.** Blood and urine assays are not routinely available and are not useful for emergency management. These drugs may or may not appear on routine or even comprehensive toxicology screening.
B. **Other useful laboratory studies** include electrolytes, glucose, arterial blood gases or pulse oximetry, and ECG monitoring.
V. **Treatment.**
A. **Emergency and supportive measures**
1. Maintain an open airway and assist ventilation if needed (see pp 1–7). Administer supplemental oxygen.
2. Treat coma (p 18), hypotension (p 15), and seizures (p 21) if they occur.
B. **Specific drugs and antidotes.** For suspected serotonin syndrome, anecdotal reports claim benefit from methysergide (Sansert), 2 mg orally every 6 hours for 3 doses (1 case report), and cyproheptadine (Periactin), 4 mg orally every hour for 3 doses (1 case report), presumably because of the serotonin antagonist effects of these drugs.
C. **Decontamination** (see p 43)
1. **Prehospital.** Administer activated charcoal if available.
2. **Hospital.** Administer activated charcoal. Gastric emptying is not necessary if activated charcoal can be given promptly.
D. **Enhanced elimination.** Owing to extensive protein binding and large volumes of distribution, dialysis, hemoperfusion, peritoneal dialysis, and repeat-dose charcoal are not effective.

▶ ANTIDIABETIC AGENTS

Susan Kim, PharmD

Agents used to lower blood glucose are divided into two main groups: oral drugs and insulin products. The oral agents include sulfonylureas, biguanides, acarbose, and troglitazone, each with a different mechanism of action, potency, and duration of activity. All **insulin** products are given by the parenteral route, and all produce effects similar to those of endogenous insulin; they differ by antigenicity and by onset and duration of effect. Table II–7 lists the various available antidiabetic agents. Other drugs and poisons can also cause hypoglycemia (see Table I–25).
I. **Mechanism of toxicity.**
A. **Oral agents**
1. **Sulfonylureas** lower blood glucose primarily by stimulating endogenous pancreatic insulin secretion and secondarily by enhancing peripheral insulin receptor sensitivity and reducing glycogenolysis.
2. **Biguanides.** Metformin decreases hepatic glucose production and intestinal absorption of glucose, while increasing peripheral glucose uptake and utilization. It does not stimulate insulin release, and is not likely to produce acute hypoglycemia. Severe **lactic acidosis** is a rare but potentially fatal side effect of metformin (and its predecessor phenformin, no longer available in the United States). It occurs mainly in patients with renal insufficiency, alcoholism, and advanced age, and has occurred after injection of iodinated contrast agents resulted in acute renal failure.
3. **Acarbose** is an alpha-glucosidase inhibitor that delays the digestion of ingested carbohydrates, reducing postprandial blood glucose concentrations.
4. **Troglitazone** decreases hepatic glucose output and improves target cell response to insulin.
5. While metformin, acarbose, and troglitazone are not likely to cause hypoglycemia after acute overdose, they may contribute to the hypoglycemic effects of sulfonylureas or insulin (eg, by limiting glucose uptake from the intestinal tract or decreasing hepatic glucose production).

TABLE II–7. ANTIDIABETIC AGENTS[a]

Agent	Onset (h)	Peak (h)	Duration[b] (h)
Insulins			
Insulin zinc	1–2	8–12	18–24
Isophane insulin (NPH)	1–2	8–12	18–24
Lispro		0.25	0.5–1 3–4
Prolonged insulin zinc	4–8	16–18	36
Protamine zinc	4–8	14–20	36
Rapid insulin zinc	0.5	4–7	12–16
Regular insulin	0.5–1	2–3	5–7
Oral Sulfonylureas			
Acetohexamide	2	4	12–24
Chlorpropamide	1	3–6	24–72[b]
Glimepiride		2–3	24
Glipizide	0.25–0.5	0.5–2	<24
Glyburide	0.25–1	4	24[b]
Tolazamide	1	4–6	14–20
Tolbutamide	1	5–8	6–12
Other oral agents			
Acarbose	N/A (less then 2% of an oral dose absorbed systemically)		
Metformin		2	2.5–6
Troglitazone		3	0.16–0.34

[a]See also Table II–55 (p 319).
[b]Duration of hypoglycemic effects after overdose may be much longer, especially with glyburide and chlorpropamide.

B. **Insulin.** Blood glucose is lowered directly by the stimulation of cellular uptake and metabolism of glucose. Cellular glucose uptake is accompanied by an intracellular shift of potassium and magnesium. Insulin also promotes glycogen formation and lipogenesis.

C. **Pharmacokinetics** (See Table II–7 and Table II–55).

II. **Toxic dose.**

A. **Sulfonylureas.** Toxicity depends on the agent and the total amount ingested. Toxicity may also occur owing to drug interactions, resulting in impaired elimination of the oral agent.

1. **Acetohexamide.** Two 500-mg tablets have caused hypoglycemic coma in an adult.

2. **Chlorpropamide**, 500–750 mg/d for 2 weeks has caused hypoglycemia in adults.

3. **Glyburide.** Acute overdose (10–15 mg) in a child produced profound hypoglycemic coma. In a 79-year-old nondiabetic person, 5 mg caused hypoglycemic coma.

4. **Interactions** with the following drugs may increase the risk of hypoglycemia: other hypoglycemics, sulfonamides, propranolol, salicylates, clofibrate, probenecid, pentamidine, valproic acid, dicumarol, cimetidine, MAO inhibitors, and alcohol. In addition, co-ingestion of alcohol may occasionally produce a disulfiramlike interaction (see p 158).

5. **Hepatic** or **renal insufficiency** may impair drug elimination and result in hypoglycemia.

    B. Metformin. Lactic acidosis occurred 9 hours after ingestion of 25 g of metformin by an 83-year-old patient.

    C. Insulin. Severe hypoglycemic coma and permanent neurologic sequelae have occurred after injections of 800–3200 units of insulin. Orally administered insulin is not absorbed and is not toxic.

III. Clinical presentation.

    A. Hypoglycemia may be delayed in onset depending on the agent used and the route of administration (ie, subcutaneous versus intravenous). Manifestations of hypoglycemia include agitation, confusion, coma, seizures, tachycardia, and diaphoresis. The serum potassium and magnesium levels may also be depressed. Note that in patients receiving beta-adrenergic blocking agents (see p 107), many of the manifestations of hypoglycemia (tachycardia, diaphoresis) may be blunted or absent.

    B. Lactic acidosis from metformin or phenformin may begin with nonspecific symptoms such as malaise, vomiting, myalgias, and respiratory distress. The mortality rate for severe lactic acidosis is reportedly as high as 50%.

IV. Diagnosis. Overdose involving a sulfonylurea or insulin should be suspected in any patient with hypoglycemia. Other causes of hypoglycemia that should be considered include alcohol ingestion (especially in children) and fulminant hepatic failure.

    A. Specific levels

      1. Serum concentrations of many agents can be determined in regional commercial toxicology laboratories, but have little utility in acute clinical management.

      2. Exogenously administered animal insulin can be distinguished from endogenous insulin (ie, in a patient with hypoglycemia caused by insulinoma) by determination of C peptide (present with endogenous insulin secretion).

    B. Other useful laboratory studies include glucose, electrolytes, magnesium, and ethanol. If metformin or phenformin is suspected, obtain a venous blood lactate level (grey top tube).

V. Treatment.

    A. Emergency and supportive measures

      1. Maintain an open airway and assist ventilation if necessary (see pp 1–7).

      2. Treat coma (p 18) and seizures (p 21) if they occur.

    B. Specific drugs and antidotes

      1. Administer concentrated **glucose** (see p 372) as soon as possible after drawing a baseline blood sample for later blood glucose determination. In adults, give 50% dextrose ($D_{50}W$), 1–2 mL/kg; in children, use 25% dextrose ($D_{25}W$), 2–4 mL/kg.

      2. Follow serum glucose levels closely for several hours after the last dose of dextrose. Give repeated glucose boluses and administer 5–10% dextrose (D_5–D_{10}) as needed to maintain the serum glucose level at or above 100 mg/dL.

      3. For patients with a **sulfonylurea overdose**, consider intravenous **octreotide** (see p 394) or **diazoxide** (see p 356) if 5% dextrose infusions do not maintain satisfactory glucose concentrations.

      4. Lactic acidosis may be treated with judicious doses of sodium bicarbonate. Excessive bicarbonate administration may worsen intracellular acidosis.

    C. Decontamination (see p 43)

      1. Sulfonylureas

        a. Prehospital. Administer activated charcoal if available.

        b. Hospital. Administer activated charcoal. Gastric emptying is not necessary if activated charcoal can be given promptly.

      2. Metformin, acarbose, and troglitazone. Because there is limited experience with the effects of acute overdoses of these agents, ingestion of a large or unknown amount should be treated with oral activated charcoal.

      3. Insulin

        a. Orally ingested insulin is not absorbed and produces no toxicity, so gut decontamination is not necessary.

      b. Local excision of tissue at the site of massive intradermal injection has been performed, but the general utility of this procedure has not been established.

D. Enhanced elimination

  1. Sulfonylureas. Alkalinization of the urine (pH 8 or greater) increases the renal elimination of chlorpropamide. Forced diuresis and dialysis procedures are of no known value for other hypoglycemic agents. The high degree of protein binding of the sulfonylureas suggests that dialysis procedures would not generally be effective. However, charcoal hemoperfusion reduced the serum half-life of chlorpropamide in a patient with renal failure.

  2. Metformin is effectively removed by hemodialysis, which can also help correct severe lactic acidosis.

▶ ANTIHISTAMINES

S. Alan Tani, PharmD

Antihistamines (H_1 receptor antagonists) are commonly found in over-the-counter and prescription medications used for motion sickness, control of allergy-related itching, and cough and cold palliation and as sleep aids (Table II–8). Acute intoxication with antihistamines results in symptoms very similar to those of anticholinergic poisoning. H_2 receptor blockers (cimetidine, ranitidine, and famotidine) inhibit gastric acid secretion but otherwise share no effects with H_1 agents, do not produce significant intoxication, and are not discussed here. *Common combination products containing antihistamines* include Actifed, Allerest, Contac, Coricidin, Dimetapp, Dristan, Drixoral, Excedrin PM, Nyquil, Nytol, Pamprin, Pediacare, Tavist, Triaminic, Triaminicol, Unisom Dual Relief Formula, and Vicks Pediatric Formula 44.

  I. Mechanism of toxicity. H_1 blocker antihistamines are structurally related to histamine and antagonize the effects of histamine on H_1 receptor sites. They possess anticholinergic effects (except the "nonsedating" agents: astemizole, azatadine, fexofenadine, loratadine, and terfenadine). They may also stimulate or

TABLE II–8. COMMON H_1 RECEPTOR ANTAGONIST ANTIHISTAMINES

Drug	Usual Duration of Action (hr)	Usual Single Adult Dose (mg)	Sedation
Ethanolamines			
Bromdiphenhydramine	4–6	12.5–25	+++
Carbinoxamine	3–4	4–8	++
Clemastine	10–12	0.67–2.68	++
Dimenhydrinate	4–6	50–100	+++
Diphenhydramine	4–6	25–50	+++
Diphenylpyraline	6–8	5	++
Doxylamine	4–6	25	+++
Phenyltoloxamine	6–8	50	+++
Ethylenediamines			
Pyrilamine	4–6	25–50	++
Thenyldiamine	8	10	++
Tripelennamine	4–6	25–50	++

(continued)

TABLE II–8. COMMON H$_1$ RECEPTOR ANTAGONIST ANTIHISTAMINES (CONTINUED)

Drug	Usual Duration of Action (hr)	Usual Single Adult Dose (mg)	Sedation
Alkylamines			
Acrivastine	6–8	8	+
Brompheniramine	4–6	4–8	+
Chlorpheniramine	4–6	4–8	+
Dexbrompheniramine	6–8	2–4	+
Dexchlorpheniramine	6–8	2–4	+
Dimethindene	8	1–2	+
Pheniramine	8–12	25–50	+
Pyrrobutamine	8–12	15	+
Triprolidine	4–6	2.5	+
Piperazines			
Buclizine	8	50	
Cetrizine	24	5–10	+/–
Cinnarizine	8	15–30	+
Cyclizine	4–6	25–50	+
Flunarizine	24	5–10	+
Hydroxyzine	20–25	25–50	+++
Meclizine	12–24	25–50	+
Phenothiazines			
Methdilazine	6–12	4–8	+++
Promethazine	4–8	25–50	+++
Trimeprazine	6	2.5	+++
Others			
Astemizole	30–60 days	10	+/–
Azatidine	12	1–2	++
Cyproheptadine	8	2–4	+
Fexofenadine	24	60	+/–
Loratadine	>24	10	+/–
Phenindamine	4–6	25	+/–
Terfenadine	12	60	+/–

depress the CNS, and some agents (eg, diphenhydramine) have local anesthetic and membrane-depressant effects in large doses.

    Pharmacokinetics. Drug absorption may be delayed because of the pharmacologic effects of these agents on the gastrointestinal tract. Volumes of distribution are generally large (3–20 L/kg). Elimination half-lives are highly variable, ranging for 1–4 hours for diphenhydramine to 7–24 hours for many of the others. The half-life of astemizole is 7–19 days. (See also Table II–55, p 319)

II. **Toxic dose.** The estimated fatal oral dose of diphenhydramine is 20–40 mg/kg. In general, toxicity occurs after ingestion of 3–5 times the usual daily dose. Children are more sensitive to the toxic effects of antihistamines than adults.

III. Clinical presentation.

A. An overdose results in many symptoms similar to anticholinergic poisoning: drowsiness, dilated pupils, flushed dry skin, fever, tachycardia, delirium, hallucinations, and myoclonic or choreoathetoid movements. Convulsions, rhabdomyolysis and hyperthermia may occur with a serious overdose.

B. Massive **diphenhydramine** overdoses have been reported to cause QRS widening and myocardial depression similar to tricyclic antidepressant overdoses (see p 310).

C. QT interval prolongation and torsades-type atypical ventricular tachycardia (see p 14) have been associated with elevated serum levels of **terfenadine** or **astemizole**. These have occurred after an overdose, excessive daily dosing, or use of an interacting drug (eg, erythromycin, ketoconazole, or itraconazole).

IV. Diagnosis is generally based on the history of ingestion and can usually be readily confirmed by the presence of typical anticholinergic syndrome. Comprehensive urine toxicology screening will detect most common antihistamines.

A. **Specific levels** are not generally available or useful. Common over-the-counter antihistamines are usually detectable on general urine toxicology screening.

B. **Other useful laboratory studies** include electrolytes, glucose, arterial blood gases or pulse oximetry, and ECG and ECG monitoring (diphenhydramine, terfenadine, and astemizole).

V. Treatment.

A. **Emergency and supportive measures**
  1. Maintain an open airway and assist ventilation if necessary (see pp 1–7).
  2. Treat coma (p 18), seizures (p 21), hyperthermia (p 20), and atypical ventricular tachycardia (p 14) if they occur.
  3. Monitor the patient for at least 6–8 hours after ingestion. For terfenadine or astemizole, consider monitoring for at least 18–24 hours.

B. **Specific drugs and antidotes.** There is no specific antidote for antihistamine overdose. As for anticholinergic poisoning (see p 78), physostigmine has been used for treatment of severe delirium or tachycardia. However, because antihistamine overdoses carry a greater risk for seizures, physostigmine is not routinely recommended. **Sodium bicarbonate** (see p 345), 1–2 meq/kg IV, may be useful for myocardial depression and QRS interval prolongation after a massive diphenhydramine overdose.

C. **Decontamination** (see p 43)
  1. **Prehospital.** Administer activated charcoal if available.
  2. **Hospital.** Administer activated charcoal. Consider gastric lavage for massive ingestions.

D. **Enhanced elimination.** Hemodialysis, hemoperfusion, peritoneal dialysis, and repeat-dose activated charcoal are not effective in removing antihistamines.

▶ ANTIMONY AND STIBINE

Peter Wald, MD, MPH

Antimony is widely used as a hardening agent in soft metal alloys and alloys of lead; for compounding rubber; in flameproofing compounds; and as a coloring agent in dyes, varnishes, paints, and glazes. Exposure to antimony dusts and fumes may also occur during mining and refining of ores and from the discharge of firearms. Organic antimony compounds are used as antiparasitic drugs. **Stibine** (antimony hydride, SbH_3) is a colorless gas with the odor of rotten eggs that is produced as a by-product when antimony-containing ores or furnace slag is treated with acid.

I. **Mechanism of toxicity.** The mechanism of antimony and stibine toxicity is not known. Because these compounds are chemically related to arsenic and arsine, their modes of action may be similar.
   A. **Antimony** compounds probably act by binding to sulfhydryl groups and inactivating key enzymes.
   B. **Stibine**, like arsine, may cause hemolysis. It is also an irritant gas.

II. **Toxic dose.**
   A. The lethal oral dose of **antimony** in mice is 100 mg/kg; at these doses mice developed eosinophilia and cardiac failure. The recommended workplace limit (ACGIH TLV-TWA) for antimony is 0.5 mg/m^3 as an 8-hour time-weighted average.
   B. The recommended workplace limit (ACGIH TLV-TWA) for **stibine** is 0.1 ppm as an 8-hour time-weighted average. The air level considered immediately dangerous to life or health (IDLH) is 5 ppm.

III. **Clinical presentation.**
   A. **Acute ingestion of antimony** causes nausea, vomiting, and diarrhea (often bloody). Hepatitis and renal insufficiency may occur. Death is rare if the patient survives the initial gastroenteritis.
   B. **Acute stibine inhalation** causes acute hemolysis, resulting in anemia, jaundice, hemoglobinuria, and renal failure.
   C. **Chronic exposure to antimony dusts and fumes** in the workplace is the most common type of exposure and may result in headache, anorexia, pneumonitis, peptic ulcers, and dermatitis (antimony spots). Sudden death presumably resulting from a direct cardiotoxic effect has been reported in workers exposed to antimony trisulfide.

IV. **Diagnosis** is based on a history of exposure and typical clinical presentation.
   A. **Specific levels.** Normal serum and urine antimony levels are below 10 μg/L. Serum and urine concentrations correlate poorly with workplace exposure, but exposure to air concentrations greater than the TLV-TWA will increase urinary levels. Urinary antimony is increased after firearm discharge exposure. There is no established toxic antimony level after stibine exposure.
   B. **Other useful laboratory studies** include CBC, plasma-free hemoglobin, electrolytes, BUN, creatinine, urinalysis for free hemoglobin, liver transaminases, bilirubin, and prothrombin time (PT).

V. **Treatment.**
   A. **Emergency and supportive measures**
      1. **Antimony.** Large-volume intravenous fluid resuscitation may be necessary for shock caused by gastroenteritis (see p 15).
      2. **Stibine.** Blood transfusion may be necessary after massive hemolysis. Treat hemoglobinuria with fluids and bicarbonate as for rhabdomyolysis (see p 25).
   B. **Specific drugs and antidotes.** There is no specific antidote. BAL (dimercaprol) and penicillamine are not effective chelators for antimony, nor are they expected to be effective for stibine.
   C. **Decontamination** (see p 43)
      1. **Inhalation.** Remove the patient from exposure, and give supplemental oxygen if available. Protect rescuers from exposure.
      2. **Ingestion** of antimony salts
         a. **Prehospital.** Administer activated charcoal if available (although there is no evidence for its effectiveness). Ipecac-induced vomiting may be useful for initial treatment at the scene (eg, children at home) if it can be given within a few minutes of exposure.
         b. **Hospital.** Perform gastric lavage, and administer activated charcoal. Do *not* use cathartics.
   D. **Enhanced elimination.** Hemodialysis, hemoperfusion, and forced diuresis are *not* effective at removing antimony or stibine. Exchange transfusion may be effective in treating massive hemolysis caused by stibine.

▶ ANTINEOPLASTIC AGENTS

Susan Kim, PharmD

Because of the inherently cytotoxic nature of most chemotherapeutic antineoplastic agents, overdoses are likely to be extremely serious. These agents are classified into six categories (Table II–9). Other than iatrogenic errors, relatively few acute overdoses have been reported for these agents.

I. **Mechanism of toxicity.** In general, toxic effects are extensions of the pharmacologic properties of these drugs.
   A. **Alkylating agents.** These drugs provide highly charged carbon atoms that attack nucleophilic sites on DNA, resulting in alkylation and cross-linking and thus inhibiting replication and transcription. Binding to RNA or protein moieties appears to contribute little to cytotoxic effects.
   B. **Antibiotics.** These drugs intercalate within base pairs in DNA, inhibiting DNA-directed RNA synthesis. Another potential mechanism may be the generation of cytotoxic free radicals.
   C. **Antimetabolites.** These agents interfere with DNA synthesis at various stages. For example, methotrexate binds reversibly to dihydrofolate reductase, preventing synthesis of purine and pyrimidine nucleotides.
   D. **Hormones.** Steroid hormones regulate the synthesis of steroid-specific proteins. The exact mechanism of antineoplastic action is unknown.
   E. **Mitotic inhibitors.** These agents act in various ways to inhibit orderly mitosis, thereby arresting cell division.
   F. **Others.** The cytotoxic actions of other antineoplastic drugs result from a variety of mechanisms, including DNA alkylation, blockade of protein synthesis, and inhibition of hormone release.
   G. **Pharmacokinetics.** Most oral antineoplastic agents are readily absorbed, with peak levels reached within 1–2 hours of ingestion. Due to rapid intracellular incorporation and the delayed onset of toxicity, pharmacokinetic values are usually of little utility in managing acute overdose. (See also Table II–55.)

II. **Toxic dose.** Because of the highly toxic nature of these agents (except for hormones), exposure to even therapeutic amounts should be considered potentially serious.

III. **Clinical presentation.** The organ systems affected by the various agents are listed in Table II–9. The most common sites of toxicity are the hematopoietic and gastrointestinal systems.
   A. **Leukopenia** is the most common manifestation of bone marrow depression. Thrombocytopenia and anemia may also occur. Death may result from overwhelming infections or hemorrhagic diathesis. With alkylating agents, nadirs occur 1–4 weeks after exposure, whereas with antibiotics, antimetabolites, and mitotic inhibitors, the nadirs occur 1–2 weeks after exposure.
   B. **Gastrointestinal** toxicity is also very common. Nausea, vomiting, and diarrhea often accompany therapeutic administration, and severe ulcerative gastroenteritis and extensive fluid loss may occur.
   C. **Extravasation** of some antineoplastic drugs at the intravenous injection site may cause severe local injury, with skin necrosis and sloughing.

IV. **Diagnosis** is usually based on the history. Because some of the most serious toxic effects may be delayed until several days after exposure, early clinical symptoms and signs may not be dramatic.
   A. **Specific levels.** Not generally available. For methotrexate, see Table III–7, p 379.
   B. **Other useful laboratory studies** include CBC with differential, platelet count, electrolytes, glucose, BUN and creatinine, liver enzymes, and prothrombin time (PT). ECG may be indicated for cardiotoxic agents, and pulmonary function tests are indicated for agents with known pulmonary toxicity.

V. **Treatment.**
   A. **Emergency and supportive measures**
      1. Maintain an open airway and assist ventilation if necessary (see pp 1–7).

TABLE II–9. COMMON ANTINEOPLASTIC AGENTS AND THEIR TOXICITIES

Drug	Major Site(s) of Toxicity[a]	Comments
Alkylating agents		
Busulfan	D+, En+, M+, P++	Pulmonary fibrosis, adrenal insufficiency with chronic use.
Carboplatin	G++, An+, M++	Peripheral neuropathy in 4% of patients.
Carmustine (BCNU)	D+, G+, H+, M+, Ex+, P+	Flushing, hypotension, and tachycardia with rapid IV injection.
Chlorambucil	D+, G+, H+, M+ N++	Seizures, confusion, coma reported after overdose. Acute ODs of 1.5–6.8 mg/kg in children caused seizures up to 3–4 hours post ingestion. Not dialyzable.
Cisplatin	An+, G++, M+, N+, P+, R++	Ototoxic, nephrotoxic. Good hydration essential. Hemodialysis not effective.
Cyclophosphamide	Al++, C+, D+, En+, G++, M++, R+	Hemodialysis effective. Acetylcysteine and 2 mercaptoethanesulfonate have been used investigationally to reduce hemorrhagic cystitis.
Ifosfamide	M++, N+, Al++, G+	Urotoxic. Hemorrhagic cystitis, somnolence, confusion, hallucinations, status epilepticus, coma seen during therapy.
Lomustine (CCNU)	Al+, G+, H+, M+, P+	Thrombocytopenia, leukopenia, liver and lymph node enlargement after overdose.
Mechlorethamine	D+, G++, M++, N+, Ex+	Lymphocytopenia may occur within 24 hours. Watch for hyperuricemia.
Melphalan	An+, G+, M+	Hemodialysis effective although of questionable need (half-life only 90 minutes).
Pipobroman	G+, M+	Discontinued in the United States.
Thiotepa	An+, G++, M++	Bone marrow suppression usually very severe.
Uracil mustard	G+, M++	Bone marrow suppression first noted as thrombocytopenia, leukopenia. Discontinued in the United States.
Antibiotics		
Bleomycin	An++, D++, G+, P++	Pulmonary fibrosis with chronic use. Febrile reaction in 20–25% of patients.
Dactinomycin	Al++, D+, G++, M++, Ex++	Severe inflammatory reaction may occur at previously irradiated sites. Highly corrosive to soft tissue.
Daunorubicin	Al++, An+, C++, G++, M++, Ex++	Congestive cardiomyopathy may occur after total cumulative dose > 600 mg/m².

(continued)

TABLE II–9. COMMON ANTINEOPLASTIC AGENTS AND THEIR TOXICITIES (CONTINUED)

Drug	Major Site(s) of Toxicity[a]	Comments
Doxorubicin	Al++, An+, C++, D+, G++, M++, Ex++	Cardiotoxicity and cardiomyopathy may occur after total cumulative dose > 550 mg/m^2. Arrhythmias after acute overdose. Hemoperfusion may be effective.
Idarubicin	C++, G+, M++, Ex++	Congestive heart failure, acute life-threatening arrhythmias may occur.
Mitomycin	Al+, D+, G++, H+, M+, P+, R+, Ex++	Hemolytic uremic syndrome reported with therapeutic doses.
Mitoxantrone	An+, C+, G++, M++	Four reported overdosed patients died from severe leukopenia and infection.
Pentostatin	D+, G+, M+, N++, R++,	Central nervous system depression, convulsions, coma seen at high doses.
Plicamycin (mithramycin)	An+, D+, G++, H++, M++, N+, Ex+	Coagulopathy, electrolyte disturbances may occur. Check calcium frequently.
Antimetabolites		
Cytarabine	An+, En+, G+, H+, M+	"Cytarabine syndrome": fever myalgia, bone pain, rash, malaise.
Floxuridine	Al+, G++, M++	
Fludarabine	G+, M++, N++, R+	Blindness, coma, death at high doses.
5-Fluorouracil	Al+, D+, G++, M++, N+	Acute cerebellar syndrome seen. Coronary vasospasm with angina may occur.
6-Mercaptopurine	G+, H++, M+	Hemodialysis removes drug but of questionable need (half-life 20–60 minutes).
Methotrexate	Al+, D+, G++, H+, M++, N+, P+, R+	Peak serum level 1–2 hours after oral dose. Folinic acid (leucovorin; see p 378) is specific antidote. Hemoperfusion questionably effective. Urinary alkalinization and repeat dose charcoal may be helpful.
6-Thioguanine	G+, H+, M+, R+	Hemodialysis probably ineffective owing to rapid intracellular incorporation.
Hormones		
Androgens		
Testolactone	En+, G±	Toxicity unlikely after single acute overdose.
Antiandrogens		
Flutamide, bicalutamide, nilutamide	G+	Gynecomastia. Aniline metabolite of flutamide has caused methemoglobinemia (see p 220). Nilutamide 13g ingestion resulted in no evidence of toxicity.
Estrogens		
Diethylstilbestrol	En+, G±	Possible carcinogenic effect on fetus if taken during early pregnancy.
Estramustine	En±, G±, H±, M±	Has both weak estrogenic and alkylating activity.

Polyestradiol	En±, G±	Toxicity unlikely after single acute overdose.
Antiestrogens		
Tamoxifen	Al±, D±, En±, G±	Acute toxic effects unlikely. Tremors, hyperreflexia, unsteady gait, QT prolongation with high doses.
Progestins		
Medroxyprogesterone	An±, En±, G±	Acute toxic effects unlikely. May induce porphyria in susceptible patients.
Megestrol	En±, G±	Acute toxic effects unlikely. May induce porphyria in susceptible patients.
Aromatase Inhibitor		
Anastrozole	G±	Acute toxic effects unlikely.
Other hormones		
Leuprolide, Goserelin	En+	Acute toxic effects unlikely. Initial increase in luteinizing hormone, follicle-stimulating hormone levels.
Mitotic inhibitors		
Etoposide	An+, G+, M++	Myelosuppression major toxicity. Dystonic reaction reported.
Teniposide	An+, G+, M++, Ex++	One report of sudden death from hypotension, cardiac arrhythmias. Hypotension from rapid IV injection.
Vinblastine	G+, M++, N+, Ex++	Myelosuppression, ileus, syndrome of inappropriate antidiuretic hormone reported after overdose. Fatal if given intrathecally.
Vincristine sulfate	G+, M±, N++, Ex++	Delayed (up to 9 days) seizures, delirium, coma reported after overdoses. Fatal if given intrathecally. Glutamic acid 500 mg TID orally may reduce the incidence of neurotoxicity.
Vinorelbine	G+, M++, N+, Ex++	Severe granulocytopenia
Miscellaneous		
Aldesleukin (Interleukin 2)	C++, G+, H+, M+, N+, P+, R+	Commonly causes capillary leak syndrome resulting in severe hypotension.
Altretamine	G+, N+, M+	Reversible peripheral sensory neuropathy.
Asparaginase	An++, En+, G+, H++, N++, R+	Bleeding diathesis, hyperglycemia, pancreatitis.
BCG (Intravesical)	G+	Attenuated mycobacterium bovis. Bladder irritation common. Risk of sepsis in immunocompromised patients.
Cladribine	M++, N++, R++	Irreversible paraparesis/quadriparesis seen in high doses.
Dacarbazine	Al+, An+, En+, G++, H+, M+, N+, Ex±	May produce flulike syndrome. Photosensitivity reported.

(continued)

TABLE II–9. COMMON ANTINEOPLASTIC AGENTS AND THEIR TOXICITIES (CONTINUED)

Drug	Major Site(s) of Toxicity[a]	Comments
Docetaxel	An+, D+, M++, N+	Severe fluid retention in 6% of patients.
Hydroxyurea	D+, G+, M++	Leukopenia, anemia more common than thrombocytopenia. Peak serum level within 2 h of oral dose.
Interferon alpha 2a	G+, H+, M++, N+	Flulike symptoms common. Severe hypotension from inadvertent IV reported.
Interferon alpha 2b	G+, M+	Flulike symptoms common.
Levamisole	G+, N+	May have nicotinic and muscarinic effects at cholinergic receptors. Gastroenteritis, dizziness, headache after 2.5 mg/kg dose reported. Disulfiram-like ethanol interaction.
Mitotane	Al+, D+, En++, G++, N++	Adrenal suppression; glucocorticoid replacement essential during stress.
Paclitaxel	An++, C+, M+, N+	Severe hypersensitivity reactions, including death, reported. Hypotension, bradycardia, ECG abnormalities, conduction abnormalities may occur. Fatal myocardial infarction 15 h into infusion reported.
Pegaspargase	An++, G+, H+, N+	Bleeding diathesis.
Procarbazine hydrochloride	An+, D+, En+, G++, M++, N++	Monoamine oxidase inhibitor activity. Disulfiramlike ethanol interaction.
Streptozocin	En+, G+, H+, M+, R++	Destroys pancreatic beta islet cells, may produce acute diabetes mellitus. Niacinamide (see p 389) may be effective in preventing islet cell destruction. Renal toxicity in two-thirds of patients.
Tretinoin	C+, D+, G+, N+, P+	Retinoic acid-APL syndrome seen in ~25% of patients with acute promyelocytic leukemia: fever, dyspnea, pulmonary infiltrates, and pleural or pericardial effusions.
Topoisomerase inhibitors		
Irinotecan	G++, M+	Severe diarrhea.
Topotecan	G+, M++	Severe thrombocytopenia, anemia common.

[a]Al = alopecia; An = anaphalaxis, allergy or drug fever; C = cardiac; D = dermatologic; En = endocrine; Ex = extravasation risk; G = gastrointestinal; H = hepatic; M = myelosuppressive; N = neurologic; P = pulmonary; R = renal; + = mild to moderate severity; ++ = severe toxicity; ± = minimal.

2. Treat coma (p 18), seizures (p 21), hypotension (p 15), and arrhythmias (pp 10–14) if they occur.
3. Treat nausea and vomiting with metoclopramide (p 382) and fluid loss caused by gastroenteritis with intravenous crystalloid fluids.
4. **Bone marrow depression** should be treated with the assistance of an experienced hematologist or oncologist.
5. **Extravasation.** Immediately stop the infusion and withdraw as much fluid as possible by negative pressure on the syringe. Then give the following specific treatment:
    a. **Dactinomycin, daunorubicin, doxorubicin, idarubicin, mitomycin-C, mitoxantrone, and plicamycin.** Apply ice compresses to the extravasation site for 15 minutes 4 times daily for 3 days. Topical application of dimethyl sulfoxide (DMSO) may be beneficial (commercially available 50% solution is less concentrated than those used in experimental studies, but may be tried). There is no justification for injection of hydrocortisone or sodium bicarbonate.
    b. **Mechlorethamine** (and concentrated **dacarbazine** and **cisplatin**). Infiltrate the site of extravasation with 10–15 mL of sterile 0.15 M sodium thiosulfate (dilute 4 mL of 10% thiosulfate with sterile water to a volume of 15 mL); apply ice compresses for 6–12 hours.
    c. **Vincristine** or **vinblastine.** Place a heating pad over the area and apply heat intermittently for 24 hours; elevate the limb. Local injection of hyaluronidase (150–900 units) may be beneficial. Do not use ice packs.
B. **Specific drugs and antidotes.** Very few specific treatments or antidotes are available (Table II–9).
C. **Decontamination** (see p 43)
    1. **Prehospital.** Administer activated charcoal, if available. Ipecac-induced vomiting may be useful for initial treatment at the scene (eg, children at home) if it can be given within a few minutes of exposure.
    2. **Hospital.** Administer activated charcoal. Gastric emptying is not necessary after a small ingestion if activated charcoal can be given promptly.
D. **Enhanced elimination.** Because of the rapid intracellular incorporation of most agents, dialysis and other extracorporeal removal procedures are generally not effective (see Table II–9 for exceptions).

▶ ANTISEPTICS AND DISINFECTANTS

Olga F. Woo, PharmD

Antiseptics are applied to living tissue to kill or prevent the growth of microorganisms. **Disinfectants** are applied to inanimate objects to destroy pathogenic microorganisms. Despite their unproved worth, they are widely used in the household, food industry, and hospitals. This chapter describes toxicity caused by **hydrogen peroxide, potassium permanganate, hexylresorcinol,** and **ichthammol.** All these agents are generally used as dilute solutions and cause little or no toxicity. Hexylresorcinol is commonly found in throat lozenges. Ichthammol is found in many topical salves. Descriptions of the toxicity of other antiseptics and disinfectants can be found elsewhere in this book, including the following: hypochlorite (p 134), iodine (p 190), isopropyl alcohol (p 197), mercurochrome (p 213), phenol (p 255), and pine oil (p 183).
I. **Mechanism of toxicity.**
    A. **Hydrogen peroxide** is an oxidizing agent, but it is very unstable and readily breaks down to oxygen and water. Generation of oxygen gas in closed body cavities can potentially cause mechanical distention resulting in gastric or intestinal perforation, as well as venous or arterial gas embolization.

B. Potassium permanganate is an oxidant, and the crystalline form or concentrated solutions are corrosive.

C. Hexylresorcinol is related to phenol but is much less toxic, although alcohol-based solutions possess vesicant properties.

D. Ichthammol (ichthyol, ammonium ichthosulfonate) contains about 10% sulfur in the form of organic sulfonates, and it is keratolytic to tissues.

II. Toxic dose.

A. Hydrogen peroxide for household use is available in 3–5% solutions and it causes only mild throat and gastric irritation with ingestion of less than 1 oz. Concentrations above 10% are found in some hair-bleaching solutions and are potentially corrosive. Most reported deaths have been associated with ingestion of undiluted 35% hydrogen peroxide, sold in some health food stores as "hyperoxygen therapy."

B. Potassium permanganate solutions of greater than 1:5000 strength may cause corrosive burns.

C. Hexylresorcinol is used in some antihelminthics, in doses of 400 mg (for children aged 1–7 years) to 1 g (older children and adults). Most lozenges contain only about 2–4 mg.

III. Clinical presentation. Most antiseptic ingestions are benign, and mild irritation is self-limited. Spontaneous vomiting and diarrhea may occur, especially after a large-volume ingestion.

A. Exposure to **concentrated** solutions may cause corrosive burns on the skin and mucous membranes, and oropharyngeal, esophageal, or gastric injury may occur. Glottic edema has been reported after ingestion of concentrated potassium permanganate.

B. Permanganate may also cause **methemoglobinemia** (see p 220).

C. Hydrogen peroxide ingestion may cause gastric distention and, rarely, perforation. Severe corrosive injury and air emboli have been reported with the concentrated forms and may be caused by the entry of gas through damaged gastric mucosa or gas production within the venous or arterial circulation.

IV. Diagnosis is based on a history of exposure and the presence of mild gastrointestinal upset or frank corrosive injury. Solutions of potassium permanganate are dark purple, and skin and mucous membranes are often characteristically stained.

A. Specific levels. Drug levels in body fluids are not generally useful or available.

B. Other useful laboratory studies include electrolytes, glucose, methemoglobin level (for potassium permanganate exposure), and upright chest x-ray (for suspected gastric perforation).

V. Treatment.

A. Emergency and supportive measures

1. In patients who have ingested concentrated solutions, monitor the airway for swelling and intubate if necessary.

2. Consult a gastroenterologist for possible endoscopy after ingestions of corrosive agents such as concentrated hydrogen peroxide or potassium permanganate. Most ingestions are benign, and mild irritation is self-limited.

3. Consider **hyperbaric oxygen** treatment for gas emboli associated with concentrated peroxide ingestion.

B. Specific drugs and antidotes. No specific antidotes are available for irritant or corrosive effects. If **methemoglobinemia** occurs, administer methylene blue (see p 381).

C. Decontamination

1. **Ingestion** of concentrated corrosive agents (see p 45)

   a. Dilute immediately with water or milk.

   b. Do *not* induce vomiting because of the risk of corrosive injury. Perform gastric lavage cautiously.

   c. Activated charcoal and cathartics are not effective.

    2. **Eyes and skin.** Irrigate the eyes and skin with copious amounts of tepid water. Remove contaminated clothing.

  D. Enhanced elimination. Enhanced elimination methods are neither necessary nor effective.

▶ ARSENIC

Saralyn R. Williams, MD

Many inorganic and organic arsenic compounds are used in a variety of industries and commercial products, including wood preservatives, weed killers, herbicides, glass manufacturing, nonferrous alloys, and semiconductors. Arsenic is recovered as a by-product in copper and lead smelting. Natural soil deposits may contaminate artesian well water, particularly in regions of geothermal activity. Some commercial household ant stakes (eg, Grant's Ant Control Ant Stakes) contain arsenic-impregnated gels. Arsenic compounds are used in some veterinary pharmaceuticals and may also occur in some folk remedies and tonics. Arsine gas, a hydride of arsenic, is discussed on p 97.

  I. Mechanism of toxicity. Arsenic compounds may be organic or inorganic and may contain arsenic in either a pentavalent (arsenate) or trivalent (arsenite) form. Once absorbed, arsenicals disrupt enzymatic reactions vital to cellular metabolism by interacting with sulfhydryl groups (trivalent arsenic) or substituting for phosphate (pentavalent arsenic).

    A. Soluble arsenic compounds, which are well absorbed after ingestion or inhalation, pose the greatest risk for human intoxication.

    B. Inorganic arsenic dusts (such as arsenic trioxide) are also irritants of the skin, mucous membranes, and respiratory and gastrointestinal tracts. Systemic poisoning can occur after percutaneous absorption.

    C. Arsenic exerts clastogenic effects and is a known human carcinogen. Although arsenic compounds of low solubility (eg, gallium arsenide, calcium arsenate, or elemental arsenic) have low acute toxicity, they may be retained in the lungs after inhalation, possibly increasing cancer risk.

  II. Toxic dose. The toxicity of arsenic compounds varies considerably based on the valence state, physical state, solubility, and the animal species exposed.

    A. Inorganic arsenic compounds. In general, trivalent arsenic (As^{+3}) is 2–10 times more toxic than pentavalent arsenic (As^{+5}).

      1. Acute ingestion of as little as 100–300 mg of a trivalent arsenic compound (eg, sodium arsenite) could be fatal.

      2. In sensitive populations, repeated ingestion of 20–60 µg/kg/d (roughly 1–4 mg/d in an adult) may be associated with signs of chronic poisoning.

      3. A two- to threefold elevation in lung cancer mortality has been detected after 15–25 years of occupational exposure to airborne arsenic concentrations of 300–600 µg/m³. The Occupational Safety and Health Administration (OSHA) regulates arsenic as a workplace carcinogen.

    B. Organic arsenic. In general, pentavalent organic arsenate compounds are less toxic than trivalent inorganic compounds. Marine organisms may contain large quantities of arsenobetaine, an organic trimethylated compound, which is excreted unchanged in the urine and produces no known toxic effects.

  III. Clinical presentation.

    A. Acute exposure most commonly occurs after accidental, suicidal, or deliberate poisoning by ingestion.

      1. Gastrointestinal effects. After a delay of minutes to hours, diffuse capillary damage results in hemorrhagic gastroenteritis. Nausea, vomiting, abdominal pain, and watery diarrhea are common. In severe cases, extensive tissue third-spacing of fluids combined with fluid loss from gastroenteritis may lead to hypotension, shock, and death.

2. **Cardiopulmonary effects.** Congestive cardiomyopathy, cardiogenic or noncardiogenic pulmonary edema, cardiac conduction abnormalities, and QT interval prolongation with polymorphous ventricular tachycardia (see p 14) may occur promptly or after a delay of several days.

3. **Neurologic effects.** Acute poisoning can cause delirium, encephalopathy, seizures, and coma. A delayed sensorimotor peripheral neuropathy may appear 2–6 weeks after acute ingestion. Sensory effects, particularly painful dysesthesias, occur early and more commonly in moderate poisoning, while ascending weakness and paralysis may predominate in severe poisoning. Neuromuscular respiratory failure has occurred.

4. **Other effects.** Transverse white striae in the nails (Aldrich-Mees lines) may become apparent months after an acute intoxication. Hair loss may also occur. Pancytopenia, particularly leukopenia, reaches a nadir at 1–3 weeks. Basophilic stippling of red cells may also be present.

B. **Chronic intoxication** is also associated with multisystemic effects, which may include fatigue and malaise, gastroenteritis, leukopenia and anemia (occasionally megaloblastic), sensorimotor peripheral neuropathy, hepatic transaminase elevation, noncirrhotic portal hypertension, and peripheral vascular insufficiency. In addition, skin disorders and cancer may occur.

1. **Skin lesions** take years to manifest (3–7 years for a characteristic pattern of hypo- and hyperpigmentation and hyperkeratoses; up to 40 years for skin cancer) and may occur after lower doses than those causing neuropathy or anemia.

2. **Cancer.** Chronic inhalation is associated with lung cancer. Chronic ingestion may also increase the risk of lung, liver, kidney, and bladder cancer.

IV. **Diagnosis** is usually based on a history of exposure combined with a typical presentation. Suspect acute arsenic poisoning in a patient with abrupt onset of abdominal pain, vomiting, watery diarrhea, and hypotension, possibly in association with multisystem signs and symptoms described above. A garlicky odor on the breath has been described but often is not present. Some arsenic compounds, particularly those of lower solubility, are radiopaque and may be visible on a plain abdominal x-ray.

A. **Specific levels.** In the first 2–3 days after acute symptomatic poisoning, total 24-hour urinary excretion is typically in excess of several thousand micrograms (spot urine > 1000 µg/L) and, depending on the severity of poisoning, may not return to background levels (< 50 µg in a 24-hr specimen) for several weeks.

1. Ingestion of **seafood**, which may contain very large amounts of nontoxic arsenobetaine and arsenocholine, can "falsely" elevate total urinary arsenic for 2–3 days. Speciation of urinary arsenic into inorganic and organic forms may be helpful in ruling out toxic arsenic exposure; in such cases the urinary inorganic arsenic should not exceed 25 µg/L or 25 µg/24 hours.

2. **Blood levels** are highly variable and are rarely of value in management. Although whole-blood arsenic, normally less than 3 µg/dL, may be elevated early in acute intoxication, it may decline rapidly to the normal range despite persistent elevated urinary excretion and continuing symptoms.

3. **Elevated concentrations of arsenic in nails or hair** (normally < 1 ppm) may persist for months after urine levels normalize, but should be interpreted cautiously owing to the possibility of external contamination.

B. **Other useful laboratory studies** include CBC and smear for basophilic stippling, electrolytes, glucose, BUN and creatinine, liver enzymes, CPK, urinalysis, ECG and ECG monitoring, and abdominal and chest x-rays.

V. **Treatment.**

A. **Emergency and supportive measures**

1. Maintain an open airway and assist ventilation if necessary (see pp 1–7).

2. Treat coma (p 18), shock (p 15), and arrhythmias (pp 10–14) if they occur. Because of the association of arsenic with prolonged QT intervals, avoid quinidine, procainamide, and other type Ia antiarrhythmic agents.

3. Treat hypotension and fluid loss with aggressive use of intravenous crystalloid solutions.
4. Prolonged inpatient support and observation are indicated for patients with significant acute intoxication because cardiopulmonary complications may be delayed for several days.

B. Specific drugs and antidotes

1. In symptomatic patients, administer **BAL** (dimercaprol; see p 341), 3–5 mg/kg intramuscularly (IM) every 4–6 hours. The antidotal efficacy of BAL has been demonstrated in animals when it is administered promptly (ie, minutes to hours) after exposure. Treatment should not be delayed during the several days commonly required to obtain specific laboratory confirmation.
2. **Dimercaptosuccinic acid** (2,3-DMSA, succimer [p 360]), a water-soluble analog of BAL, is also effective. However, it is available in the United States only as an oral formulation, which precludes its use early in acute poisoning, when gastroenteritis and splanchnic edema may limit gut absorption. It may be used for oral treatment after the patient has stabilized or in patients with chronic intoxication.
3. The therapeutic end points of chelation are poorly defined; however, once urinary arsenic levels are less than 500 µg/L, endogenous biomethylation and detoxification may obviate the need for further chelation. The value of chelation for treatment of an established neuropathy (or prevention of an incipient neuropathy) has not been proved.

C. Decontamination (see p 43)

1. **Prehospital.** Administer activated charcoal if available. Ipecac-induced vomiting may be useful for initial treatment at the scene (eg, children at home) if it can be given within a few minutes of exposure.
2. **Hospital.** Administer activated charcoal. However, note that animal and in vitro studies suggest that activated charcoal has a relatively poor affinity for inorganic arsenic salts. Consider gastric lavage for large ingestions.

D. Enhanced elimination. Hemodialysis may be of possible benefit in patients with concomitant renal failure, but otherwise contributes minimally to arsenic clearance. There is no known role for diuresis, hemoperfusion, or repeat-dose charcoal.

▶ ARSINE

Peter Wald, MD, MPH

Arsine is a colorless gas formed when arsenic comes into contact with hydrogen or with reducing agents in aqueous solution. Typically, exposure occurs in metal smelting and refining industries when metals containing arsenic as an alloy react with an acid. Arsine is also used as a dopant in the microelectronics industry.

I. **Mechanism of toxicity.** Arsine enters red blood cells and forms a complex that results in massive intravascular hemolysis. Several explanations are postulated for the hemolysis, including liberation of elemental arsenic and the formation of complexes with sulfhydryl groups essential to erythrocyte enzymes. **Renal failure** is the most common cause of death after arsine exposure. Renal failure is probably secondary to massive hemolysis and hemoglobinuria, but it may also be caused by direct toxic effects on renal tubular cells or deposition of the arsine-hemoglobin-haptoglobin complex.

II. **Toxic dose.** Arsine is the most toxic form of arsenic. The air level considered immediately dangerous to life or health (IDLH) is 3 ppm. Exposure to 250 ppm may be instantly lethal, and exposure to 25–50 ppm for 30 minutes is usually lethal. The recommended workplace limit (ACGIH TLV-TWA) is 0.05 ppm (0.16 mg/m^3) as an 8-hour time-weighted average. The odor threshold is approximately 0.5 ppm.

III. Clinical presentation.

A. Because arsine gas is not acutely irritating, inhalation causes **no immediate symptoms**. Those exposed to high concentrations may describe a garliclike odor in the air but more typically are unaware that significant exposure has occurred.

B. After a **latent period of 2–24 hours** (depending on the intensity of exposure), massive hemolysis occurs, with early symptoms of malaise, headache, weakness, dyspnea, nausea, vomiting, abdominal pain, hemoglobinuria, and jaundice. Oliguria and acute renal failure often occur 1–3 days after exposure.

IV. Diagnosis is based on a history of exposure; it should be suspected in any worker potentially exposed to arsine who develops acute hemolysis. Laboratory evidence of hemolysis includes acute anemia, anisocytosis, and fragmented red cells. Plasma-free hemoglobin levels may exceed 2 g/dL, and haptoglobin levels are lowered. Routine urinalysis reveals hemoglobinuria but few intact red blood cells.

A. Specific levels. The urine arsenic concentration may be elevated, but this does not assist in emergency management. Whole-blood arsenic concentrations of greater than 0.4 mg/L are associated with fatal cases.

B. Other useful laboratory studies include CBC, plasma-free hemoglobin, haptoglobin, blood type and screen (cross-match if needed), BUN and creatinine, and urinalysis for free hemoglobin.

V. Treatment.

A. Emergency and supportive measures
1. Treat hemolysis with blood transfusions as needed.
2. Prevent deposition of hemoglobin and arsine complex in the kidney tubules by intravenously administering bicarbonate, fluids, and mannitol, if needed, to maintain an adequate (2–3 mL/kg/h) alkaline urine flow. (See discussion of treatment of rhabdomyolysis, p 25.)

B. Specific drugs and antidotes. BAL and other chelators are *not* effective for arsine-induced intoxication.

C. Decontamination. Remove victim from area. Rescuers should wear self-contained breathing apparatus to protect themselves from exposure.

D. Enhanced elimination. The arsine-haptoglobin-hemoglobin complex is not significantly removed by hemodialysis. Forced alkaline diuresis may prevent renal tubular necrosis but does not enhance removal of the complex.

▶ **ASBESTOS**

John Balmes, MD

Asbestos is the name given to a group of naturally occurring silicates, chrysotile, amosite, and crocidolite, and the asbestiform types of tremolite, actinolite, and anthophylite. Exposure to asbestos is a well-documented cause of pulmonary and pleural fibrosis, lung cancer, and mesothelioma, illnesses that may appear many years after exposure.

I. Mechanism of toxicity. Inhalation of thin fibers longer than 5 microns (μ) produces lung fibrosis and cancer in animals (shorter fibers are generally phagocytosed by macrophages and cleared from the lungs). The exact mechanism of toxicity is unknown. Smoking cigarettes appears to enhance the likelihood of developing lung disease and malignancy.

II. Toxic dose. A safe threshold of exposure to asbestos has not been established. Balancing potential health risks against feasibility of workplace control, the 1986 OSHA federal asbestos standard set a permissible exposure limit (PEL) of 0.2 fibers per cubic centimeter (fibers/cc) as an 8-hour time-weighted average.

III. Clinical presentation. After a latent period of 15–20 years, the patient may develop one or more of the following clinical syndromes:

A. **Asbestosis** is a slowly progressive fibrosing disease of the lungs. Pulmonary impairment resulting from lung restriction and decreased gas exchange is common.

B. **Pleural plaques** typically involve only the parietal pleura and are usually asymptomatic but provide a marker of asbestos exposure. Rarely, significant lung restriction occurs as a result of severe pleural fibrosis involving both parietal and visceral surfaces.

C. **Pleural effusions** may occur as early as 5–10 years after the onset of exposure and are often not recognized as asbestos related.

D. **Lung cancer** is a common cause of death in patients with asbestos exposure, especially in cigarette smokers. **Mesothelioma** is a malignancy that may affect the pleura or the peritoneum. The incidence of **gastrointestinal cancer** may be increased in asbestos-exposed workers.

IV. **Diagnosis** is based on a history of exposure to asbestos (usually at least 15–20 years before onset of symptoms) and clinical presentation of one or more of the syndromes described above. Chest x-ray typically shows small, irregular, round opacities distributed primarily in the lower lung fields. Pleural plaques, diffuse thickening, or calcification may be present. Pulmonary function tests reveal decreased vital capacity and total lung capacity and impairment of carbon monoxide diffusion.

A. **Specific tests.** There are no specific blood or urine tests.

B. **Other useful laboratory studies** include chest x-ray, arterial blood gases, and pulmonary function tests.

V. **Treatment.**

A. **Emergency and supportive measures.** Emphasis should be placed on **prevention** of exposure. All asbestos workers should be encouraged to stop smoking and to observe workplace control measures stringently.

B. **Specific drugs and antidotes.** There are none.

C. **Decontamination**

1. **Inhalation.** Persons exposed to asbestos dust and those assisting victims should wear protective equipment, including appropriate respirators and disposable gowns and caps. Watering down any dried material will help to prevent its dispersion into the air as dust.

2. **Skin exposure.** Asbestos is not absorbed through the skin. However, it may be inhaled from skin and clothes, so removal of clothes and washing the skin are recommended.

3. **Ingestion.** Asbestos is not known to be harmful by ingestion, so no decontamination is necessary.

D. **Enhanced elimination.** There is no role for these procedures.

▶ AZIDE, SODIUM

Jo Ellen Dyer, PharmD

Sodium azide is a highly toxic, white crystalline solid. It has come into widespread use in automobile airbags: its explosive decomposition to nitrogen gas provides rapid inflation of the airbag. In addition, sodium azide is used in the production of metallic azide explosives and as a preservative in laboratories. It has no current medical uses, but because of its potent vasodilatory effects, it has been evaluated as an antihypertensive agent.

I. **Mechanism of toxicity.**

A. The mechanism of azide toxicity is unclear. Like cyanide and hydrogen sulfide, azide inhibits iron-containing respiratory enzymes such as cytochrome oxidase, resulting in cellular asphyxiation. Azide is also a potent, direct-acting vasodilator.

B. Although neutral solutions are stable, acidification rapidly converts the azide salt to **hydrazoic acid**, particularly in the presence of solid metals (eg, drain pipes). Hydrazoic acid vapors are pungent and (at high concentrations) explosive. The acute toxicity of hydrazoic acid has been compared with that of hydrogen cyanide and hydrogen sulfide.

II. Toxic dose. Although several grams of azide are found in an automobile airbag, it is completely consumed and converted to nitrogen during the explosive inflation process, and toxicity has not been reported from exposure to spent airbags.

A. Inhalation. Irritation symptoms or pungent odor do not give adequate warning of toxicity. The recommended workplace ceiling limit (ACGIH TLV-C) is 0.29 mg/m^3 for sodium azide and 0.11 ppm for hydrazoic acid. Air concentrations as low as 0.5 ppm may result in mucous membrane irritation, hypotension, and headache. A chemist who intentionally sniffed the vapor above a 1% hydrazoic acid solution became hypotensive, collapsed, and recovered 15 minutes later with residual headache. Workers in a lead azide plant exposed to air concentrations of 0.3–3.9 ppm experienced symptoms of headache, weakness, palpitations, mild smarting of the eyes and nose, and a drop in blood pressure. Laboratory workers adjacent to a sulfur analyzer emitting vapor concentrations of 0.5 ppm experienced symptoms of nasal stuffiness without detecting a pungent odor.

B. Dermal. Industrial workers handling bulk sodium azide experienced headache, nausea, faintness, and hypotension, but it is unclear whether the exposure occurred via dermal absorption or inhalation. An explosion of a metal waste drum containing a 1% sodium azide solution caused burns over a 45% body surface area and led to typical azide toxicity with a time course similar to oral ingestion; coma and hypotension developed within one hour followed by refractory metabolic acidosis, shock, and death 14 hours later.

C. Ingestion. Several serious or fatal poisonings occurred as a result of drinking large quantities of laboratory saline or distilled water containing 0.1–0.2% sodium azide as a preservative.

1. Ingestion of several grams can cause death within 1–2 hours.

2. Ingestion of 700 mg resulted in myocardial failure after 72 hours. Ingestion of 150 mg produced shortness of breath, tachycardia, restlessness, nausea, vomiting, and diarrhea within 15 minutes. Later, polydipsia, T-wave changes on ECG, leukocytosis, and numbness occurred, lasting 10 days.

3. Doses of 0.65–3.9 mg/d given for up to 2.5 years have been used experimentally as an antihypertensive. The hypotensive effect occurred within 1 minute. Headache was the only complaint noted in these patients.

III. Clinical presentation.

A. Irritation. Exposure to dust or gas may produce reddened conjunctivas and nasal and bronchial irritation that may progress to pulmonary edema.

B. Systemic toxicity. Both inhalation and ingestion are associated with a variety of dose-dependent systemic symptoms. Early in the course, hypotension and tachycardia occur that can evolve to bradycardia, ventricular fibrillation, and myocardial failure. Neurologic symptoms include headache, restlessness, facial flushing, loss of vision, faintness, weakness, hyporeflexia, seizures, coma, and respiratory failure. Nausea, vomiting, diarrhea, diaphoresis, and lactic acidosis also appear during the course.

IV. Diagnosis is based on the history of exposure and clinical presentation.

A. Specific levels. Specific blood or serum levels are not routinely available. A simple qualitative test can be used on powders and solid materials: azide forms a red precipitate in the presence of ferric chloride (use gloves and respiratory protection when handling the azide).

B. Other useful laboratory studies include electrolytes, glucose, arterial blood gases or pulse oximetry, and ECG.

V. Treatment. *Caution:* Cases involving severe azide ingestion are potentially dangerous to health care providers. In the acidic environment of the stomach, azide salts are converted to hydrazoic acid, which is highly volatile. Quickly isolate all vomitus or gastric washings, and keep the patient in a well-ventilated area. Wear appropriate respiratory protective gear if available and personnel are trained to use it. Dispose of azide with care. Contact with heavy metals, including copper or lead found in water pipes, forms metal azides that may explode.

A. Emergency and supportive measures
  1. Protect the airway and assist ventilation (see pp 1–7) if necessary. Insert an intravenous line and monitor the ECG and vital signs.
  2. Treat coma (p 18), hypotension (p 15), seizures (p 21), and arrhythmias (pp 10–14) if they occur.

B. Specific drugs and antidotes. There is no specific antidote.

C. Decontamination (see p 43)
  1. **Inhalation.** Remove the victim from exposure and give supplemental oxygen if available. Rescuers should wear self-contained breathing apparatus and appropriate chemical-protective clothing.
  2. **Skin.** Remove and bag contaminated clothing and wash affected areas copiously with soap and water.
  3. **Ingestion.** See caution statement above; isolate all vomitus or gastric washings to avoid exposure to volatile hydrazoic acid.
     a. **Prehospital.** Administer activated charcoal if available. Do *not* induce vomiting because of the risk of abrupt onset of hypotension or seizures.
     b. **Hospital.** Perform gastric lavage, and administer activated charcoal. The affinity of charcoal for azide is not known.

D. Enhanced elimination. There is no role for dialysis or hemoperfusion in acute azide poisoning.

▶ BARBITURATES

Timothy E. Albertson, MD, PhD

Barbiturates are used as hypnotic and sedative agents, for the induction of anesthesia, and for the treatment of epilepsy and status epilepticus. They are often divided into four major groups by their pharmacologic activity and clinical use: **ultrashort-acting, short-acting, intermediate-acting,** and **long-acting** (Table II–10). *Common combination products* containing small amounts of barbiturates include Fiorinal and Donnatal.

I. Mechanism of toxicity.
  A. All barbiturates cause generalized **depression of neuronal activity** in the brain. Interaction with a barbiturate receptor leads to enhanced γ-aminobutyric acid (GABA)-mediated chloride currents and results in synaptic inhibition. Hypotension that occurs with large doses is caused by depression of central sympathetic tone as well as by direct depression of cardiac contractility.
  B. **Pharmacokinetics** vary by agent and group (see Tables II–10 and II–55).
     1. **Ultrashort-acting** barbiturates are highly lipid-soluble and rapidly penetrate the brain to induce anesthesia, then are quickly redistributed to other tissues. For this reason, the clinical duration of effect is much shorter than the elimination half-life for these compounds.
     2. **Long-acting barbiturates** are distributed more evenly and have long elimination half-lives, making them useful for once-daily treatment of epilepsy. Primidone (Mysoline) is metabolized to phenobarbital and phenylethylmalonamide (PEMA); although phenobarbital accounts for only about 25% of the metabolites, it has the greatest anticonvulsant activity.

II. Toxic dose. The toxic dose of barbiturates varies widely and depends on the drug, the route and rate of administration, and individual patient tolerance. In general, toxicity is likely when the dose exceeds 5–10 times the hypnotic dose. Chronic users or abusers may have striking tolerance to depressant effects.

TABLE II-10. COMMON BARBITURATES[a]

Drug	Normal Terminal Elimination Half-Life (h)	Usual Duration of Effect (h)	Usual Hypnotic Dose (Adult) (mg)	Minimum Toxic Level (mg/L)
Ultrashort-acting				
Methohexital	3–5	< 0.5	50–120	>5
Thiopental	8–10	< 0.5	50–75	>5
Short-acting				
Pentobarbital	15–50	> 3–4	50–200	>10
Secobarbital	15–40	> 3–4	100–200	>10
Intermediate-acting				
Amobarbital	10–40	> 4–6	65–200	>10
Aprobarbital	14–34	> 4–6	40–160	>10
Butabarbital	35–50	> 4–6	100–200	>10
Long-acting				
Mephobarbital	10–70	> 6–12	50–100	>30
Phenobarbital	80–120	> 6–12	100–320	>30

[a]References: Hobbs WR, Rall TW, Verdoorn TA: Hypnotics and Sedatives, Chapter 17, pp 361–396, in: *Goodman & Gilman's The Pharmacological Basis of Therapeutics,* 9th ed. Hardman JG, et al. (editors), McGraw-Hill, 1996; and El-lenhorn MJ et al. (editors): Sedative-Hypnotic Drugs, Chapter 41, pp. 684–711, in *Medical Toxicology,* 2nd ed. Williams & Wilkins, 1997.

    A. The potentially fatal **oral dose** of the shorter-acting agents is 2–3 g, compared with 6–10 g for phenobarbital.

    B. Several deaths were reported in young women undergoing therapeutic abortion after they received rapid **intravenous injections** of as little as 1–3 mg/kg of methohexital.

III. Clinical presentation. The onset of symptoms depends on the drug and the route of administration.

    A. Lethargy, slurred speech, nystagmus, and ataxia are common with mild to moderate intoxication. With higher doses, hypotension, coma, and respiratory arrest commonly occur. With deep coma, the pupils are usually small or mid-position; the patient may lose all reflex activity and appear to be dead.

    B. Hypothermia is common in patients with deep coma, especially if the victim has suffered exposure to a cool environment. Hypotension and bradycardia commonly accompany hypothermia.

IV. Diagnosis is usually based on a history of ingestion and should be suspected in any epileptic patient with stupor or coma. Although skin bullae are sometimes seen with barbiturate overdose, these are not specific for barbiturates. Other causes of coma should also be considered (see p 18).

    A. Specific levels of phenobarbital are usually readily available from hospital clinical laboratories; concentrations greater than 60–80 mg/L are usually associated with coma and those greater than 150–200 mg/L with severe hypotension. For short- and intermediate-acting barbiturates, coma is likely when the serum concentration exceeds 20–30 mg/L. Barbiturates are easily detected in routine urine toxicologic screening.

    B. Other useful laboratory studies include electrolytes, glucose, BUN, creatinine, arterial blood gases or pulse oximetry, and chest x-ray.

V. Treatment.

    A. Emergency and supportive measures

        1. Protect the airway and assist ventilation (see pp 1–7) if necessary.

    2. Treat coma (p 18), hypothermia (p 19), and hypotension (p 15) if they occur.

B. Specific drugs and antidotes. There is no specific antidote.

C. Decontamination (see p 43)

    1. Prehospital. Administer activated charcoal, if available.

    2. Hospital. Administer activated charcoal. Consider gastric lavage for massive ingestion.

D. Enhanced elimination

    1. Alkalinization of the urine (p 346) increases the urinary elimination of phenobarbital but not other barbiturates. Its value in acute overdose is unproved, and it may potentially contribute to fluid overload and pulmonary edema.

    2. Repeat-dose activated charcoal has been shown to decrease the half-life of phenobarbital, but it has not been shown to actually shorten the duration of coma.

    3. Hemoperfusion or hemodialysis may be necessary for severely intoxicated patients not responding to supportive care (ie, with intractable hypotension).

▶ BARIUM

Olga F. Woo, PharmD

Barium poisonings are uncommon and usually result from accidental contamination of food sources, suicidal ingestion, or occupational inhalation exposure. The water-soluble barium salts (acetate, carbonate, chloride, hydroxide, nitrate, and sulfide) are highly toxic, whereas the insoluble salt, barium sulfate, is nontoxic because it is not absorbed. Soluble barium salts are found in depilatories, fireworks, ceramic glazes, and rodenticides and are used in the manufacture of glass and in dyeing textiles. Barium sulfide and polysulfide may also produce hydrogen sulfide toxicity (see p 188).

I. Mechanism of toxicity.

    A. Systemic barium poisoning is characterized by profound hypokalemia, leading to respiratory and cardiac arrest. The mechanism for the rapid onset of severe hypokalemia is not known; studies have excluded intracellular sequestration of potassium, enhanced renal elimination, and adrenergic stimulation. It is proposed that barium ions have a direct action on muscle cell potassium permeability, which stimulates smooth, striated, and cardiac muscles resulting in peristalsis, arterial hypertension, muscle twitching, and cardiac arrhythmias.

    B. Inhalation of insoluble inorganic barium salts can cause baritosis, a benign pneumoconiosis.

    C. Pharmacokinetics. Barium is stored in bone and slowly excreted via the feces. Tissue distribution follows a three-compartment model with half-lives of 3.6, 34, and 1033 days.

II. Toxic dose. The minimum oral toxic dose of soluble barium salts is undetermined but may be as low as 200 mg. Lethal doses range from 1–30 g for various barium salts because absorption is influenced by gastric pH and foods high in sulfate.

III. Clinical presentation. Within minutes to a few hours after ingestion, victims develop profound hypokalemia and skeletal muscle weakness progressing to flaccid paralysis of the limbs and respiratory muscles. Ventricular arrhythmias also occur. Gastroenteritis with severe watery diarrhea, mydriasis with impaired visual accommodation, and CNS depression are sometimes present. More often, patients remain conscious even when severely intoxicated.

IV. Diagnosis is based on a history of exposure, accompanied by rapidly progressive hypokalemia and muscle weakness.

    A. Specific levels. Blood barium levels are not routinely available.

    B. Other useful laboratory studies include electrolytes (potassium), BUN, creatinine, phosphorus, arterial blood gases or pulse oximetry, and ECG.

V. Treatment.

    A. Emergency and supportive measures

        1. Maintain an open airway and assist ventilation if necessary (see pp 1–7).

        2. Treat fluid losses from gastroenteritis with intravenous crystalloids.

        3. Attach a cardiac monitor and observe patient closely for several hours after ingestion.

    B. Specific drugs and antidotes. Administer **potassium chloride** (KCl) at 10–15 meq/h IV to treat symptomatic or severe hypokalemia. Large doses of potassium may be necessary (doses as high as 420 meq over 24 hours have been given).

    C. Decontamination (see p 43)

        1. Prehospital. Ipecac-induced vomiting may be useful for initial treatment at the scene (eg, children at home) if it can be given within a few minutes of exposure.

        2. Hospital.

            a. Perform gastric lavage. *Caution:* Rapidly progressive weakness may increase the risk of pulmonary aspiration.

            b. Magnesium sulfate or sodium sulfate (30 g; children 250 mg/kg) should be administered orally to precipitate ingested barium as the insoluble sulfate salt.

            c. The efficacy of activated charcoal is not known.

    D. Enhanced elimination

        1. Diuresis with saline and furosemide to obtain a urine flow of 4–6 mL/kg/h may enhance barium elimination.

        2. Hemodialysis and hemoperfusion have not been evaluated in the treatment of serious barium poisoning.

▶ BENZENE

Alan Buchwald, MD

Benzene, a clear volatile liquid with an acrid aromatic odor, is one of the most widely used industrial chemicals. It is used as a constituent in gasoline; as a solvent for fats, inks, paints, and plastics; and as a chemical intermediate in the synthesis of a variety of materials. It is generally not present in household products.

  I. Mechanism of toxicity. Like other hydrocarbons, benzene can cause a chemical pneumonia if it is aspirated. See p 183 for a general discussion of hydrocarbon toxicity.

    A. Once absorbed, benzene causes CNS depression and may sensitize the myocardium to the arrhythmogenic effects of catecholamines.

    B. Benzene is also known for its chronic effects on the hematopoietic system, which are thought to be mediated by a reactive toxic intermediate metabolite.

    C. Benzene is a known human carcinogen (ACGIH category Al).

  II. Toxic dose. Benzene is rapidly absorbed by inhalation and ingestion and, to a limited extent, percutaneously.

    A. The estimated lethal **oral** dose is 100 mL, but as little as 15 mL has caused death.

    B. The recommended workplace limit (ACGIH TLV-TWA) for benzene **vapor** is 0.5 ppm (1.6 mg/m^3) as an 8-hour time-weighted average. The short-term exposure limit (STEL) is 2.5 ppm. The level considered immediately dangerous to life or health (IDLH) is 500 ppm. A single exposure to 7,500–20,000 ppm

can be fatal. Chronic exposure to air concentrations well below the threshold for smell (2 ppm) are associated with hematopoietic toxicity.
  C. The Environmental Protection Agency (EPA) Maximum Contaminant Level (MCL) in water is 5 ppb.
III. **Clinical presentation.**
  A. **Acute exposure** may cause immediate CNS effects, including headache, nausea, dizziness, convulsions, and coma. Symptoms of CNS toxicity should be apparent immediately after inhalation or within 30–60 minutes after ingestion. Severe inhalation may result in noncardiogenic pulmonary edema. Ventricular arrhythmias may result from increased sensitivity of the myocardium to catecholamines. Benzene can cause chemical burns to the skin with prolonged or massive exposure.
  B. After **chronic exposure**, hematologic disorders such as pancytopenia, aplastic anemia, acute myelogenous leukemia, and its variants may occur. Causality is suspected for chronic myelogenous leukemia, chronic lymphocytic leukemia, multiple myeloma, Hodgkin's disease, and paroxysmal nocturnal hemoglobinuria. There is unproven association between benzene exposure and acute lymphoblastic leukemia, myelofibrosis, and lymphomas. Chromosomal abnormalities have been reported, although no effects on fertility have been described in women after occupational exposure.
IV. **Diagnosis** of benzene poisoning is based on a history of exposure and typical clinical findings. With chronic hematologic toxicity, erythrocyte, leukocyte, and thrombocyte counts may first increase and then decrease before the onset of aplastic anemia.
  A. **Specific levels.** *Note:* smoke from one cigarette contains 60–80 µg of benzene; a typical smoker inhales 1–2 mg of benzene daily. This may confound measurements of low-level benzene exposures.
    1. Increased urine phenol levels may be useful indicators for monitoring workers' exposure (if diet is carefully controlled for phenol products). A spot urine phenol measurement higher than 20 mg/L suggests excessive occupational exposure. Urinary *trans*-muconic acid and *S*-phenylmercapturic acid (S-PMA) are more sensitive and specific tests for the measurement of low levels of benzene exposure.
    2. Benzene can also be measured in expired air for up to 2 days after exposure.
    3. Blood levels of benzene or metabolites are not clinically useful.
  B. **Other useful laboratory studies** include CBC, electrolytes, BUN, creatinine, liver function tests, ECG monitoring, and chest x-ray (if aspiration is suspected).
V. **Treatment.**
  A. **Emergency and supportive measures**
    1. Maintain an open airway and assist ventilation if necessary (see pp 1–7).
    2. Treat coma (p 18), seizures (p 21), arrhythmias (pp 10–14), and other complications if they occur.
    3. Be cautious with use of any adrenergic agents (eg, epinephrine, metoproterenol, albuterol) because of the possibility of myocardial sensitization.
    4. Monitor vital signs and ECG for 12–24 hours after significant exposure.
  B. **Specific drugs and antidotes.** There is no specific antidote.
  C. **Decontamination** (see p 43)
    1. **Inhalation.** Immediately move the victim to fresh air and administer oxygen if available.
    2. **Skin and eyes.** Remove clothing and wash the skin; irrigate exposed eyes with copious amounts of water or saline.
    3. **Ingestion** (see p 45)
      a. **Prehospital.** Administer activated charcoal if available. Do *not* induce vomiting because of the risk of abrupt onset of coma or convulsions.
      b. **Hospital.** Administer activated charcoal. Consider gastric lavage for a recent (less than 30 minutes), large ingestion.
  D. **Enhanced elimination.** Dialysis and hemoperfusion are not effective.

▶ BENZODIAZEPINES

Karl A. Sporer, MD

The drug class of benzodiazepines contains many compounds that vary widely in potency, duration of effect, presence or absence of active metabolites, and clinical use (Table II–11). In general, death from benzodiazepine overdose is rare, unless the drugs are combined with other CNS-depressant agents such as ethanol or barbiturates. Newer potent, short-acting agents have been considered the sole cause of death in recent forensic cases.

I. **Mechanism of toxicity.** Benzodiazepines enhance the action of the inhibitory neurotransmitter γ-aminobutyric acid (GABA). They also inhibit other neuronal systems by poorly defined mechanisms. The result is generalized depression of spinal reflexes and the reticular activating system. This may cause coma and respiratory arrest.

   A. Respiratory arrest is more likely with newer short-acting triazolobenzodiazepines such as triazolam (Halcion), alprazolam (Xanax), and midazolam (Versed).

   B. Cardiopulmonary arrest has occurred after rapid injection of diazepam, possibly because of CNS-depressant effects or because of the toxic effects of the diluent propylene glycol.

   C. **Pharmacokinetics.** Most agents are highly protein bound (90–100%). Volumes of distribution and elimination half-lives are given in Table II–55, p 319.

II. **Toxic dose.** In general, the toxic: therapeutic ratio for benzodiazepines is very high. For example, oral overdoses of diazepam have been reported in excess of 15–20 times the therapeutic dose without serious depression of consciousness. On the other hand, respiratory arrest has been reported after ingestion of 5 mg of triazolam and after rapid intravenous injection of diazepam, midazolam, and many other benzodiazepines. Also, ingestion of another drug with CNS-depressant properties (eg, ethanol, barbiturates, opioids, etc) will likely produce additive effects.

TABLE II–11. BENZODIAZEPINES FOR ORAL USE

Drug	Half-Life(h)	Active Metabolite	Oral Adult Dose (mg)
Alprazolam	6–15	Yes	0.25–0.5
Chlordiazepoxide	5–30	Yes	5–50
Clonazepam	20–60	Yes	0.5–2
Clorazepate	50–100[a]	Yes	3.75–30
Diazepam	50–100[a]	Yes	5–20
Estazolam	10–24	Slight	1–2
Flunitrazepam	8–10	Slight	1–2
Flurazepam	50–100[a]	Yes	15–30
Lorazepam	9–20	No	2–4
Midazolam	1–5	Yes	1–5[b]
Oxazepam	5–20	No	15–30
Prazepam	5–10[a]	Yes	20–60
Temazepam	10–12	Slight	15–30
Triazolam	1–6	?	0.125–0.5
Zolpidem	2–3	No	10–20

[a]Half-life of active metabolite, to which effects can be attributed.
[b]IM or IV.

III. Clinical presentation. Onset of CNS depression may be observed within 30–120 minutes of ingestion, depending on the compound. Lethargy, slurred speech, ataxia, coma, and respiratory arrest may occur. Generally, patients with benzodiazepine-induced coma have hyporeflexia and mid-position or small pupils. Hypothermia may occur. Serious complications are more likely when newer short-acting agents are involved or when other depressant drugs have been ingested.

IV. Diagnosis is usually based on the history of ingestion or recent injection. The differential diagnosis should include other sedative-hypnotic agents, antidepressants, antipsychotics, and narcotics. Coma and small pupils do not respond to naloxone but will reverse with administration of flumazenil (see below).

    A. Specific levels. Serum drug levels are often available from regional commercial toxicology laboratories but are rarely of value in emergency management. Urine and blood qualitative screening may provide rapid confirmation of exposure. Certain immunoassays may not detect newer benzodiazepines or those in low concentrations. Triazolam and prazepam are rarely detectable.

    B. Other useful laboratory studies include glucose, arterial blood gases, or pulse oximetry.

V. Treatment.

    A. Emergency and supportive measures

        1. Protect the airway and assist ventilation if necessary (see pp 1–7).

        2. Treat coma (p 18), hypotension (p 15), and hypothermia (p 19) if they occur. Hypotension usually responds promptly to supine position and intravenous fluids.

    B. Specific drugs and antidotes. Flumazenil (see p 369) is a specific benzodiazepine receptor antagonist that can rapidly reverse coma. However, because benzodiazepine overdose by itself is rarely fatal, the role of flumazenil in routine management has yet to be established. It is administered intravenously with a starting dose of 0.1–0.2 mg, repeated as needed up to a total of no more than 3 mg. It has some important potential drawbacks:

        1. It may induce seizures in patients with tricyclic antidepressant overdose.

        2. It may induce acute withdrawal, including seizures and autonomic instability, in patients who are addicted to benzodiazepines.

        3. Resedation is common when the drug wears off after 1–2 hours, and repeated dosing is usually required.

    C. Decontamination (see p 43)

        1. Prehospital. Administer activated charcoal if available.

        2. Hospital. Administer activated charcoal. Gastric emptying is not necessary if activated charcoal can be given promptly.

    D. Enhanced elimination. There is no role for diuresis, dialysis, or hemoperfusion. Repeat-dose charcoal has not been studied.

▶ BETA-ADRENERGIC BLOCKERS

Neal L. Benowitz, MD

Beta-adrenergic blocking agents are widely used for the treatment of hypertension, arrhythmias, angina pectoris, migraine headaches, and glaucoma. Many patients with beta-blocker overdose will have underlying cardiovascular diseases or will be taking other cardioactive medications, both of which may aggravate beta-blocker overdose. A variety of beta blockers are available, with various pharmacologic effects and clinical uses (Table II–12).

I. Mechanism of toxicity. Excessive beta-adrenergic blockade is common to overdose with all drugs in this category. Although beta-receptor specificity is seen at low doses, it is lost in overdose.

    A. Propranolol and other agents with membrane-depressant (quinidinelike) effects further depress myocardial contractility and conduction. Propranolol is

TABLE II–12. COMPARISON OF BETA-ADRENERGIC BLOCKING AGENTS

Drug	Usual Daily Adult Dose (mg/24 h)	Cardio-selective	Membrane Depression	Partial Agonist	Normal Half-life (h)
Acebutolol	400–800	+	+	+	3–6
Alprenolol	200–800	0	+	++	2–3
Atenolol	50–100	+	0	0	4–10
Betaxolol[a]	10–20	+	0	0	12–22
Bisoprolol	5–20	+	0	0	8–12
Carteolol	2.5–10	0	0	+	6
Carvedilol[c]	6.25–50	0	0	0	6–10
Esmolol[b]		+	0	0	9 min
Labetalol[c]	200–800	0	+	0	6–8
Levobunolol[a]		0	0	0	5–6
Metoprolol	100–450	+	+/–	0	3–7
Nadolol	80–240	0	0	0	10–24
Oxyprenolol	40–480	0	+	++	1–3
Penbutolol	20–40	0	0	+	17–26
Pindolol	5–60	0	+	+++	3–4
Propranolol	40–360	0	++	0	2–6
Sotalol[d]	160–480	0	0	0	5–15
Timolol[a]	20–80	0	0	+/–	2–4

[a]Also available as ophthalmic preparation.
[b]Intravenous infusion 50–200 μg/kg/min.
[c]Alpha-adrenergic blocking activity.
[d]Class III antiarrhythmic activity.

also lipid soluble, which enhances brain penetration and can cause seizures and coma.

B. **Pindolol** and other agents with partial beta-agonist activity may cause hypertension.

C. **Sotalol**, which also has type III antiarrhythmic activity, prolongs the QT interval in a dose-dependent manner and may cause torsades de pointes (see p 14) and ventricular fibrillation.

D. **Pharmacokinetics.** Peak absorption occurs within 1–4 hours but may be much longer with sustained-release preparations. Volumes of distribution are generally large. Elimination of most agents is by hepatic metabolism, although nadolol is excreted unchanged in the urine and esmolol is rapidly inactivated by red blood cell esterases. (See also Table II–55, p 319)

II. **Toxic dose.** The response to beta-blocker overdose is highly variable depending on underlying medical disease or other medications. Susceptible patients may have severe or even fatal reactions to therapeutic doses. There are no clear guidelines, but ingestion of only 2–3 times the therapeutic dose (Table II–12) should be considered potentially life-threatening in all patients. Atenolol and pindolol appear to be less toxic than other agents.

III. **Clinical presentation.** The pharmacokinetics of beta blockers vary considerably, and duration of poisoning may range from minutes to days.

A. **Cardiac disturbances**, including hypotension and bradycardia, are the most common manifestations of poisoning. Atrioventricular block, intraventricular conduction disturbances, cardiogenic shock, and asystole may occur with severe overdose, especially with membrane-depressant drugs such as propranolol. The ECG usually shows a normal QRS duration with increased PR intervals; QRS widening occurs with massive intoxication.

B. **CNS toxicity**, including convulsions, coma, and respiratory arrest, is commonly seen with propranolol and other membrane-depressant and lipid-soluble drugs.

C. **Bronchospasm** is most common in patients with preexisting asthma or chronic bronchospastic disease.

D. **Hypoglycemia** and **hyperkalemia** may occur.

IV. **Diagnosis** is based on the history of ingestion, accompanied by bradycardia and hypotension. Other drugs that may cause a similar presentation after overdose include sympatholytic and antihypertensive drugs, digitalis, and calcium channel blockers.

A. **Specific levels.** Measurement of beta-blocker serum levels may confirm the diagnosis but does not contribute to emergency management. Metoprolol and propranolol may be detected in comprehensive urine toxicology screening.

B. **Other useful laboratory studies** include electrolytes, glucose, BUN, creatinine, arterial blood gases, and 12-lead ECG and ECG monitoring.

V. **Treatment.**

A. **Emergency and supportive measures**
1. Maintain an open airway and assist ventilation if necessary (see pp 1–7).
2. Treat coma (p 18), seizures (p 21), hypotension (p 15), hyperkalemia (p 36), and hypoglycemia (p 33) if they occur.
3. Treat bradycardia with atropine, 0.01–0.03 mg/kg IV; isoproterenol (start with 4 μg/min and increase infusion as needed); or cardiac pacing.
4. Treat bronchospasm with nebulized bronchodilators (p 9).
5. Continuously monitor the vital signs and ECG for at least 6 hours after ingestion.

B. **Specific drugs and antidotes**
1. Bradycardia and hypotension resistant to the above measures should be treated with **glucagon**, 5–10 mg IV bolus, repeated as needed and followed by an infusion of 1–5 mg/h (see p 371). **Epinephrine** (intravenous infusion starting at 1–4 μg/min and titrating to effect; see p 365 may also be useful.
2. Wide complex conduction defects caused by membrane-depressant poisoning may respond to **sodium bicarbonate**, 1–2 meq/kg, as given for tricyclic antidepressant overdose (see p 345).
3. Torsades de pointes polymorphous ventricular tachycardia associated with QT prolongation resulting from sotalol poisoning can be treated with **isoproterenol** infusion, **magnesium**, or **overdrive pacing** (see p 14). Correction of hypokalemia may also be useful.

C. **Decontamination** (see p 43)
1. **Prehospital.** Administer activated charcoal if available.
2. **Hospital.** Administer activated charcoal. Consider gastric lavage for large ingestions, especially involving propranolol. Gastric emptying is not necessary for small ingestions if activated charcoal can be given promptly.

D. **Enhanced elimination.** Most beta blockers, especially the more toxic drugs such as propranolol, are highly lipophilic and have a large volume of distribution (Vd). For those with a relatively small volume of distribution coupled with a long half-life or low intrinsic clearance (eg, acebutolol, atenolol, nadolol, or sotalol), hemoperfusion, hemodialysis, or repeat-dose charcoal may be effective.

▶ BETA-2-ADRENERGIC STIMULANTS

Susan Kim, PharmD

Beta-adrenergic agonists can be broadly categorized as having β_1 and β_2 receptor activity. This section describes the toxicity of several β_2-selective agonists that are commonly available for oral use: albuterol (salbutamol), metaproterenol, and terbu-

TABLE II–13. COMMONLY AVAILABLE β₂ SELECTIVE AGONISTS

Drug	Adult Dose (mg/d)	Pediatric Dose (mg/kg/d)	Duration (h)
Albuterol	8–16	0.3–0.8	4–8
Metaproterenol	60–80	0.9–2.0	4
Ritodrine[a]	40–120	N/A	4–6
Terbutaline	7.5–20	0.15–0.6	4–8

[a]No longer available as an oral formulation in the United States.

taline (see Table II–13). Nylidrin, a peripheral vasodilator with mixed β_1 and β_2 activity, would be expected to have a similar toxicity profile.

I. **Mechanism of toxicity.** Stimulation of β_2 receptors results in relaxation of smooth muscles in the bronchi, uterus, and skeletal muscle vessels. At high toxic doses, selectivity for β_2 receptors may be lost, and β_1 effects may be seen.

Pharmacokinetics. Readily absorbed orally or by inhalation. Volumes of distribution (Vd) are approximately 0.7–1.8 L/kg. Half-lives and other pharmacokinetic parameters are described in Table II–55 (p 319).

II. **Toxic dose.** Generally, a single ingestion of more than the total daily dose (see Table II–13) is expected to produce signs and symptoms of toxicity. Dangerously exaggerated responses to therapeutic doses of terbutaline have been reported in pregnant women, presumably as a result of pregnancy-induced hemodynamic changes.

III. **Clinical presentation.** Overdoses of these drugs affect primarily the cardiovascular system. Most overdoses, especially in children, result in only mild toxicity.

A. **Vasodilation** results in reduced peripheral vascular resistance and can lead to significant hypotension. The diastolic pressure is usually reduced to a greater extent than the systolic pressure, resulting in a wide pulse pressure and bounding pulse.

B. **Tachycardia** is a common reflex response to vasodilation and may also be caused by direct stimulation of β_1 receptors as β_2 selectivity is lost in high doses. Supraventricular tachycardia or ventricular extrasystoles are occasionally reported.

C. **Agitation and skeletal muscle tremors** are common. Seizures are rare.

D. **Metabolic effects** include hypokalemia, hyperglycemia, and lactic acidosis. Hypokalemia is caused by an intracellular shift of potassium rather than true depletion.

IV. **Diagnosis** is based on the history of ingestion. The findings of tachycardia, hypotension with a wide pulse pressure, tremor, and hypokalemia are strongly suggestive. Theophylline overdose (see p 303) may present with similar manifestations.

A. **Specific levels** are not generally available and do not contribute to emergency management. These drugs are not usually detectable on comprehensive urine toxicology screening.

B. **Other useful laboratory studies** include electrolytes, glucose, BUN, creatinine, CPK (if excessive muscle activity suggests rhabdomyolysis), and ECG monitoring.

V. **Treatment.** Most overdoses are mild and do not require aggressive treatment.

A. **Emergency and supportive measures**

1. Maintain an open airway and assist ventilation if necessary (see pp 1–7).

2. Monitor the vital signs and ECG for about 4–6 hours after ingestion.

3. If seizures or altered mental status occurs, it is most likely caused by cerebral hypoperfusion and should respond to treatment of hypotension (see below).

4. Treat hypotension initially with boluses of intravenous crystalloid, 10–30 mL/kg. If this fails to improve the blood pressure, use a beta-adrenergic blocker (see **B**, below).
5. Sinus tachycardia rarely requires treatment, especially in children, unless accompanied by hypotension or ventricular dysrhythmias. If treatment is necessary, use beta-adrenergic blockers (see **B**, below).
6. Hypokalemia does not usually require treatment, since it is transient and does not reflect a total body potassium deficit.

B. Specific drugs and antidotes. Hypotension, tachycardia, and ventricular arrhythmias are caused by excessive beta-adrenergic stimulation, and beta blockers are specific antagonists. Give **propranolol** (see p 405), 0.01–0.02 mg/kg IV, or **esmolol** (see p 366), 25–50 µg/kg/min IV. Use beta blockers cautiously in patients with a prior history of asthma or wheezing.

C. Decontamination (see p 43)
1. **Prehospital.** Administer activated charcoal, if available. Ipecac-induced vomiting may be useful for initial treatment at the scene (eg, children at home) if it can be given within a few minutes of exposure.
2. **Hospital.** Administer activated charcoal. Gastric emptying is not necessary if activated charcoal can be given promptly.

D. Enhanced elimination. There is no role for these procedures.

▶ BORIC ACID, BORATES, AND BORON

Olga F. Woo, PharmD

Boric acid and sodium borate have been used for many years in a variety of products as antiseptics and fungistatic agents in baby talcum powder. Boric acid powder (99%) is still used as a pesticide against ants and cockroaches. In the past, repeated and indiscriminate application of boric acid to broken or abraded skin resulted in many cases of severe poisoning. Epidemics have also occurred after boric acid was mistakenly added to infant formula or used in food preparation. Although chronic toxicity seldom occurs now, acute ingestion by children at home is common.

Other boron-containing compounds with similar toxicity include boron oxide and orthoboric acid (sassolite).

I. Mechanism of toxicity. The mechanism of borate poisoning is unknown. Boric acid is not highly corrosive, but is irritating to mucous membranes. It probably acts as a general cellular poison. Organ systems most commonly affected are the gastrointestinal tract, brain, liver, and kidneys.

Pharmacokinetics. The volume of distribution (Vd) is 0.17–0.50 L/kg. Elimination is mainly through the kidneys, and 85–100% of a dose may be found in the urine over 5–7 days. The elimination half-life is 12–27 hours.

II. Toxic dose.
A. The **acute** single oral toxic dose is highly variable, but serious poisoning is reported to occur with 1–3 g in newborns, 5 g in infants, and 20 g in adults. A teaspoon of 99% boric acid contains 3–4 g. Most accidental ingestions in children result in minimal or no toxicity.
B. Chronic ingestion or application to abraded skin is much more serious than acute single ingestion. Serious toxicity and death occurred in infants ingesting 5–15 g in formula over several days; serum borate levels were 400–1600 mg/L.

III. Clinical presentation.
A. After oral or dermal absorption, the earliest symptoms are gastrointestinal with vomiting and diarrhea. Vomiting and diarrhea may have a blue-green color. Significant dehydration and renal failure can occur, with death caused by profound shock.

B. Neurologic symptoms of hyperactivity, agitation, and seizures may occur early.

C. An erythrodermic rash (boiled-lobster appearance) is followed by exfoliation after 2–5 days. Alopecia totalis has been reported.

IV. Diagnosis is based on a history of exposure, the presence of gastroenteritis (possibly with blue-green emesis), erythematous rash, acute renal failure, and elevated serum borate levels.

    A. Specific levels. Serum or blood borate levels are not generally available and may not correlate accurately with the level of intoxication. Analysis of serum for borates can be obtained from National Medical Services, Inc., telephone (215) 657-4900, or consult a local laboratory. Normal serum or blood levels vary with diet, but are usually less than 7 mg/L. The serum boron level can be estimated by dividing the serum borate by 5.72.

    B. Other useful laboratory studies include electrolytes, glucose, BUN, creatinine, and urinalysis.

V. Treatment.

    A. Emergency and supportive measures

        1. Maintain an open airway and assist ventilation if necessary (see pp 1–7).

        2. Treat coma (p 18), seizures (p 21), hypotension (p 15), and renal failure (p 37) if they occur.

    B. Specific drugs and antidotes. There is no specific antidote.

    C. Decontamination (see p 43)

        1. Prehospital. Administer activated charcoal, if available. Ipecac-induced vomiting may be useful for initial treatment at the scene (eg, children at home) if it can be given within a few minutes of exposure.

        2. Hospital. Administer activated charcoal (although boric acid is not well adsorbed). Consider gastric lavage for large ingestions.

    D. Enhanced elimination. Hemodialysis is effective and is indicated after massive ingestions and for supportive care of renal failure. Peritoneal dialysis has not proved effective in enhancing elimination in infants.

▶ BOTULISM

Olga F. Woo, PharmD

As early as the 1700s, botulism was a recognized cause of fatal food poisoning. Classically, botulism has been associated with ingestion of **preformed toxin** from improperly preserved (eg, canned, fermented, or smoked) foods. Newer sources continue to be discovered, such as improperly prepared or stored pot pies, fried onions, baked potatoes, potato salad, chopped garlic in oil, yogurt with conserve sweetened with aspartame instead of sugar, and turkey stuffing. **Wound botulism** and **infant botulism** are other recognized syndromes.

I. Mechanism of toxicity.

    A. Botulism is caused by a heat-labile neurotoxin (botulin) produced by the bacteria *Clostridium botulinum*. Different strains of the bacterium produce seven distinct exotoxins: A, B, C, D, E, F, and G; types A, B, and E are most frequently involved in human disease. Botulin toxin irreversibly binds to cholinergic nerve terminals and prevents acetylcholine release from the axon. Severe muscle weakness results, and death is caused by respiratory failure. The toxin does not cross the blood-brain barrier.

    B. Botulinum spores are ubiquitous in nature but are not dangerous unless they are allowed to germinate in an anaerobic environment with a pH greater than 4.6. Incompletely cooked foods left out at ambient temperatures for several hours may produce lethal amounts of botulin toxin. The spores can be destroyed by pressure cooking at a temperature of at least 120 °C (250 °F) for 30 minutes. The toxin can be destroyed by boiling at 100 °C (212 °F) for 1 minute or heating at 80 °C (176 °F) for 20 minutes. Nitrites added to meats and canned foods inhibit clostridium growth.

II. Toxic dose. Botulin toxin is extremely potent; as little as one taste of botulin-contaminated food (approximately 0.05 μg of toxin) may be fatal.

III. Clinical presentation.
  A. **Classic botulism** occurs after ingestion of preformed toxin in contaminated food. The incubation period is usually 18–36 hours after ingestion but can vary from a few hours to 8 days. The earlier the onset of symptoms, the more severe the illness. Initial symptoms are nonspecific and may suggest a flulike syndrome (eg, sore throat, dry mouth, and gastrointestinal upset). Later, diplopia, ptosis, dysarthria, and other cranial nerve weaknesses occur, followed by progressive symmetric descending paralysis and finally respiratory arrest. The patient's mentation is clear, and there is no sensory loss. Pupils may be either dilated and unreactive or normal. Constipation may occur.
  B. **Infant botulism** is not caused by ingestion of preformed toxin but by in vivo production of toxin (typically types A or B) in the immature infant gut. Infants 1 week to 6 months old (most cases are in infants 2–6 months old), breast-fed infants, and those given honey may have a higher risk of developing the disease, which is characterized by hypotonia, constipation, tachycardia, difficulty in feeding, head lag, and diminished gag reflex. It is rarely fatal, and infants usually recover strength within 4–6 weeks.
  C. **Wound botulism** occurs mostly in intravenous drug abusers who "skin pop" (inject the drug subcutaneously rather than intravenously), and occasionally results from infected surgical or traumatic wounds. The organism germinates in an infected injection site and produces toxin in vivo. Typical manifestations of botulism occur after an incubation period of 4–14 days.

IV. Diagnosis is based on a high index of suspicion in any patient with a dry sore throat, clinical findings of descending cranial nerve palsies or gastroenteritis, and a history of ingestion of home-canned food. Symptoms may be slow in onset but are sometimes rapidly progressive. Electromyography may reveal normal conduction velocity but decreased motor action potential and no incremental response to repetitive stimulation.

The *differential diagnosis* includes myasthenia gravis, sudden infant death syndrome (SIDS), Eaton-Lambert syndrome, and the Fisher variant of Guillain-Barré syndrome.
  A. **Specific levels.** Diagnosis is confirmed by determination of the toxin in serum, stool, or a wound; although these tests are useful for public health investigation, they cannot be used to determine initial treatment because the analysis takes more than 24 hours to perform. Obtain serum, stool, wound pus, vomitus, gastric contents, and suspect food for toxin analysis by the local or state health department. The results may be negative if the samples were collected late or the quantity of toxin is small.
  B. **Other useful laboratory studies** include electrolytes, blood sugar, arterial blood gases, electromyogram, and cerebrospinal fluid (CSF) if CNS infection is suspected.

V. Treatment.
  A. **Emergency and supportive measures**
    1. Maintain an open airway and assist ventilation if necessary (see pp 1–7).
    2. Obtain arterial blood gases and observe closely for respiratory weakness; respiratory arrest can occur abruptly.
  B. **Specific drugs and antidotes**
    1. **Classic and wound botulism**
      a. **Botulin antitoxin** (see p 346) binds the circulating free toxin and prevents the progression of illness; however, it does not reverse established neurologic manifestations. It is most effective when given within 24 hours of the onset of symptoms. Available antitoxins are bivalent (AB) and trivalent (ABE); trivalent antitoxin is preferred unless the exact toxin is known.

    (1) Contact the local or state health department or the Centers for Disease Control, Atlanta, GA; telephone (404) 329-2888 (24-hour number) to obtain antivenin.

    (2) Determine sensitivity to horse serum prior to treatment.

    (3) The empiric dose for suspected botulism is one to two vials. For confirmed illness, administer one vial every 4 hours for at least 4–5 doses.

  b. Guanidine increases the release of acetylcholine at the nerve terminal, but has not been shown to be clinically effective.

  c. For wound botulism, antibiotic (penicillin) treatment is indicated, along with wound debridement and irrigation.

2. Infant botulism

  a. Trivalent antitoxin is not recommended for infant botulism, but recent clinical trials showed the effectiveness of **human tissue-derived botulism immune globulin (BIG)**; U.S. Food and Drug Administration (FDA) approval is pending. To obtain BIG in California, contact the state Department of Health Services, telephone (510) 540-2646.

    Antibiotics are not recommended except for treament of secondary infections. Cathartics are not recommended.

C. Decontamination (see p 45)

  1. Prehospital. Administer activated charcoal or induce vomiting if recent ingestion of known or suspected contaminated material has occurred.

  2. Hospital. If recent ingestion is suspected, perform gastric lavage and administer activated charcoal.

D. Enhanced elimination. There is no role for enhanced elimination; the toxin binds rapidly to nerve endings, and any free toxin can be readily detoxified with antitoxin.

▶ BROMATES

Kathryn H. Keller, PharmD

Bromate poisoning was most common during the 1940s and 1950s when it was a popular ingredient in home permanent neutralizers. Less toxic substances have been substituted for bromates in kits for home use, but poisonings still occur occasionally from professional products (bromate-containing permanent wave neutralizers have been ingested in suicide attempts by professional hairdressers). Commercial bakeries often use bromate salts to improve bread texture, and bromates are components of fusing material for some explosives. Bromates were previously used in matchstick heads. Bromate-contaminated sugar was the cause of one reported epidemic of bromate poisoning.

I. Mechanism of toxicity. The mechanism is not known. The bromate ion is toxic to the cochlea, causing irreversible hearing loss, and nephrotoxic, causing acute tubular necrosis. Bromates may be converted to hydrobromic acid in the stomach, causing gastritis. Bromates are also strong oxidizing agents, capable of oxidizing hemoglobin to methemoglobin.

II. Toxic dose. The acute ingestion of 200–500 mg/kg of potassium bromate is likely to cause serious poisoning. Ingestion of 2–4 oz of 2% potassium bromate solution caused serious toxicity in children. The sodium salt is believed to be less toxic.

III. Clinical presentation.

  A. Within 2 hours of ingestion, victims develop gastrointestinal symptoms, including vomiting (occasionally with hematemesis), diarrhea, and epigastric pain. This may be accompanied by restlessness, lethargy, coma, and convulsions.

  B. An asymptomatic phase of a few hours may follow before overt renal failure develops. Anuria is usually apparent within 1–2 days of ingestion; renal failure may be irreversible.

    C. Tinnitus and irreversible sensorineural deafness occurs between 4–16 hours after ingestion in adults, but deafness may be delayed for several days in children.

    D. Hemolysis and thrombocytopenia have been reported in some pediatric cases.

    E. Methemoglobinemia (see p 220) has been reported, but is rare.

IV. Diagnosis is based on a history of ingestion, especially if accompanied by gastroenteritis, hearing loss, or renal failure.

    A. **Specific levels.** Bromates may be reduced to bromide in the serum, but bromide levels do not correlate with the severity of poisoning. There are qualitative tests for bromates, but serum concentrations are not available.

    B. **Other useful laboratory studies** include CBC, electrolytes, glucose, BUN, creatinine, urinalysis, audiometry, and methemoglobin.

V. Treatment.

    A. **Emergency and supportive measures**

        1. Maintain an open airway and assist ventilation if necessary (see pp 1–7).

        2. Treat coma (p 18) and seizures (p 21) if they occur.

        3. Replace fluid losses, treat electrolyte disturbances caused by vomiting and diarrhea, and monitor renal function. Perform hemodialysis as needed for support of renal failure.

    B. **Specific drugs and antidotes**

        1. **Sodium thiosulfate** (see p 408) may theoretically reduce bromate to the less toxic bromide ion. There are few data to support the use of thiosulfate, but in the recommended dose it is benign. Administer 10% thiosulfate solution, 10–50 mL (0.2–1 mL/kg) IV.

        2. Treat methemoglobinemia with **methylene blue** (see p 381).

    C. **Decontamination** (see p 43)

        1. **Prehospital**

            a. Sodium bicarbonate (baking soda), 1 tsp in 8 oz of water PO may prevent formation of hydrobromic acid in the stomach.

            b. Administer activated charcoal if available. Ipecac-induced vomiting may be useful for initial treatment at the scene (eg, children at home) if it can be given within a few minutes of exposure.

        2. **Hospital**

            a. For large recent ingestions, consider gastric lavage with a 2% sodium bicarbonate solution to prevent formation of hydrobromic acid in the stomach.

            b. Administer activated charcoal.

    D. **Enhanced elimination.** The bromate ion may be removed by hemodialysis, but this treatment has not been carefully evaluated. Since bromates are primarily excreted renally, initiating hemodialysis early in the course of a documented large ingestion may be prudent therapy to prevent irreversible hearing loss and renal failure.

▶ BROMIDES

Delia A. Dempsey, MD

Bromide was once used as a sedative and an effective anticonvulsant, and until 1975 it was the major ingredient in a variety of over-the-counter products such as Bromo-Seltzer and Dr. Miles' Nervine. Currently, bromide is still found in photographic chemicals and as the bromide salt or other constituent of numerous medications. Bromism (chronic bromide intoxication) has been reported with some bromide-containing drugs (halothane and pyridostigmine), but not others (eg, dextromethorphan hydrobromide, brompheniramine, and ipratropium bromide). Bromide is also found in some sources of well water, and it may be released from some bromide-containing hydrocarbons (eg, methyl bromide, ethylene dibromide, and halothane). Brominated vegetable oil added to some soft drinks caused bromism after excessive consumption. Foodstuff fumigated with methyl bromide may contain residual bromide, but the amounts are too small to cause toxicity.

I. **Mechanism of toxicity.** Bromide ions substitute for chloride in various membrane transport systems, particularly within the nervous system. It is preferentially reabsorbed over chloride by the kidney. Up to 30% of chloride may be replaced in the body. With high bromide levels, the membrane-depressant effect progressively impairs neuronal transmission.

   Pharmacokinetics. The Volume of Distribution (Vd) of bromide is 0.35–0.48 L/kg. The half-life is 9–12 days, and bioaccumulation occurs with chronic exposure. Clearance is about 26 mL/kg/d and elimination is renal. Bromide is excreted in breast milk. It crosses the placenta, and neonatal bromism has been described.

II. **Toxic dose.** The adult therapeutic dose of bromide is 3–5 g. One death has been reported after ingestion of 100 g of sodium bromide. Chronic consumption of 0.5–1 g per day may cause bromism.

III. **Clinical presentation.** Death is rare. Acute oral overdose usually causes nausea and vomiting from gastric irritation. Chronic intoxication can result in a variety of neurologic, psychiatric, gastrointestinal, and dermatologic effects.

   A. **Neurologic** and **psychiatric** manifestations are protean and include restlessness, irritability, ataxia, confusion, hallucinations, psychosis, weakness, stupor, and coma. At one time bromism was responsible for 5–10% of admissions to psychiatric facilities.

   B. **Gastrointestinal** effects include nausea and vomiting (acute ingestion) and anorexia and constipation (chronic use).

   C. **Dermatologic** effects include acneiform, pustular, or erythematous rashes. Up to 25% of patients are affected.

IV. **Diagnosis.** Consider bromism in any confused or psychotic patient with a high serum chloride level and a low or negative anion gap. The serum chloride level is often falsely elevated owing to interference by bromide in the analytic test; the serum chloride is elevated by 0.8 meq/L for each 1 meq/L (or 8 mg/dL) of bromide present.

   A. **Specific levels.** A specific serum bromide level may be obtained. *Check units carefully* (80 mg/L = 1 meq/L = 8 mg/dL = 8 mg% = 0.08 mg/mL). The threshold for detection by usual methods is 50 mg/L. Therapeutic levels are 50–100 mg/L (0.6–1.2 meq/L); sedation may occur with levels of 100–500 mg/L (1.2–6 meq/L); bromide levels above 500 mg/dL (6 meq/L) are common in patients with severe bromism; and levels above 3000 mg/L (40 meq/L) may be fatal.

   B. **Other useful laboratory studies** include electrolytes, glucose, BUN, creatinine, and abdominal x-ray (bromide is radiopaque).

V. **Treatment.**

   A. **Emergency and supportive measures**
      1. Protect the airway and assist ventilation if needed (see pp 1–7).
      2. Treat coma if it occurs (see p 18).

   B. **Specific drugs and antidotes.** There is no specific antidote. However, administering chloride will promote bromide excretion (see below).

   C. **Decontamination** (see p 43)
      1. **Prehospital.** Ipecac-induced vomiting may be useful for initial treatment at the scene (eg, children at home) if it can be given within a few minutes of exposure.
      2. **Hospital.** After recent ingestion, induce vomiting or perform gastric lavage, and administer a cathartic. Activated charcoal does not adsorb inorganic bromide ions, but it may adsorb organic bromides, and should also be used if other drug ingestion is suspected.

   D. **Enhanced elimination.** Bromide is eliminated entirely by the kidney. The serum half-life can be dramatically reduced with fluids and chloride loading. Administer **sodium chloride** intravenously as half-normal saline (D50/0.5 NS) at a rate sufficient to obtain a urine output of 4–6 mL/kg/h. **Furosemide**, 1 mg/kg, may assist urinary excretion. Hemodialysis may rarely be indicated in patients with renal insufficiency or severe toxicity. Hemoperfusion is not effective.

▶ CADMIUM

Kent R. Olson, MD

Cadmium (Cd) is found in sulfide ores, along with zinc and lead. Exposure is common during the mining and smelting of zinc, copper, and lead. The metallic form of Cd is used in electroplating because of its anticorrosive properties; the metallic salts are used as pigments and stabilizers in plastics; and Cd alloys are used in soldering and welding and in nickel-cadmium batteries. Cd solder in water pipes and Cd pigments in pottery can be sources of contamination of water and acidic foods.

I. **Mechanism of toxicity.** Inhaled Cd is at least 60 times more toxic than the ingested form. Fumes and dust may cause delayed chemical pneumonitis and resultant pulmonary edema and hemorrhage. Ingested Cd is a gastrointestinal tract irritant. Once absorbed, Cd is bound to metallothionein and filtered by the kidney, where renal tubule damage may occur.

II. **Toxic dose.**
   A. **Inhalation.** The ACGIH-recommended threshold limit value (TLV-TWA) for air exposure to Cd dusts and fumes is 0.01 (inhalable fraction)–0.002 (respirable dusts) mg/m^3 as an 8-hour time-weighted average. Exposure to 5 mg/m^3 inhaled for 8 hours may be lethal. The level considered immediately hazardous to life or health (IDLH) for Cd dusts or fumes is 9 mg Cd/m^3.
   B. **Ingestion.** Cd salts in solutions of greater than 15 mg/L may induce vomiting. The lethal oral dose ranges from 350 to 8900 mg.

III. **Clinical presentation.**
   A. **Acute inhalation** may cause cough, wheezing, headache, fever, and, if severe, chemical pneumonitis and noncardiogenic pulmonary edema within 12–24 hours after exposure.
   B. **Acute oral ingestion** of Cd salts causes nausea, vomiting, abdominal cramps, and diarrhea, sometimes bloody, within minutes after exposure. Deaths after oral ingestion result from shock or acute renal failure.
   C. **Chronic** accumulation of Cd in bones causes painful *itai-itai* ("ouch-ouch") disease.

IV. **Diagnosis** is based on a history of exposure and the presence of respiratory complaints (after inhalation) or gastroenteritis (after ingestion).
   A. **Specific levels.** Whole-blood Cd levels may confirm the exposure. Very little Cd is excreted in the urine, and urine determinations are of little value. Measures of tubular microproteinuria (beta-microglobulin, retinol-binding protein, albumin, and metallothionein) are used to monitor the early and toxic effects of Cd on the kidney.
   B. **Other useful laboratory studies** include CBC, electrolytes, glucose, BUN, creatinine, arterial blood gases or oximetry, and chest x-ray.

V. **Treatment.**
   A. **Emergency and supportive measures**
      1. **Inhalation.** Monitor arterial blood gases and obtain chest x-ray. Observe for at least 6–8 hours and treat wheezing and pulmonary edema (see pp 7–9) if they occur. After significant exposure, it may be necessary to observe for 1–2 days for delayed-onset noncardiogenic pulmonary edema.
      2. **Ingestion.** Treat fluid loss caused by gastroenteritis with intravenous crystalloid fluids (see p 15).
   B. **Specific drugs and antidotes.** There is no evidence that chelation therapy (eg, with BAL, EDTA, or penicillamine) is effective, although various chelating agents have been used.

C. **Decontamination**
1. **Inhalation.** Remove the victim from exposure and give supplemental oxygen if available.
2. **Ingestion** (see p 45)
   a. **Prehospital.** Administer activated charcoal, if available (uncertain benefit). Do *not* induce vomiting because of the corrosive and irritant nature of Cd salts.
   b. **Hospital.** Perform gastric lavage. Administer activated charcoal, although the efficacy of charcoal is unknown. Do not give cathartics if the patient has diarrhea.
D. **Enhanced elimination.** There is no role for dialysis, hemoperfusion, or repeat-dose charcoal.

▶ CAFFEINE

Christopher R. Brown, MD

Caffeine is the most widely used psychoactive substance. Besides its well-known presence in coffee, it is available in many over-the-counter and prescription oral medications and as injectable caffeine sodium benzoate (occasionally used for neonatal apnea). Caffeine is widely used as an anorexiant, a coanalgesic, a diuretic, and a sleep suppressant. Although caffeine has a wide therapeutic index and rarely causes serious toxicity, there are many documented cases of accidental, suicidal, and iatrogenic intoxication, some resulting in death.

I. **Mechanism of toxicity.** Caffeine is a trimethylxanthine closely related to theophylline. It acts primarily through inhibition of the adenosine receptor. In addition, with overdose there is considerable β_1- and β_2-adrenergic stimulation secondary to release of endogenous catecholamines.

   Pharmacokinetics. Caffeine is rapidly and completely absorbed orally with a volume of distribution of 0.7–0.8 L/kg. Its elimination half-life ranges from 3 hours in healthy smokers to 10 hours in nonsmokers; after overdose the half-life may be as long as 15 hours. In infants less than 2–3 months old, metabolism is extremely slow and the half-life may exceed 24 hours. (See also Table II–55.)

II. **Toxic dose.** The reported lethal oral dose is 10 g (150–200 mg/kg), although one case report documents survival after a 24-g ingestion. In children, ingestion of 35 mg/kg may lead to moderate toxicity. Coffee contains 50–200 mg (tea, 40–100 mg) of caffeine per cup depending on how it is brewed. No-Doz and other sleep suppressants usually contain about 200 mg each. Infants younger than 2–3 months of age metabolize caffeine very slowly and may become toxic after repeated doses. As with theophylline, chronic administration of excessive doses may cause serious toxicity with relatively low serum concentrations compared with an acute single ingestion.

III. **Clinical presentation.**
   A. The earliest symptoms of **acute** caffeine poisoning are usually anorexia, tremor, and restlessness. These are followed by nausea, vomiting, tachycardia, and confusion. With serious intoxication, delirium, seizures, supraventricular and ventricular tachyarrhythmias, hypokalemia, and hyperglycemia may occur. Hypotension is caused by excessive β_2-mediated vasodilation and is characterized by a low diastolic pressure and a wide pulse pressure.
   B. **Chronic** high-dose caffeine intake can lead to "caffeinism" (nervousness, irritability, anxiety, tremulousness, muscle twitching, insomnia, palpitations, and hyperreflexia).

IV. **Diagnosis** is suggested by the history of caffeine exposure or the constellation of nausea, vomiting, tremor, tachycardia, seizures, and hypokalemia (also consider theophylline; see p 303).

A. **Specific levels.** Serum caffeine levels are not routinely available in hospital laboratories but can be determined at regional commercial toxicology laboratories. Toxic concentrations may be detected by cross-reaction with theophylline assays (see Table I–33, p 42). Coffee drinkers have caffeine levels of 1–10 mg/L, while levels of 80 mg/L have been associated with death. The level associated with a high likelihood of seizures is unknown.
B. **Other useful laboratory studies** include electrolytes, glucose, and ECG monitoring.
V. **Treatment.**
A. **Emergency and supportive measures**
1. Maintain an open airway and assist ventilation if necessary (see pp 1–7).
2. Treat seizures (p 21) and hypotension (p 15) if they occur.
3. Hypokalemia usually resolves without aggressive treatment.
4. Monitor ECG and vital signs for at least 6 hours after ingestion or until the serum level is documented to be decreasing.
B. **Specific drugs and antidotes.** Beta blockers effectively reverse cardiotoxic effects mediated by excessive beta-adrenergic stimulation. Treat tachyarrhythmias or hypotension with intravenous **propranolol**, 0.01–0.02 mg/kg (see p 405), or **esmolol**, 25–100 µg/kg/min (see p 366), beginning with low doses and titrating to effect. Because of its short half-life and cardioselectivity, esmolol is preferred.
C. **Decontamination** (see p 45)
1. **Prehospital.** Administer activated charcoal if available.
2. **Hospital.** Administer activated charcoal. Gastric emptying is not necessary if activated charcoal can be given promptly, although gastric lavage should be considered for massive ingestion.
D. **Enhanced elimination.** Repeat-dose activated charcoal (see p 54) may enhance caffeine elimination. Seriously intoxicated patients (with multiple seizures, significant tachyarrhythmias, or intractable hypotension) may require charcoal hemoperfusion (see p 52).

▶ **CALCIUM ANTAGONISTS**

Neal L. Benowitz, MD

Calcium antagonists (also known as calcium channel blockers or calcium blockers) are widely used to treat angina pectoris, coronary spasm, hypertension, hypertrophic cardiomyopathy, supraventricular cardiac arrhythmias, and migraine headache. Toxicity from calcium antagonists may occur with therapeutic use (often owing to drug interactions) or as a result of accidental or intentional overdose. Overdoses of calcium antagonists are frequently life-threatening and represent an increasingly important source of drug-induced mortality.
I. **Mechanism of toxicity.** Calcium antagonists slow the influx of calcium through cellular calcium channels. Currently marketed agents act primarily on vascular smooth muscle and the heart. They result in coronary and peripheral vasodilation, reduced cardiac contractility, slowed (AV) nodal conduction, and depressed sinus node activity. Lowering of blood pressure through a fall in peripheral vascular resistance may be offset by reflex tachycardia, although this reflex response may be blunted by depressant effects on contractility and sinus node activity. Table II–14 summarizes usual doses, sites of activity, and half-lives of common calcium antagonists.
A. In usual therapeutic doses, amlodipine, felodipine, isradipine, nicardipine, nifedipine, and nitrendipine act primarily on blood vessels, whereas verapamil, diltiazem, and mibefradil act on both the heart and blood vessels. In overdose, however, this selectivity may be lost.

TABLE II–14. COMMON CALCIUM ANTAGONISTS

Drug	Usual Adult Daily Dose (mg)	Elimination Half-Life (h)	Primary Site(s) of activity[a]
Amlodipine	2.5–10	30–50	V
Bepridil	200–400	24	M,V
Diltiazem	90–360 (PO) 0.25 mg/kg (IV)	4–6	M,V
Felodipine	5–30	11–16	V
Isradipine	5–25	8	V
Mibefradil	50–100	17–25	M[b], V
Nicardipine	60–120	8	V
Nifedipine	30–120	2–5	V
Nisoldipine	20–40	4	V
Nitrendipine	40–80	2–20	V
Verapamil	120–480 (PO) 0.075–0.15 mg/kg (IV)	2–8	M,V

[a]Major toxicity: M = myocardial (decreased contractility, AV block); V = vascular (vasodilation).
[b]Myocardial effect limited to bradycardia and AV blocks.

B. **Bepridil,** used primarily for refractory angina pectoris, has verapamil-like effects on the heart, inhibits the fast sodium channel, and has type III antiarrhythmic activity. Bepridil also has proarrhythmic effects, especially in the presence of hypokalemia.

C. **Nimodipine** has a greater action on cerebral arteries and is used to reduce vasospasm after recent subarachnoid hemorrhage.

D. Important **drug interactions** may result in toxicity. Hypotension is more likely to occur in patients taking beta blockers, nitrates, or both, especially if they are hypovolemic after diuretic therapy. Patients taking disopyramide or other depressant cardioactive drugs and those with severe underlying myocardial disease are also at risk for hypotension. Life-threatening bradyarrhythmias, including asystole, may occur when beta blockers and verapamil are given together parenterally. Propranolol also inhibits the metabolism of verapamil.

E. **Pharmacokinetics.** Absorption may be delayed with sustained-release preparations. Most agents are highly protein bound and have large volumes of distribution (Vd). Eliminated mainly via extensive hepatic metabolism. In a report on two patients with verapamil overdoses (serum levels 2,200 and 2,700 ng/mL), the elimination half-lives were 7.8 and 15.2 hours. (See also Table II–55, p 319)

II. **Toxic dose.** Usual therapeutic daily doses for each agent are listed in Table II–14. The toxic/therapeutic ratio is relatively small, and serious toxicity may occur with therapeutic doses. For example, severe bradycardia can occur with therapeutic doses of mibefradil. Any dose greater than the usual therapeutic range should be considered potentially life-threatening. Note that many of the common agents are available in sustained-release formulations, which can result in delayed onset or sustained toxicity.

III. **Clinical presentation.**

A. The primary features of calcium antagonist intoxication are **hypotension** and **bradycardia.**

1. Hypotension may be caused by peripheral vasodilation, reduced cardiac contractility, slowed heart rate, or a combination of all of these.

    2. Bradycardia may result from sinus bradycardia, second- or third-degree AV block, or sinus arrest with junctional rhythm.

    3. Most calcium antagonists do not affect intraventricular conduction, so the QRS duration is usually unaffected. The PR interval is prolonged even with therapeutic doses of verapamil. Bepridil prolongs the QT interval and may cause ventricular arrhythmias, including torsades de pointes (see p 14). Mibefradil also causes QT prolongation, but has not been associated with arrhythmias.

  B. **Noncardiac manifestations** of intoxication include nausea and vomiting, abnormal mental status (stupor and confusion), metabolic acidosis (probably resulting from hypotension), and hyperglycemia (owing to blockade of insulin release).

IV. Diagnosis. The findings of hypotension and bradycardia, particularly with sinus arrest or AV block, in the absence of QRS interval prolongation should suggest calcium antagonist intoxication. The differential diagnosis should include beta blockers and other sympatholytic drugs.

  A. **Specific levels.** Serum or blood drug levels are not widely available. Diltiazem and verapamil may be detectable in comprehensive urine toxicology screening.

  B. **Other useful laboratory studies** include electrolytes, glucose, BUN, creatinine, arterial blood gases or oximetry, and ECG and ECG monitoring.

V. Treatment.

  A. **Emergency and supportive measures**

    1. Maintain an open airway and assist ventilation if necessary (see pp 1–7).

    2. Treat coma (p 18), hypotension (p 15), and bradyarrhythmias (p 10) if they occur. The use of cardiopulmonary bypass to allow time for liver metabolism has been reported in a patient with massive verapamil poisoning. Cardiac pacing should be considered for bradyarrhythmias that are contributing to hypotension.

    3. Monitor the vital signs and ECG for at least 6 hours after alleged ingestion. Admit symptomatic patients for at least 24 hours.

  B. **Specific drugs and antidotes**

    1. **Calcium** (see p 350) usually promptly reverses the depression of cardiac contractility, but it does not affect sinus node depression or peripheral vasodilation and has variable effects on AV nodal conduction. Administer **calcium chloride** 10%, 10 mL (0.1–0.2 mL/kg) IV, or **calcium gluconate** 10%, 20 mL (0.3–0.4 mL/kg) IV. Repeat every 5–10 minutes as needed. In case reports, doses as high as 10–15 g over 1–2 hours and 30 g over 12 hours have been administered without apparent calcium toxicity.

    2. **Glucagon** (see p 371), **epinephrine** (see p 365), and amrinone (Inocor, 0.75 mg/kg IV followed by infusion of 5–10 µg/kg/min) have been reported to increase blood pressure in patients with refractory hypotension. Glucagon and epinephrine can also increase the heart rate.

    3. Outside the United States, **4-aminopyridine** may be available as an antidote for calcium antagonist intoxication.

  C. **Decontamination** (see p 43)

    1. **Prehospital.** Administer activated charcoal if available.

    2. **Hospital.** Administer activated charcoal. Consider gastric lavage for all but the most trivial ingestions. For large ingestions of a sustained-release preparation, consider whole bowel irrigation (see p 50) in addition to repeated doses of charcoal (see p 54). Continue charcoal administration for up to 48–72 hours.

  D. **Enhanced elimination.** Owing to extensive protein binding, dialysis and hemoperfusion are not effective. Repeat-dose activated charcoal has not been evaluated, but may serve as an adjunct to gastrointestinal decontamination after overdose with sustained-release preparations.

► CAMPHOR AND OTHER ESSENTIAL OILS

Ilene B. Anderson, PharmD

Camphor is one of several essential oils (volatile oils) derived from natural plant products that have been used for centuries as topical rubefacients and counterirritant agents for analgesic and antipruritic purposes (Table II–15). Camphor and other essential oils are found in many over-the-counter remedies such as Campho-Phenique (10.8% camphor, 4.66% phenol), Vicks Vaporub (4.73% camphor, 2.6% menthol, 1.2% eucalyptus oil, 4.5% turpentine spirits), camphorated oil (20% camphor), and Mentholatum (9% camphor, 1.35% menthol, 1.96% eucalyptus oil, 1.4% turpentine spirits). Toxic effects have occurred primarily when camphorated oil was mistakenly administered instead of castor oil, and in accidental pediatric ingestions.

I. **Mechanism of toxicity.** After topical application, essential oils produce dermal hyperemia followed by a feeling of comfort, but if ingested they can cause systemic toxicity. Most essential oils cause CNS stimulation or depression. **Camphor** is a CNS stimulant that causes seizures shortly after ingestion. The underlying mechanism is unknown. Camphor is rapidly absorbed from the gastrointestinal tract and is metabolized by the liver. It is not known whether metabolites contribute to toxicity.

II. **Toxic dose.** Serious poisonings and death have occurred in children after ingestion of as little as 1 g of camphor. This is equivalent to just 10 mL of Campho-Phenique or 5 mL of camphorated oil. Recovery after ingestion of 42 g in an adult has been reported. The concentrations of other essential oils range from 1 to 20%; doses of 5–15 mL are considered potentially toxic.

TABLE II–15. SOME ESSENTIAL OILS

Name	Comments
Birch oil	Contains 98% methyl salicylate (equivalent to 1.4 g aspirin per mL; see Salicylates, p 284)
Camphor	Pediatric toxic dose 1 g (see text).
Cinnamon oil	Stomatitis and skin burns can result from prolonged contact. Potent antigen. Smoked as a hallucinogen.
Clove oil	Contains 80–90% eugenol. Clove cigarettes may cause irritant tracheobronchitis, hemoptysis.
Eucalyptus oil	Contains 70% eucalyptol. Toxic dose is 5 mL; may cause rapid CNS depression.
Eugenol	A phenol derived from clove oil; used in dentistry for its disinfectant property.
Guaiacol	Nontoxic.
Lavender oil	Used in doses of 0.1 mL as a carminative. Contains trace amounts of coumarin (see p 148). May cause photosensitization.
Menthol	An alcohol derived from various mint oils. Toxic dose is 2 g.
Myristica oil	Nutmeg oil. A carminative in a dose of 0.03 mL. Used as a hallucinogen (2–4 tbsp of ground nutmeg can cause psychogenic effects).
Pennyroyal oil	Fatal coma and hepatic necrosis occurred after ingestion of 30 mL by an 18-year-old woman. N-acetylcysteine may be effective in preventing hepatic necrosis.
Peppermint oil	Contains 50% menthol. Toxic dose is 5–10 g.
Thymol	Used as an antiseptic (see phenol. p 255).
Turpentine oils	Toxic dose 15 mL in children; 140 mL in adults may be fatal. Can cause pneumonitis if aspirated.
Wintergreen oil	Contains methyl salicylate 98% (equivalent to 1.4 g of aspirin per mL; see Salicylates, p 284).

III. Clinical presentation.

  A. Oral. Manifestations of **acute** oral overdose usually occur within 5–30 minutes after ingestion. Burning in the mouth and throat occurs immediately, followed by nausea and vomiting. Ataxia, drowsiness, confusion, restlessness, delirium, muscle twitching, and coma may occur. Camphor typically causes abrupt onset of seizures about 20–30 minutes after ingestion. Death may result from CNS depression and respiratory arrest or may be secondary to status epilepticus. **Chronic** camphor intoxication may produce symptoms similar to Reye's syndrome.

  B. Prolonged **skin contact** may result in a burn.

  C. Smoking (eg, clove cigarettes) or inhaling essential oils may cause tracheobronchitis.

IV. Diagnosis is usually based on a history of exposure. The pungent odor of camphor and other volatile oils is usually apparent.

  A. Specific levels are not available.

  B. Other useful laboratory studies include electrolytes, glucose, liver transaminases, arterial blood gases (if the patient is comatose or in status epilepticus).

V. Treatment.

  A. Emergency and supportive measures

  1. Maintain an open airway and assist ventilation if necessary (see pp 1–7).

  2. Treat seizures (p 21) and coma (p 18) if they occur.

  B. Specific drugs and antidotes. There are no specific antidotes for camphor. **N-acetylcysteine** (see p 334) may be effective for preventing hepatic injury after pennyroyal oil ingestion.

  C. Decontamination (see p 43)

  1. Prehospital. Administer activated charcoal, if available. Do **not** induce vomiting because of the risk of abrupt onset of seizures.

  2. Hospital. Administer activated charcoal. Gastric emptying is not necessary for small ingestions if activated charcoal can be given promptly.

  D. Enhanced elimination. The volumes of distribution of camphor and other essential oils are extremely large, and it is unlikely that any enhanced removal procedure will remove significant amounts of camphor. Poorly substantiated case reports have recommended hemoperfusion.

▶ **CARBAMAZEPINE**

Olga F. Woo, PharmD

Carbamazepine was introduced in the United States in 1974 for the treatment of trigeminal neuralgia. Since then it has become a first-line drug for the treatment of temporal lobe epilepsies and a variety of other seizure disorders and has found expanded use for neurogenic pain and psychiatric illnesses.

  I. Mechanism of toxicity. Most toxic manifestations appear to be related to its anticholinergic effects. In addition, presumably because its chemical structure is similar to that of the tricyclic antidepressant imipramine, acute carbamazepine overdose can cause seizures and cardiac conduction disturbances (although this is rare).

  Pharmacokinetics: Carbamazepine is slowly and erratically absorbed from the gastrointestinal tract, and peak levels may be delayed for 6–24 hours, particularly after an overdose (continued absorption for up to 72 hours has been reported). The volume of distribution (Vd) is 1.4 L/kg, and up to 3 L/kg after overdose. Up to 28% of a dose is eliminated in the feces, and there is enterohepatic recycling. The parent drug is metabolized to its 10,11-epoxide, which is as active as the parent compound. The normal elimination half-life is approximately 15–24 hours for carbamazepine and 5–10 hours for the epoxide.

II. Toxic dose. Acute ingestion of over 10 mg/kg may result in a blood level above the therapeutic range of 4–8 mg/L. The recommended maximum dose is 1600 mg/d in adults (30 mg/kg/d in children, to a maximum of 1 g). Death has occurred after adult ingestion of 6–60 g, but survival has been reported after an 80-g ingestion. Life-threatening toxicity occurred after ingestion of 5.8–10 g in adults and 2 g (148 mg/kg) in a 23-month-old child.

III. Clinical presentation.

  A. Ataxia, nystagmus, ophthalmoplegia, dystonia, mydriasis, and sinus tachycardia are common with mild to moderate overdose. With more serious intoxication, myoclonus, seizures, hyperthermia, coma, and respiratory arrest may occur. Atrioventricular (AV) block and bradycardia have been reported. Based on its structural similarity to tricyclic antidepressants, carbamazepine may cause QRS and QT interval prolongation; however, in case reports of overdose, QRS widening rarely exceeds 100–120 ms and is usually transient.

  B. After an acute overdose, manifestations of intoxication may be delayed for several hours because of erratic absorption. Cyclic coma and rebound relapse of symptoms may be caused by continued absorption from a tablet mass as well as enterohepatic circulation of the drug.

  C. Chronic use has been associated with mild leukopenia and thrombocytopenia. Aplastic anemia is extremely rare. Hyponatremia occasionally occurs.

IV. Diagnosis is based on a history of exposure and clinical signs such as ataxia, stupor, and tachycardia, along with elevated serum levels.

  A. Specific levels. Obtain a stat serum carbamazepine level and repeat levels every 4–6 hours to rule out delayed or prolonged absorption.

    1. Serum levels greater than 10 mg/L are associated with ataxia and nystagmus. Serious intoxication may occur with serum levels greater than 20 mg/L, although there is poor correlation between levels and severity of clinical effects. Serious cardiac toxicity has not been reported with levels less than 40 mg/L. Death occurred in a patient who had a peak concentration of 120 mg/L.

    2. The epoxide metabolite may be produced in high concentrations after overdose. It is nearly equipotent, and may cross-react with some carbamazepine immunoassays to a variable extent.

  B. Other useful laboratory studies include CBC, electrolytes, glucose, arterial blood gases or oximetry, and ECG monitoring.

V. Treatment.

  A. Emergency and supportive measures

    1. Maintain an open airway and assist ventilation if necessary (see pp 1–7). Administer supplemental oxygen.

    2. Treat seizures (p 21), coma (p 18), and arrhythmias (pp 10–14) if they occur.

    3. Asymptomatic patients should be observed for a minimum of 6 hours after ingestion.

  B. Specific drugs and antidotes. There is no specific antidote. Sodium bicarbonate (see p 345) is of unknown value for QRS prolongation. Physostigmine is **not** recommended for anticholinergic toxicity.

  C. Decontamination (see p 43)

    1. Prehospital. Administer activated charcoal if available.

    2. Hospital. Administer activated charcoal. Gastric lavage is not necessary after small to moderate ingestions if activated charcoal can be given promptly. For massive ingestions, consider repeated doses of activated charcoal and possibly whole bowel irrigation (see p 50).

  D. Enhanced elimination. In contrast to tricyclic antidepressants, the volume of distribution of carbamazepine is small, making it accessible to enhanced removal procedures.

    1. Repeat-dose activated charcoal is effective and may increase clearance by up to 50%. However, it may be difficult to perform safely in a patient with obtundation and ileus, and there is no demonstrated benefit on morbidity or mortality.

2. **Charcoal hemoperfusion** is highly effective and may be indicated for severe intoxication (eg, status epilepticus, cardiotoxicity, serum level > 60 mg/L) unresponsive to standard treatment.

3. Peritoneal dialysis and hemodialysis do not effectively remove carbamazepine.

▶ CARBON MONOXIDE

Kent R. Olson, MD

Carbon monoxide (CO) is a colorless, odorless, tasteless, and nonirritating gas produced by the incomplete combustion of any carbon-containing material. Common sources of human exposure include smoke inhalation in fires, automobile exhaust fumes, faulty or poorly ventilated charcoal, kerosene or gas stoves, and, to a lesser extent, cigarette smoke and methylene chloride (see p 224).

I. **Mechanism of toxicity.** Toxicity is a consequence of cellular hypoxia and ischemia.

A. CO binds to hemoglobin with an affinity 250 times that of oxygen, resulting in reduced oxyhemoglobin saturation and decreased blood oxygen-carrying capacity. In addition, the oxyhemoglobin dissociation curve is displaced to the left, impairing oxygen delivery at the tissues.

B. CO may also directly inhibit cytochrome oxidase, further disrupting cellular function, and it is known to bind to myoglobin, possibly contributing to impaired myocardial contractility.

C. In animal models of intoxication, damage is most severe in areas of the brain that are highly sensitive to ischemia and often correlates with the severity of systemic hypotension.

D. Fetal hemoglobin is more sensitive to binding by CO, and fetal or neonatal levels may be higher than maternal levels.

II. **Toxic dose.** The recommended workplace limit (ACGIH TLV-TWA) for carbon monoxide is 25 ppm as an 8-hour time-weighted average. The level considered immediately dangerous to life or health (IDLH) is 1200 ppm (0.12%). Several minutes of exposure to 1000 ppm (0.1%) may result in 50% saturation of carboxyhemoglobin.

III. **Clinical presentation.** Symptoms of intoxication are predominantly in organs with high oxygen consumption such as the brain and heart.

A. The majority of patients complain of headache, dizziness, and nausea. Patients with coronary disease may experience angina or myocardial infarction. With more severe exposures, impaired thinking, syncope, coma, convulsions, cardiac arrhythmias, hypotension, and death may occur. Although blood carboxyhemoglobin levels may not correlate reliably with the severity of intoxication, levels greater than 40 are usually associated with obvious intoxication (Table II–16).

B. Survivors of serious poisoning may suffer numerous overt neurologic sequelae consistent with an hypoxic-ischemic insult, ranging from gross deficits such as parkinsonism and a persistent vegetative state to subtler personality and memory disorders.

C. Exposure during pregnancy may result in fetal demise.

IV. **Diagnosis** is not difficult if there is a history of exposure (eg, the patient was found in a car in a locked garage) but may be elusive if not suspected in less obvious cases. There are no specific reliable clinical findings; cherry red skin coloration or bright-red venous blood is highly suggestive but not frequently noted. The routine arterial blood gas machine measures the partial pressure of oxygen dissolved in plasma (pO_2), but oxygen saturation is calculated from the pO_2 and

TABLE II–16. CARBON MONOXIDE POISONING[a]

Carbon Monoxide Concentration	Carboxyhemo-globin (%)	Symptoms[b]
Less than 35 ppm (cigarette smoking)	5	None, or mild headache.
0.005% (50 ppm)	10	Slight headache, dyspnea on vigorous exertion.
0.01% (100 ppm)	20	Throbbing headache, dyspnea with moderate exertion.
0.02% (200 ppm)	30	Severe headache, irritability, fatigue, dimness of vision.
0.03–0.05% (300–500 ppm)	40–50	Headache, tachycardia, confusion, lethargy, collapse.
0.08–0.12% (800–1200 ppm)	60–70	Coma, convulsions.
0.19% (1900 ppm)	80	Rapidly fatal.

[a]Reproduced, with permission, from *Current Emergency Diagnosis & Treatment*, 3rd ed. Ho MT, Saunders CE (editors). Appleton & Lange, 1990.
[b]Symptoms and signs of toxicity do not always correlate with measured carboxyhemoglobin level.

is therefore unreliable in patients with CO poisoning. Pulse oximetry also gives falsely normal readings, because it is unable to distinguish between oxyhemoglobin and carboxyhemoglobin.

A. Specific levels. Obtain a specific carboxyhemoglobin concentration (see Table II–16). Persistence of fetal hemoglobin may produce falsely elevated carboxyhemoglobin levels in young infants.

B. Other useful laboratory studies include electrolytes, glucose, BUN, creatinine, ECG, and pregnancy tests.

V. Treatment.

A. Emergency and supportive measures

1. Maintain an open airway and assist ventilation if necessary (see pp 1–7). If smoke inhalation has also occurred, consider early intubation for airway protection.
2. Treat coma (p 18) and seizures (p 21) if they occur.
3. Continuously monitor the ECG for several hours after exposure.
4. Because smoke often contains other toxic gases, consider the possibility of cyanide poisoning (p 150), methemoglobinemia (p 220), and irritant gas injury (p 181).

B. Specific drugs and antidotes. Administer **oxygen** in the highest possible concentration (100%). Breathing 100% oxygen speeds the elimination of CO from hemoglobin to approximately 1 hour, compared with 6 hours in room air. Use a tight-fitting mask and high-flow oxygen with a reservoir (nonrebreather) or administer the oxygen by endotracheal tube. Treat until the carboxyhemoglobin level is less than 5%.

C. Decontamination. Remove the patient immediately from exposure and give supplemental oxygen. Rescuers exposed to potentially high concentrations of CO should wear self-contained breathing apparatus.

D. Enhanced elimination. Hyperbaric oxygen provides 100% oxygen under 2–3 atm of pressure and can enhance elimination of CO (half-life reduced to 20–30 minutes). It may be useful in patients with severe intoxication who do not respond rapidly to oxygen at atmospheric pressure, or for pregnant women or newborns, when there is ready access to a chamber. However, long-distance transport of an unstable patient for hyperbaric treatment may be risky, and it remains controversial whether hyperbaric oxygen is clinically more effective than 100% oxygen administered at atmospheric pressure. Consult a regional poison control center (see p 55) for advice and for the location of nearby hyperbaric chambers.

▶ CARBON TETRACHLORIDE

Randall G. Browning, MD, MPH

Carbon tetrachloride (CCl_4, tetrachloromethane) was once widely used as a dry cleaning solvent, degreaser, spot remover, fire extinguisher agent, and anthelmintic. Because of its liver toxicity and known carcinogenicity in animals, its role has become limited; it is now used mainly as an intermediate in chemical manufacturing.

I. **Mechanism of toxicity.** Carbon tetrachloride is a CNS depressant and a potent hepatic and renal toxin. It may also increase the sensitivity of the myocardium to arrhythmogenic effects of catecholamines. The mechanism of hepatic and renal toxicity is thought to be a result of a toxic free-radical intermediate of metabolism. Chronic use of metabolic enzyme inducers such as phenobarbital and ethanol increase the toxicity of carbon tetrachloride. Carbon tetrachloride is a known animal and suspected human carcinogen.

II. **Toxic dose.**
   A. Toxicity from **inhalation** is dependent on the concentration in air and the duration of exposure. Symptoms have occurred after exposure to 160 ppm for 30 minutes. The recommended workplace limit (ACGIH TLV-TWA) is 5 ppm as an 8-hour time-weighted average, and the air level considered immediately dangerous to life or health (IDLH) is 200 ppm.
   B. **Ingestion** of as little as 5 mL has been reported to be fatal.

III. **Clinical presentation.**
   A. Persons exposed to carbon tetrachloride from acute inhalation, skin absorption, or ingestion may present with nausea, vomiting, dizziness, and confusion. With serious intoxication, coma and cardiac arrhythmias may occur.
   B. Severe and sometimes fatal renal and hepatic damage may become apparent after 1–3 days.
   C. Skin exposure can cause dermatitis from defatting of the outer skin layers.

IV. **Diagnosis** is based on a history of exposure and the clinical presentation of CNS depression, arrhythmias, and hepatic necrosis. The liquid is radiopaque and may be visible on abdominal x-ray after acute ingestion.
   A. **Specific levels.** Blood levels are not available in most commercial laboratories. Qualitative urine screening for chlorinated hydrocarbons (Fujiwara test) may be positive after massive overdose.
   B. **Other useful laboratory studies** include electrolytes, glucose, BUN, creatinine, liver transaminases, prothrombin time (PT), and ECG monitoring.

V. **Treatment.**
   A. **Emergency and supportive measures**
      1. Maintain an open airway and assist ventilation if necessary (see pp 1–7).
      2. Treat coma (p 18) and arrhythmias (pp 10–14) if they occur. *Caution:* avoid use of epinephrine because it may induce or aggravate arrhythmias. Tachyarrhythmias caused by increased myocardial sensitivity may be treated with **propranolol**, 1–2 mg IV (see p 405), or **esmolol**, 25–100 µg/kg/min IV (see p 366).
   B. **Specific treatment.** *N*-acetylcysteine (NAC; see p 334) may minimize hepatic and renal toxicity by providing a scavenger for the toxic intermediate. Although its use for carbon tetrachloride poisoning has not been studied in humans, acetylcysteine is widely used without serious side effects for treatment of acetaminophen overdose. If possible, it should be given within the first 12 hours after exposure. Animal studies also suggest possible roles for cimetidine, calcium channel blockers, and hyperbaric oxygen in reducing hepatic injury, but there is insufficient human experience with these treatments.
   C. **Decontamination** (see p 43)
      1. **Inhalation.** Remove from exposure and give supplemental oxygen, if available.
      2. **Skin and eyes.** Remove contaminated clothing and wash affected skin with copious soap and water. Irrigate exposed eyes with copious saline or water.

3. **Ingestion**
   a. **Prehospital.** Administer activated charcoal if available. Ipecac-induced vomiting may be useful for initial treatment if it can be given immediately after the ingestion, but is generally avoided because of the risk of abrupt onset of coma.
   b. **Hospital.** Perform gastric lavage, and administer activated charcoal.
D. **Enhanced elimination.** There is no role for dialysis, hemoperfusion, or other enhanced removal procedures.

▶ CARDIAC GLYCOSIDES

Neal L. Benowitz, MD

Cardiac glycosides are found in several plants, including oleander, foxglove, lily of the valley, red squill, and rhododendron, and in toad venom (*Bufo* spp, which may be found in some Chinese herbal medications). Cardiac glycosides are used therapeutically in tablet form as digoxin and digitoxin. Digoxin is also available in liquid-filled capsules with greater bioavailability.

I. **Mechanism of toxicity.** Cardiac glycosides inhibit the function of the sodium potassium-ATPase pump. After acute overdose, this results in hyperkalemia (with chronic intoxication, the serum potassium level is usually normal or low owing to concurrent diuretic therapy). Vagal tone is potentiated, and sinus and atrioventricular (AV) node conduction velocity is decreased. Automaticity in Purkinje fibers is increased.

   Pharmacokinetics. The bioavailability of digoxin ranges from 60–80%; for digitoxin more than 90% is absorbed. The volume of distribution (Vd) of digoxin is very large (5–10 L/kg), whereas for digitoxin the Vd is small (about 0.5 L/kg). Peak effects occur after a delay of 6–12 hours. The elimination half-life of digoxin is 30–50 hours, and for digitoxin is 5–8 days (owing to enterohepatic recirculation). (See also Table II–55, p 319)

II. **Toxic dose.** Acute ingestion of as little as 1 mg of digoxin in a child or 3 mg of digoxin in an adult can result in serum concentrations well above the therapeutic range. More than these amounts of digoxin and other cardiac glycosides may be found in just a few leaves of oleander or foxglove. Generally, children appear to be more resistant than adults to the cardiotoxic effects of cardiac glycosides.

III. **Clinical presentation.** Intoxication may occur after acute accidental or suicidal ingestion or with chronic therapy. Signs and symptoms depend on the chronicity of the intoxication.
   A. With **acute overdose**, vomiting, hyperkalemia, sinus bradycardia, sinoatrial arrest, and second- or third-degree AV block are common. Ventricular tachycardia or fibrillation may occur.
   B. With **chronic intoxication**, visual disturbances, weakness, sinus bradycardia, atrial fibrillation with slowed ventricular response rate or junctional escape rhythm, and ventricular arrhythmias (ventricular bigeminy or trigeminy, ventricular tachycardia, bidirectional tachycardia, and ventricular fibrillation) are common. Accelerated junctional tachycardia and paroxysmal atrial tachycardia with block are frequently seen. Hypokalemia and hypomagnesemia from chronic diuretic use may be evident and appear to worsen the tachyarrhythmias.

IV. **Diagnosis** is based on a history of recent overdose or characteristic arrhythmias (eg, bidirectional tachycardia and accelerated junctional rhythm) in a patient receiving chronic therapy. Hyperkalemia suggests acute ingestion but may also be seen with very severe chronic poisoning. Serum potassium levels higher than 5.5 meq/L are associated with severe poisoning.
   A. **Specific levels.** Stat serum digoxin or digitoxin levels are recommended, although they may not correlate accurately with severity of intoxication. This is

especially true after acute ingestion, when the serum level is high for 6–12 hours before tissue distribution is complete. After use of digitalis-specific antibodies, the radioimmunoassay digoxin level is falsely markedly elevated. Therapeutic levels of digoxin are 0.5–2 ng/mL; of digitoxin, 10–30 ng/mL.

   B. Other useful laboratory studies include electrolytes, BUN, creatinine, serum magnesium, and ECG and ECG monitoring.

V. Treatment.

   A. Emergency and supportive measures

     1. Maintain an open airway and assist ventilation if necessary (see pp 1–7).

     2. Monitor the patient closely for at least 12–24 hours after significant ingestion because of delayed tissue distribution.

     3. Treat **hyperkalemia** (p 36), if greater than 5.5 meq/L, with sodium bicarbonate (1 meq/kg), glucose (0.5 g/kg IV) with insulin (0.1 U/kg IV), or sodium polystyrene sulfonate (Kayexalate, 0.5 g/kg PO). Do *not* use calcium; it may worsen ventricular arrhythmias. Mild hyperkalemia may actually protect against tachyarrhythmias.

     4. Treat **bradycardia** or **heart block** with atropine, 0.5–2 mg IV (p 340); a temporary pacemaker may be needed for persistent symptomatic bradycardia.

     5. Ventricular tachyarrhythmias may respond to lidocaine (p 379) or phenytoin (p 401), or to correction of low potassium or magnesium. Avoid quinidine, procainamide, and bretylium.

   B. Specific drugs and antidotes. Fab fragments of **digoxin-specific antibodies** (Digibind) are indicated for significant poisoning (eg, severe hyperkalemia and symptomatic arrhythmias not responsive to drugs described above) and possibly for prophylactic treatment in a massive oral overdose with high serum levels. Digibind rapidly binds to digoxin and, to a lesser extent, digitoxin and other cardiac glycosides. The inactive complex that is formed is rapidly excreted in the urine. Details of dose calculation and infusion rate are given on p 357.

   C. Decontamination (see p 45)

     1. Prehospital. Administer activated charcoal, if available. Ipecac-induced vomiting may be useful for initial treatment at the scene (eg, children at home) if it can be given within a few minutes of exposure.

     2. Hospital. Administer activated charcoal. Gastric emptying is not necessary if activated charcoal can be given promptly.

   D. Enhanced elimination (see p 51)

     1. Because of its large volume of distribution, **digoxin** is not effectively removed by dialysis or hemoperfusion. Repeat-dose activated charcoal may be useful in patients with severe renal insufficiency, in whom clearance of digoxin is markedly diminished.

     2. Digitoxin has a small volume of distribution and also undergoes extensive enterohepatic recirculation, and its elimination can be markedly enhanced by repeat-dose charcoal.

▶ CAUSTIC AND CORROSIVE AGENTS

Walter H. Mullen, PharmD

A wide variety of chemical and physical agents may cause corrosive injury. These include mineral and organic acids, alkalies, oxidizing agents, denaturants, some hydrocarbons, and agents causing exothermic reactions. Although the mechanism and the severity of injury may vary, the consequences of mucosal damage and permanent scarring are shared by all agents.

   Button batteries are small disk-shaped batteries used in watches, calculators, and cameras. They contain caustic metal salts such as mercuric chloride that may cause corrosive injury.

I. **Mechanism of toxicity.**
   A. **Acids** cause an immediate coagulation-type necrosis that creates an eschar, which tends to self-limit further damage.
   B. In contrast, **alkalies** (eg, Drano) cause a liquefactive necrosis with saponification and continued penetration into deeper tissues, resulting in extensive damage.
   C. **Other agents** may act by alkylating, oxidizing, reducing, or denaturing cellular proteins or by defatting surface tissues.
   D. **Button batteries** cause injury by corrosive effects resulting from leakage of the corrosive metal salts, by direct impaction of the disk-shaped foreign body, and possibly by local discharge of electrical current at the site of impaction.
II. **Toxic dose.** There is no specific toxic dose or level, because the concentration of corrosive solutions and the potency of caustic effects vary widely. The concentration or the pH of the solution may indicate the potential for serious injury. For alkalies, the titratable alkalinity (concentration of the base) is a better predictor of corrosive effect than the pH.
III. **Clinical presentation.**
   A. **Inhalation** of corrosive gases (eg, chlorine or ammonia) may cause upper respiratory tract injury, with stridor, hoarseness, wheezing, and noncardiogenic pulmonary edema. Pulmonary symptoms may be delayed after exposure to gases with low water solubility (eg, nitrogen dioxide or phosgene; see p 181).
   B. **Eye or skin** exposure to corrosive agents usually results in immediate pain and redness, followed by blistering. Conjunctivitis and lacrimation are common. Serious full-thickness burns and blindness can occur.
   C. **Ingestion** of corrosives can cause oral pain, dysphagia, drooling, and pain in the throat, chest, or abdomen. Esophageal or gastric perforation may occur, manifested by severe chest or abdominal pain, signs of peritoneal irritation, or pancreatitis. Free air may be visible in the mediastinum or abdomen on x-ray. Hematemesis and shock may occur. Systemic acidosis has been reported after acid ingestion and may be partly caused by absorption of hydrogen ions. Scarring of the esophagus or stomach may result in permanent stricture formation and chronic dysphagia.
   D. **Systemic toxicity** can occur after inhalation, skin exposure, or ingestion of a variety of agents (Table II–17).

TABLE II–17. EXAMPLES OF SYSTEMIC SYMPTOMS FROM CORROSIVE AGENTS[a]

Corrosive Agent	Systemic Symptoms
Formaldehyde	Metabolic acidosis; formate poisoning
Hydrofluoric acid	Hypocalcemia; hyperkalemia
Methylene chloride	CNS depression; cardiac arrhythmias; converted to carbon monoxide
Oxalic acid	Hypocalcemia; renal failure
Paraquat	Pulmonary fibrosis
Permanganate	Methemoglobinemia
Phenol	Seizures; coma; hepatic and renal damage
Phosphorus	Hepatic and renal injury
Picric acid	Renal injury
Silver nitrate	Methemoglobinemia
Tannic acid	Hepatic injury

[a]Reference: Edelman PA: Chemical and electrical burns, pages 183–202. In *Management of the Burned Patient*, Achauer BM (editor). Appleton & Lange, 1987.

  E. Button batteries usually cause serious injury only if they become impacted in the esophagus, leading to perforation into the aorta or mediastinum. Most cases involve large (25-mm diameter) batteries. If button batteries reach the stomach without impaction in the esophagus, they nearly always pass uneventfully via the stools within several days.

IV. Diagnosis is based on a history of exposure to a corrosive agent and characteristic findings of skin, eye, or mucosal irritation or redness and the presence of injury to the gastrointestinal tract. Victims with oral or esophageal injury nearly always have drooling or pain on swallowing.

  A. Endoscopy. Esophageal or gastric injury is unlikely after ingestion if the patient is completely asymptomatic, but studies have repeatedly shown that a small number of patients will have injury in the absence of oral burns or obvious dysphagia. For this reason, many authorities recommend endoscopy for all patients regardless of symptoms.

  B. X-rays of the chest and abdomen will usually reveal impacted button batteries. X-rays may also demonstrate air in the mediastinum from esophageal perforation or free abdominal air from gastric perforation.

  C. Specific levels. See specific chemical. Urine mercury levels have been reported to be elevated after button battery ingestion.

  D. Other useful laboratory studies include CBC, electrolytes, glucose, arterial blood gases, chest x-ray, and upright abdominal x-ray.

V. Treatment.

  A. Emergency and supportive measures

   1. Inhalation. Give supplemental oxygen, and observe closely for signs of progressive airway obstruction or noncardiogenic pulmonary edema (see pp 1–7).

   2. Ingestion

    a. Immediately give water or milk to drink.

    b. If esophageal or gastric perforation is suspected, obtain immediate surgical or endoscopic consultation.

  B. Specific drugs and antidotes. For most agents, there is no specific antidote. (See p 186 for hydrofluoric acid burns and p 255 for phenol burns.) In the past, corticosteroids were used by many clinicians in the hope of reducing scarring, but this treatment has been proved ineffective. Moreover, steroids may be harmful in the patient with perforation because they mask early signs of inflammation and inhibit resistance to infection.

  C. Decontamination (see p 43). *Caution:* Rescuers should use appropriate respiratory and skin-protective equipment.

   1. Inhalation. Remove from exposure; give supplemental oxygen if available.

   2. Skin and eyes. Remove all clothing; wash skin and irrigate eyes with copious water or saline.

   3. Ingestion

    a. Prehospital. Immediately give water or milk to drink. Do *not* induce vomiting or give pH-neutralizing solutions (eg, dilute vinegar or bicarbonate).

    b. Hospital. Gastric lavage to remove the corrosive material is controversial but is probably beneficial in acute liquid corrosive ingestion, and it will be required before endoscopy anyway. Use a soft flexible tube and lavage with repeated aliquots of water or saline, frequently checking the pH of the washings.

    c. In general, do *not* give activated charcoal, as it may interfere with visibility at endoscopy. Charcoal may be appropriate if the ingested agent can cause significant systemic toxicity.

    d. Button batteries lodged in the esophagus must be removed immediately by endoscopy to prevent rapid perforation. Batteries in the stomach or intestine should not be removed unless signs of perforation or obstruction develop.

  D. Enhanced elimination. In general, there is no role for any of these procedures (see specific chemical).

▶ CHLORATES

Kathryn H. Keller, PharmD

Potassium chlorate is a component of some match heads; barium chlorate (see also p 103) is used in the manufacture of fireworks and explosives; sodium chlorate is still a major ingredient of some weed killers used in commercial agriculture; and other chlorate salts are used in dye production. Safer and more effective compounds have replaced chlorate in toothpaste and antiseptic mouthwashes. Chlorate poisoning is similar to bromate intoxication (see p 114), but chlorates are more likely to cause intravascular hemolysis and methemoglobinemia.

I. **Mechanism of toxicity.** Chlorates are potent oxidizing agents and also attack sulfhydryl groups, particularly in red blood cells and the kidneys. Chlorates cause methemoglobin formation as well as increased red blood cell membrane fragility, which may result in intravascular hemolysis. Renal failure is probably caused by a combination of direct cellular toxicity and hemolysis.

II. **Toxic dose.** The minimum toxic dose in children is not established, but is estimated to range from 1 g in infants to 5 g in older children. Children may ingest up to 1–2 matchbooks without toxic effect (each match head may contain 10–12 mg of chlorate). The adult lethal dose was estimated to be 7.5 g in one case but is probably closer to 20–35 g. A 26-year-old woman survived a 150- to 200-g ingestion.

III. **Clinical presentation.** Within a few minutes to hours after ingestion, abdominal pain, vomiting, and diarrhea may occur. Methemoglobinemia is common (see p 220). Massive hemolysis, hemoglobinuria, and acute tubular necrosis may occur over 1–2 days after ingestion. Coagulopathy and hepatic injury have been described.

IV. **Diagnosis** is usually based on a history of exposure and the presence of methemoglobinemia and hemolysis.
   A. **Specific levels.** Blood levels are not available, nor are they useful.
   B. **Other useful laboratory studies** include CBC, haptoglobin, plasma free hemoglobin, electrolytes, glucose, BUN, creatinine, bilirubin, methemoglobin level, prothrombin time (PT), liver transaminases, and urinalysis.

V. **Treatment.**
   A. **Emergency and supportive measures**
      1. Maintain an open airway and assist ventilation if necessary (see pp 1–7).
      2. Treat coma (p 18), hemolysis, hyperkalemia (p 36), and renal (p 37) or hepatic failure (p 38) if they occur.
      3. Massive hemolysis may require blood transfusions. To prevent renal failure resulting from deposition of free hemoglobin in the kidney tubules, administer intravenous fluids and sodium bicarbonate.
   B. **Specific drugs and antidotes**
      1. Treat methemoglobinemia with **methylene blue** (see p 381), 1–2 mg/kg (0.1–0.2 mL/kg) of 1% solution. Methylene blue is reportedly most effective when used early in mild cases, but has poor effectiveness in severe cases where hemolysis has already occurred.
      2. Intravenous **sodium thiosulfate** (see p 408) may inactivate the chlorate ion and has been reported successful in anecdotal reports. However, this treatment has not been clinically tested. Administration as a lavage fluid may potentially produce some hydrogen sulfide, and so is contraindicated.
   C. **Decontamination** (see p 43)
      1. **Prehospital.** Administer activated charcoal, if available. Ipecac-induced vomiting may be useful for initial treatment at the scene (eg, children at home) if it can be given within a few minutes of exposure. *Note:* Spontaneous vomiting is common after significant ingestion.
      2. **Hospital.** Administer activated charcoal. Gastric emptying is not necessary after small ingestions if activated charcoal can be given promptly.

D. Enhanced elimination. Chlorates are eliminated mainly through the kidney; elimination may be hastened by hemodialysis, especially in patients with renal insufficiency. Exchange transfusion and peritoneal dialysis have been used in a few cases.

▶ CHLORINATED HYDROCARBON PESTICIDES

Brent R. Ekins, PharmD

Chlorinated hydrocarbon pesticides are widely used in agriculture, structural pest control, and malaria control programs around the world. Lindane is used medicinally for the treatment of lice and scabies. Chlorinated hydrocarbons are of major toxicologic concern, and many (eg, DDT and chlordane) are now banned from commercial use because they persist in the environment and accumulate in biologic systems.

I. **Mechanism of toxicity.** Chlorinated hydrocarbons are neurotoxins that interfere with transmission of nerve impulses, especially in the brain, resulting in behavioral changes, involuntary muscle activity, and depression of the respiratory center. They may also sensitize the myocardium to arrhythmogenic effects of catecholamines, and many can cause liver or renal injury, possibly owing to generation of toxic metabolites. In addition, some chlorinated hydrocarbons may be carcinogenic.

Pharmacokinetics. Chlorinated hydrocarbons are well absorbed from the gastrointestinal tract, across the skin, and by inhalation. They are highly lipid-soluble and accumulate with repeated exposure. Elimination does not follow first-order kinetics; compounds are slowly released from body stores over days to several months or years.

II. **Toxic dose.** The acute toxic doses of these compounds are highly variable, and reports of acute human poisonings are limited. Table II–18 ranks the relative toxicity of several common compounds.

A. **Ingestion** of as little as 1 g of lindane can produce seizures in a child, and 10–30 g is considered lethal in an adult. The estimated adult lethal oral doses of aldrin and chlordane are 3–7 g each; of dieldrin, 2–5 g. A 49-year-old man died after ingesting 12 g of endrin. A 20-year-old man survived a 60-g endosulfan ingestion but was left with a chronic seizure disorder.

III. **Clinical presentation.** Shortly after acute ingestion, nausea and vomiting occur, followed by paresthesias of the tongue, lips, and face; confusion; tremor; obtundation; coma; seizures; and respiratory depression. Because chlorinated hydrocarbons are highly lipid-soluble, the duration of toxicity may be prolonged.

A. Recurrent or delayed-onset seizures have been reported.

B. Arrhythmias may occur owing to myocardial sensitivity to catecholamines.

C. Metabolic acidosis may occur.

TABLE II–18. COMMON CHLORINATED HYDROCARBONS

Low Toxicity (animal oral LD_{50} > 1g/kg)	Moderately Toxic (animal oral LD_{50} > 50 mg/kg)	Highly Toxic (animal oral LD_{50} < 50 mg/kg)
Ethylan (Perthane)	Chlordane	Aldrin
Hexachlorobenzene	DDT	Dieldrin
Methoxychlor	Heptachlor	Endrin
	Kepone	Endosulfan
	Lindane	
	Mirex	
	Toxaphene	

D. Signs of hepatitis or renal injury may develop.

E. Hematopoietic dyscrasias can develop late.

IV. Diagnosis is based on the history of exposure and clinical presentation.

  A. Specific levels. Chlorinated hydrocarbons can be measured in the serum, but levels are not routinely available.

  B. Other useful laboratory studies include electrolytes, glucose, BUN, creatinine, hepatic transaminases, prothrombin time (PT), and ECG monitoring.

V. Treatment.

  A. Emergency and supportive measures

    1. Maintain an open airway and assist ventilation if necessary (see pp 1–7). Administer supplemental oxygen. As most liquid products are formulated in organic solvents, observe for evidence of pulmonary aspiration (see Hydrocarbons, p 183).

    2. Treat seizures (p 21), coma (p 18), and respiratory depression (p 6) if they occur. Ventricular arrhythmias may respond to beta-adrenergic blockers such as propranolol (p 405) or esmolol (see p 366).

    3. Attach an electrocardiographic monitor, and observe the patient for at least 6–8 hours.

  B. Specific drugs and antidotes. There is no specific antidote.

  C. Decontamination (see p 43)

    1. Skin and eyes. Remove contaminated clothing and wash affected skin with copious soap and water, including hair and nails. Irrigate exposed eyes with copious tepid water or saline. Rescuers must take precautions to avoid personal exposure.

    2. Ingestion

      a. Prehospital. Administer activated charcoal if available. Do *not* induce vomiting because of the risk of an abrupt onset of seizures.

      b. Hospital. Administer activated charcoal. Consider gastric lavage for large ingestions.

  D. Enhanced elimination (see p 51)

    1. Repeat-dose activated charcoal or cholestyramine resin may be administered to enhance elimination by interrupting enterohepatic circulation.

    2. Exchange transfusion, peritoneal dialysis, hemodialysis, and hemoperfusion are not likely to be beneficial because of the large volume of distribution of these chemicals.

▶ CHLORINE

R. Steven Tharratt, MD

Chlorine is a heavier-than-air, yellowish-green gas with an irritating odor. It is used widely in chemical manufacturing, bleaching, and (as hypochlorite) in swimming pool disinfectant and cleaning agents. **Hypochlorite** is an aqueous solution produced by the reaction of chlorine gas with water; most household bleach solutions contain 3–5% hypochlorite; swimming pool disinfectants and industrial strength cleaners may contain up to 20% hypochlorite. The addition of acid to hypochlorite solution may release chlorine gas. The addition of ammonia to hypochlorite solution may release chloramine, a gas with properties similar to those of chlorine.

I. Mechanism of toxicity. Chlorine gas produces a corrosive effect on contact with moist tissues such as the eyes and upper respiratory tract. Exposure to aqueous solutions causes corrosive injury to the eyes, skin, or gastrointestinal tract (see p 129). Chloramine is less water-soluble and may produce more indolent or delayed irritation.

II. Toxic dose.

  A. Chlorine gas. The recommended workplace limit (ACGIH TLV-TWA) for chlorine gas is 0.5 ppm (1.5 mg/m^3) as an 8-hour time-weighted average. The

short-term exposure limit (STEL) is 1 ppm. The level considered immediately dangerous to life or health (IDLH) is 10 ppm.
  B. **Aqueous solutions.** Dilute aqueous hypochlorite solutions (3–5%) commonly found in homes rarely cause serious burns but are moderately irritating. However, more concentrated industrial cleaners (20% hypochlorite) are much more likely to cause serious corrosive injury.
III. **Clinical presentation.**
  A. **Inhalation of chlorine gas.** Symptoms are rapid in onset owing to the relatively high water solubility of chlorine. Immediate burning of the eyes, nose, and throat occurs, accompanied by coughing. Wheezing may also occur, especially in patients with pre-existing bronchospastic disease. With serious exposure, upper-airway swelling may rapidly cause airway obstruction, preceded by croupy cough, hoarseness, and stridor. With massive exposure, noncardiogenic pulmonary edema (chemical pneumonitis) may also occur.
  B. **Skin or eye contact with gas or concentrated solution.** Serious corrosive burns may occur. Manifestations are similar to those of other corrosive exposures (see p 129).
  C. **Ingestion of aqueous solutions.** Immediate burning in the mouth and throat is common, but no further injury is expected after ingestion of 3–5% hypochlorite. With more concentrated solutions, serious esophageal and gastric burns may occur, and victims often have dysphagia, drooling, and severe throat, chest, and abdominal pain. Hematemesis and perforation of the esophagus or stomach may occur.
IV. **Diagnosis** is based on a history of exposure and description of the typical irritating odor, accompanied by irritative or corrosive effects on the eyes, skin, or upper respiratory or gastrointestinal tract.
  A. **Specific levels** are not available.
  B. **Other useful laboratory studies** include, with **ingestion**, CBC, electrolytes, and chest and abdominal x-rays; with **inhalation**, arterial blood gases or oximetry and chest x-ray.
V. **Treatment.**
  A. **Emergency and supportive measures**
    1. **Inhalation of chlorine gas**
      a. Immediately give humidified supplemental oxygen. Observe carefully for signs of progressive upper-airway obstruction, and intubate the trachea if necessary (see pp 1–6).
      b. Use bronchodilators for wheezing (p 8), and treat noncardiogenic pulmonary edema (p 7) if it occurs.
    2. **Ingestion of hypochlorite solution.** If a solution of 10% or greater has been ingested, or if there are any symptoms of corrosive injury (dysphagia, drooling, or pain), flexible endoscopy is recommended to evaluate for serious esophageal or gastric injury. Obtain chest and abdominal x-rays to look for mediastinal or intra-abdominal air, which suggests perforation.
  B. **Specific drugs and antidotes.** There is no proved specific treatment for this or other common caustic burns or inhalations. The administration of corticosteroids is unproved and may be harmful in patients with perforation or serious infection.
  C. **Decontamination** (see p 43)
    1. **Inhalation.** Remove immediately from exposure, and give supplemental oxygen if available.
    2. **Skin and eyes.** Remove contaminated clothing, and flush exposed skin immediately with copious water. Irrigate exposed eyes with water or saline.
    3. **Ingestion of hypochlorite solution**
      a. **Prehospital.** Immediately give water by mouth. Do *not* induce vomiting.
      b. **Hospital.** Gastric lavage is recommended after concentrated liquid ingestion, in order to remove any corrosive material in the stomach and to prepare for endoscopy; use a small flexible tube to avoid injury to damaged mucosa.

c. Do *not* use activated charcoal; it may obscure the endoscopist's view.

D. Enhanced elimination. There is no role for enhanced elimination.

▶ CHLOROFORM

Randall G. Browning, MD, MPH

Chloroform (trichloromethane) is a chlorinated hydrocarbon solvent used as a raw material in the production of freon and as an extractant and solvent in the chemical and pharmaceutical industry. Because of its hepatic toxicity, it is no longer used as a general anesthetic or anthelmintic agent. Chronic low-level exposure may occur in some municipal water supplies owing to chlorination of biologic methanes.

I. **Mechanism of toxicity.** Chloroform is a direct CNS depressant. In addition, as with other chlorinated hydrocarbons, it may potentiate cardiac arrhythmias by sensitizing the myocardium to catecholamines. Hepatic and renal toxicity is probably caused by metabolism to a highly reactive intermediate, possibly a free radical or phosgene. Chloroform is embryotoxic and is an animal carcinogen.

II. **Toxic dose.**
   A. The fatal **oral** dose of chloroform may be as little as 10 mL, although survival after ingestion of more than 100 mL has been reported. The oral LD_{50} in rats is 2000 mg/kg.
   B. The **air level** considered immediately dangerous to life or health (IDLH) is 500 ppm. The recommended workplace limit (ACGIH TLV-TWA) is 10 ppm as an 8-hour time-weighted average.

III. **Clinical presentation.**
   A. **Skin or eye contact** results in irritation and a defatting dermatitis. Mucous membrane irritation is also seen with ingestion or inhalation.
   B. **Inhalation or ingestion.** Mild to moderate systemic toxicity includes headache, nausea, vomiting, confusion, and drunkenness. More severe exposures may cause coma, respiratory arrest, and ventricular arrhythmias. Hepatic and renal injury may be apparent 1–3 days after exposure.

IV. **Diagnosis** is based on history and clinical presentation. Be aware that hepatic and renal toxicity may be delayed.
   A. **Specific levels.** Blood, urine, or breath concentrations may document exposure but are rarely available and are not useful for acute management.
   B. **Other useful laboratory studies** include electrolytes, BUN, creatinine, liver transaminases, prothrombin time (PT), and ECG monitoring.

V. **Treatment.**
   A. **Emergency and supportive measures**
      1. Maintain an open airway and assist ventilation if necessary (see pp 1–7).
      2. Treat coma (p 18) and arrhythmias (p 10–14) if they occur. Avoid use of epinephrine or other sympathomimetic amines, which may precipitate arrhythmias. Tachyarrhythmias caused by myocardial sensitization may be treated with **propranolol**, 1–2 mg IV (see p 405), or **esmolol**, 25–100 μg/kg/min IV (see p 366).
      3. Monitor by ECG for at least 4–6 hours after exposure.
   B. **Specific drugs and antidotes.** *N*-acetylcysteine (NAC; see p 334) may be helpful in preventing hepatic and renal damage by scavenging toxic metabolic intermediates, but no controlled study has been performed.
   C. **Decontamination** (see p 43)
      1. **Inhalation.** Remove the victim from exposure and give supplemental oxygen if available.
      2. **Skin and eyes.** Remove contaminated clothing and wash exposed skin with soap and water. Irrigate exposed eyes with copious tepid water or saline.

3. **Ingestion**
    a. **Prehospital.** Administer activated charcoal, if available. Do **not** induce vomiting with ipecac because of the risk of abrupt onset of coma.
    b. **Hospital.** Perform gastric lavage, and administer activated charcoal.
D. **Enhanced elimination.** There is no documented efficacy for forced diuresis, hemodialysis, hemoperfusion, or repeat-dose charcoal.

▶ CHLOROPHENOXY HERBICIDES

Michael A. O'Malley, MD, MPH

Chlorophenoxy compounds have been widely used as herbicides. Agent Orange was a mixture of the chlorophenoxy herbicides 2,4-D (dichlorophenoxyacetic acid) and 2,4,5-T (trichlorophenoxyacetic acid) that also contained small amounts of the highly toxic contaminant TCDD (2,3,7,8-tetrachlorodibenzo-*p*-dioxin; see p 156) derived from the process of manufacturing 2,4,5-T. Commercially available 2,4-D does not contain TCDD. Concentrated formulations of 2,4-D are likely to contain petroleum solvents; while these are considered "inert" ingredients because they are not pesticides, they may have their own innate toxicity (see Toluene and Xylene, p 307; and Hydrocarbons, p 183).

I. **Mechanism of toxicity.** In plants, the compounds act as growth hormone stimulators. Their mechanism of toxicity in animals is not known. In animal studies, widespread muscle damage occurs, and the cause of death is usually ventricular fibrillation. Massive rhabdomyolysis has been described in human cases.

II. **Toxic dose.** The minimum toxic dose of 2,4-D in humans is 3–4 g or 40–50 mg/kg, and death has occurred after adult ingestion of 6.5 g. Less than 6% of 2,4-D applied to the skin is absorbed systemically, although dermal exposure may produce skin irritation.

III. **Clinical presentation.** Tachycardia, muscle weakness, and muscle spasms occur shortly after ingestion and may progress to profound muscle weakness and coma. Massive rhabdomyolysis, metabolic acidosis, and severe and intractable hypotension have been reported, resulting in death within 24 hours. Hepatitis and renal injury may occur.

IV. **Diagnosis** depends on a history of exposure and the presence of muscle weakness and elevated serum CPK.
    A. **Specific levels** of urinary 2,4-D can be measured but may not be available in a timely enough fashion to be of help in establishing the diagnosis.
    B. **Other useful laboratory studies** include electrolytes, glucose, BUN, creatinine, CPK, urinalysis (occult heme test positive in the presence of myoglobin), liver enzymes, 12-lead ECG and ECG monitoring.

V. **Treatment.**
    A. **Emergency and supportive measures**
        1. Maintain an open airway and assist ventilation if necessary (see pp 1–7).
        2. Treat coma (p 18), hypotension (p 15), and rhabdomyolysis (p 25) if they occur.
        3. Monitor the patient closely for at least 6–12 hours after ingestion because of the potential for delayed onset of symptoms.
    B. **Specific drugs and antidotes.** There is no specific antidote.
    C. **Decontamination** (see p 43)
        1. **Prehospital.** Administer activated charcoal if available. Ipecac-induced vomiting may be useful for initial treatment at the scene (eg, children at home) if it can be given within a few minutes of exposure.
        2. **Hospital.** Administer activated charcoal, then perform gastric lavage. After lavage, give an additional dose of charcoal.
    D. **Enhanced elimination.** There is no proven role for these procedures, although alkalinization of the urine may promote excretion of 2,4-D.

▶ CHLOROQUINE AND OTHER AMINOQUINOLINES

Neal L. Benowitz, MD

Chloroquine and other aminoquinolines are used in the prophylaxis or therapy of malaria and other parasitic diseases. Chloroquine and hydroxychloroquine are also used in the treatment of rheumatoid arthritis. Drugs in this class include chloroquine phosphate (Aralen), amodiaquine hydrochloride (Camoquin), hydroxychloroquine sulfate (Plaquenil), mefloquine (Lariam), primaquine phosphate, and quinacrine hydrochloride (Atabrine). Chloroquine overdose is common, especially in countries where malaria is prevalent, and the mortality rate is 10–30%. Quinine toxicity is described on p 279.

I. **Mechanism of toxicity.**
   A. **Chloroquine** blocks the synthesis of DNA and RNA and also has some quinidinelike cardiotoxicity. Hydroxychloroquine has similar actions but is considerably less potent.
   B. **Primaquine** and **quinacrine** are oxidizing agents and can cause methemoglobinemia or hemolytic anemia (especially in patients with glucose-6-phosphate dehydrogenase [G6PD] deficiency).
   C. **Pharmacokinetics.** Chloroquine and related drugs are highly tissue-bound (volume of distribution (Vd) = 150–250 L/kg) and are eliminated very slowly from the body. The terminal half-life of chloroquine is 2 months. Primaquine is extensively metabolized with a half-life of 3–8 hours to an active metabolite that is eliminated much more slowly (half-life 22–30 hours) and can accumulate with chronic dosing. (See also Table II–55.)

II. **Toxic dose.** The therapeutic dose of chloroquine phosphate is 500 mg once a week for malaria prophylaxis or 2.5 g over 2 days for treatment of malaria. Deaths have been reported in children after doses as low as 300 mg; the lethal dose of chloroquine for an adult is estimated at 30–50 mg/kg.

III. **Clinical presentation.**
   A. **Mild to moderate chloroquine overdose** results in dizziness, nausea and vomiting, abdominal pain, headache and visual disturbances (sometimes including irreversible blindness), auditory disturbances (sometimes leading to deafness), agitation, and neuromuscular excitability.
   B. **Severe chloroquine overdose** may cause convulsions, coma, shock, and respiratory or cardiac arrest. Quinidinelike cardiotoxicity may be seen, including sinoatrial arrest, depressed myocardial contractility, QRS or QT interval prolongation, heart block, and ventricular arrhythmias. Severe hypokalemia sometimes occurs and may contribute to arrhythmias.
   C. **Primaquine** and **quinacrine** intoxication commonly cause gastrointestinal upset and may also cause severe methemoglobinemia (see p 220) or hemolysis; chronic treatment can cause ototoxicity and retinopathy.
   D. **Amodiaquine** in therapeutic doses has caused severe and even fatal neutropenia.
   E. **Mefloquine** in therapeutic use or overdose may cause dizziness, vertigo, hallucinations, psychosis, and seizures.

IV. **Diagnosis.** The findings of gastritis, visual disturbances, and neuromuscular excitability, especially if accompanied by hypotension, QRS or QT interval widening, or ventricular arrhythmias, should suggest chloroquine overdose. Hemolysis or methemoglobinemia should suggest primaquine or quinacrine overdose.
   A. **Specific levels.** Chloroquine levels can be measured in blood but are not generally available. Because chloroquine is concentrated intracellularly, whole blood measurements are fivefold higher than serum or plasma levels.
      1. Plasma (trough) concentrations of 10–20 ng/mL (0.01–0.02 mg/L) are effective in the treatment of various types of malaria.
      2. Cardiotoxicity may be seen with serum levels of 1 mg/L (1000 ng/mL); serum levels reported in fatal cases have ranged from 1–210 mg/L (average, 55 mg/L).

B. **Other useful laboratory studies** include electrolytes, glucose, BUN, creatinine, and ECG and ECG monitoring. With **primaquine** or **quinacrine**, also include CBC, free plasma hemoglobin, and methemoglobin.

V. Treatment.
A. **Emergency and supportive measures**
  1. Maintain an open airway and assist ventilation if necessary (see pp 1–7).
  2. Treat seizures (p 21), coma (p 18), hypotension (p 15), and methemoglobinemia (p 220) if they occur.
  3. Treat massive hemolysis with blood transfusions if needed, and prevent hemoglobin deposition in the kidney tubules by alkaline diuresis (as for rhabdomyolysis; see p 25).
  4. Continuously monitor the ECG for at least 6–8 hours.
B. **Specific drugs and antidotes**
  1. Treat cardiotoxicity as for quinidine poisoning (see p 277) with **sodium bicarbonate** (see p 345), 1–2 meq/kg IV.
  2. **Epinephrine** infusion (see p 365) may be useful in treating hypotension via combined vasoconstrictor and inotropic actions. Dosing recommendations in one study were 0.25 µg/kg/min, increasing by increments of 0.25 µg/kg/min until adequate blood pressure was obtained, along with administration of high-dose diazepam (see below) and mechanical ventilation.
  3. High-dose **diazepam** (2 mg/kg IV, given over 30 minutes after endotracheal intubation and mechanical ventilation) has been reported to reduce mortality in animals and to ameliorate cardiotoxicity in human chloroquine poisonings. The mechanism of protection is unknown.
C. **Decontamination** (see p 43)
  1. **Prehospital.** Administer activated charcoal if available.
  2. **Hospital.** Administer activated charcoal. Perform gastric lavage for significant ingestions (eg, > 30–50 mg/kg). Gastric emptying is probably not necessary after small ingestions if activated charcoal can be given promptly.
D. **Enhanced elimination.** Because of extensive tissue distribution, enhanced removal procedures are ineffective.

▶ CHROMIUM

Thomas J. Ferguson, MD, PhD

Chromium is a durable metal used in electroplating, paint pigments (chrome yellow), primers and corrosion inhibitors, wood preservatives, textile preservatives, and leather tanning agents. Chromium exposure may occur by inhalation, ingestion, or skin exposure. Although chromium can exist in a variety of oxidation states, most human exposures involve one of two types: trivalent (eg, chromic oxide, chromic sulfate) or hexavalent (eg, chromium trioxide, chromic anhydride, chromic acid, dichromate salts). Toxicity is most commonly associated with hexavalent compounds; however, fatalities have occurred after ingestion of compounds of either type, and chronic skin sensitivity is probably related to the trivalent form. Chromium picolinate is a trivalent chromium compound often used as a body-building agent.

I. **Mechanism of toxicity.**
A. **Trivalent chromium** compounds are relatively insoluble and noncorrosive, and are less likely to be absorbed through intact skin. Biological toxicity is estimated to be 10- to 100-fold lower than for the hexavalent compounds.
B. **Hexavalent compounds** are powerful oxidizing agents and are corrosive to the airway, skin, mucous membranes, and gastrointestinal tract. Acute hemolysis and renal tubular necrosis may also occur. Chronic occupational exposure to less soluble hexavalent forms is associated with chronic bronchitis, dermatitis, and lung cancer.
C. **Chromic acid** is a strong acid, while some chromate salts are strong bases.

II. Toxic dose.
   A. Inhalation. The OSHA workplace Permissible Exposure Limit (PEL, 8-hour time-weighted average) for chromic acid and hexavalent compounds is 0.001 mg/m^3 (carcinogen). For bivalent and trivalent chromium the PEL is 0.5 mg/m^3.
   B. Skin. Chromium salts can cause skin burns, which may enhance systemic absorption, and death has occurred after a 10% surface area burn.
   C. Ingestion. Life-threatening toxicity has occurred from ingestion of as little as 500 mg of hexavalent chromium. The estimated lethal dose of chromic acid is 1–2 g and of potassium dichromate, 6–8 g. Drinking water standards are set at 50 µg/L (1 µmol/L) total chromium.

III. Clinical presentation.
   A. Inhalation. Acute inhalation can cause upper respiratory tract irritation, wheezing, and noncardiogenic pulmonary edema (which may be delayed for several hours to days after exposure). Chronic expsoure to hexavalent compounds may lead to pulmonary sensitization, asthma, and cancer.
   B. Skin and eyes. Acute contact may cause severe corneal injury, deep skin burns, and oral or esophageal burns. Hypersensitivity dermatitis may result. It has been estimated that chronic chromium exposure is responsible for about 8% of all cases of contact dermatitis. Nasal ulcers may also occur after chronic exposure.
   C. Ingestion. Ingestion may cause acute hemorrhagic gastroenteritis; the resulting massive fluid and blood loss may cause shock and oliguric renal failure. Hemolysis, hepatitis, and cerebral edema have been reported. Chromates are capable of oxidizing hemoglobin, but clinically significant methemoglobinemia is relatively uncommon after acute overdose.

IV. Diagnosis is based on a history of exposure and clinical manifestations such as skin and mucous membrane burns, gastroenteritis, renal failure, or shock.
   A. Specific levels. Blood levels are not useful in emergency management, nor are they widely available. Detection in the urine may confirm exposure; normal urine levels are less than 1 µg/L.
   B. Other useful laboratory studies include CBC, plasma free hemoglobin and haptoglobin (if hemolysis is suspected), electrolytes, glucose, BUN, creatinine, liver transaminases, urinalysis (for hemoglobin), arterial blood gas or pulse oximetry, methemoglobin, and chest x-ray.

V. Treatment.
   A. Emergency and supportive measures
      1. Inhalation. Give supplemental oxygen. Treat wheezing (see p 8), and monitor the victim closely for delayed-onset noncardiogenic pulmonary edema (p 7). Delays in the onset of pulmonary edema of up to 72 hours have been reported after inhalation of concentrated solutions of chromic acid.
      2. Ingestion
         a. Dilute immediately with water. Treat hemorrhagic gastroenteritis with aggressive fluid and blood replacement (p 15). Consider early endoscopy to assess the extent of esophageal or gastric injury.
         b. Treat hemoglobinuria resulting from hemolysis with alkaline diuresis as for rhabdomyolysis (p 25). Treat methemoglobinemia (p 220) if it occurs.
   B. Specific drugs and antidotes
      1. Chelation therapy (eg, with BAL) is not effective.
      2. After oral ingestion of hexavalent compounds, **ascorbic acid** has been suggested to assist the conversion of hexavalent to less toxic trivalent compounds. While no definitive studies exist, the treatment is benign and may be helpful. In animal studies the effective dose was 2–4 g of ascorbic acid orally per g of hexavalent chromium compound ingested.
      3. Acetylcysteine (see p 334) has been used in several animal studies and one human case of dichromate poisoning.

    C. Decontamination (see p 43)

      1. Inhalation. Remove the victim from exposure and give supplemental oxygen if available.

      2. Skin. Remove contaminated clothing and wash exposed areas immediately with copious soap and water. EDTA (see p 363) 10% ointment may facilitate removal of chromate scabs. A 10% topical solution of ascorbic acid has been advocated to enhance the conversion of hexavalent chromium to the less toxic trivalent state.

      3. Eyes. Irrigate copiously with tepid water or saline and perform fluorescein examination to rule out corneal injury if pain or irritation persists.

      4. Ingestion

        a. Prehospital. Give milk or water to dilute corrosive effects. Do *not* induce vomiting owing to the potential for corrosive injury.

        b. Hospital. Perform gastric lavage. Activated charcoal is of uncertain benefit in adsorbing chromium and may obscure the view if endoscopy is performed.

    D. Enhanced elimination. There is no evidence for the efficacy of enhanced removal procedures such as dialysis or hemoperfusion.

▶ CLONIDINE AND RELATED DRUGS

Olga F. Woo, PharmD

Clonidine and the related centrally acting adrenergic inhibitors **guanabenz, guanfacine,** and **methyldopa** are commonly used for the treatment of hypertension. Clonidine has also been used to alleviate opioid and nicotine withdrawal symptoms. Clonidine overdose may occur after ingestion of pills or ingestion of the long-acting skin patches. **Oxymetazoline** and **tetrahydrozoline** are nasal decongestants that may cause toxicity identical to that of clonidine. **Tizanidine** is a chemically related agent used for the treatment of muscle spasticity.

  I. Mechanism of toxicity. All of these agents decrease central sympathetic outflow by stimulating α_2-adrenergic presynaptic (inhibitory) receptors in the brain.

    A. Clonidine, oxymetazoline, and **tetrahydrozoline** may also stimulate peripheral α_1-receptors, resulting in vasoconstriction and transient hypertension.

    B. Guanabenz is structurally similar to guanethidine, a ganglionic blocker. **Guanfacine** is related closely to guanabenz and has more selective α_2-agonist activity than clonidine.

    C. Methyldopa may further decrease sympathetic outflow by metabolism to a false neurotransmitter (alpha-methylnorepinephrine) or by decreasing plasma renin activity.

    D. Tizanidine is structurally related to clonidine but has low affinity for α_1 receptors.

    E. Pharmacokinetics. The onset of effects is rapid (30 min) after oral administration of clonidine. Other than methyldopa, the drugs are widely distributed with large volumes of distribution (see also Table II–55).

  II. Toxic dose.

    A. Clonidine. As little as one tablet of 0.1-mg clonidine has produced toxic effects in children; however, 10 mg shared by twin 34-month-old girls was not lethal. Adults have survived acute ingestions with as much as 100 mg. No fatalities from acute overdoses have been reported.

    B. Guanabenz. Mild toxicity developed in adults who ingested 160–320 mg and in a 3-year-old who ingested 12 mg. Severe toxicity developed in a 19-month-old who ingested 28 mg. A 3-year-old child had moderate symptoms after ingesting 480 mg. All these children had recovered by 24 hours.

    C. Guanfacine. Severe toxicity developed in a 25-year-old woman who ingested 60 mg. A 2-year-old boy ingested 4 mg and became lethargic within 20 minutes, but the peak hypotensive effect occurred 20 hours later.

D. Methyldopa. More than 2 g in adults is considered a toxic dose, and death was reported in an adult after an ingestion of 25 g. However, survival was reported after ingestion of 45 g. The therapeutic dose of methyldopa for children is 10–65 mg/kg/d, and the higher dose is expected to cause mild symptoms.

III. Clinical presentation. Manifestations of intoxication result from generalized sympathetic depression and include pupillary constriction, lethargy, coma, apnea, bradycardia, hypotension, and hypothermia. Paradoxic hypertension, caused by stimulation of peripheral α_1 receptors, may occur with clonidine, oxymetazoline, and tetrahydrozoline (and possibly guanabenz) and is usually transient. The onset of symptoms is usually within 30–60 minutes, although peak effects may occur more than 6–12 hours after ingestion. Full recovery is usual within 24 hours. In an unusual massive overdose, a 28-year-old man who accidentally ingested 100 mg of clonidine powder had a 3-phase intoxication over 4 days: initial hypertension, followed by hypotension, and then a withdrawal reaction with hypertension.

IV. Diagnosis. Poisoning should be suspected in patients with pinpoint pupils, respiratory depression, hypotension, and bradycardia. Although clonidine overdose may mimic an opioid overdose, it does not usually respond to administration of naloxone.

A. Specific levels. Serum drug levels are not routinely available or clinically useful. These drugs are not usually detectable on comprehensive urine toxicology screening.

B. Other useful laboratory studies include electrolytes, glucose, and arterial blood gases or oximetry.

V. Treatment. Patients usually recover within 24 hours with supportive care.

A. Emergency and supportive measures
1. Protect the airway and assist ventilation if necessary (see pp 1–7).
2. Treat coma (p 18), hypotension (p 15), and bradycardia (p 10), if they occur. These usually resolve with supportive measures such as fluids, atropine, and dopamine. Hypertension is usually transient and does not require treatment.

B. Specific drugs and antidotes
1. **Naloxone** (see p 384) has been reported to reverse signs and symptoms of clonidine overdose, but this has not been confirmed. However, because the overdose mimics opioid intoxication, naloxone is indicated because of the possibility that narcotics may also have been ingested.
2. **Tolazoline,** a central α_2-receptor antagonist, was previously recommended but the response has been highly variable and it should *not* be used.

C. Decontamination (see p 43)
1. **Prehospital.** Administer activated charcoal, if available. Do *not* induce vomiting because of the risk of abrupt onset of coma and altered blood pressure.
2. **Hospital.** Administer activated charcoal. Gastric emptying is not necessary if activated charcoal can be given promptly.

D. Enhanced elimination. There is no evidence that enhanced removal procedures are effective.

► **COCAINE**

Neal L. Benowitz, MD

Cocaine is one of the most popular drugs of abuse. It may be sniffed into the nose (snorted), smoked, or injected intravenously. Occasionally it is combined with heroin and injected (speedball). Cocaine purchased on the street is usually of high purity, but it may occasionally contain substitute drugs such as lidocaine (see p 70) or stimulants such as caffeine (see p 118), phenylpropanolamine (p 259), ephedrine (p 259), or phencyclidine (p 254).

The **"free base"** form of cocaine is preferred for smoking because it volatilizes at a lower temperature and is not as easily destroyed by heat as the crystalline hydrochloride salt. Free base is made by dissolving cocaine salt in an aqueous alkaline solution and then extracting the free base form with a solvent such as ether. Heat is sometimes applied to hasten solvent evaporation, creating a fire hazard. **"Crack"** is a free base form of cocaine produced by using sodium bicarbonate to create the alkaline aqueous solution, which is then dried.

I. **Mechanism of toxicity.** The primary actions of cocaine are local anesthetic effects (see p 70), CNS stimulation, and inhibition of neuronal uptake of catecholamines.

   A. CNS stimulation and inhibition of catecholamine uptake result in a state of generalized sympathetic stimulation very similar to that of amphetamine intoxication (see p 68).

   B. Cardiovascular effects of high doses of cocaine, presumably related to blockade of cardiac-cell sodium channels, include depression of conduction and contractility.

   C. **Pharmacokinetics.** Cocaine is well absorbed from all routes, and toxicity has been described after mucosal application as a local anesthetic. Smoking and intravenous injection produce maximum effects within 1–2 minutes, while oral or mucosal absorption may take up to 20–30 minutes. Once absorbed, cocaine is eliminated by metabolism and hydrolysis with a half-life of about 60 minutes. In the presence of ethanol, cocaine is transesterified to **cocaethylene**, which has similar pharmacologic effects and a longer half-life than cocaine. (See also Table II–55.)

II. **Toxic dose.** The toxic dose is highly variable and depends on individual tolerance, the route of administration, and the presence of other drugs, as well as other factors. Rapid intravenous injection or smoking may produce transient high brain and heart levels resulting in convulsions or cardiac arrhythmias, whereas the same dose swallowed or snorted may produce only euphoria.

   A. The usual maximum recommended dose for intranasal local anesthesia is 100–200 mg (1–2 mL of 10% solution).

   B. A typical "line" of cocaine to be snorted contains 20–30 mg or more. Crack is usually sold in pellets or "rocks" containing 100–150 mg.

   C. Ingestion of 1 g or more of cocaine is very likely to be fatal.

III. **Clinical presentation.**

   A. **CNS manifestations** of toxicity may occur within minutes after smoking or intravenous injection or may be delayed for 30–60 minutes after snorting, mucosal application, or oral ingestion.

      1. Initial euphoria may be followed by anxiety, agitation, delirium, psychosis, tremulousness, muscle rigidity or hyperactivity, and seizures. High doses may cause respiratory arrest.

      2. Seizures are usually brief and self-limited; status epilepticus should suggest continued drug absorption (as from ruptured cocaine-filled condoms in the gastrointestinal tract) or hyperthermia.

      3. Coma may be caused by a postictal state, hyperthermia, or intracranial hemorrhage resulting from cocaine-induced hypertension.

      4. With chronic cocaine use, insomnia, weight loss, and paranoid psychosis may occur. A "washed-out" syndrome has been observed in cocaine abusers after a prolonged binge, consisting of profound lethargy and deep sleep that may last for several hours to days, followed by spontaneous recovery.

   B. **Cardiovascular toxicity** may also occur rapidly after smoking or intravenous injection and is mediated by sympathetic overactivity.

      1. Fatal ventricular tachycardia or fibrillation may occur.

      2. Severe hypertension may cause hemorrhagic stroke or aortic dissection.

      3. Coronary artery spasm and/or thrombosis may result in myocardial infarction, even in patients with no coronary disease. Diffuse myocardial necrosis similar to catecholamine myocarditis and chronic cardiomyopathy have been described.

   4. Shock may be caused by myocardial, intestinal, or brain infarction, hyper-
      thermia, tachyarrhythmias, or hypovolemia produced by extravascular fluid
      sequestration owing to vasoconstriction.
   5. Renal failure may result from shock, renal arterial spasm, or rhabdomyoly-
      sis with myoglobinuria.
C. **Death** is usually caused by a sudden fatal arrhythmia, status epilepticus, intracranial hemorrhage, or hyperthermia. Hyperthermia is usually caused by
   seizures, muscular hyperactivity, or rigidity and is typically associated with
   rhabdomyolysis, myoglobinuric renal failure, coagulopathy, and multiple
   organ failure.
D. A variety of **other effects** have occurred after smoking or snorting cocaine.
   1. Chest pain without ECG evidence of myocardial ischemia is common. The
      presumed basis is musculoskeletal and may be associated with chest wall
      muscle rhabdomyolysis.
   2. Pneumothorax and pneumomediastinum cause pleuritic chest pain, and
      the latter is often recognized by a "crunching" sound ("Hammond's
      crunch") heard over the anterior chest.
   3. Nasal septal perforation may occur after chronic snorting.
   4. Accidental subcutaneous injection of cocaine may cause localized necrotic
      ulcers ("coke burns"), and wound botulism (see p 112) has been reported.
E. **Body "packers"** or **"stuffers."** Persons attempting to smuggle cocaine may
   swallow large numbers of tightly packed cocaine-filled condoms ("body packers"). Street vendors suddenly surprised by a police raid may quickly swallow
   their wares, often without carefully wrapping or closing the packets or vials
   ("body stuffers"). The swallowed condoms, packets, or vials may break open,
   releasing massive quantities of cocaine. The packages are sometimes, but
   not always, visible on plain abdominal x-ray.
IV. **Diagnosis** is based on a history of cocaine use or typical features of sympathomimetic intoxication. Skin marks of chronic intravenous drug abuse, especially
   with scarring from coke burns, and nasal septal perforation after chronic snorting
   suggest cocaine use. Chest pain with electrocardiographic evidence of ischemia
   or infarction in a young, otherwise healthy person also suggests cocaine use.
   Note that young adults, particularly young African-American men, have a high
   prevalence of normal J-point elevation on ECG, which can be mistaken for acute
   myocardial infarction.
   A. **Specific levels.** Blood cocaine levels are not routinely available and do not
      assist in emergency management. Cocaine and its metabolite benzoylecgo-
      nine are easily detected in the urine and provide qualitative confirmation of
      cocaine use.
   B. **Other useful laboratory studies** include electrolytes, glucose, BUN, creati-
      nine, CPK, urinalysis, urine myoglobin, ECG and ECG monitoring, CT head
      scan (if hemorrhage is suspected), and abdominal x-ray (if cocaine-filled con-
      dom or packet ingestion is suspected).
V. **Treatment.**
   A. **Emergency and supportive measures**
      1. Maintain an open airway and assist ventilation if necessary (see pp 1–7).
      2. Treat coma (p 18), agitation (p 23), seizures (p 21), hyperthermia
         (p 20), arrhythmias (pp 10–14), and hypotension (p 15) if they occur.
      3. Angina pectoris may be treated with nitrates or calcium channel blockers.
         For acute myocardial infarction, thrombolysis has been recommended but
         is controversial. Supporting its use is the high prevalence of acute throm-
         bosis, often superimposed on coronary spasm. Against its use are the ex-
         cellent prognosis for patients with cocaine-induced infarction, even without
         thrombolysis, and concerns about increased risks of bleeding caused by
         intracranial hemorrhage or aortic dissection.
      4. Monitor vital signs and ECG for several hours. Patients with suspected
         coronary artery spasm should be admitted to a coronary care unit, and be-
         cause of reports of persistent or recurrent coronary spasm up to several

days after initial exposure, consider use of an oral calcium antagonist and/or cardiac nitrates for 2–4 weeks after discharge.
B. **Specific drugs and antidotes.** There is no specific antidote. Although propranolol was previously recommended as the drug of choice for treatment of cocaine-induced hypertension, it may in fact produce paradoxic worsening of hypertension because of blockade of β_2-mediated vasodilation; **propranolol** (p 405) or **esmolol** (p 366) may be used **in combination** with a vasodilator such as **phentolamine** (p 400). Beta blockers may be used alone for treatment of tachyarrhythmias.
C. **Decontamination** (see p 43). Decontamination is not necessary after smoking, snorting, or intravenous injection. After **ingestion**, perform the following steps:
1. **Prehospital.** Administer activated charcoal if available. Do *not* induce vomiting because of the risk of abrupt onset of seizures.
2. **Hospital.** Administer activated charcoal. Gastric emptying is not necessary if activated charcoal can be given promptly.
3. For ingestion of cocaine-filled condoms or packets, give repeated doses of activated charcoal and consider whole bowel irrigation (see p 50). If large ingested packets (ie, Ziploc bags) are not removed by these procedures, laparotomy and surgical removal may be necessary.
D. **Enhanced elimination.** Because cocaine is extensively distributed to tissues and rapidly metabolized, dialysis and hemoperfusion procedures are not effective. Acidification of the urine does not significantly enhance cocaine elimination and may aggravate myoglobinuric renal failure.

▶ COLCHICINE

Neal L. Benowitz, MD

Colchicine is marketed in tablets used for treatment of gout and familial Mediterranean fever and is found in certain plants: autumn crocus or meadow saffron (*Colchicum autumnale*) and glory lily (*Gloriosa superba*). A colchicine overdose is extremely serious, with considerable mortality that is often delayed.
I. **Mechanism of toxicity.** Colchicine inhibits mitosis of dividing cells and, in high concentrations, is a general cellular poison. Colchicine is rapidly absorbed and extensively distributed to body tissues (volume of distribution 2–20 L/kg). (See also Table II–55.)
II. **Toxic dose.** The maximum therapeutic dose of colchicine is 8–10 mg in 1 day. Tablets contain 0.5–0.6 mg. Fatalities have been reported with single ingestions of as little as 7 mg. In a series of 150 cases, doses of 0.5 mg/kg were associated with diarrhea and vomiting but not death; 0.5–0.8 mg/kg with marrow aplasia and 10% mortality. Ingestions of parts of colchicine-containing plants have resulted in severe toxicity and death.
III. **Clinical presentation.** Colchicine poisoning affects many organ systems, with toxic effects occurring over days to weeks.
A. After an **acute overdose**, symptoms are typically delayed for 2–12 hours and include nausea, vomiting, abdominal pain, and severe bloody diarrhea. Shock results from depressed cardiac contractility and fluid loss into the gastrointestinal tract and other tissues. Delirium, seizures or coma may occur. Lactic acidosis related to shock and inhibition of cellular metabolism is common. Other manifestations of acute colchicine poisoning include acute myocardial injury, rhabdomyolysis with myoglobinuria, disseminated intravascular coagulation, and acute renal failure.
B. **Death** usually occurs after 8–36 hours and is caused by respiratory failure, intractable shock, and cardiac arrhythmias or sudden cardiac arrest.

C. **Late complications** include bone marrow suppression, particularly leukopenia and thrombocytopenia (4–5 days) and alopecia (2–3 weeks). Chronic colchicine therapy may produce myopathy (proximal muscle weakness and elevated creatinine kinase levels) and polyneuropathy. This has also occurred after acute poisoning.

IV. **Diagnosis.** A syndrome beginning with severe gastroenteritis, shock, rhabdomyolysis, and acute renal failure and, several days later, leukopenia and thrombocytopenia should suggest colchicine poisoning. A history of gout or familial Mediterranean fever in the patient or a family member is also suggestive.

A. **Specific levels.** Measurement of levels in blood and urine is neither available nor clinically useful.

B. **Other useful laboratory studies** include CBC, electrolytes, glucose, BUN, creatinine, CPK, urinalysis, and ECG monitoring.

V. **Treatment.**

A. **Emergency and supportive measures.** Provide aggressive supportive care, with careful monitoring and treatment of fluid and electrolyte disturbances.

1. Anticipate sudden respiratory or cardiac arrest, and maintain an open airway and assist ventilation if necessary (see pp 1–7).
2. Treatment of shock (p 15) may require large amounts of crystalloid fluids, possibly blood (to replace loss from hemorrhagic gastroenteritis), and pressor agents such as dopamine (p 362).
3. Infusion of sodium bicarbonate and mannitol is recommended if there is evidence of rhabdomyolysis (p 25).
4. Bone marrow depression requires specialized intensive care. Severe neutropenia requires patient isolation and management of febrile episodes as for other neutropenic conditions. Platelet transfusions may be required to control bleeding.

B. **Specific drugs and antidotes.** Colchicine-specific antibodies (Fab fragments) are under investigation but not yet available in the United States. Granulocyte colony-stimulating factor (G-CSF) has been used for the treatment of severe leukopenia.

C. **Decontamination** (see p 43).

1. **Prehospital.** Administer activated charcoal if available. Ipecac-induced vomiting may be useful for initial treatment at the scene (eg, children at home) if it can be given within a few minutes of exposure.
2. **Hospital.** Administer activated charcoal. Consider gastric lavage for large ingestions.

D. **Enhanced elimination.** Because colchicine is highly bound to tissues, with a large volume of distribution, hemodialysis and hemoperfusion are ineffective. Colchicine undergoes enterohepatic recirculation, so **repeat-dose charcoal** might be expected to accelerate elimination, although this has not been documented.

▶ COPPER

B. Zane Horowitz, MD

Copper is widely used in its elemental metallic form, in metal alloys, and in the form of copper salts. Elemental metallic copper is used in electrical wiring and plumbing materials and was formerly the main consituent of pennies (now mostly zinc). Copper salts such as copper sulfate, copper oxide, copper chloride, copper nitrate, copper cyanide, and copper acetate are used as pesticides and algicides and in a variety of industrial processes. Because of its toxicity, copper sulfate is no longer used as an emetic. Copper levels may be elevated in persons drinking from copper containers or using copper plumbing. The increased acidity of beverages stored in copper alloy (eg, brass or bronze) containers enhances leaching of copper into the liquid.

I. **Mechanism of toxicity.**
   A. **Elemental metallic copper** is poorly absorbed orally and is essentially non-toxic. However, inhalation of copper dust, or metallic fumes created when welding or brazing copper alloys, may cause chemical pneumonitis or a syndrome similar to metal fume fever (see p 217). Metallic copper dust in the eye (chalcosis) may lead to corneal opacification, uveitis, ocular necrosis, and blindness unless the dust is removed quickly.
   B. **Copper sulfate** salt is highly irritating, depending on the concentration, and may produce mucous membrane irritation and severe gastroenteritis.
   C. **Systemic absorption** can produce hepatic and renal tubular injury. Hemolysis has been associated with copper exposure from hemodialysis equipment or absorption through burned skin.

II. **Toxic dose.**
   A. **Inhalation.** The recommended workplace limit (ACGIH TLV-TWA) for copper fumes is 0.2 mg/m^3; for dusts and mists, it is 1 mg/m^3. The air level considered immediately dangerous to life or health for dusts or fumes is 100 mg Cu/m^3.
   B. **Ingestion** of more than 250 mg of copper sulfate can produce vomiting, and larger ingestions can potentially cause hepatic and renal injury.
   C. **Water.** The United States Environmental Protection Agency (EPA) has established a safe limit of 1.3 mg/L in drinking water.

III. **Clinical presentation.**
   A. **Inhalation of copper fumes** or **dusts** initially produces a metallic taste and upper respiratory irritation (dry cough, sore throat, and eye irritation). Large exposures may cause severe cough, dyspnea, fever, leukocytosis, and pulmonary infiltrates (see also metal fume fever, p 217).
   B. **Ingestion of copper sulfate or other salts** causes the rapid onset of nausea and vomiting with characteristic blue-green emesis. Gastrointestinal bleeding may occur. Fluid and blood loss from gastroenteritis may lead to hypotension and oliguria. Intravascular hemolysis can result in acute tubular necrosis. Hepatitis has been reported, due to centrilobular necrosis. Multisystem failure, shock and death may occur.
   C. **Chronic** exposure to Bordeaux mixture (copper sulfate with hydrated lime) may occur in vineyard workers. Pulmonary fibrosis, lung cancer, liver fibrosis, cirrhosis, angiosarcoma, and portal hypertension have been associated with this occupational exposure.
   D. **Swimming** in water contaminated with copper-based algicides can cause green discoloration of the hair.

IV. **Diagnosis** is based on a history of acute ingestion or occupational exposure. Occupations at risk include those associated with handling algicides, herbicides, wood preservatives, pyrotechnics, ceramic glazes, electrical wiring, and welding or brazing copper alloys.
   A. **Specific levels.** If copper salt ingestion is suspected, a serum copper level should be obtained. Normal serum copper concentrations average 1 mg/L, and this doubles during pregnancy. Serum copper levels above 5 mg/L are considered very toxic. Whole blood copper levels may correlate better with acute intoxication because acute excess copper is carried in the red blood cells; however, whole blood copper levels are not as widely available.
   B. **Other useful laboratory studies** include CBC, electrolytes, BUN, creatinine, hepatic transaminases, arterial blood gases or oximetry, and chest x-ray. If hemolysis is suspected, send blood for type and cross-match, plasma free hemoglobin, and haptoglobin, and check urinalysis for occult blood (hemoglobinuria).

V. **Treatment.**
   A. **Emergency and supportive measures**
      1. **Inhalation of copper fumes** or **dusts.** Give supplemental oxygen if indicated by arterial blood gases or oximetry, and treat bronchospasm (see p 8) and chemical pneumonitis (p 7) if they occur. Symptoms are usually short-lived and resolve without specific treatment.

2. Ingestion of copper salts
  a. Treat shock caused by gastroenteritis with aggressive intravenous fluid replacement and, if necessary, pressor drugs (p 15).
  b. Consider endoscopy to rule out corrosive esophageal or stomach injury, depending on the concentration of the solution and the patient's symptoms.
  c. Blood transfusion may be needed if significant hemolysis or gastrointestinal bleeding occurs.
B. Specific drugs and antidotes. BAL (dimercaprol; see p 341) and **penicillamine** (see p 397) are effective chelating agents and should be used in seriously ill patients with large ingestions. Triethyl tetramine dihydrochloride (Trien or Cuprid) is a specific copper chelator approved for use in Wilson's Disease; although it is better tolerated than penicillamine, its role in acute ingestion or chronic environmental exposure has not been established.
C. Decontamination (p 43)
  1. Inhalation. Remove the victim from exposure and give supplemental oxygen if available.
  2. Eyes. Irrigate copiously and attempt to remove all copper from the surface; perform a careful slit-lamp exam and refer the case to an ophthalmologist urgently if any residual material remains.
  3. Ingestion
    a. Prehospital. Do *not* induce vomiting because it may worsen gastroenteritis.
    b. Hospital. Perform gastric lavage if there has been a recent ingestion of a large quantity of copper salts. There is no proven benefit for activated charcoal, and its use may obscure the view if endoscopy is performed.
D. Enhanced elimination. There is no role for hemodialysis, hemoperfusion, repeat-dose charcoal, hemodiafiltration, or other enhanced elimination techniques. Hemodialysis may be required for supportive care of patients with acute renal failure, and it can marginally increase the elimination of the copper-chelator complex.

▶ COUMARIN AND RELATED RODENTICIDES

Ilene B. Anderson, PharmD

Dicumarol and other natural anticoagulants are found in sweet clover. Coumarin derivatives are used both therapeutically and as rodenticides. Warfarin (Coumadin) is widely used as a therapeutic anticoagulant, but is no longer popular as a rodenticide because rats and mice have become resistant. The most common anticoagulant rodenticides available today contain long-acting **"superwarfarins"** such as brodifacoum, diphacinone, bromadiolone, chlorophacinone, difenacoum, pindone, and valone, which have profound and prolonged anticoagulant effects.
I. Mechanism of toxicity. All these compounds inhibit hepatic synthesis of the vitamin K-dependent coagulation factors II, VII, IX, and X. Only the synthesis of new factors is affected, and the anticoagulant effect is delayed until currently circulating factors have been degraded. Peak effects are usually not observed for 2–3 days because of the long half-lives of factors IX and X (24–60 hours).
  A. The duration of anticoagulant effect after a single dose of **warfarin** is usually 2–7 days. (See also Table II–55, p 322)
  B. Superwarfarin products may continue to produce significant anticoagulation for weeks to months after a single ingestion.
II. Toxic dose. The toxic dose is highly variable.
  A. Generally, a single small ingestion of **warfarin** (eg, 10–20 mg) will not cause serious intoxication (most warfarin-based rodenticides contain 0.05% warfarin). In contrast, chronic or repeated ingestion of even small amounts (eg, 2

mg/d) can produce significant anticoagulation. Patients with hepatic dysfunction, malnutrition, or a bleeding diathesis are at greater risk.
   B. Superwarfarins are extremely potent and have prolonged effects even after a single small ingestion (ie, as little as 1 mg in an adult).
   C. Multiple **drug interactions** are known to alter the anticoagulant effect of warfarin (Table II–19).
III. Clinical presentation. Excessive anticoagulation may cause ecchymoses, subconjunctival hemorrhage, bleeding gums, or evidence of internal hemorrhage (eg, hematemesis, melena, or hematuria). The most immediately life-threatening complications are massive gastrointestinal bleeding and intracranial hemorrhage.
   A. Anticoagulant effects may be apparent within 8–12 hours, but most commonly they are delayed for at least 1–2 days after ingestion.
   B. Evidence of continuing anticoagulant effects may persist for days, weeks, or even months with superwarfarin products.
IV. Diagnosis is based on the history and evidence of anticoagulant effects. It is important to identify the exact product ingested to ascertain whether a superwarfarin is involved.
   A. Specific levels. Blood levels of anticoagulants are not available, nor are they helpful.
      1. An anticoagulant effect is best quantified by baseline and daily repeated measurement of the **prothrombin time** (PT) and calculation of the International Normalized Ratio (INR), which may not be elevated until 1–2 days after ingestion. A normal PT 48 hours after exposure rules out significant ingestion.
      2. Blood levels of clotting factors II, VII, IX, and X will be decreased, but these measurements are not routinely available.
   B. Other useful laboratory studies include CBC and blood type and cross-match. The partial thromboplastin time (PTT), bleeding time, and platelet count may be used to rule out other causes of bleeding.
V. Treatment.
   A. Emergency and supportive measures. If significant bleeding occurs, be prepared to treat shock with transfusions and fresh-frozen plasma, and obtain immediate neurosurgical consultation if intracranial bleeding is suspected.
      1. Take care not to precipitate hemorrhage in severely anticoagulated patients; prevent falls and other trauma. If possible, avoid use of nasogastric or endotracheal tubes or central intravenous lines.
      2. Avoid drugs that may enhance bleeding or decrease metabolism of the anticoagulant (Table II–19).
   B. Specific drugs and antidotes. Vitamin K$_1$ (phytonadione), but **not vitamin K$_3$** (menadione), effectively restores the production of clotting factors. It should be given if there is evidence of significant anticoagulation. *Note*, however, that if it is given prophylactically after an acute ingestion, the 48-hour

TABLE II–19. EXAMPLES OF DRUG INTERACTIONS WITH WARFARIN

Increased anticoagulant effect	Decreased anticoagulant effect
Allopurinol	Barbiturates
Amiodarone	Carbamazepine
Anabolic steroids	Cholestyramine
Chloral hydrate	Glutethimide
Cimetidine	Nafcillin
Disulfiram	Oral contraceptives
Indomethacin and other nonsteroidal anti-inflammatory agents	Rifampin
Quinidine	
Salicylates	
Sulfonamides	

prothrombin time cannot be used to determine the severity of the overdose, and the patient will have to be monitored for a minimum of 5 days after the last vitamin K₁ dose.

1. Give 5–10 mg of **vitamin K₁** very slowly IV or subcutaneously (SC) (see p 409). *Caution*: Vitamin K-mediated reversal of anticoagulation may be dangerous for patients who require constant anticoagulation (eg, for prosthetic heart valves). Very minute doses should be given to titrate for partial effect. **Repeated doses** of vitamin K may be required, especially in patients who have ingested a long-acting superwarfarin product. Doses as high as 200 mg/d have been used.

2. Because vitamin K will not begin to restore clotting factors for 6 or more hours (peak effect 24 hours), patients with active hemorrhage may require **fresh-frozen plasma** or **fresh whole blood**.

C. **Decontamination** (see p 43)
1. **Prehospital.** Administer activated charcoal if available. Ipecac-induced vomiting may be useful for initial treatment at the scene (eg, children at home) if it can be given within 30 minutes of exposure.
2. **Hospital.** Administer activated charcoal. Gastric emptying is not necessary if activated charcoal can be given promptly, and should be avoided in the person who is already anticoagulated.

D. **Enhanced elimination.** There is no role for enhanced elimination procedures.

▶ CYANIDE

Paul D. Blanc, MD, MSPH

Cyanide is a highly reactive chemical with a variety of uses, including chemical synthesis, laboratory analysis, and metal plating. Aliphatic nitriles (acrylonitrile and propionitrile) used in plastics manufacturing are metabolized to cyanide. The vasodilator drug nitroprusside releases cyanide on exposure to light or through metabolism. Natural sources of cyanide (amygdalin and many other cyanogenic glycosides) are found in apricot pits, cassava, and many other plants and seeds, some of which may be important depending on ethnobotanical practices. Acetonitrile, a component of some artificial nail glue removers, has caused several pediatric deaths.

Hydrogen cyanide is a gas easily generated by mixing acid with cyanide salts and is a common combustion byproduct of burning plastics, wool, and many other natural and synthetic products. Hydrogen cyanide poisoning is an important cause of death from structural fires, and deliberate cyanide exposure remains an important instrument of homicide and suicide.

I. **Mechanism of toxicity.** Cyanide is a chemical asphyxiant; binding to cellular cytochrome oxidase, it blocks the aerobic utilization of oxygen. Unbound cyanide is detoxified by metabolism to thiocyanate, a much less toxic compound that is excreted in the urine.

II. **Toxic dose.**
A. Exposure to **hydrogen cyanide gas** (HCN) even at low levels (150–200 ppm) can be fatal. The air level considered immediately dangerous to life or health (IDLH) is 50 ppm. The recommended workplace ceiling limit (ACGIH TLV-C) for HCN is 4.7 ppm (5 mg/m³). HCN is well-absorbed across the skin.
B. Adult **ingestion** of as little as 200 mg of the sodium or potassium salt may be fatal. Solutions of cyanide salts can be absorbed through intact skin.
C. Acute cyanide poisoning is relatively rare with nitroprusside infusion (at normal infusion rates) or after ingestion of amygdalin-containing seeds (unless they have been pulverized).

III. **Clinical presentation.** Abrupt onset of profound toxic effects shortly after exposure is the hallmark of cyanide poisoning. Symptoms include headache, nausea, dyspnea, and confusion. Syncope, seizures, coma, agonal respirations, and cardiovascular collapse ensue rapidly after heavy exposure.

A. Brief delay may occur if the cyanide is ingested as a salt, especially if it is in a capsule or if there is food in the stomach.

B. Delayed onset (minutes to hours) may also occur after ingestion of nitriles and plant-derived cyanogenic glycosides, because metabolism to cyanide is required.

C. Chronic neurologic sequelae may follow severe cyanide poisoning.

IV. Diagnosis is based on a history of exposure or the presence of rapidly progressive symptoms and signs. Severe lactic acidosis is usually present with significant exposure. The **measured venous oxygen saturation** may be elevated owing to blocked cellular oxygen consumption. The classic "bitter almond" odor of hydrogen cyanide may or may not be noted, because of genetic variability in the ability to detect the smell.

A. Specific levels. Cyanide determinations are rarely of use in emergency management because they cannot be performed rapidly enough to influence initial treatment. In addition, they must be interpreted with caution because of a variety of complicating technical factors.

1. Whole blood levels higher than 0.5–1 mg/L are considered toxic.
2. Cigarette smokers may have levels up to 0.1 mg/L.
3. Rapid nitroprusside infusion may produce levels as high as 1 mg/L, accompanied by metabolic acidosis.

B. Other useful laboratory studies include electrolytes, glucose, serum lactate, arterial blood gas, mixed venous oxygen saturation, and carboxyhemoglobin (if smoke inhalation exposure).

V. Treatment.

A. Emergency and supportive measures. Treat all cyanide exposures as potentially lethal.

1. Maintain an open airway and assist ventilation if necessary (see pp 1–7). Administer supplemental oxygen.
2. Treat coma (p 18), hypotension (p 15), and seizures (p 21) if they occur.
3. Start an intravenous line and monitor the patient's vital signs and ECG closely.

B. Specific drugs and antidotes

1. The **cyanide antidote package** (Taylor Pharmaceuticals) consists of amyl and sodium **nitrites** (see p 390), which produce cyanide-scavenging methemoglobinemia, and sodium **thiosulfate** (see p 408), which accelerates the conversion of cyanide to thiocyanate.

   a. Break a pearl of **amyl nitrite** under the nose of the victim; and administer **sodium nitrite**, 300 mg IV (6 mg/kg for children). *Caution*: Nitrite-induced methemoglobinemia can be extremely dangerous and even lethal. Nitrite should not be given if the symptoms are mild or if the diagnosis is uncertain, especially if concomitant carbon monoxide poisoning is suspected.

   b. Administer **sodium thiosulfate**, 12.5 g IV. Thiosulfate is relatively benign and may be given empirically even if the diagnosis is uncertain. It may also be useful in mitigating nitroprusside toxicity (see p 235).

2. The most promising alternative antidote is **hydroxocobalamin** (see p 374). Unfortunately, it remains an investigational drug in the United States.

3. **Hyperbaric oxygen** has no proven role in cyanide poisoning treatment.

C. Decontamination (see p 43). *Caution*: Avoid contact with cyanide-containing salts or solutions, and avoid inhaling vapors from vomitus (which may give off hydrogen cyanide gas).

1. **Inhalation.** Remove victims from hydrogen cyanide exposure and give supplemental oxygen if available. Each rescuer should wear a positive-pressure, self-contained breathing apparatus and, if possible, chemical-protective clothing.

2. **Skin.** Remove and isolate all contaminated clothing and wash affected areas with copious soap and water.
3. **Ingestion** (see p 45). Even though charcoal has a relatively low affinity for cyanide, it will effectively bind the doses typically ingested (eg, 100–500 mg).
   a. **Prehospital.** Immediately administer activated charcoal if available. Do *not* induce vomiting unless victim is more than 20 minutes from a medical facility and charcoal is not available.
   b. **Hospital.** Immediately place a gastric tube and administer activated charcoal, then perform gastric lavage. Give additional activated charcoal and a cathartic after the lavage.
D. **Enhanced elimination.** There is no role for hemodialysis or hemoperfusion in cyanide poisoning treatment. Hemodialysis may be indicated in patients with renal insufficiency who develop high thiocyanate levels while on extended nitroprusside therapy.

▶ DAPSONE

Kathryn Meier, PharmD

Dapsone is an antibiotic used for many years to treat leprosy and rare dermatologic conditions. Recently, its major use is for prophylaxis against *Pneumocystis carinii* infections in patients with AIDS and other immunodeficiency disorders. Absorption of dapsone is delayed; peak plasma levels occur between 4 and 8 hours after ingestion. Dapsone is metabolized by two primary routes, acetylation and P-450 oxidation. Acetylated dapsone can be metabolized back to dapsone or oxidized by the P-450 system. Both dapsone and its acetylated metabolite undergo enterohepatic recirculation. The average elimination half-life is 30 hours after a therapeutic dose and as long as 77 hours after an overdose.

I. **Mechanism of toxicity.** Toxic effects are caused by the P-450 metabolites and include methemoglobinemia, sulfhemoglobinemia, and Heinz body hemolytic anemia—all of which decrease the oxygen-carrying capacity of the blood.
   A. Dapsone metabolites oxidize the ferrous iron hemoglobin complex to the ferric state, resulting in methemoglobinemia.
   B. Sulfhemoglobinemia occurs when dapsone metabolites sulfate the pyrrole hemoglobin ring; this is an irreversible reaction, and there is no antidote.
   C. Hemolysis may occur owing to depletion of intracellular glutathione by oxidative metabolites.
   D. **Pharmacokinetics.** Peak absorption occurs in 2–6 hours. The volume of distribution (Vd) is 1.5 L/kg. Protein binding is approximately 70–90%. The drug undergoes enterohepatic recirculation. The half-life is approximately 30 hours (up to 77 hours after overdose). (See also Table II–55.)

II. **Toxic dose.** The therapeutic dose ranges from 50 to 300 mg/d. Chronic daily dosing of 100 mg has resulted in methemoglobin levels of 5–8%. Hemolysis has not been reported at doses less than 300 mg/d. Persons with glucose-6-phosphate dehydrogenase (G6PD) deficiency, congenital hemoglobin abnormalities, and underlying hypoxemia may experience greater toxicity at lower doses. Death has occurred with overdoses of 1.4 g and greater.

III. **Clinical presentation** includes methemoglobinemia, sulfhemoglobinemia, and intravascular hemolysis. Clinical manifestations are more severe in patients with underlying medical conditions that may contribute to hypoxemia.
   A. **Methemoglobinemia** (see p 220) causes cyanosis and dyspnea. Drawn blood may appear dark "chocolate" brown when the methemoglobin level is greater than 15–20%. Because of the long half-life of dapsone and its metabolites, methemoglobinemia may persist for several days, requiring repeated antidotal treatment.

B. **Sulfhemoglobinemia** also decreases oxyhemoglobin saturation and is unresponsive to methylene blue, so patients may rarely continue to appear cyanotic even after receiving antidotal treatment (uncommon because the amount of sulfhemoglobin generated is rarely more than 5%).

C. **Hemolysis.** Heinz bodies may be seen, but hemolysis may be delayed in onset 2–3 days after the ingestion.

IV. **Diagnosis** is based on a history of dapsone use and should be suspected in any immunocompromised patient with a suspected drug overdose, particularly since manifestations of toxicity may be delayed. Although there are many agents that can cause methemoglobinemia, there are very few that produce both detectable sulfhemoglobin and a prolonged, recurrent methemoglobinemia.

A. **Specific levels.** Dapsone levels are not routinely available.

1. **Methemoglobinemia** (see p 220) is suspected when a cyanotic patient fails to respond to high-flow oxygen or cyanosis persists despite a normal arterial PO_2 (note that pulse oximetry is not a reliable indicator of oxygen saturation in patients with methemoglobinemia). Specific methemoglobin concentrations can be measured using a multiwave cooximeter. Qualitatively, a drop of blood on white filter paper will appear brown (when directly compared with normal blood) if the methemoglobin level is greater than 15–20%.

2. *Note:* administration of the antidote methylene blue (see V.B.1. below) can cause transient false elevation of the measured methemoglobin level (up to 15%).

3. Sulfhemoglobin is difficult to detect, in part because its spectrophotometric absorbance is similar to methemoglobin on the cooximeter. If a crystal of potassium cyanide is added to a blood sample, methemoglobin will become red, but not if significant sulfhemoglobin is present.

B. **Other useful laboratory studies** include CBC (with differential smear to look for reticulocytes and Heinz bodies), glucose, electrolytes, liver transaminases, bilirubin, and arterial blood gases.

V. **Treatment.**

A. **Emergency and supportive measures**

1. Maintain an open airway and assist ventilation if needed (pp 1–7). Administer supplemental oxygen.

2. If hemolysis occurs, administer intravenous fluids and alkalinize the urine, as for rhabdomyolysis (see p 25), to prevent acute renal tubular necrosis. For severe hemolysis, blood transfusions may be required.

3. Mild symptoms may resolve without intervention, although it may take 2–3 days.

B. **Specific drugs and antidotes**

1. **Methylene blue** (see p 381) is indicated in the symptomatic patient with a methemoglobin level greater than 15% or with lower levels if even minimal compromise of oxygen-carrying capacity is potentially harmful (eg, severe pneumonia, anemia, or myocardial ischemia).

   a. Give 1–2 mg/kg (0.1–0.2 mL/kg of 1% solution) over several minutes. Therapeutic response may be delayed up to 30 minutes.

   b. Serious overdoses usually require repeated dosing every 6–8 hours for 2–3 days because of the prolonged half-life of dapsone and its metabolites.

   c. Methylene blue is ineffective for sulfhemoglobin, and can cause hemolysis in patients with G6PD deficiency. Excessive doses may worsen methemoglobinemia.

2. Other therapies such as ascorbic acid, cimetidine, and vitamin E have been proposed, but their efficacy is unproven.

C. **Decontamination** (see p 43)

1. **Prehospital.** Administer activated charcoal if available. Ipecac-induced vomiting may be useful for initial treatment at the scene (eg, children at home) if it can be given within a few minutes of exposure.

2. **Hospital.** Administer activated charcoal. Gastric emptying is not necessary after a small ingestion if activated charcoal can be given promptly, but

it should be considered for a large overdose, even if it has been more than 60 minutes since the ingestion (one report documented tablet fragment return 5 hours after ingestion).

D. **Enhanced elimination** (see p 51)
1. **Repeat-dose activated charcoal** interrupts enterohepatic recirculation and is very effective, reducing the half-life from 77 to 13.5 hours in one report. Continue charcoal for at least 48–72 hours.
2. **Charcoal hemoperfusion** can reduce the half-life to 1.5 hours and might be considered in a severe intoxication unresponsive to conventional treatment. Hemodialysis is ineffective because dapsone and its metabolites are highly protein bound.

▶ DETERGENTS

Gary J Ordog, MD and Jonathan Wasserberger, MD

Detergents, familiar and indispensable products in the home, are synthetic surface-active agents chemically classified as **anionic, nonionic**, or **cationic** (Table II–20). Most products also contain bleaching (chlorine-releasing), bacteriostatic (having a low concentration of quaternary ammonium compound), or enzymatic agents. Accidental ingestion of detergents by children is very common, but severe toxicity rarely occurs.

I. **Mechanism of toxicity.** Detergents may precipitate and denature protein, are irritating to tissues, and possess keratolytic and corrosive actions.
   A. **Anionic** and **nonionic** detergents are only mildly irritating, but **cationic** detergents are more hazardous because quaternary ammonium compounds may be caustic (benzalkonium chloride solutions of 10% have been reported to cause corrosive burns).
   B. **Low-phosphate** detergents and **electric dishwasher** soaps often contain alkaline corrosive agents such as sodium metasilicate, sodium carbonate, and sodium tripolyphosphate.
   C. The **enzyme-containing** detergents may cause skin irritation and have sensitizing properties; they may release bradykinin and histamine, causing bronchospasm.
II. **Toxic dose.** No minimum or lethal toxic doses have been established. Mortality and serious morbidity are rare. Cationic and dishwasher detergents are more dangerous than anionic and nonionic products.
III. **Clinical presentation.** Immediate spontaneous vomiting often occurs after oral ingestion. Large ingestions may produce intractable vomiting, diarrhea, and hematemesis. Exposure to the eye may cause mild to serious corrosive injury depending on the specific product. Dermal contact generally causes a mild erythema or rash.
   A. Phosphate-containing products may produce hypocalcemia and tetany.
   B. Methemoglobinemia was reported in a 45-year-old woman after copious irrigation of a hydatid cyst with a 0.1% solution of cetrimide, a cationic detergent.
IV. **Diagnosis** is based on a history of exposure and prompt onset of vomiting. A sudsy or foaming mouth may also suggest exposure.

TABLE II–20. COMMON CATIONIC DETERGENTS

Pyridinium compounds	Quaternary ammonium compounds	Quinolinium compounds
Cetalkonium chloride	Benzalkonium chloride	Dequalinium chloride
Cetrimide	Benzethonium chloride	
Cetrimonium bromide		
Cetylpyridinium chloride		
Stearalkonium chloride		

A. **Specific levels.** There are no specific blood or urine levels.
B. **Other useful laboratory studies** include electrolytes, glucose, calcium and phosphate (after ingestion of phosphate-containing products), and methemoglobin (cationic detergents).
V. **Treatment.**
  A. **Emergency and supportive measures**
    1. In patients with protracted vomiting or diarrhea, administer intravenous fluids to correct dehydration and electrolyte imbalance (see p 15).
    2. If corrosive injury is suspected, consult a gastroenterologist for possible endoscopy. Ingestion of products containing greater than 5–10% cationic detergents is more likely to cause corrosive injury.
  B. **Specific drugs and antidotes.** If symptomatic hypocalcemia occurs after ingestion of a phosphate-containing product, administer intravenous **calcium** (see p 350). If methemoglobinemia occurs, administer **methylene blue** (see p 381).
  C. **Decontamination** (see p 43)
    1. **Ingestion.** Dilute orally with small amounts of water or milk. A significant ingestion is unlikely if spontaneous vomiting has not already occurred.
      a. Do **not** induce vomiting because of the risk for corrosive injury.
      b. Consider gastric lavage after large ingestions of cationic, corrosive, or phosphate-containing detergents.
      c. Activated charcoal is not effective.
    2. **Eyes and skin.** Irrigate with copious amounts of tepid water or saline. Consult an ophthalmologist if eye pain persists or if there is significant corneal injury on fluorescein examination.
  D. **Enhanced elimination.** There is no role for these procedures.

▶ DEXTROMETHORPHAN

Timothy E. Albertson, MD, PhD

Dextromethorphan is a common antitussive agent found in many over-the-counter cough and cold preparations. Many ingestions occur in children, but severe intoxication is rare. Dextromethorphan is often found in combination products containing antihistamines (see p 84), decongestants (p 259), ethanol (p 162), or acetaminophen (p 62). *Common combination products containing dextromethorphan* include Nyquil Nighttime Cold Medicine, Triaminic Nite Lite, Pediacare 1, Pediacare 3, Robitussin DM, Robitussin CF, Triaminic DM, and Vicks Pediatric Formula 44.

I. **Mechanism of toxicity.** Dextromethorphan is the d-isomer of 3-methoxy-*N*-methylmorphinan, a synthetic analogue of codeine. (The l-isomer is the opioid analgesic levorphanol.) Although it has approximately equal antitussive efficacy as codeine, dextromethorphan has no apparent analgesic or addictive properties and produces relatively mild opioid effects in overdose.
  A. Both dextromethorphan and its o-demethylated metabolite appear to antagonize *N*-methyl-D-aspartate (NMDA) glutamate receptors, which may explain anticonvulsant properties and protection against hypoxia-ischemia observed in animal models.
  B. Dextromethorphan inhibits reuptake of serotonin, and may lead to the **serotonin syndrome** (p 21) in patients taking monoamine oxidase inhibitors (p 225). Serotoninergic effects, as well as NMDA glutatmate receptor inhibition, may explain the acute and chronic abuse potential of dextromethorphan.
  C. Dextromethorphan hydrobromide can cause bromide poisoning (p 115).
  D. **Pharmacokinetics.** Dextromethorphan is well absorbed orally, and effects are often apparent within 15–30 minutes (peak 2.5 hours). The volume of distribution is approximately 5–6 L/kg. The duration of effect is normally 3–6 hours. A genetic polymorphism exists for the debrisoquin hydroxylase enzyme (P450IIDC). Dextromethorphan is a high-affinity substrate for this enzyme.

Rapid metabolizers have a plasma half-life of about 3–4 hours, but in slow metabolizers (about 10% of the population) the half-life may exceed 24 hours. In addition, dextromethorphan competitively inhibits P-450IIID6-mediated metabolism, leading to many potential drug interactions. (See also Table II–55.)

II. **Toxic dose.** The toxic dose is highly variable and depends largely on other ingredients in the ingested product. Symptoms usually occur when the amount of dextromethorphan ingested exceeds 10 mg/kg. The usual recommended adult daily dose of dextromethorphan is 60–120 mg/d; in children age 2–5 years, up to 30 mg/d.

III. **Clinical presentation.**
  A. **Mild intoxication** produces clumsiness, ataxia, nystagmus, and restlessness. Visual and auditory hallucinations have been reported.
  B. With **severe poisoning**, stupor, coma, and respiratory depression may occur, especially if alcohol has been co-ingested. The pupils may be constricted or dilated. A few cases of seizures have been reported after ingestions of more than 20–30 mg/kg.
  C. **Serotonin syndrome** (see p 21). Severe hyperthermia, muscle rigidity, and hypertension may occur with therapeutic doses in patients taking **monoamine oxidase inhibitors** (see p 225).

IV. **Diagnosis** should be considered with ingestion of any over-the-counter cough suppressant, especially when there is nystagmus, ataxia, and lethargy. Because dextromethorphan is often combined with other ingredients (eg, antihistamines, phenylpropanolamine, or acetaminophen), suspect mixed ingestion.
  A. **Specific levels.** Both gas chromatography (GC) and high-performance liquid chromatography (HPLC) assays exist for serum and urine analysis, but are not generally available, nor are they clinically useful. Despite its structural similarity to opioids, even twice therapeutic doses of dextromethorphan are not likely to produce a false-positive urine opioid EMIT screen. Dextromethorphan is readily detected by comprehensive urine toxicology screening.
  B. **Other useful laboratory studies** include electrolytes, glucose, and arterial blood gases (if respiratory depression is suspected). Blood ethanol and acetaminophen levels should be obtained if those drugs are contained in the ingested product.

V. **Treatment.**
  A. **Emergency and supportive measures.** Most patients with mild symptoms (ie, restlessness, ataxia, or mild drowsiness) can be observed for 4–6 hours and discharged if they are improving.
    1. Maintain an open airway and assist ventilation if needed (see pp 1–7).
    2. Treat seizures (p 21) and coma (p 18) if they occur.
  B. **Specific drugs and antidotes.** Although **naloxone** (see p 384) has been reported effective in doses of 0.06–0.4 mg, other cases have failed to respond to as much as 2.4 mg.
  C. **Decontamination** (see p 43)
    1. **Prehospital.** Administer activated charcoal if available. Do **not** induce vomiting, because signs of intoxication can develop rapidly.
    2. **Hospital.** Administer activated charcoal. Gastric emptying is not necessary if activated charcoal can be given promptly.
  D. **Enhanced elimination.** The volume of distribution of dextromethorphan is very large, and there is no role for enhanced removal procedures.

▶ **DIOXINS**

Paul D. Blanc, MD, MSPH

Polychlorinated dibenzodioxins (PCDDs) and dibenzofurans (PCDFs) are a group of highly toxic substances commonly known as dioxins. PCDDs are formed during the production of certain organochlorines (trichlorophenoxyacetic acid [2,4,5-T], silvex, hexachlorophene, pentachlorophenol, etc), and PCDFs are formed by the combustion of these and other compounds such as polychlorinated biphenyls (PCBs; see p 274). Agent Orange, a herbicide used by the United States against Vietnam during the Vietnam War, contained dioxins (most importantly, 2,3,7,8-tetrachlorodibenzo-*p*-dioxin [TCDD]) as contaminants.

I. **Mechanism of toxicity.** Dioxins are highly lipid-soluble and are concentrated in fat and the thymus. Dioxins are known to induce porphyrinogen synthesis and oxidative cytochrome P-450 metabolism and have a variety of effects on various organ systems. The actual mechanism of toxicity is unknown. They are mutagenic and are suspected human carcinogens.

II. **Toxic dose.** Dioxins are extremely potent animal toxins. The FDA-suggested "no effect" level for inhalation is 70 ng/d per person. The oral 50% lethal dose (LD_{50}) in animals varies from 0.0006 to 0.045 mg/kg. Daily dermal exposure to 10–30 ppm in oil or 100–3000 ppm in soil produces toxicity in animals. Chloracne is likely with daily dermal exposure exceeding 100 ppm.

III. **Clinical presentation.**
   A. **Acute symptoms** after exposure include irritation of the skin, eyes, and mucous membranes and nausea, vomiting, and myalgias.
   B. **After a latency period** which may be prolonged (up to several weeks or more), chloracne, porphyria cutanea tarda, hirsutism, or hyperpigmentation may occur. Elevated levels of hepatic transaminases and blood lipids may be found. Polyneuropathies with sensory impairment and lower-extremity motor weakness have been reported.
   C. **Death** in laboratory animals occurs a few weeks after a lethal dose and is caused by a "wasting syndrome" characterized by reduced food intake and loss of body weight.

IV. **Diagnosis** is difficult and rests mainly on history of exposure; the presence of chloracne (which is considered pathognomonic for exposure to dioxins and related compounds) provides strong supporting evidence. Although 2,4,5-T no longer contains TCDD as a contaminant, possible exposures to PCDDs and PCDFs occur during many types of chemical fires (eg, PCBs), and the possibility of exposure can cause considerable public and individual anxiety.
   A. **Specific levels.** It is difficult and expensive to detect dioxins in human blood or tissue, and there is no established correlation with symptoms. Unexposed persons have a mean of 7 pg of 2,3,7,8-TCDD per g of serum lipid, compared with workers producing trichlorophenols, who had a mean of 220 pg/g.
   B. **Other useful laboratory studies** include glucose, electrolytes, BUN, creatinine, liver transaminases and liver function tests, and uroporphyrins (if porphyria suspected).

V. **Treatment.**
   A. **Emergency and supportive measures.** Treat skin, eye, and respiratory irritation symptomatically.
   B. **Specific drugs and antidotes.** There is no specific antidote.
   C. **Decontamination** (see p 43)
      1. **Inhalation.** Remove victims from exposure and give supplemental oxygen if available.
      2. **Eyes and skin.** Remove contaminated clothing and wash affected skin with copious soap and water; irrigate exposed eyes with copious tepid water or saline. Personnel involved in decontamination should wear protective gear appropriate to the suspected level of contamination.
      3. **Ingestion**
         a. **Prehospital.** Administer activated charcoal if available. Ipecac-induced vomiting may be useful for initial treatment at the scene (eg, children at home) if it can be given within a few minutes of exposure.
         b. **Hospital.** Administer activated charcoal. Gastric emptying is not necessary if activated charcoal can be given promptly.
   D. **Enhanced elimination.** There is no known role for these procedures.

▶ DISULFIRAM

Richard J. Geller, MD

Disulfiram (tetraethylthiuram disulfide or Antabuse) is an antioxidant industrial chemical also used as a drug in the treatment of alcoholism. Ingestion of ethanol while taking disulfiram causes a well-defined unpleasant reaction, the fear of which provides a negative incentive to drink.

I. **Mechanism of toxicity.** Disulfiram inhibits aldehyde dehydrogenase, leading to accumulation of acetaldehyde after ethanol ingestion. In addition, it inhibits dopamine betahydroxylase (necessary for norepinephrine synthesis), resulting in norepinephrine depletion at pre-synaptic sympathetic nerve endings and leading to vasodilation and orthostatic hypotension.

   Pharmacokinetics. Disulfiram is rapidly and completely absorbed, but peak effects require 8–12 hours. Although the elimination half-life is 7–8 hours, clinical actions may persist for several days. Disulfiram is metabolized in the liver; it inhibits the metabolism of many other drugs, including isoniazid, phenytoin, theophylline, phenytoin, warfarin, and many benzodiazepines. (See also Table II–55.)

II. **Toxic dose.**
   A. **Disulfiram overdose.** Ingestion of 2.5 g or more has caused toxicity in children after a delay of 3–12 hours.
   B. **Disulfiram-ethanol interaction.** Ingestion of as little as 7 mL of ethanol can cause a severe reaction in patients taking as little as 200 mg/d of disulfiram. Mild reactions have been reported after use of cough syrup, after-shave lotions, and other alcohol-containing products.

III. **Clinical presentation.**
   A. **Acute disulfiram overdose (without ethanol)** may cause vomiting, ataxia, confusion, lethargy, seizures, and coma. Hypersensitivity hepatitis has occurred, including several deaths resulting from hepatic failure.
   B. **Disulfiram-ethanol interaction.** Shortly after ingestion of ethanol, the patient receiving chronic disulfiram therapy develops flushing, throbbing headache, dyspnea, anxiety, vertigo, vomiting, and confusion. Orthostatic hypotension with warm extremities is very common.

   The severity of the reaction usually depends on the dose of disulfiram and ethanol. Reactions do not usually occur unless the patient has been on oral disulfiram therapy for at least 1 day; the reaction may occur up to several days after the last dose of disulfiram. Disulfiram has been implanted subcutaneously in Europe, leading to reactions after alcohol consumption that are milder but of longer duration.

IV. **Diagnosis** of disulfiram overdose is based on a history of acute ingestion and the presence of CNS symptoms. The disulfiram-ethanol interaction is diagnosed in a patient with a history of chronic disulfiram use and possible exposure to ethanol who exhibits a characteristic hypotensive flushing reaction.
   A. **Specific levels.** Blood disulfiram levels are not of value in diagnosis or treatment. Blood acetaldehyde levels may be elevated during the disulfiram-ethanol reaction, but this information is of little value in acute management.
   B. **Other useful laboratory studies** include electrolytes, glucose, BUN, creatinine, liver transaminases, and ethanol level.

V. **Treatment.**
   A. **Emergency and supportive measures**
      1. **Acute disulfiram overdose**
         a. Maintain an open airway and assist ventilation if necessary (see pp 1–7).
         b. Treat coma (p 18) and seizures (p 21) if they occur.
      2. **Disulfiram-ethanol interaction**
         a. Maintain an open airway and assist ventilation if necessary (see pp 1–7).
         b. Treat hypotension with supine position and intravenous fluids (eg, saline), and treat vomiting with metoclopramide (see p 382). If a pres-

sor agent is needed, a direct-acting agent such as norepinephrine (see
p 393) is preferred over indirect-acting drugs such as dopamine.
   c. Administer benzodiazepine anxiolytics (eg, diazepam or lorazepam,
   p 342) and reassurance as needed.
B. Specific drugs and antidotes. There is no specific antidote.
C. Decontamination (see p 43)
   1. Acute disulfiram overdose
      a. Prehospital. Administer activated charcoal, if available. Do **not** induce
      vomiting.
      b. Hospital. Administer activated charcoal. Gastric emptying is not neces-
      sary if activated charcoal can be given promptly.
   2. Disulfiram-ethanol interaction. Decontamination procedures are not
   likely to be of benefit once the reaction begins
D. Enhanced elimination. Hemodialysis is not indicated for disulfiram overdose, but it may remove ethanol and acetaldehyde and has been reported to
   be effective in treating the acute disulfiram-ethanol interaction. This is not
   likely to be necessary in patients receiving adequate fluid and pressor support. There are no data to support the use of repeat-dose activated charcoal
   for any of the disulfiram syndromes.

▶ DIURETICS

Shoshana Zevin, MD

Diuretics are commonly prescribed for the management of essential hypertension.
Adverse effects from chronic use or misuse are more frequently encountered than
those from acute overdose. Overdoses are generally benign, and no serious outcomes have resulted from acute ingestion. Common currently available diuretics are
listed in Table II–21.
   I. Mechanism of toxicity. The toxicity of these drugs is associated with their phar-
      macologic effects to decrease fluid volume and promote electrolyte loss, includ-
      ing dehydration, hypokalemia (or hyperkalemia, with spironolactone), hypomag-
      nesemia, hyponatremia, and hypochloremic alkalosis. Electrolyte imbalance may
      lead to cardiac arrhythmias and may enhance digitalis toxicity (see p 128). Di-

TABLE II–21. COMMON DIURETICS

Drug	Maximum Adult Daily Dose (mg)	Drug	Maximum Adult Daily Dose (mg)
Carbonic anhydrase inhibitors		**Thiazides**	
Acetazolamide	1000	Bendroflumethiazide	20
Dichlorphenamide	200	Chlorothiazide	2000
Methazolamide	300	Chlorthalidone	200
Loop diuretics		Cyclothiazide	6
Bumetanide	2	Flumethiazide	2000
Ethacrynic acid	200	Hydrochlorothiazide	200
Furosemide	600	Hydroflumethiazide	200
Mercurial		Indapamide	5
Mersalyl	200	Methyclothiazide	10
Potassium-sparing		Metolazone	20
Amiloride	20	Polythiazide	4
Spironolactone	200	Quinethazone	200
Triamterene	300	Trichlormethiazide	4

uretics are classified based on the pharmacologic mechanisms by which they affect solute and water loss (Table II–21).
   Pharmacokinetics. See Table II–55, p 319.
II. Toxic dose. Minimum toxic doses have not been established. Significant dehydration or electrolyte imbalance is unlikely if the amount ingested is less than the usual recommended daily dose (Table II–21). High doses of intravenous ethacrynic acid and furosemide can cause ototoxicity, especially when administered rapidly and in patients with renal failure.
III. Clinical presentation. Gastrointestinal symptoms including nausea, vomiting, and diarrhea are common after acute oral overdose. Lethargy, weakness, hyporeflexia, and dehydration (and occasionally hypotension) may be present if volume loss and electrolyte disturbances are present, although the onset of symptoms may be delayed for 2–4 hours or more until diuretic action is obtained. Spironolactone is very slow, with maximal effects after the third day.
   A. Hypokalemia may cause muscle weakness, cramps, and tetany. Severe hypokalemia may result in flaccid paralysis and rhabdomyolysis. Cardiac rhythm disturbances may also occur.
   B. Spironolactone and other potassium-sparing agents may cause hyperkalemia.
   C. Hypocalcemia and hypomagnesemia may also cause tetany.
   D. Hyperglycemia, hypercalcemia, and hyperuricemia may occur, especially with thiazide diuretics.
   E. Carbonic anhydrase inhibitors may induce metabolic acidosis.
IV. Diagnosis is based on a history of exposure and evidence of dehydration and acid-base or electrolyte imbalance. Note that patients on diuretics may also be taking other cardiac and antihypertensive medications.
   A. Specific levels are not routinely available nor clinically useful.
   B. Other useful laboratory studies include electrolytes (including calcium and magnesium), glucose, BUN, creatinine, and ECG.
V. Treatment.
   A. Emergency and supportive measures
      1. Replace fluid loss with intravenous crystalloid solutions, and correct electrolyte abnormalities (see Potassium, p 36).
      2. Monitor the ECG until the potassium level is normalized.
   B. Specific drugs and antidotes. There are no specific antidotes.
   C. Decontamination (see p 43)
      1. Prehospital. Administer activated charcoal if available.
      2. Hospital. Administer activated charcoal. Do not use a cathartic if the patient appears dehydrated. Gastric emptying is not necessary if activated charcoal can be given promptly.
   D. Enhanced elimination. No experience with extracorporeal removal of diuretics has been reported.

▶ ERGOT DERIVATIVES

Neal L. Benowitz, MD

Ergot derivatives are used primarily to treat migraine headache and to a lesser extent to enhance uterine contraction postpartum. Ergots are produced by the fungus *Claviceps purpurea*, which may grow on rye and other grains. Specific ergot-containing drugs include ergotamine (Cafergot, Ergomar, Gynergen, and Ergostat), methysergide (Sansert), dihydroergotamine (DHE-45), and ergonovine (Ergotrate). Some ergoloid derivatives (dihydroergocornine, dihydroergocristine, and dihydroergocryptine) have been used in combination (Hydergine and Deapril-ST) for the treatment of dementia. Bromocriptine (Parlodel, see p 348) and pergolide (Permax) are ergot derivatives with dopamine agonist activity used to treat Parkinson's disease. Bromocriptine is also used to treat hyperprolactinemic states.

I. **Mechanism of toxicity.** Ergot derivatives directly stimulate vasoconstriction and uterine contraction, antagonize alpha-adrenergic and serotonin receptors, and may also dilate some blood vessels via a CNS sympatholytic action. The relative contribution of each of these mechanisms to toxicity depends on the particular ergot alkaloid and its dose. **Sustained vasoconstriction** causes most of the serious toxicity; reduced blood flow causes local tissue hypoxia and ischemic injury, resulting in tissue edema and local thrombosis, worsening ischemia and causing further injury. At a certain point, reversible vasospasm progresses to irreversible vascular insufficiency and limb gangrene.

    Pharmacokinetics. See Table II–55, p 319.

II. **Toxic dose.** Death has been reported in a 14-month-old child after acute ingestion of 12 mg of ergotamine. However, most cases of severe poisoning occur with chronic overmedication for migraine headaches rather than acute single overdoses. Daily doses of 10 mg or more of ergotamine are usually associated with toxicity. There are many case reports of vasospastic complications with normal therapeutic dosing.

III. **Clinical presentation.**
    A. **Ergotamine and related agents.** Mild intoxication causes nausea and vomiting. Serious poisoning results in vasoconstriction that may involve many parts of the body. Owing to persistence of ergots in tissues, vasospasm may continue for up to 10–14 days.
        1. Involvement of the extremities causes paresthesias, pain, pallor, coolness, and loss of peripheral pulses in the hands and feet; gangrene may ensue.
        2. Other complications of vasospasm include coronary ischemia and myocardial infarction, abdominal angina and bowel infarction, renal infarction and failure, visual disturbances and blindness, and stroke. Psychosis, seizures, and coma occur rarely.
    B. **Bromocriptine** intoxication may present with hallucinations, paranoid behavior, hypertension and tachycardia. Involuntary movements, hallucinations, and hypotension are reported with **pergolide**.
    C. Chronic use of **methysergide** occasionally causes retroperitoneal fibrosis.

IV. **Diagnosis** is based on a history of ergot use and clinical findings of vasospasm.
    A. **Specific levels.** Ergotamine levels are not widely available, and blood concentrations do not correlate well with toxicity.
    B. **Other useful laboratory studies** include CBC, electrolytes, BUN, creatinine, and ECG. Arteriography of the affected vascular bed is occasionally indicated.

V. **Treatment.**
    A. **Emergency and supportive measures**
        1. Maintain an open airway and assist ventilation if necessary (see pp 1–7).
        2. Treat coma (p 18) and convulsions (p 21) if they occur.
        3. Immediately discontinue ergot treatment. Hospitalize patients with vasospastic symptoms and treat promptly to prevent complications.
    B. **Specific drugs and antidotes**
        1. **Peripheral ischemia** requires prompt vasodilator therapy and anticoagulation to prevent local thrombosis.
            a. Administer intravenous **nitroprusside** (see p 392), starting with 1–2 μg/kg/min, or intravenous **phentolamine** (p 400), starting with 0.5 mg/min, increasing the infusion rate until ischemia is improved or systemic hypotension occurs. Intra-arterial infusion is occasionally required. **Nifedipine** (p 389) or other calcium antagonists may also enhance peripheral blood flow.
            b. Administer **heparin**, 5000 units IV followed by 1000 units/h (in adults), with adjustments in the infusion rate to maintain the activated coagulation time (ACT) or the activated partial thromboplastin time (APTT) at approximately 2 times the baseline.
        2. **Coronary spasm.** Administer **nitroglycerin**, 0.15–0.6 mg sublingually or 5–20 μg/min IV; or **nifedipine** (p 389), 10–20 mg PO (adult doses). Intra-

coronary artery nitroglycerin may be required if there is no response to intravenous infusion.

C. **Decontamination** after acute ingestion (see p 45).
   1. **Prehospital.** Administer activated charcoal if available. Ipecac-induced vomiting may be useful for initial treatment at the scene (eg, children at home) if it can be given within a few minutes of exposure.
   2. **Hospital.** Administer activated charcoal. Gastric emptying is not necessary if activated charcoal can be given promptly.
D. **Enhanced elimination.** Dialysis and hemoperfusion are not effective. Repeat-dose charcoal has not been studied, but because of extensive tissue distribution of ergots it is not likely to be useful.

▶ ETHANOL

B. Zane Horowitz, MD

Commercial beer, wine, and liquors contain various amounts of ethanol. Ethanol is also found in a variety of colognes, perfumes, after-shaves, mouthwashes, some rubbing alcohols, many food flavorings (eg, vanilla, almond, and lemon extracts), pharmaceutical preparations (eg, elixirs), and many other products. Ethanol is frequently ingested recreationally and is the most common co-ingestant with other drugs in suicide attempts. Ethanol may also serve as an antidote in the emergency treatment of methanol and ethylene glycol poisonings (see p 367).

I. **Mechanism of toxicity.**
   A. **CNS depression** is the principal effect of acute ethanol intoxication. Ethanol has additive effects with other CNS depressants such as barbiturates, benzodiazepines, opioids, antidepressants, and antipsychotics.
   B. **Hypoglycemia** may be caused by impaired gluconeogenesis in patients with depleted glycogen stores (particularly small children and poorly nourished persons).
   C. Ethanol intoxication and chronic alcoholism also predispose patients to trauma, exposure-induced hypothermia, injurious effects of alcohol on the gastrointestinal tract and nervous system, and a number of nutritional disorders and metabolic derangements.
   D. **Pharmacokinetics.** Ethanol is readily absorbed (peak 30–120 min) and distributed into the body water (volume of distribution 0.5–0.7 L/kg or about 50 liters in the average adult). Elimination is mainly by oxidation in the liver and follows zero-order kinetics. The average adult can metabolize about 7–10 g of alcohol per hour; or about 12–25 mg/dL/h (this rate is highly variable depending on the individual and the blood alcohol level).
II. **Toxic dose.** Generally, 0.7 g/kg pure ethanol (approximately 3–4 drinks) will produce a blood ethanol concentration of 100 mg/dL (0.1 g/dL), legally considered intoxicated in many states.
   A. A level of 100 mg/dL decreases reaction time and judgment and may be enough to inhibit gluconeogenesis and cause hypoglycemia in children and patients with liver disease, but by itself is not enough to cause coma.
   B. The level sufficient to cause deep coma or respiratory depression is highly variable, depending on the individual's degree of tolerance to ethanol. Although levels above 300 mg/dL usually cause coma in novice drinkers, chronic alcoholics may be awake with levels of 500–600 mg/dL or higher.
III. **Clinical presentation.**
   A. **Acute intoxication**
      1. With **mild** to moderate intoxication, patients exhibit euphoria, mild incoordination, ataxia, nystagmus, and impaired judgment and reflexes. Social inhibitions are loosened, and boisterous or aggressive behavior is com-

mon. Hypoglycemia may occur, especially in children and in persons with reduced hepatic glycogen stores

2. With **deep intoxication**, coma, respiratory depression, and pulmonary aspiration may occur. In these patients, the pupils are usually small and the temperature, blood pressure, and pulse rate are often decreased. Rhabdomyolysis may result from prolonged immobilization on a hard floor.

B. **Chronic ethanol abuse** is associated with numerous complications:

1. **Hepatic toxicity** includes fatty infiltration of the liver, alcoholic hepatitis, and cirrhosis. Liver scarring leads to portal hypertension, ascites, and bleeding from esophageal varices and hemorrhoids; hyponatremia from fluid retention; and bacterial peritonitis. Production of clotting factors is impaired, leading to prolonged prothrombin time (PT). Hepatic metabolism of drugs and endogenous toxins is impaired and may contribute to hepatic encephalopathy.

2. **Gastrointestinal** bleeding may result from alcohol-induced gastritis, esophagitis, and duodenitis. Other causes of massive bleeding include Mallory-Weiss tears of the esophagus and esophageal varices. Acute pancreatitis is a common cause of abdominal pain and vomiting.

3. **Cardiac** disorders include various dysrhythmias associated with potassium and magnesium depletion and poor caloric intake ("Holiday heart") and cardiomyopathy, which has been associated with long-term alcohol use as well as with ingestion of cobalt (which was once used to stabilize beer).

4. **Neurologic** toxicity includes cerebral atrophy; cerebellar degeneration; and peripheral stocking-glove sensory neuropathy. Nutritional disorders such as thiamine (Vitamin B-1) deficiency can cause Wernicke's encephalopathy or Korsakoff's psychosis.

5. **Alcoholic ketoacidosis** is characterized by anion gap metabolic acidosis and elevated levels of betahydroxybutyrate and, to a lesser extent, acetoacetate. The osmolar gap may also be elevated, causing this condition to be mistaken for methanol or ethylene glycol poisoning.

C. **Alcohol withdrawal.** Sudden discontinuation after chronic high-level alcohol use often causes headache, tremulousness, anxiety, palpitations, and insomnia. Brief, generalized seizures may occur, usually within 6–12 hours. Sympathetic nervous system overactivity may progress to **delirium tremens**, a life-threatening syndrome charcaterized by tacycardia, diaphoresis, hyperthermia, and delirium, which usually manifests 48–72 hours after cessation of heavy alcohol use. The "DTs" may cause significant morbidity and mortality if untreated.

D. **Other problems.** Ethanol abusers sometimes intentionally or accidentally ingest ethanol substitutes such as isopropyl alcohol (see p 197), methanol (p 218), or ethylene glycol (p 166). In addition, ethanol may serve as the vehicle for swallowing large numbers of pills in a suicide attempt. Disulfiram (Antabuse, p 158) use can cause a serious acute reaction with ethanol.

IV. **Diagnosis** of ethanol intoxication is usually simple, based on the history of ingestion, the characteristic smell of fresh alcohol or the fetid odor of acetaldehyde and other metabolic products, and the presence of nystagmus, ataxia, and altered mental status. It is imperative to consider other etiologies that may accompany or mimic intoxication, such as hypoglycemia, head trauma, hypothermia, meningitis, or intoxication with other drugs or poisons.

A. **Specific levels.** Serum ethanol levels are easily and rapidly determined by most hospital laboratories and, depending on the method used, are accurate and specific.

1. In general, there is only rough correlation between blood levels and clinical presentation; however, an ethanol level below 300 mg/dL in a comatose patient should initiate a search for alternative causes.

2. If ethanol levels are not readily available, the ethanol concentration may be estimated by calculating the osmolar gap (see p 30).

B. **Suggested laboratory studies** include glucose, electrolytes, BUN, creatinine, liver transaminases, prothrombin time (PT), magnesium, arterial blood gases or oximetry, and chest x-ray (if pulmonary aspiration is suspected). Consider CT scan of the head if the patient has focal neurological deficits or altered mental status inconsistent with the degree of blood alcohol elevation.

V. **Treatment.**

A. **Emergency and supportive measures**

   1. **Acute intoxication.** Treatment is mainly supportive.

      a. Protect the airway to prevent aspiration and intubate and assist ventilation if needed (pp 1–7).

      b. Give glucose and thiamine (pp 372 and 408), and treat coma (p 18) and seizures (p 21) if they occur. Glucagon is not effective for alcohol-induced hypoglycemia.

      c. Correct hypothermia with gradual rewarming (p 19).

      d. Most patients will recover within 4–6 hours. Observe children until their blood alcohol level is below 50 mg/dL and there is no evidence of hypoglycemia.

   2. **Alcoholic ketoacidosis.** Treat with volume replacement, thiamine (p 408), and supplemental glucose (p 372). Most patients recover rapidly.

   3. **Alcohol withdrawal.** Treat with benzodiazepines (eg, diazepam, 2–10 mg IV initially, repeated as needed; see p 342).

B. **Specific drugs and antidotes.** There is no available specific ethanol receptor antagonist, despite anecdotal reports of arousal after administration of naloxone.

C. **Decontamination** (see p 43)

   2. **Prehospital.** Do not induce vomiting or administer activated charcoal.

   2. **Hospital.** Because ethanol is rapidly absorbed, gastric lavage is usually not indicated unless other drug ingestion is suspected. Consider lavage only if the alcohol ingestion was massive and recent (within 30–45 minutes). Activated charcoal does not effectively adsorb ethanol but may be given if other toxins were ingested.

D. **Enhanced elimination.** Metabolism of ethanol normally occurs at a fixed rate of approximately 20–30 mg/dL/h. Elimination rates are faster in chronic alcoholics and at serum levels above 300 mg/dL. Hemodialysis efficiently removes ethanol, but enhanced removal is rarely needed because supportive care is usually sufficient. Hemoperfusion and forced diuresis are not effective.

▶ ETHYLENE DIBROMIDE

Janet Weiss, MD

Ethylene dibromide (EDB or dibromoethane) is a volatile liquid produced by the bromination of ethylene. EDB is used as a lead scavenger in leaded gasoline and as a pesticide and fumigant in soil and on grain, fruits, and vegetables. Because EDB has been classified as a suspected human carcinogen and is a male reproductive toxin, its use as a pesticide has been restricted since 1984.

I. **Mechanism of toxicity.**

A. **Liquid EDB is an irritant** capable of causing chemical burns. Inhalation of EDB vapor produces respiratory tract irritation and delayed-onset pulmonary edema.

B. **Once absorbed systemically,** EDB is converted to active metabolites that become irreversibly bound to macromolecules, including DNA, and inhibit enzymes. Metabolism of EDB involves an oxidative pathway (cytochrome p-450) and a conjugation pathway (glutathione). The liver is a principal target organ for toxicity.

II. Toxic dose.
    A. Inhalation. Because EDB is a suspected carcinogen (ACGIH category A2), no "safe" workplace exposure limit has been determined. Although the current OSHA legal Permissible Exposure Limit (PEL) is 20 ppm as an 8-hour time-weighted average with a ceiling of 30 ppm, the National Institute for Occupational Safety and Health (NIOSH) recommends a ceiling exposure of no more than 0.13 ppm. Exposure to vapor concentrations greater than 200 ppm can produce lung irritation, and 400 ppm is the air level considered immediately dangerous to life or health (IDLH).
    B. Ingestion of 4.5 mL of liquid EDB (160 mg/kg) resulted in death.
    C. Dermal application of as little as 16 mg/kg caused systemic intoxication.
    D. The Environmental Protection Agency (EPA) drinking-water Maximum Contaminant Limit (MCL) for EDB is 0.00005 mg/L.
III. Clinical presentation.
    A. Inhalation of EDB vapor causes irritation of the eyes and upper respiratory tract. Pulmonary edema usually occurs within 1–6 hours but may be delayed as long as 48 hours after exposure.
    B. Skin exposure produces painful local inflammation, swelling, and blistering.
    C. Oral ingestion causes prompt vomiting and diarrhea.
    D. Systemic manifestations of intoxication include CNS depression, delirium, seizures, and metabolic acidosis. Skeletal muscle necrosis, acute renal failure, and hepatic necrosis have also been reported in fatal cases.
IV. Diagnosis of EDB poisoning is based on a history of exposure and evidence of upper-airway and eye irritation (in cases of inhalation) or gastroenteritis (after ingestion). EDB vapor has a strong chemical odor.
    A. Specific levels. EDB is detectable in expired air, blood, and tissues, although levels are not useful in emergency management. Serum bromide levels may be elevated (> 0.1 mEq/L) in severe cases, because bromide is released from EDB in the body.
    B. Other useful laboratory studies include electrolytes, glucose, BUN, creatinine, liver transaminases, CPK, arterial blood gases, and chest x-ray.
V. Treatment.
    A. Emergency and supportive measures
       1. Maintain an open airway and assist ventilation if necessary (see pp 1–7).
       2. After inhalation exposure, anticipate and treat wheezing, airway obstruction, and pulmonary edema (pp 7–8). Monitor blood gases, provide supplemental oxygen if needed, and avoid fluid overload.
       3. Treat coma (p 18), seizures (p 21), rhabdomyolysis (p 25), and metabolic acidosis (p 31) if they occur.
    B. Specific drugs and antidotes. There is no specific antidote.
    C. Decontamination (see p 43). *Caution*: Rescuers should use self-contained breathing apparatus and wear protective clothing to avoid personal exposure.
       1. Inhalation. Remove the victim from exposure and provide supplemental oxygen if available.
       2. Skin and eyes. Remove and safely discard all contaminated clothing, and wash exposed skin with copious soap and water. Irrigate exposed eyes with tepid saline or water.
       3. Ingestion
          a. Prehospital. Administer activated charcoal if available. Do **not** induce vomiting, because of corrosive effects and the risk of rapid onset of coma or seizures.
          b. Hospital. Perform gastric lavage if the patient presents within 30 minutes of ingestion or has ingested a large quantity (more than 1–2 oz). Administer activated charcoal.
    D. Enhanced elimination. There is no role for dialysis or hemoperfusion, diuresis, or repeat-dose charcoal.

▶ ETHYLENE GLYCOL AND OTHER GLYCOLS

Ilene B. Anderson, PharmD

Ethylene glycol is the primary ingredient (up to 95%) in antifreeze. It is sometimes intentionally consumed as an alcohol substitute by alcoholics and is tempting to children because of its sweet taste. Intoxication by ethylene glycol itself causes inebriation and mild gastritis; in addition, its metabolic products cause metabolic acidosis, renal failure, and death. Other glycols may also produce toxicity (Table II–22).

I. **Mechanism of toxicity.**
   A. **Ethylene glycol** is metabolized by alcohol dehydrogenase to glycoaldehyde, which is then metabolized to glycolic, glyoxylic, and oxalic acids. These acids, along with excess lactic acid, are responsible for the anion gap metabolic acidosis. Oxalate readily precipitates with calcium to form insoluble calcium oxalate crystals. Tissue injury is caused by widespread deposition of oxalate crystals and the toxic effects of glycolic and glyoxylic acids.
   B. **Pharmacokinetics.** Ethylene glycol is well-absorbed. The volume of distribution (Vd) is about 0.8 L/kg. It is not protein bound. Metabolism is by alcohol dehydrogenase with a half-life of about 3–5 hours. In the presence of ethanol or fomepizole (see below), which block ethylene glycol metabolism, elimination is entirely renal with a half-life of about 17 hours.
   B. **Other glycols** (Table II–22). Propylene and dipropylene glycols are of relatively low toxicity. Polypropylene glycol and other high-molecular-weight polyethylene glycols are poorly absorbed and virtually nontoxic. However, diethylene glycol and glycol ethers produce toxic metabolites with toxicity similar to that of ethylene glycol.
II. **Toxic dose.** The approximate lethal oral dose of 95% ethylene glycol (eg, antifreeze) is 1.5 mL/kg; however, survival has been reported after an ingestion of 2 L in a patient who received treatment within 1 hour of ingestion.
III. **Clinical presentation.**
   A. **Ethylene glycol**
      1. **During the first 3–4 hours** after acute ingestion, the victim may appear intoxicated as if by ethanol. The osmolar gap (see p 30) is increased, but there is no initial acidosis. Gastritis with vomiting may also occur.
      2. **After a delay of 4–12 hours,** evidence of intoxication by metabolic products occurs, with anion gap acidosis, hyperventilation, convulsions, coma, cardiac conduction disturbances, and arrhythmias. Renal failure is common but usually reversible. Pulmonary edema and cerebral edema may also occur. Hypocalcemia with tetany has been reported.
   B. **Other glycols** (Table II–22). Diethylene glycol and glycol ethers are extremely toxic and may produce acute renal failure and metabolic acidosis. Calcium oxalate crystals may or may not be present.
IV. **Diagnosis** of ethylene glycol poisoning is usually based on the history of antifreeze ingestion, typical symptoms, and elevation of the osmolar and anion gaps. Oxalate or hippurate crystals may be present in the urine (crystals may be cuboidal or elongate in form). Because many antifreeze products contain fluorescein, the urine may fluoresce under Wood's lamp, depending on the amount ingested, the time since ingestion, and the urine concentration.
   A. **Specific levels.** Tests for ethylene glycol levels are usually available from regional commercial toxicology laboratories but are difficult to obtain quickly.
      1. Serum levels higher than 50 mg/dL are usually associated with serious intoxication, although lower levels do not rule out poisoning if the parent compound has already been metabolized (in such a case, the anion gap should be markedly elevated). Calculation of the osmolar gap (see p 30) may be used to estimate the ethylene glycol level.
      2. False-positive ethylene glycol levels can be caused by elevated triglycerides (see Table I–33, p 41).

TABLE II–22. TOXICITY OF OTHER GLYCOLS

Compounds	Toxicity and Comments	Treatment
Propylene glycol	Relatively low toxicity. Lactic acidosis, central nervous system depression, coma, hypoglycemia, seizures, and hemolysis have been reported rarely after massive exposures or chronic exposures in high-risk patients. Risk factors include: renal insufficiency, small infants, epilepsy, or burn patients with extensive dermal application of propylene glycol. Osmolar gap, anion gap, and lactate may be elevated. Levels: 70 mg/dL resulted in lactic acidosis and central nervous system depression in a patient with azotemia; 6–42 mg/dL did not result in toxicity after acute infusion; 70 mg/dL resulted in lactic acidosis with a lactate level equal to 24 meq/L without an osmolar gap following chronic infusion; 1059 mg/dL was reported in an 8-month-old with extensive burn injuries after repeated dermal application (the child experienced cardiopulmonary arrest); 400 mg/dL was measured in an epileptic patient who experienced status epilepticus, respiratory depression, elevated osmolar gap, and metabolic acidosis. Metabolites are lactate and pyruvate. Molecular weight is 76.	Supportive care, sodium bicarbonate. There is no role for ethanol therapy. Hemodialysis is effective but rarely indicated.
Dipropylene glycol	Relatively low toxicity. Central nervous system depression, hepatic injury, and renal damage have occurred in animal studies after massive exposures. There are no reports of acidosis or lactate elevation. Molecular weight is 134.	Supportive care. There is no role for ethanol therapy.
Polyethylene glycols	Very low toxicity. A group of compounds with molecular weights ranging from 200 to more than 4000. High-molecular-weight compounds (>500) are poorly absorbed and are rapidly excreted by the kidneys. Low-molecular-weight compounds (200–400) may result in metabolic acidosis, renal failure, hypercalcemia, and elevation in the osmolar gap after massive oral ingestions or repeated dermal applications in patients with extensive burn injuries. Alcohol dehydrogenase metabolizes polyethylene glycols.	Supportive care.
Diethylene glycol	Highly nephrotoxic: similar to ethylene glycol. Renal failure, coma, acidosis, and death have been reported in 5 patients with extensive burn injuries after repeated dermal application. Calcium oxalate crystals have not been reported in human poisoning but have been seen in animal studies. Molecular weight is 106.	Supportive care. The role of ethanol therapy is unknown. In animal studies, bicarbonate therapy was as effective as ethanol therapy.

(continued)

TABLE II–22. TOXICITY OF OTHER GLYCOLS (CONTINUED)

Compounds	Toxicity and Comments	Treatment
Ethylene glycol mono butyl ether (EGBE, 2-butoxy-ethanol, butyl cellosolve).	Oxalate crystals, renal dysfunction, and increased osmolar gap may or may not occur. Levels of 432 μg/mL have been associated with coma, hypertension, and acidosis without an osmolar gap, oxalate crystals, or renal dysfunction. ARDS has been reported in one patient. Animal studies indicate that EGBE is metabolized in part to ethylene glycol and that pyrazole (an alcohol dehydrogenase blocker) prevents toxicity, but the affinity of alcohol dehydrogenase for EGBE is unknown. Molecular weight is 118.	Ethanol may be effective.
Ethylene glycol mono ethyl ether (EGEE, ethyl cello-solve)	Calcium oxalate crystals have been reported in animals. Animal studies indicate that EGEE is metabolized in part to ethylene glycol; however, the affinity of alcohol dehydrogenase is higher for EGEE than for ethanol. Teratogenic effect has been reported in humans and animals. Molecular weight is 90.	Ethanol may be effective.
Ethylene glycol mono methyl ether (EGME, methyl cello-solve)	Delayed toxic effects (8 and 18 hours postingestion) similar to ethylene glycol have been reported. Calcium oxalate crystals may or may not occur. Cerebral edema, hemorrhagic gastritis, and degeneration of the liver and kidneys were reported in one autopsy. Animal studies indicate that EGME is metabolized in part to ethyl-ene glycol; however, the affinity of alcohol dehydrogenase is about the same for EGME as for ethanol. Oligospermia has been reported with chronic exposure in humans. Teratogenic effects have been reported in animals. Molecular weight is 76.	Ethanol may be effective.
Dioxane (dimer of ethylene glycol)	May cause coma, liver and kidney damage. The vapor (> 300 ppm) may cause mucous membrane irritation. Dermal exposure to the liquid may have a defatting action. Metabolites unknown. Molecular weight is 88.	Role of ethanol is unknown, but it may be effective.

      3. In the absence of a serum ethylene glycol level, if the osmolar and anion gaps are both normal and the patient is asymptomatic, then serious ingestion is not likely to have occurred.

    B. **Other useful laboratory studies** include electrolytes, glucose, BUN, creatinine, calcium, hepatic transaminases, urinalysis (for crystals and Wood's lamp examination), measured osmolality, arterial blood gases, and ECG monitoring. Serum betahydroxybutyrate levels may help distinguish ethylene glycol poisoning from **alcoholic ketoacidosis**, which may also cause increased anion and osmolar gaps. (Patients with alcoholic ketoacidosis may not have markedly positive tests for ketones, but the betahydroxybutyrate level will usually be elevated.)

V. Treatment.

  A. **Emergency and supportive measures**

    1. Maintain an open airway and assist ventilation if necessary (see pp 1–7). Administer supplemental oxygen.

    2. Treat coma (p 18), convulsions (p 21), cardiac arrhythmias (pp 10–14), and metabolic acidosis (p 31) if they occur. Observe the patient for several hours to monitor for development of metabolic acidosis, especially if the patient is symptomatic or there is known co-ingestion of ethanol.

    3. Treat hypocalcemia with intravenous calcium gluconate or calcium chloride (p 350).

  B. **Specific drugs and antidotes**

    1. Administer **fomepizole** (see p 370) or **ethanol** (see p 367) to saturate the enzyme alcohol dehydrogenase and prevent metabolism of ethylene glycol to its toxic metabolites. Indications for therapy include the following:

      a. Ethylene glycol level higher than 20 mg/dL.

      b. History of ethylene glycol ingestion accompanied by an osmolar gap greater than 5 mOsm/L not accounted for by ethanol or other alcohols.

      c. Anion gap acidosis accompanied by a history of glycol ingestion or presence of oxalate crystalluria or positive Wood's lamp examination of urine.

    2. Administer **pyridoxine** (see p 407), **folate** (p 370), and **thiamine** (p 408), cofactors required for the metabolism of ethylene glycol that may alleviate toxicity by enhancing metabolism of glyoxylic acid to nontoxic metabolites.

  C. **Decontamination** (see p 43)

    1. **Prehospital.** Do not induce vomiting or administer activated charcoal.

    2. **Hospital.** Perform gastric lavage as quickly as possible. Activated charcoal has not been shown to effectively adsorb glycols.

  D. **Enhanced elimination.** The volume of distribution of ethylene glycol is 0.7–0.8 L/kg, making it accessible to enhanced elimination procedures. **Hemodialysis** efficiently removes ethylene glycol and its toxic metabolites and rapidly corrects acidosis and electrolyte and fluid abnormalities.

    1. Indications for hemodialysis include:

      a. Suspected ethylene glycol poisoning with an osmolar gap greater than 10 mOsm/L not accounted for by ethanol or other alcohols.

      b. Any ethylene glycol intoxication accompanied by renal failure.

      c. An ethylene glycol serum concentration greater than 20–50 mg/dL.

    2. The minimum serum concentration of ethylene glycol associated with serious toxicity is not known; dialysis should be continued until the osmolar and anion gaps are normalized.

▶ ETHYLENE OXIDE

Gary J Ordog, MD and Jonathon Wasserberger, MD

Ethylene oxide is a highly penetrating gas, widely used in hospitals as a sterilizer of medical equipment and supplies. It is also an important industrial chemical, used as a solvent, plasticizer, and chemical intermediate.

I. **Mechanism of toxicity.** Ethylene oxide is an alkylating agent and reacts directly with proteins and DNA to cause cell death. Direct contact with the gas causes irritation of the eyes, mucous membranes, and lungs. Ethylene oxide is mutagenic, teratogenic, and carcinogenic (regulated as a carcinogen by OSHA; ACGIH classification A2 [suspected carcinogen]).

II. **Toxic dose.** The recommended workplace limit (ACGIH TLV-TWA) in air is 1 ppm (1.8 mg/m^3) as an 8-hour time-weighted average. The air level immediately dangerous to life or health (IDLH) is 800 ppm. The odor threshold is approximately 700 ppm, giving the gas poor warning properties. High levels of ethylene oxide can occur when sterilizers malfunction or with the opening or replacing of ethylene oxide tanks.

III. **Clinical presentation.**
   A. Ethylene oxide is a potent mucous membrane irritant and can cause eye and oropharyngeal irritation, bronchospasm, and pulmonary edema. Cataract formation has been described after significant eye exposure. Exposure to the liquid can cause vesicant injury to the skin.
   B. Neurotoxicity, including convulsions and delayed peripheral neuropathy, may occur after exposure.
   C. Other systemic effects include cardiac arrhythmias when ethylene oxide is used in combination with freon (see p 178) as carrier gas.
   D. Leukemia has been described in workers chronically exposed to relatively low levels of ethylene oxide.

IV. **Diagnosis** is based on a history of exposure and typical upper-airway irritant effects. Detection of ethylene oxide odor indicates significant exposure. Industrial hygiene sampling is necessary to document air levels of exposure.
   A. **Specific levels.** Blood levels are not available. Ethylene oxide DNA adducts may indicate exposure but are not available for clinical use.
   B. **Other useful laboratory studies** include arterial blood gases or pulse oximetry and chest x-ray.

V. **Treatment.**
   A. **Emergency and supportive measures.** Monitor closely for several hours after exposure.
      1. Maintain an open airway and assist ventilation if necessary (see pp 1–7). Treat bronchospasm (p 8) and pulmonary edema (p 7) if they occur.
      2. Treat coma (p 18), convulsions (p 21), and arrhythmias (pp 10–14) if they occur.
   B. **Specific drugs and antidotes.** There is no specific antidote.
   C. **Decontamination** (see p 43)
      1. Remove the victim from the contaminated environment immediately and administer oxygen. Rescuers should wear self-contained breathing apparatus and chemical-protective clothing.
      2. Remove all contaminated clothing and wash exposed skin. For eye exposures, irrigate copiously with tepid water or saline.
   D. **Enhanced elimination.** There is no role for these procedures.

▶ FLUORIDE

Kathryn H. Meier, PharmD

Fluoride-liberating chemicals are used in some insecticides, rodenticides, aluminum production, vitamins or dietary supplements, and various products to prevent dental caries (eg, Luride drops and Listermint with Fluoride). Toothpaste contains up to about 5 mg fluoride per teaspoon. Fluoride is commonly added to community drinking water. It is also found in hydrofluoric acid (see p 186). Soluble fluoride salts are rapidly absorbed within 30 minutes and are more toxic (see Table II–23). Fluoride is slowly eliminated in urine and sweat.

TABLE II–23. FLUORIDE-CONTAINING COMPOUNDS

Compound	Elemental Fluoride (%)
Soluble salts	
Hydrogen fluoride	95
Sodium fluoride	45
Sodium fluosilicate	61
Less soluble salts	
Cryolite	54
Sodium monofluorophosphate	13
Stannous fluoride	24

I. **Mechanism of toxicity.** Toxicity results from direct cytotoxic and metabolic effects as well as binding to calcium and magnesium causing hypocalcemia and hypomagnesemia. Specific effects include: impaired oxidative phosphorylation and glycolysis, enhanced proteolytic processes, impaired blood coagulation (in vitro), myocardial irritability, impaired neurotransmission, and tetany.

Pharmacokinetics. Peak absorption occurs in about 1 hour. The volume of distribution is 0.5–0.7 L/kg. Fluoride is not protein bound. The elimination half-life is 2–9 hours and is prolonged in patients with renal failure.

II. **Toxic dose.** Vomiting and abdominal pain are common with ingestions of 3–5 mg/kg elemental fluoride (see Table II–23); hypocalcemia and muscular symptoms appear with ingestions of 5–10 mg/kg. Death has been reported in a 3-year-old child after ingestion of 16 mg/kg and in adults with doses in excess of 32 mg/kg.

III. **Clinical presentation.** Nausea and vomiting frequently occur within 30–60 minutes of ingestion. Symptoms of more serious intoxication include skeletal muscle weakness, tetanic contractions, respiratory muscle weakness, and respiratory arrest. Cardiac dysrhythmias may be associated with hypocalcemia, hypomagnesemia, and hyperkalemia.

IV. **Diagnosis** is usually based on a history of ingestion. Symptoms of abdominal distress, muscle weakness, hypocalcemia, and hyperkalemia suggest fluoride intoxication.

A. **Specific levels.** The normal serum fluoride concentration is less than 20 µg/L (ng/mL) but varies considerably with diet and water source. Serum fluoride concentrations are generally difficult to obtain and thus are of limited utility for acute overdose management.

B. **Other useful laboratory studies** include electrolytes, glucose, BUN, creatinine, calcium, albumin (to assess free calcium), magnesium, and ECG.

V. **Treatment.**

A. **Emergency and supportive measures**
1. Maintain an open airway and assist ventilation if necessary (see pp 1–7).
2. Monitor ECG and serum calcium for at least 4–6 hours, and admit symptomatic patients to an intensive care setting.

B. **Specific drugs and antidotes.** When clinically significant hypocalcemia is present, administer **intravenous calcium gluconate** (p 350), 10–20 mL (children: 0.2–0.3 mL/kg). Treat hypomagnesemia with intravenous **magnesium sulfate**, 1–2 g given over 10–15 min (children: 25–50 mg/kg diluted to less than 10 mg/mL).

C. **Decontamination** (see p 43)
1. **Prehospital.** Administer **calcium** salts (eg, calcium carbonate [Tums], calcium lactate, or milk) to form insoluble complexes with fluoride, minimizing absorption. Magnesium-containing antacids may also bind fluoride, although there are no reports of their use. Do **not** induce vomiting because of the risk of abrupt onset of seizures and arrhythmias.

    2. **Hospital.** After recent ingestion, perform gastric lavage. Administer **calcium** salts as discussed above. Activated charcoal does not adsorb fluoride and is not likely to be beneficial.

  D. Enhanced elimination. Although fluoride is a small ion with minimal protein binding, it rapidly binds to free calcium and bone and has a short elimination half-life (2–9 hours); therefore, hemodialysis and hemoperfusion are unlikely to be beneficial.

▶ FLUOROACETATE

Gerald Joe, PharmD

Fluoroacetate, also known as compound 1080, sodium monofluoroacetate (SMFA), and sodium fluoroacetate, is one of the most toxic substances known. In the past, it was used primarily as a rodenticide by licensed pest control companies, but it has been removed from the U.S. market because of its hazard. It is a tasteless, odorless, water-soluble white crystalline powder. Fluoroacetamide (compound 1081) is a similar compound with similar toxicity.

  I. Mechanism of Toxicity. Fluoroacetate is metabolized to the toxic compound fluorocitrate, which blocks cellular metabolism by inhibiting the Krebs cycle. Clinical effects of poisoning are delayed (from 30 minutes to several hours) until fluoroacetate is metabolized to fluorocitrate.

    Pharmacokinetics. The onset of effect is reported to be 30 minutes to several hours after ingestion. The time to peak effect, volume of distribution (Vd), duration of action, and elimination half-life in humans are unknown. In rats, only 1% of an oral dose is excreted in the urine and feces within 5 hours and only 12% by 48 hours.

  II. Toxic dose. Inhalation or ingestion of as little as 1 mg of fluoroacetate is sufficient to cause serious toxicity. Death is likely after ingestion of more than 5 mg/kg.

  III. Clinical presentation. After a delay of minutes to several hours, manifestations of diffuse cellular poisoning become apparent; nausea, vomiting, diarrhea, metabolic acidosis, renal failure, agitation, confusion, seizures, coma, respiratory arrest, pulmonary edema, and ventricular arrhythmias may occur.

  IV. Diagnosis is based on a history of ingestion and clinical findings, which may be delayed for several hours. Poisoning with fluoroacetate may mimic poisoning with other cellular toxins such as hydrogen cyanide and hydrogen sulfide, although with these poisons the onset of symptoms is usually more rapid.

    A. Specific levels. There is no assay available.

    B. Other useful laboratory studies include electrolytes, glucose, BUN, creatinine, arterial blood gases, and chest x-ray.

  V. Treatment.

    A. Emergency and supportive measures

      1. Maintain an open airway and assist ventilation if necessary (see pp 1–7). Administer supplemental oxygen.

      2. Replace fluid losses from gastroenteritis with intravenous saline or other crystalloids.

      3. Treat shock (p 15), seizures (p 21), and coma (p 18) if they occur. Monitor the ECG for at least 4–6 hours.

    B. Specific drugs and antidotes. There is no available antidote. Monoacetin (glyceryl monoacetate) has been used experimentally in monkeys, but is not available or recommended for human use.

    C. Decontamination (see p 43)

      1. **Prehospital.** If it is available, immediately administer activated charcoal. Do *not* induce vomiting unless the victim is more than 30 minutes from a medical facility.

2. **Hospital.** Immediately place a gastric tube and administer activated charcoal, then perform gastric lavage. After lavage, give an additional dose of activated charcoal.
3. **Skin exposure.** Remove contaminated clothing and wash exposed skin thoroughly.
D. **Enhanced elimination.** There is no role for any enhanced removal procedure.

▶ FOOD POISONING: BACTERIAL

Susan Kim, PharmD

Food-borne bacteria and bacterial toxins are the most common causes of epidemic food-borne gastroenteritis. In general, the illness is relatively mild and self-limited, with recovery within 24 hours. However, severe and even fatal poisoning may occur with listeriosis, salmonellosis, or **botulism** (see p 112), and with certain strains of *Escherichia coli*. Poisoning after the consumption of **fish and shellfish** is discussed on p 175. **Mushroom** poisoning is discussed on p 227. Viruses such as the Norwalk agent and rotaviruses can also be transmitted through food and are the causative agent in as many as 40% of group-related diarrhea epidemics. Other microbes that can cause food-borne illness include cryptosporidium and cyclospora, which can cause serious illness in immunocompromised patients.

I. **Mechanism of toxicity.** Gastroenteritis may be caused by invasive bacterial infection of the intestinal mucosa or by a toxin elaborated by bacteria. Bacterial toxins may be preformed in food that is improperly prepared and improperly stored before use, or may be produced in the gut by the bacteria after they are ingested (Table II–24).

TABLE II–24. SUMMARY OF BACTERIAL FOOD POISONING

Organism	Incubation Period	Mechanism	Common Foods
Bacillus cereus	1–6 h (emesis) 8–16 h (diarrhea)	Toxins produced in food and patient	Reheated fried rice.
Campylobacter	1–2 d	Invasive	Water, direct contact.
Clostridium perfringens	6–16 h	Toxin produced in food and patient	Meats, gravy.
Escherichia coli (enterotoxigenic)	12–72 h	Toxin produced in patient	Water, meats.
Listeria monocytogenes	9–32	Invasive	Milk, soft cheeses
Salmonella	12–36 h	Invasive	Meat, dairy, bakery foods; water; direct contact.
Shigella	1–7 d	Invasive	Water, fruits, vegetables.
Staphylococcus aureus	1–6 h	Toxin preformed in food; heat-resistant	Very common: meats, dairy, bakery foods.
Vibrio parahemolyticus	8–30 h	Invasive *and* toxin produced in patient	Shellfish, water
Yersinia enterocolitica	3–7 d	Invasive	Water, meats, dairy.

II. **Toxic dose.** The toxic dose depends on the type of bacteria or toxin and its concentration in the ingested food, as well as individual susceptibility or resistance. Some of the preformed toxins (eg, staphylococcal toxin) are heat-resistant and once in the food are not removed by cooking or boiling.

III. **Clinical presentation.** Commonly, a delay or "incubation period" of from 2 hours to 3 days precedes the onset of symptoms (Table II–24).

A. **Gastroenteritis** is the most common finding, with nausea, vomiting, abdominal cramps, and diarrhea. Significant fluid and electrolyte abnormalities may occur, especially in young children or elderly patients.

B. **Fever**, **bloody stools**, and **fecal leukocytosis** are common with invasive bacterial infections.

C. **Systemic infection** can result from *E coli, Salmonella, Shigella,* or *Listeria.*

1. **Listeriosis** can cause sepsis and meningitis, particularly in the elderly and immunocompromised persons. Infection during pregnancy produces a mild, flulike illness in the mother but serious intrauterine infection resulting in fetal death, neonatal sepsis, or meningitis.

2. *Shigella* and *E coli* **0157:H7** strain may cause acute hemorrhagic colitis complicated by hemolytic-uremic syndrome, renal failure and death, especially in children or immunocompromised adults.

IV. **Diagnosis.** Bacterial food poisoning is often difficult to distinguish from common viral gastroenteritis, unless the incubation period is short and there are multiple victims who ate similar foods at one large gathering. The presence of many white blood cells in a stool smear suggests invasive bacterial infection. With any epidemic gastroenteritis, consider other food-borne illnesses, such as those caused by viruses (eg, Norwalk agent), illnesses associated with seafood (see next section), botulism (p 112), and illnesses related to ingestions of certain mushrooms (p 227).

A. **Specific levels.** There are no specific assays that will assist clinical management.

1. **Stool culture** may differentiate *Salmonella, Shigella*, and *Campylobacter* infections. An ELISA test can detect Norwalk agent in stools.

2. **Blood** and **CSF** may grow invasive organisms, especially *Listeria* (and rarely, *Salmonella* or *Shigella*).

3. **Food samples** should be saved for bacterial culture and toxin analysis, primarily for use by public health investigators.

B. **Other useful laboratory studies** include CBC, electrolytes, glucose, BUN, and creatinine.

V. **Treatment.**

A. **Emergency and supportive measures**

1. Replace fluid and electrolyte losses with intravenous saline or other crystalloid solutions (patients with mild illness may tolerate oral rehydration). Patients with hypotension may require large-volume intravenous fluid resuscitation.

2. Antiemetic agents are acceptable for symptomatic treatment, but strong antidiarrheal agents such as Lomotil (diphenoxylate plus atropine) should not be used in patients with suspected invasive bacterial infection (fever and bloody stools).

B. **Specific drugs and antidotes.** There are no specific antidotes.

1. In patients with invasive bacterial infection, antibiotics may be used once the stool culture reveals the specific bacteria responsible. Empiric treatment with ciprofloxacin or trimethoprim-sulfamethoxazole is commonly given while awaiting culture results.

2. Pregnant women who have eaten *Listeria*-contaminated foods should be treated empirically, even if only mildly symptomatic, to prevent serious intrauterine infection. The antibiotic of choice is ampicillin, with gentamicin added for severe infection.

C. **Decontamination.** There is no role for gut decontamination.

D. **Enhanced elimination.** There is no role for enhanced removal procedures.

► FOOD POISONING: FISH AND SHELLFISH

Susan Kim, PharmD

A variety of toxins may produce illness after ingestion of fish or shellfish. The most common types of seafood-related toxins include **ciguatera, scombroid, neurotoxic shellfish poisoning, paralytic shellfish poisoning, tetrodotoxin,** and **domoic acid.** Shellfish-induced bacterial diarrhea is described in the previous section (see p 173).

I. **Mechanism of Toxicity.** The mechanism varies with each toxin. The toxins are all heat-stable; therefore, cooking the seafood does not prevent illness.

   A. **Ciguatera.** The toxin is produced by dinoflagellates, which are then consumed by reef fish. The mechanism of intoxication is uncertain, but may involve increased sodium permeability in sodium channels and stimulation of central or ganglionic cholinergic receptors.

   B. **Scombroid.** Scombrotoxin is a mixture of histamine and other histaminelike compounds produced when histidine in fish tissue decomposes.

   C. **Neurotoxic shellfish.** The mechanism appears to involve stimulation of sodium channels, resulting in depolarization of nerve fibers.

   D. **Paralytic shellfish.** Dinoflagellates ("red tide") produce saxitoxin, which is concentrated by filter-feeding clams and mussels. Saxitoxin blocks sodium conductance and neuronal transmission in skeletal muscles.

   E. **Tetrodotoxin,** found in puffer fish, California newts, and some South American frogs, blocks the voltage-dependent sodium channel in nerve cell membranes.

   F. **Domoic acid** is produced by phytoplanktons, which are concentrated by filter-feeding fish and shellfish. The toxin is thought to bind to glutamate receptors, causing neuroexcitatory responses.

II. **Toxic dose.** The concentration of toxin varies widely depending on geographic and seasonal factors. The amount of toxin necessary to produce symptoms is unknown. Saxitoxin is extremely potent; the estimated lethal dose in humans is 0.3–1 mg, and contaminated mussels may contain 15–20 mg.

III. **Clinical presentation.** The onset of symptoms and clinical manifestations vary with each toxin (Table II–25). In the majority of cases, the seafood appears normal with no adverse smell or taste (scombroid may have a peppery taste).

   A. **Ciguatera.** Intoxication produces vomiting and watery diarrhea 1–6 hours after ingestion, followed by headache, malaise, myalgias, paresthesias of the mouth and extremities, ataxia, blurred vision, photophobia, reversal of hot and cold sensation, extreme pruritus, hypotension, bradycardia, and rarely, seizures and respiratory arrest.

   B. **Scombroid.** Symptoms begin rapidly (minutes to 3 hours) after ingestion. Gastroenteritis, headache, and skin flushing are sometimes accompanied by urticaria and bronchospasm.

   C. **Neurotoxic shellfish.** Onset is within a few minutes to 3 hours. Gastroenteritis is accompanied by paresthesias of the mouth, face, and extremities; muscular weakness; and respiratory arrest.

   D. **Paralytic shellfish.** Vomiting, diarrhea, and facial paresthesias usually begin within 30 minutes of ingestion. Headache, myalgias, dysphagia, weakness, and ataxia have been reported. In serious cases respiratory arrest may occur after 1–12 hours.

   E. **Tetrodotoxin.** Symptoms occur within 30–40 minutes after ingestion and include vomiting, paresthesias, salivation, twitching, diaphoresis, weakness, and dysphagia. Hypotension, bradycardia, and respiratory arrest may occur up to 6–24 hours after ingestion.

   F. **Domoic acid.** Symptoms begin from 15 minutes to 38 hours after ingestion and consist of gastroenteritis accompanied by unusual neurologic toxicity including fasciculations, mutism, severe headache, hemiparesis, and my-

TABLE II-25. SUMMARY OF FISH AND SHELLFISH INTOXICATIONS

Type	Onset	Common Sources	Syndrome
Ciguatera	1–6 h	Barracuda, red snapper, grouper	Gastroenteritis, hot and cold reversal, paresthesias, myalgias, weakness.
Domoic acid (amnestic shellfish poisoning)	Minutes to hours	Mussels, clams, anchovies	Gastroenteritis, headache, myoclonus, seizures, coma. Persistent neuropathy and memory impairment.
Neurotoxic shellfish	Minutes to 3 h	Bivalve shellfish	Gastroenteritis, ataxia, paresthesias.
Paralytic shellfish	Within 30 min	Bivalve shellfish, "red tide"	Gastroenteritis, paresthesias, ataxia, respiratory paralysis.
Scombroid	Minutes to hours	Tuna, mahi mahi, bonita, mackerel	Gastroenteritis, flushed skin, urticaria, wheezing.
Tetrodotoxin	Within 30–40 min	Puffer fish ("fugu"), sun fish, porcupine fish, California newt	Vomiting, paresthesias, muscle twitching, diaphoresis, weakness, respiratory paralysis.

oclonus. Coma, seizures, hypotension, and profuse bronchial secretions have been reported with severe intoxication. Long-term sequelae include persistent severe anterograde memory loss (amnesic shellfish poisoning), motor neuropathy, and axonopathy.

IV. **Diagnosis** depends on a history of ingestion and is more likely to be recognized when multiple victims present after consumption of a common meal. Scombroid may be confused with an allergic reaction because of the histamine-induced urticaria.

    A. **Specific levels** are not generally available. However, when epidemic poisoning is suspected, state public health departments or the Centers for Disease Control may be able to analyze suspect food for toxins.

    B. **Other useful laboratory studies** include electrolytes, glucose, BUN, creatinine, arterial blood gases, ECG monitoring, and stool for bacterial culture.

V. **Treatment.**

    A. **Emergency and supportive measures.** Most cases are mild and self-limited and require no specific treatment. However, because of the risk of respiratory arrest, all patients should be observed for several hours.

      1. Maintain an open airway and assist ventilation if necessary (see pp 1–7).

      2. Replace fluid and electrolyte losses from gastroenteritis with intravenous crystalloid fluids.

    B. **Specific drugs and antidotes**

      1. **Scombroid** intoxication can be treated symptomatically with antihistamines, including diphenhydramine (see p 359) and cimetidine, 300 mg IV. Rarely, bronchodilators may also be required.

      2. **Ciguatera.** There are anecdotal reports of successful treatment with intravenous mannitol, 0.5–1 g/kg infused IV over 30 minutes.

    C. **Decontamination** (see p 43)

      1. **Prehospital.** Administer activated charcoal if available.

      2. **Hospital.** Administer activated charcoal. Consider gastric lavage if ingestion occurred within the preceding hour.

    D. **Enhanced elimination.** There is no role for these procedures.

▶ FORMALDEHYDE

John Balmes, MD

Formaldehyde is a gas with a pungent odor commonly used in the processing of paper, fabrics, and wood products and for the production of urea foam insulation. Low-level formaldehyde exposure has been found in stores selling clothing treated with formaldehyde-containing crease-resistant resins, in mobile homes, and in tightly enclosed rooms built with large quantities of formaldehyde-containing products used in construction materials. Formaldehyde aqueous solution (formalin) is used in varying concentrations (usually 37%) as a disinfectant and tissue fixative. Stabilized formalin may also contain 6–15% methanol.

I. **Mechanism of toxicity.**
   A. Formaldehyde causes precipitation of proteins and will cause coagulation necrosis of exposed tissue. The gas is highly water-soluble and when inhaled produces immediate local irritation of the upper respiratory tract and has been reported to cause spasm and edema of the larynx.
   B. Metabolism of formaldehyde produces formic acid, which may accumulate and produce metabolic acidosis.
   C. Formaldehyde is a known animal and suspected human carcinogen.

II. **Toxic dose.**
   A. **Inhalation.** The recommended workplace ceiling limit (ACGIH TLV-C) is 0.3 ppm (0.37 mg/m^3), which should not be exceeded at any time. The air level considered immediately dangerous to life or health (IDLH) is 20 ppm.
   B. **Ingestion** of as little as 30 mL of 37% formaldehyde solution has been reported to have caused death in an adult.

III. **Clinical presentation.**
   A. **Formaldehyde gas** exposure produces irritation of the eyes, and inhalation can produce cough, wheezing, and noncardiogenic pulmonary edema.
   B. **Ingestion** of formaldehyde solutions may cause severe corrosive esophageal and gastric injury, depending on the concentration. Lethargy and coma have been reported. Metabolic (anion gap) acidosis may be caused by formic acid accumulation from metabolism of formaldehyde or methanol.
   C. Hemolysis has occurred when formalin was accidentally introduced into the blood through contaminated hemodialysis equipment.

IV. **Diagnosis** is based on a history of exposure and evidence of mucous membrane, respiratory, or gastrointestinal tract irritation.
   A. **Specific levels**
      1. Plasma formaldehyde levels are not useful, but formate levels may indicate severity of intoxication.
      2. Methanol (see p 218) and formate levels may be helpful in cases of intoxication by formalin solutions containing methanol.
   B. **Other useful laboratory studies** include electrolytes, glucose, BUN, creatinine, and osmolar gap (see p 30).

V. **Treatment.**
   A. **Emergency and supportive measures**
      1. Maintain an open airway and assist ventilation if necessary (see pp 1–7).
      2. **Inhalation.** Treat bronchospasm (p 8) and pulmonary edema (p 7) if they occur. Administer supplemental oxygen, and observe for at least 4–6 hours.
      3. **Ingestion**
         a. Treat coma (p 18) and shock (p 15) if they occur.
         b. Administer intravenous saline or other crystalloids to replace fluid losses caused by gastroenteritis. Avoid fluid overload in patients with inhalation exposure because of the risk of pulmonary edema.
         c. Treat metabolic acidosis with sodium bicarbonate (p 345).
   B. **Specific drugs and antidotes**

1. If a **methanol**-containing solution has been ingested, then evaluate and treat with **ethanol** and **folic acid** as for methanol poisoning (see p 218).
2. **Formate** intoxication caused by formaldehyde alone should be treated with **folic acid** (see p 370), but ethanol infusion is not effective.
C. **Decontamination** (see p 43). Rescuers should wear self-contained breathing apparatus and appropriate chemical-protective clothing if handling a heavily contaminated patient.
   1. **Inhalation.** Remove victims from exposure and give supplemental oxygen if available.
   2. **Skin and eyes.** Remove contaminated clothing and wash exposed skin with soap and water. Irrigate exposed eyes with copious tepid water or saline; perform fluorescein examination to rule out corneal injury if pain and lacrimation persist.
   3. **Ingestion** (see p 45). Depending on the concentration of solution and patient symptoms, consider endoscopy to rule out esophageal or gastric injury.
      a. **Prehospital.** Administer activated charcoal if available. Do *not* induce vomiting because of the risk of corrosive injury.
      b. **Hospital.** Perform gastric lavage. Administer activated charcoal (although note that charcoal may obscure view during endoscopy).
D. **Enhanced elimination**
   1. **Hemodialysis** is effective in removing methanol and formate and in correcting severe metabolic acidosis. Indications for hemodialysis include severe acidosis or osmolar gap (see p 30) greater than 10 mOsm/L.
   2. **Alkalinization** of the urine helps promote excretion of formate.

▶ FREONS AND HALONS

Dennis Shusterman, MD, MPH

Freons (fluorocarbons and chlorofluorocarbons [CFCs]) have historically been widely used as aerosol propellants, in refrigeration units, and as degreasing agents. Under provisions of the Montreal Protocol of 1987, the use of CFCs is being phased out to avoid further depletion of stratospheric ozone. Nevertheless, freons remain in older refrigeration and air conditioning systems, and illicit import of freons is common. Most freons are gases at room temperature, but some are liquids (Freons 11, 21, 113, and 114) and may be ingested. Some fire extinguishers contain closely related compounds known as **halons**, which contain bromine, fluorine, and (variably) chlorine.

I. **Mechanism of toxicity.**
   A. Freons are mild CNS depressants. They may also displace oxygen from the air, causing hypoxemia. Freons are well-absorbed by inhalation or ingestion and are usually rapidly excreted in the breath within 15–60 minutes.
   B. As with chlorinated hydrocarbons, Freons may potentiate cardiac arrhythmias by increasing the sensitivity of the myocardium to the effects of catecholamines.
   C. Direct freezing of the skin, with frostbite, may occur if the skin is exposed to rapidly expanding gas as it escapes from a pressurized tank.
   D. Freons and halons may produce potent irritant gases and vapors (eg, phosgene, hydrochloric acid, hydrofluoric acid, and carbonyl fluoride) when heated to high temperatures, as might happen in a fire or if a refrigeration line is cut by a welding torch or electric arc.
   E. Some agents are hepatotoxic after large acute or chronic exposure.
II. **Toxic dose.**
   A. **Inhalation.** The toxic air level is quite variable, depending on the specific agent (see Table IV–4, p 434). Freon 21 (dichlorofluoromethane; TLV 10 ppm

[42 mg/m³]) is much more toxic that Freons 12 and 22 (TLV 1000 ppm). In general, anesthetic or CNS-depressant doses require fairly large air concentrations, which can also displace oxygen leading to asphyxia. The air level of dichloromonofluoromethane considered immediately dangerous to life or health (IDLH) is 5000. Other TLV and IDLH values can be found in Table IV–4 (p 434).

B. Ingestion. The toxic dose by ingestion is not known.

III. Clinical presentation.
  A. Skin or mucous membrane exposure may result in skin defatting and erythema. Frostbite may occur after exposure to rapidly expanding compressed gas.
  B. Systemic effects of moderate exposure include headache, nausea and vomiting, confusion, and drunkenness. More severe intoxication may result in coma or respiratory arrest. Ventricular arrhythmias may occur even with moderate exposures. A number of deaths, presumably caused by ventricular fibrillation, have been reported after freon abuse by "sniffing" or "huffing" freon products from plastic bags. Hepatic injury may occur.

IV. Diagnosis is based on a history of exposure and clinical presentation. Many chlorinated and aromatic hydrocarbon solvents may cause identical symptoms.
  A. Specific levels. Expired-breath monitoring is possible, and blood levels may be obtained to document exposure, but these are not useful in emergency clinical management.
  B. Other useful laboratory studies include arterial blood gases or oximetry, ECG monitoring, and liver enzymes.

V. Treatment.
  A. Emergency and supportive measures
    1. Maintain an open airway and assist ventilation if necessary (see pp 1–7).
    2. Treat coma (p 18) and arrhythmias (pp 10–14) if they occur. Avoid epinephrine or other sympathomimetic amines that may precipitate ventricular arrhythmias. Tachyarrhythmias caused by increased myocardial sensitivity may be treated with **propranolol** (see p 405), 1–2 mg IV, or **esmolol** (see p 366), 25–100 µg/kg/min IV.
    3. Monitor the ECG for 4–6 hours.
  B. Specific drugs and antidotes. There is no specific antidote.
  C. Decontamination (see p 43)
    1. Inhalation. Remove victim from exposure, and give supplemental oxygen if available.
    2. Ingestion (see p 45)
      a. Prehospital. Administer activated charcoal, if available. Do **not** induce vomiting because of rapid absorption and the risk of abrupt onset of CNS depression.
      b. Hospital. Administer activated charcoal, although the efficacy of charcoal is unknown. Perform gastric lavage only if the ingestion was very large and recent (less than 30 minutes).
  D. Enhanced elimination. There is no documented efficacy for diuresis, hemodialysis, hemoperfusion, or repeat-dose charcoal.

▶ GAMMA HYDROXYBUTYRATE (GHB)

Jo Ellen Dyer, PharmD

Gamma hydroxybutyrate (GHB) was originally investigated as an anesthetic agent in the 1960s but abandoned because of side effects including myoclonus and emergence delirium. Currently it is an unapproved drug in the United States and is legally available only under an FDA Investigational New Drug (IND) exemption for treatment of narcolepsy. However, it is readily available through the illicit drug market, pharmacies filling unlawful prescriptions, and kits designed for home manufacture. As a result of increasing GHB abuse, many states are adding GHB to their controlled-drug schedules. With moves to control GHB, chemical precursors that are converted to GHB in the body are becoming popular: these include **gamma butyrolactone (GBL)** and **1,4-butanediol (1,4-BD)**.

GHB has been promoted as a growth hormone releaser, muscle builder, diet aid, soporific, euphoriant, hallucinogen, and enhancer of sexual potency. GHB use in dance clubs and at rave parties commonly involves ingestion along with ethanol and other drugs. GHB has also become known as a "date rape" drug, because it can produce a rapid loss of consciousness allowing sexual assault. Other names and slang for GHB include Cherry Meth, Easy Lay, G caps, Gamma Hydrate, Georgia Home Boy, Grievous Bodily Harm, Liquid E, Liquid Ecstasy, Natural Sleep-500, Oxy-sleep, Scoop, Soap, Somatomax PM, and Vita G. European drug names include sodium oxybate (generic name), Gamma OH (France), and Somsanit (Germany). 1,4-Butanediol is also known as Borametz, Biocopia PM, pine needle extract, Promusol, and BVM. Gamma butyrolactone has been sold as Renewtrient.

I. **Mechanism of toxicity.**
   A. **GHB** is a structural analogue of the neurotransmitter γ-aminobutyric acid (GABA). It readily crosses the blood brain barrier, resulting in general anesthesia and respiratory depression. Death results from injury secondary to abrupt loss of consciousness, apnea, or pulmonary aspiration of gastric contents. Fatal potentiation of GHB's depressant effects has occurred with ethanol and other depressant drugs.
   B. **Gamma butyrolactone (GBL)**, an uncontrolled solvent, can be purchased from chemical supply stores or catalogues and chemically converted with sodium hydroxide to GHB. In addition, GBL is rapidly converted in the body by peripheral lactonases to GHB within minutes.
   C. **1,4-Butanediol (1,4-BD)**, an intermediate in chemical synthesis also readily available through chemical supply catalogues, is converted by alcohol dehydrogenase to gamma hydroxybutyraldehyde, then by aldehyde dehydrogenase to GHB.
   D. **Pharmacokinetics.** Onset of CNS depressant effects begins within 10–15 minutes after oral ingestion of GHB and 2–8 minutes after intravenous injection. Peak effects occur within 25–45 minutes, depending on the dose. The duration of effect is 1–2.5 hours after anesthetic doses of 50–60 mg/kg and about 2.5 hours in non-intubated accidental overdoses seen in the emergency department (range 15 min–5 hours). The rate of elimination of GHB is saturable. Plasma blood levels of GHB are undetectable within 4–6 hours after therapeutic doses. The volume of distribution (Vd) is variable due to saturable absorption and elimination. GHB is not protein bound.
II. **Toxic dose.**
   A. **GHB.** Response to low oral doses of GHB is unpredictable, with variability between patients and in the same patient. Narcolepsy studies with 30 mg/kg have reported effects including abrupt onset of sleep, enuresis, hallucinations, and myoclonic movements. Anesthetic studies reported unconsciousness with 50 mg/kg and deep coma with 60 mg/kg. Fasting, ethanol, and other depressants enhance the effects of GHB.
   B. **GBL**, a nonionized molecule, has greater bioavailablity than GHB when given orally in the same doses. A dose of 1.5 g produced sleep lasting 1 hour.
   C. **1,4-BD** is equipotent to GHB, although in the presence of ethanol, competition for the metabolic enzyme alcohol dehydrogenase may delay or decrease the peak effect.
III. **Clinical presentation.** Patients with acute GHB overdose commonly present with coma, bradycardia, and myoclonic movements.
   A. Soporific effects and euphoria usually occur within 15 minutes of an oral dose; unconsciousness and deep coma may follow within 30–40 minutes. When GHB is ingested alone, the duration of coma is usually short with recovery within 2 to 4 hours and complete resolution of symptoms within 8 hours.

    B. Delirium and tonic-clonic seizures are possible. Bradypnea with increased tidal volume is frequently seen. Cheyne-Stokes respiration and loss of airway-protective reflexes occur. Vomiting is seen in 30–50% of cases, and incontinence may occur. Stimulation may cause tachycardia and mild hypertension, but bradycardia is more common.

    C. Alkaline corrosive burns result from misuse of the home manufacture kits: a dangerously basic solution is produced when excess base is added, the reaction is incomplete, or there is inadequate back titration with acid. (The solution can also be acidic from excessive back titration.)

    D. Frequent use of GHB in high doses may produce tolerance and dependence. A withdrawal syndrome has been reported when chronic use is discontinued. Symptoms include tremor, paranoia, agitation, confusion, delirium, visual and auditory hallucinations, tachycardia, and hypertension.

IV. Diagnosis is usually suspected clinically in the patient who presents with abrupt onset of coma and recovers rapidly within a few hours.

    A. **Specific levels.** Laboratory tests for GHB levels are not readily available but can be obtained from a few national reference laboratories. Serum levels greater than 50 mg/L are associated with loss of consciousness, and levels over 260 mg/L usually produce unresponsive coma. GBL and 1,4-BD are rapidly converted in vivo to GHB. The duration of detection of GHB in blood and urine is short (6 and 12 hours, respectively, after therapeutic doses).

    B. **Other useful laboratory studies** include glucose, electrolytes, and arterial blood gases or oximetry. Consider urine toxicology screening and blood ethanol to rule out other common drugs of abuse that may enhance or prolong the course of poisoning.

V. Treatment.

    A. **Emergency and supportive measures**

        1. Protect the airway and assist ventilation if needed. Note that patients who require intubation are often awake and extubated within a few hours.

        2. Treat coma (p 18), seizures (p 21), bradycardia (p 10), and corrosive burns (p 129) if they occur.

    B. **Specific drugs and antidotes.** There are no specific antidotes available. Flumazenil and naloxone are not clinically effective. GHB-withdrawal syndrome has been managed with phenobarbital or benzodiazepines.

    C. **Decontamination**

        1. **Prehospital.** Do not induce vomiting, because of the risk of rapid loss of consciousness and loss of airway-protective reflexes, which may lead to pulmonary aspiration. Consider activated charcoal (p 45) if available soon after a large ingestion.

        2. **Hospital.** The small doses of GHB usually ingested are rapidly absorbed, and gastric lavage and activated charcoal are of doubtful benefit and may increase the risk of pulmonary aspiration. Consider activated charcoal administration for recent, large ingestions or when significant co-ingestion is suspected.

    D. **Enhanced elimination.** There is no role for enhanced removal procedures such as dialysis or hemoperfusion.

▶ GASES, IRRITANT

John Balmes, MD

A vast number of compounds produce irritant effects when inhaled in their gaseous form. The most common source of exposure to irritant gases is in industry, but significant exposures may occur in a variety of circumstances, such as after mixing cleaning agents at home, with smoke inhalation in structural fires, or after highway tanker spills.

I. **Mechanism of toxicity.** Irritant gases are often divided into two major groups based on their water solubility (Table II–26).
   A. **Highly soluble gases** (eg, ammonia and chlorine) are readily adsorbed by the upper respiratory tract and rapidly produce their primary effects on moist mucous membranes in the eyes, nose, and throat.
   B. **Less soluble gases** (eg, phosgene and nitrogen dioxide) are not rapidly adsorbed by the upper respiratory tract and can be inhaled deeply into the lower respiratory tract to produce delayed-onset pulmonary toxicity.
II. **Toxic dose.** The toxic dose varies depending on the properties of the gas. Table II–26 illustrates the workplace exposure limits (TLV-TWA) and the levels immediately dangerous to life or health (IDLH) for several common irritant gases.
III. **Clinical presentation.** All of these gases may produce irritant effects to the upper and/or lower respiratory tract, but warning properties and the onset and location of primary symptoms depend largely on the water solubility of the gas and the concentration of exposure.
   A. **Highly soluble gases.** Because of the good warning properties (upper respiratory tract irritation) of highly soluble gases, voluntary prolonged exposure to even low concentrations is unlikely.
      1. Low-level exposure causes rapid onset of mucous membrane and upper respiratory tract irritation; conjunctivitis, rhinitis, skin erythema and burns, sore throat, cough, wheezing, and hoarseness are common.
      2. With high-level exposure, laryngeal edema, tracheobronchitis, and abrupt airway obstruction may occur. Irritation of the lower respiratory tract and lung parenchyma causes tracheobronchial mucosal sloughing, chemical pneumonitis, and noncardiogenic pulmonary edema.

TABLE II–26. CHARACTERISTICS OF SOME COMMON IRRITANT TOXIC GASES

Gas	TLV[a](ppm)	IDLH[b](ppm)
High water solubility		
Ammonia	25	500
Formaldehyde	0.3 (C)	30
Hydrogen chloride	5 (C)	100
Hydrogen fluoride	3 (C)	30
Nitric acid	2	100
Sulfur dioxide	2	100
Moderate water solubility		
Acrolein	0.1	5
Chlorine	0.5	30
Fluorine	1	25
Low water solubility		
Nitric oxide	25	100
Nitrogen dioxide	3	50
Ozone	0.1 (C)	10
Phosgene	0.1	2

[a]TLV = Threshold limit value, ACGIH recommended exposure limit as an 8-hour time-weighted average for a 40-hour workweek (TLV-TWA). "(C)" indicates ceiling limit, which should not be exceeded at any time (TLV-C).
[b]IDLH = Air level considered immediately dangerous to life or health, defined as the maximum air concentration from which one could reasonably escape within 30 minutes without any escape-impairing symptoms or any irreversible health effects.

B. **Less soluble gases.** Because of poor warning properties owing to minimal upper respiratory tract effects, prolonged exposure to moderate levels of these gases often occurs; therefore, chemical pneumonitis and pulmonary edema are more common. The onset of pulmonary edema may be delayed up to 12–24 hours or even longer.
C. **Sequelae.** Although most patients who suffer toxic inhalation injury will recover without any permanent impairment, bronchiectasis, bronchiolitis obliterans, persistent asthma, and pulmonary fibrosis can occur.
IV. **Diagnosis** is based on a history of exposure and the presence of typical irritant upper- or lower-respiratory effects. Arterial blood gases and chest x-ray may reveal early evidence of chemical pneumonitis or pulmonary edema. Whereas highly soluble gases have good warning properties and the diagnosis is not difficult, less soluble gases may produce minimal symptoms shortly after exposure; therefore, a high index of suspicion and repeated examinations are required.
A. **Specific levels.** There are no specific blood or serum levels available.
B. **Other useful laboratory studies** include arterial blood gases or oximetry, chest x-ray, spirometry, or peak expiratory flow measurement.
V. **Treatment.**
A. **Emergency and supportive measures**
1. Immediately assess the airway; hoarseness or stridor suggests laryngeal edema, which necessitates direct laryngoscopy and endotracheal intubation if swelling is present (see p 4). Assist ventilation if necessary (p 6).
2. Give supplemental oxygen, and treat bronchospasm with aerosolized bronchodilators (p 8).
3. Monitor arterial blood gases or oximetry, chest x-ray, and pulmonary function. Treat pulmonary edema if it occurs (p 7).
4. For victims of smoke inhalation, consider the possibility of concurrent intoxication by carbon monoxide (p 125) or cyanide (p 150).
B. **Specific drugs and antidotes.** There is no specific antidote for any of these gases.
C. **Decontamination** (see p 43). Remove victim from exposure and give supplemental oxygen if available. Rescuers should take care to avoid personal exposure; in most cases, self-contained breathing apparatus should be worn.
D. **Enhanced elimination.** There is no role for enhanced elimination.

▶ HYDROCARBONS

Gary J Ordog, MD and Jonathan Wasserberger, MD

Hydrocarbons, or petroleum distillates, are widely used in the petroleum, plastic, agricultural, and chemical industries as solvents, degreasers, fuels, and pesticides. In its broadest definition, a hydrocarbon is any chemical containing hydrogen and carbon (essentially, any organic compound). There are many subcategories of hydrocarbons, including aliphatic (saturated carbon structure), alicyclic (ring compounds), aromatic (containing one or more benzene ring structures), halogenated (containing chlorine, bromine, or fluoride atoms), alcohols and glycols, ethers, ketones, carboxylic acids, and many others. The present chapter emphasizes toxicity caused by common household hydrocarbons. See also specific chemicals elsewhere in Section II and in Section IV, Table IV–4 (p 434).
I. **Mechanism of toxicity.** Toxicity from hydrocarbons may be caused by direct injury from pulmonary aspiration or systemic intoxication after ingestion, inhalation, or skin absorption (Table II–27). Many hydrocarbons are also irritating to the eyes and skin.
A. **Pulmonary aspiration.** Most hydrocarbons are capable of inducing chemical pneumonia if aspirated. The risk of aspiration is greatest for those agents that have a low viscosity (eg, petroleum naphtha and furniture polish).

TABLE II–27. RISK OF TOXICITY FROM HYDROCARBON INGESTION

Common Compounds	Risk of Systemic Toxicity After Ingestion	Risk of Chemical Aspiration Pneumonia	Treatment
No systemic toxicity, high viscosity Petrolatum jelly, motor oil	Low	Low	None.
No systemic toxicity, low viscosity Gasoline, kerosene, petroleum naphtha, mineral seal oil, petroleum ether	Low	High	Observe for pheumonia; do **not** empty stomach.
Unknown or uncertain systemic toxicity Turpentine, pine oil	Uncertain	High	Observe for pneumonia; do **not** empty stomach if ingestion is < 2 mL/kg.
Systemic toxins Camphor, phenol, halogenated, or aromatic compounds	High	High	Observe for pneumonia; perform gastric lavage or give activated charcoal or do both.

B. **Ingestion**
1. **Aliphatic hydrocarbons** and **simple petroleum distillates** such as lighter fluid, kerosene, furniture polish, and gasoline are poorly absorbed from the gastrointestinal tract and do not pose a significant risk of systemic toxicity after ingestion, as long as they are not aspirated.
2. In contrast, many **aromatic** and **halogenated hydrocarbons, alcohols, ethers, ketones,** and other **substituted or complex hydrocarbons** are capable of causing serious systemic toxicity, such as coma, seizures, and cardiac arrhythmias.
C. **Inhalation** of any hydrocarbon vapors in an enclosed space may cause intoxication as a result of systemic absorption or by displacing oxygen from the atmosphere.
D. **Dermal** asbsorption can be significant for some agents but is insignificant for most of the simple, aliphatic compounds.
II. **Toxic dose.** The toxic dose is highly variable depending on the agent involved and whether it is aspirated, ingested, or inhaled.
A. **Pulmonary aspiration** of as little as a few milliliters may produce chemical pneumonitis.
B. **Ingestion** of as little as 10–20 mL of some systemic toxins, such as camphor or carbon tetrachloride, may cause serious or fatal poisoning.
C. For recommended **inhalation** exposure limits for common hydrocarbons, see Table IV–4, p 434.
III. **Clinical presentation.**
A. If **pulmonary aspiration** has occurred, there is usually immediate onset of coughing, gagging, or choking. This may progress within a few hours to tachypnea, wheezing, and severe chemical pneumonitis. Death may ensue from secondary bacterial infection and other respiratory complications.
B. **Ingestion** often causes abrupt nausea and vomiting, occasionally with hemorrhagic gastroenteritis. Some compounds may be absorbed and produce systemic toxicity.
C. **Systemic toxicity** caused by ingestion of a toxic hydrocarbon, or inhalation of any hydrocarbon gas or vapor, is highly variable depending on the compound but usually includes confusion, ataxia, lethargy, and headache. With significant exposure, syncope, coma, and respiratory arrest may occur. Cardiac arrhythmias may occur owing to myocardial sensitization. This is most commonly reported with chlorinated and fluorinated compounds and aromatic derivatives. With many agents, hepatic and renal injury may occur.

    D. Skin or eye contact may cause local irritation, burns, or corneal injury. Chronic exposure often causes a defatting dermatitis resulting from removal of oils from the skin. Some agents are absorbed through the skin.

IV. Diagnosis.

  A. Aspiration pneumonitis. Diagnosis is based on a history of exposure and the presence of respiratory symptoms such as coughing, choking, and wheezing. If these symptoms are not present within 6 hours of exposure, it is very unlikely that chemical pneumonitis will occur. Chest x-ray and arterial blood gases or oximetry may assist in the diagnosis of chemical pneumonitis.

  B. Systemic intoxication. Diagnosis is based on a history of ingestion or inhalation, accompanied by the appropriate systemic clinical manifestations.

  C. Specific levels. Specific levels are generally not available or useful.

  D. Other useful laboratory studies include for suspected aspiration pneumonitis, arterial blood gases or oximetry and chest x-ray; and for suspected significant inhalation or ingestion of a toxic compound, electrolytes, glucose, BUN, creatinine, liver transaminases, and ECG monitoring.

V. Treatment.

  A. Emergency and supportive measures

    1. General. Provide basic supportive care for all symptomatic patients, whether from aspiration, ingestion, or inhalation.

      a. Maintain an open airway and assist ventilation if necessary (see pp 1–7). Administer supplemental oxygen.

      b. Monitor arterial blood gases or oximetry, chest x-ray, and ECG and admit symptomatic patients to an intensive care setting.

      c. Use epinephrine and other sympathomimetic amines with caution in patients with significant hydrocarbon intoxication, because arrhythmias may be induced.

    2. Pulmonary aspiration. Patients who remain asymptomatic after 4–6 hours of observation may be discharged. In contrast, if the patient is coughing on arrival, aspiration has probably occurred.

      a. Administer supplemental oxygen, and treat bronchospasm (see p 8), hypoxia (p 7), and pneumonia (p 7) if they occur.

      b. Do *not* use steroids or prophylactic antibiotics.

    3. Ingestion. In the vast majority of accidental childhood ingestions, less than 5–10 mL is actually swallowed and systemic toxicity is rare. Treatment is primarily supportive.

  B. Specific drugs and antidotes

    1. There is no specific antidote for general hydrocarbon aspiration pneumonia; corticosteroids are of no proven value.

    2. Specific drugs or antidotes may be available for systemic toxicity of some hydrocarbons (eg, acetylcysteine for carbon tetrachloride and methylene blue for methemoglobin formers) or their solutes (eg, chelation therapy for leaded gasoline and antidotes for pesticides, etc).

  C. Decontamination

    1. Inhalation. Move the victim to fresh air and administer oxygen if available.

    2. Skin and eyes. Remove contaminated clothing and wash exposed skin with water and soap. Irrigate exposed eyes with copious tepid water or saline and perform fluorescein examination for corneal injury.

    3. Ingestion (see p 45). For agents with no known systemic toxicity, gut decontamination is neither necessary nor desirable because any gut-emptying procedure may increase the risk of aspiration. *For systemic toxins*:

      a. Prehospital. Administer activated charcoal if available. Do *not* induce vomiting, because systemic complications such as seizures and coma may occur rapidly or abruptly.

      b. Hospital. Administer activated charcoal. Consider gastric lavage for large recent ingestions.

  D. Enhanced elimination. There is no known role for any of these procedures.

▶ HYDROGEN FLUORIDE AND HYDROFLUORIC ACID

Kent R. Olson, MD

Hydrogen fluoride (HF) is an irritant gas that liquifies at 19.5 °C; in aqueous solution it produces hydrofluoric acid. HF gas is used in chemical manufacturing. In addition, it may be released from fluorosilicates, fluorocarbons, or Teflon when heated over 350 °C. Hydrofluoric acid (aqueous HF solution) is widely used as a rust remover, in glass etching, and in the manufacture of silicon semiconductor chips. Hydrofluoric acid poisoning usually occurs after skin contact, although ingestions occasionally occur. Similar toxicity can result from exposure to ammonium bifluoride.

  I. **Mechanism of toxicity.** HF is a skin and respiratory irritant. Hydrofluoric acid is actually a relatively weak acid (the dissociation constant is about 1000 times less than that of hydrochloric acid), and toxic effects result primarily from the highly reactive fluoride ion.
    A. HF is able to penetrate tissues deeply, where the highly cytotoxic fluoride ion is released and cellular destruction occurs.
    B. In addition, fluoride readily precipitates with calcium; this may cause local bone demineralization and systemic hypocalcemia.
 II. **Toxic dose.** Toxicity depends on the air levels of HF or concentration of aqueous HF solutions.
    A. **Hydrogen fluoride gas.** The recommended workplace ceiling limit (ACGIH TLV-C) for HF gas is 3 ppm (2.3 mg/m³); 30 ppm is considered immediately dangerous to life or health (IDLH). A 5-minute exposure to air concentrations of 50–250 ppm is likely to be lethal.
    B. **Aqueous solutions.** Solutions of 50–70% are highly toxic and produce immediate pain; intermediate concentrations (20–40%) may cause little pain initially but result in deep injury after a delay of 1–8 hours; weak solutions (5–15%) cause almost no pain on contact but may cause delayed serious injury after 12–24 hours. Most household products containing aqueous HF contain 5–8% or less.
III. **Clinical presentation.** Symptoms and signs depend on the type of exposure (gas or liquid) and the concentration.
    A. **Inhalation** of HF gas produces eye and nose irritation, sore throat, coughing, and bronchospasm. After a delay of up to several hours, chemical pneumonia and pulmonary edema may occur.
    B. **Skin exposure.** After acute exposure to weak (5–15%) or intermediate (20–40%) solutions, there may be no symptoms because the pH effect is relatively weak. Strong (50–70%) solutions have better warning properties because of immediate pain. After a delay of 1–12 hours, progressive redness, swelling, skin blanching, and pain occur owing to deep penetration by the fluoride ion. The exposure is typically through a pinhole-sized defect in a rubber glove, and the fingertip is the most common site of injury. The pain is progressive and unrelenting. Severe deep-tissue destruction may occur, including full-thickness skin loss and destruction of underlying bone.
    C. **Ingestion** of HF may cause corrosive injury to the mouth, esophagus, and stomach.
    D. **Systemic hypocalcemia** and **hyperkalemia** may occur after ingestion or skin burns involving a large body surface area or highly concentrated solutions.
IV. **Diagnosis** is based on a history of exposure and typical findings. Immediately after exposure to weak or intermediate solutions, there may be few or no symptoms even though potentially severe injury may develop later.
    A. **Specific levels.** Serum fluoride concentrations are not useful after acute exposure but may be used in evaluating chronic occupational exposure. Normal serum fluoride is less than 20 μg/L. Urinary fluoride levels are usually less than 5 mg/day.
    B. **Other useful laboratory studies** include electrolytes, calcium, and continuous ECG monitoring.

V. Treatment.
A. Emergency and supportive measures
1. Maintain an open airway and assist ventilation if necessary (see pp 1–7). Administer supplemental oxygen. Treat pulmonary edema (p 7) if it occurs.
2. Patients with HF ingestion should be evaluated for corrosive injury, with consultation by a gastroenterologist or surgeon for possible endoscopy (p 129).
3. Monitor the ECG and serum calcium and potassium levels; give intravenous calcium (p 350; see below) if there is evidence of hypocalcemia or severe hyperkalemia.

B. Specific drugs and antidotes.
Calcium (see p 350) rapidly precipitates fluoride ions and is an effective antidote for fluoride skin exposure and for systemic hypocalcemia resulting from absorbed fluoride.
1. **Skin burns.** For exposures involving the hands or fingers, immediately consult an experienced hand surgeon, medical toxicologist, or Poison Control Center (see Table I–42, p 54). The fingernail may need to be removed, and occasionally calcium will need to be given by the intra-arterial route. *Caution:* do *not* use calcium chloride for subcutaneous or intra-arterial injections; this form contains a larger proportion of calcium ion and may cause vasospasm and tissue necrosis.
   a. **Topical.** Apply a gel containing calcium gluconate or carbonate (see p 350), or soak in a quaternary ammonium solution such as Zephiran (1.3 g/L of water) or an Epsom salt solution. If pain is not significantly improved within 30–60 minutes, consider subcutaneous or intra-arterial injection.
   b. **Subcutaneous.** Inject calcium gluconate 5–10% subcutaneously in affected areas, using a 27- or 30-gauge needle and no more than 0.5 mL per digit or 1 mL/cm² in other regions.
   c. **Intra-arterial.** Injection of calcium by the intra-arterial route (see p 350) may be necessary for burns involving several digits or subungual areas.
2. **Systemic hypocalcemia or hyperkalemia.** Administer calcium gluconate 10%, 2–4 mL/kg IV, or calcium chloride 10%, 1–2 mL/kg IV.

C. Decontamination (see p 43).
Rescuers entering a contaminated area should wear self-contained breathing apparatus and appropriate protective clothing to avoid personal exposure.
1. **Inhalation.** Immediately remove victims from exposure and give supplemental oxygen if available. The use of 2.5% calcium gluconate by nebulization is recommended by some authorities.
2. **Skin.** Immediately flood exposed areas with water. Then soak in a solution of Epsom salts (magnesium sulfate) or calcium; immediate topical use of calcium or magnesium may prevent deep burns. Some facilities that frequently manage HF cases prepare a 2.5% calcium gluconate gel (in water-based jelly), and this is highly effective if rapidly available. After skin penetration by HF, topical treatment is relatively ineffective and calcium injections (see above) may be required. Soaking in a dilute benzalkonium chloride (Zephiran) solution has been advocated as an alternative to calcium.
3. **Eyes.** Flush with copious water or saline. The effectiveness of a weak (1–2%) calcium gluconate solution is not established.
4. **Ingestion (see p 45)**
   a. **Prehospital.** Immediately give any available magnesium-containing (Epsom salts, magnesium hydroxide, etc) or calcium-containing (calcium carbonate or milk) substance by mouth. Do *not* induce vomiting because of the risk of corrosive injury. Activated charcoal is not effective.
   b. **Hospital.** Perform gastric lavage. Administer magnesium- or calcium-containing substance as in a, above.

D. Enhanced elimination.
There is no role for enhanced elimination procedures.

► HYDROGEN SULFIDE

Brett Roth, MD

Hydrogen sulfide is a highly toxic, flammable, colorless gas that is heavier than air. It is produced naturally by decaying organic matter and is also a byproduct of many industrial processes. Hazardous levels may be found in petroleum refineries, tanneries, mines, pulp-making factories, sulfur hot springs, carbon disulfide production, commercial fishing holds, hot asphalt fumes, and pools of sewage sludge or liquid manure. It is often called "swamp gas."

I. **Mechanism of toxicity.** Hydrogen sulfide causes cellular asphyxia by inhibition of the cytochrome oxidase system, similar to the action of cyanide. Because it is rapidly absorbed by inhalation, symptoms occur nearly immediately after exposure, leading to rapid unconsciousness or "knockdown." Hydrogen sulfide is also a mucous membrane irritant.

II. **Toxic dose.** The characteristic rotten egg odor of hydrogen sulfide is detectable at concentrations as low as 0.025 ppm. The recommended workplace limit (ACGIH TLV-TWA) is 10 ppm (14 mg/m^3) as an 8-hour time-weighted average, with a short-term exposure limit (STEL) of 15 ppm (21 mg/m^3). Marked respiratory tract irritation occurs with levels of 50–100 ppm. Olfactory nerve paralysis occurs with levels of 100–150 ppm. The level considered immediately dangerous to life or health (IDLH) is 100 ppm. Pulmonary edema occurs at levels of 300–500 ppm. Levels of 600–800 ppm are rapidly fatal.

III. **Clinical presentation.**
   A. **Irritant effects.** Upper-airway irritation, burning eyes, and blepharospasm may occur at relatively low levels. Skin exposure can cause painful dermatitis. Chemical pneumonitis and noncardiogenic pulmonary edema may occur after a delay of several hours.
   B. **Acute systemic effects** include headache, nausea and vomiting, dizziness, confusion, seizures, and coma. Massive exposure may cause immediate cardiovascular collapse, respiratory arrest, and death. Survivors may be left with serious neurologic impairment.

IV. **Diagnosis** is based on a history of exposure and rapidly progressive manifestations of airway irritation and cellular asphyxia, with sudden collapse. The victim or coworkers may describe the smell of rotten eggs, but because of olfactory nerve paralysis the absence of this smell does not rule out exposure. Silver coins in the pockets of victims have been blackened (by conversion to silver sulfide).
   A. **Specific levels** are not available (sulfide is unstable in vitro). Sulfhemoglobin is not thought to be produced after hydrogen sulfide exposure.
   B. **Other useful laboratory studies** include electrolytes, glucose, arterial blood gases, and chest x-ray.

V. **Treatment.**
   A. **Emergency and supportive measures.** *Note:* Rescuers should use self-contained breathing apparatus to prevent personal exposure.
      1. Maintain an open airway and assist ventilation if necessary (see pp 1–7). Administer high-flow humidified supplemental oxygen. Observe for several hours for delayed-onset chemical pneumonia or pulmonary edema (p 7).
      2. Treat coma (p 18), seizures (p 21), and hypotension (p 15) if they occur.
   B. **Specific drugs and antidotes.** Theoretically, administration of nitrites (see p 390) to produce methemoglobinemia may promote conversion of sulfide ions to sulfhemoglobin, which is far less toxic. However, there is limited evidence for the effectiveness of nitrites, and they can cause hypotension and impaired oxygen delivery.
   C. **Decontamination** (see p 41). Remove the victim from exposure and give supplemental oxygen if available.
   D. **Enhanced elimination.** There is no role for enhanced elimination procedures. Although hyperbaric oxygen therapy has been promoted for treatment of hydrogen sulfide poisoning, this is based on anecdotal cases and there is no convincing rationale or scientific evidence for its effectiveness.

► HYMENOPTERA

Richard F. Clark, MD

Venomous insects are grouped into four families of the order Hymenoptera: Apidae (honeybees), Bombidae (bumblebees), Vespidae (wasps, hornets, and yellow jackets), and Formicidae (ants). With the exception of Vespidae, most bees sting only when disturbed or when the hive is threatened. Yellow jackets may attack without provocation and are the most common cause of insect-induced anaphylactic reactions.

I. **Mechanism of toxicity.** The venoms of the Hymenopterae are complex mixtures of enzymes and are delivered by various methods. The venom apparatus is located in the posterior abdomen of the females.

    A. The terminal end of the stinger of the **Apidae** (honeybee) is barbed, so the stinger remains in the victim and some or all of the venom apparatus will be torn from the body of the bee, resulting in its death as it flies away. The musculature surrounding the venom sac continues to contract for several minutes, causing venom to be persistently ejected. The **Bombidae** and **Vespidae** have stingers that remain functionally intact after a sting, resulting in their ability to inflict multiple stings.

    B. The envenomating **Formicidae** have secretory venom glands in the posterior abdomen and envenomate either by injecting venom through a stinger or by spraying venom from the posterior abdomen into a bite wound produced by their mandibles.

II. **Toxic dose.** The dose of venom delivered per sting may vary from none to the entire contents of the venom gland. The toxic response is highly variable depending on individual sensitivity. Some hymenoptera, such as wasps, have the ability to sting several times, increasing the venom load. Disturbing an ant nest may result in as many as 3000–5000 stings within seconds.

III. **Clinical presentation.** The patient may present with signs of envenomation or an allergic reaction.

    A. Envenomation. Once venom is injected, there is usually immediate onset of severe pain followed by a local inflammatory reaction, which may include erythema, wheal formation, ecchymosis, edema, vesiculation and blisters, itching, and a sensation of warmth. Multiple stings, and very rarely severe single stings, may also produce vomiting, diarrhea, hypotension, syncope, cyanosis, dyspnea, rhabdomyolysis, coagulopathy, and death.

    B. Allergic reactions. Numerous deaths occur annually in the United States from immediate hypersensitivity (anaphylactic) reactions characterized by urticaria, angioedema, bronchospasm, and shock. Most anaphylactic reactions occur within 15 minutes of envenomation. Rarely, delayed-onset reactions may occur, including Arthus reactions (arthralgias and fever), nephritis, transverse myelitis, and Guillain-Barré syndrome.

IV. **Diagnosis** is usually obvious from the history of exposure and typical findings.

    A. Specific levels. Not relevant.

    B. Other useful laboratory studies. None.

V. **Treatment.**

    A. Emergency and supportive measures

        1. Monitor the victim closely for at least 30–60 minutes.

        2. Treat anaphylaxis (see p 26), if it occurs, with epinephrine (p 365) and diphenhydramine (p 359). Persistent urticaria may respond to the addition of cimetidine, 300 mg PO or IV. Persons known to be sensitive to Hymenoptera venom should wear medical alert jewelry and carry an epinephrine emergency kit at all times.

        3. In most cases the painful localized tissue response will resolve in a few hours without therapy. Some symptomatic relief may be obtained by topical application of ice, papain (meat tenderizer), or creams containing corticosteroids or antihistamines.

        4. Provide tetanus prophylaxis if appropriate.

B. **Specific drugs and antidotes.** There is no available antidote.
C. **Decontamination.** Examine the sting site carefully for any retained stingers; these can be removed by gentle scraping with a sharp edge (eg, knife blade). Wash the area with soap and water.
D. **Enhanced elimination.** These procedures are not applicable.

▶ IODINE

Walter H. Mullen, PharmD

The chief use of iodine is for its antiseptic property. It is bactericidal, sporicidal, proto-zoacidal, cysticidal, and virucidal. Because it is poorly soluble in water, liquid formu-lations are usually prepared as a tincture in ethanol (50% or higher). Iodoform, iodochlorhydroxyquin, iodophors (povidine-iodine), and sodium and potassium io-dides also exert their bactericidal effect by liberating iodine. Lugol's solution (5% io-dine and 10% potassium iodide) is used in the treatment of hyperthyroidism and for the prevention of radioactive iodine absorption after nuclear accidents. The antiar-rhythmic drug amiodarone releases iodine and may cause thyrotoxicosis after pro-longed use. Iodine is also used in the manufacture of dyes and photographic reagents.

I. **Mechanism of toxicity.** Iodine is corrosive because of its oxidizing properties. When ingested, iodine is poorly absorbed but may cause severe gastroenteritis. Iodine is readily inactivated by starch to convert it to iodide, which is nontoxic. In the body, iodine is rapidly converted to iodide and stored in the thyroid gland.
II. **The toxic dose** depends on the product and the route of exposure. Iodophors and iodoform liberate only small amounts of iodine and are generally nontoxic and noncaustic.
   A. **Iodine vapor.** The ACGIH-recommended workplace ceiling limit (TLV-C) for iodine vapor is 0.1 ppm (1 mg/m^3). The air level considered immediately dan-gerous to life or health (IDLH) is 2 ppm.
   B. **Skin and mucous membranes.** Strong iodine tincture (7% iodine and 5% potassium iodide in 83% ethanol) may cause burns, but USP iodine tincture (2% iodine and 2% sodium iodide in 50% ethanol) is not likely to produce cor-rosive damage. Systemic absorption of iodine may occur after an acute appli-cation of strong iodine tincture or after chronic applications of less concen-trated products.
   C. **Ingestion.** Reported fatal doses vary from 200 mg to more than 20 g of io-dine; an estimated mean lethal dose is approximately 2–4 g of free iodine. USP iodine tincture contains 100 mg iodine per 5 mL, and strong iodine tinc-ture contains 350 mg of iodine per 5 mL. Iodine ointment contains 4% iodine. Consider ethanol toxicity with large exposures (see p 162).
III. **Clinical presentation.** The manifestations of iodine poisoning are largely related to its corrosive effect on mucous membranes.
   A. **Inhalation** of iodine vapor can cause severe pulmonary irritation leading to pulmonary edema.
   B. **Skin** and eye exposures may result in severe corrosive burns.
   C. **Ingestion** can cause corrosive gastroenteritis with vomiting, hematemesis, and diarrhea, which can result in significant volume loss and circulatory col-lapse. Pharyngeal swelling and glottic edema have been reported. Mucous membranes are usually stained brown, and the vomitus may be blue if starchy foods are already present in the stomach.
   D. **Chronic** ingestions or absorption may result in hypothyroidism and goiter. Io-dides cross the placenta, and neonatal hypothyroidism and death from respi-ratory distress secondary to goiter have been reported.
IV. **Diagnosis** is based on a history of exposure and evidence of corrosive injury. Mucous membranes are usually stained brown, and vomitus may be blue.

    A. Specific levels. Blood levels are not clinically useful but may confirm exposure.

    B. Other useful laboratory studies include, for serious corrosive injury, CBC, electrolytes, BUN, and creatinine. For serious inhalation, arterial blood gases or oximetry and chest x-ray are useful.

V. Treatment.

    A. Emergency and supportive measures

        1. Maintain an open airway and perform endotracheal intubation if airway edema is progressive (see pp 1–7). Treat bronchospasm (see p 8) and pulmonary edema (p 7) if they occur.

        2. Treat fluid loss from gastroenteritis aggressively with intravenous crystalloid solutions.

        3. If corrosive injury to the esophagus or stomach is suspected, consult a gastroenterologist to perform endoscopy.

    B. Specific drugs and antidotes. Sodium thiosulfate may convert iodine to iodide and tetrathionate, but is not recommended for intravenous use because iodine is rapidly converted to iodide in the body.

    C. Decontamination (see p 43)

        1. Inhalation. Remove the victim from exposure.

        2. Skin and eyes. Remove contaminated clothing and flush exposed skin with water. Irrigate exposed eyes copiously with tepid water or saline for at least 15 minutes.

        3. Ingestion (see p 45)

            a. Prehospital. Do *not* induce vomiting because of the corrosive effects of iodine. Administer a starchy food (potato, flour, or cornstarch) or milk to lessen gastrointestinal irritation.

            b. Hospital. For large exposures, consider gastric lavage, using milk, cornstarch, or sodium thiosulfate. Activated charcoal is of unknown efficacy.

    D. Enhanced elimination. Once absorbed into the circulation, iodine is rapidly converted to the far less toxic iodide. Therefore, there is no need for enhanced drug removal.

▶ IPECAC SYRUP

Kathryn H. Keller, PharmD

Ipecac syrup is an extract of the ipecacuanha plant. Its principle active ingredients are emetine and cephaeline. Syrup of ipecac is widely available over the counter as an effective, rapidly acting emetic agent. Presently, the major source of poisoning is chronic intoxication resulting from intentional misuse by patients with eating disorders. Cases of "Munchausen's syndrome by proxy," in which a parent repeatedly administers ipecac to a child, have also been reported.

I. Mechanism of toxicity.

    A. Acute ingestion of ipecac causes vomiting by irritation of the gastric mucosa and by stimulation of the central chemoreceptor trigger zone.

    B. Chronic repeated dosing results in interstitial edema, focal connective-tissue proliferation, and necrosis of skeletal and myocardial muscle fibers. The normal cellular architecture is disrupted, and clinical myopathy occurs.

II. Toxic dose. Toxicity depends on the formulation and whether the exposure is acute or chronic.

    A. Acute ingestion of 60–120 mL of **syrup of ipecac** is not likely to cause serious poisoning. However, the **fluid extract**, which is approximately 14 times more potent than syrup of ipecac, has caused death after ingestion of as little as 10 mL.

B. Chronic dosing results in cumulative toxicity because of the slow elimination of emetine. Daily ingestion of 90–120 mL of syrup of ipecac for 3 months has caused death from cardiomyopathy.

III. Clinical presentation.

A. Acute ingestion of ipecac causes nausea and vomiting. In patients with depressed airway-protective reflexes, pulmonary aspiration of gastric contents may occur. Prolonged or forceful vomiting may cause gastritis, gastric rupture, pneumomediastinum, retropneumoperitoneum, or Mallory-Weiss tears of the cardioesophageal junction. One fatal case of intracerebral hemorrhage was reported in an elderly patient after a single therapeutic dose of ipecac syrup.

B. Chronic intoxication. In patients with chronic misuse, dehydration and electrolyte abnormalities (eg, hypokalemia) are commonly secondary to frequent vomiting and diarrhea, and myopathy or cardiomyopathy may develop. Symptoms of myopathy include muscle weakness and tenderness, hyporeflexia, and elevated serum CPK. Cardiomyopathy, with congestive heart failure and arrhythmias, may be fatal.

IV. Diagnosis is based on a history of ingestion. Chronic ipecac poisoning should be suspected in any patient with a known eating disorder and evidence of dehydration, electrolyte imbalance, or myopathy, or in a young child with repeated unexplained episodes of vomiting, diarrhea, and failure to thrive. The electrocardiogram may show prolonged QRS and QT intervals, flat or inverted T waves, and supraventricular and ventricular arrhythmias.

A. Specific levels. Emetine may be detected in the urine for up to several weeks after ingestion, and its presence may provide qualitative confirmation of ipecac exposure but does not correlate with the degree of effect. It is not part of a routine comprehensive toxicology screen and must be specifically requested.

B. Other useful laboratory studies include electrolytes, BUN, creatinine, CPK, lactate dehydrogenase (LDH), and ECG.

V. Treatment.

A. Emergency and supportive measures

1. Correct fluid and electrolyte abnormalities with intravenous fluids and potassium as needed.
2. Diuretics and pressor support may be required in patients with congestive cardiomyopathy.
3. Monitor the ECG for 6–8 hours, and admit patients with evidence of myopathy or cardiomyopathy. Treat arrhythmias with standard drugs (see pp 10–14).

B. Specific drugs and antidotes. There is no specific antidote.

C. Decontamination (acute ingestions only; see p 45).

1. **Prehospital.** Administer activated charcoal, if available. Obviously, do not administer ipecac.
2. **Hospital.** Administer activated charcoal. Consider gastric lavage for very large ingestions.

D. Enhanced elimination. There is no known role for enhanced elimination. The alkaloids are highly bound to tissue.

▶ IRON

Olga F. Woo, PharmD

Iron is widely used for treatment of anemia, for prenatal supplementation, and as a common daily vitamin supplement. Because of its wide availability (often in large, non-childproof containers) and its presumed harmlessness as a common over-the-counter nutritional supplement, it remains one of the most common childhood ingestions and is the leading cause of fatal poisonings in children. There are many different iron preparations, containing various amounts of iron salts. Most children's preparations contain 12–18 mg of elemental iron per dose, and most adult preparations contain 60–90 mg of elemental iron per dose.

I. **Mechanism of toxicity.** Toxicity results from direct corrosive effects and cellular toxicity.

    A. Iron has a direct **corrosive effect** on mucosal tissue and may cause hemorrhagic necrosis and perforation. Fluid loss from the gastrointestinal tract results in severe hypovolemia.

    B. **Absorbed iron** in excess of protein binding capacity causes cellular dysfunction, resulting in lactic acidosis and necrosis. The exact mechanism for cellular toxicity is not known, but iron ligands can cause oxidative and free-radical injury.

II. **Toxic dose.** The acute lethal dose in animal studies is 150–200 mg/kg of elemental iron. The lowest reported lethal dose in a child was 600 mg. Symptoms are unlikely if less than 20 mg/kg of elemental iron has been ingested. Doses between 20–30 mg/kg may produce self-limited vomiting, abdominal pain, and diarrhea. Ingestion of more than 40 mg/kg is considered potentially serious and more than 60 mg/kg potentially lethal.

III. **Clinical presentation.** Iron poisoning is usually described in four stages, although the clinical manifestations may overlap.

    A. Shortly after ingestion, the corrosive effects of iron cause vomiting and diarrhea, often bloody. Massive fluid or blood loss into the gastrointestinal tract may result in shock, renal failure, and death.

    B. Victims who survive this phase may experience a latent period of apparent improvement over 12 hours.

    C. This may be followed by an abrupt relapse with coma, shock, seizures, metabolic acidosis, coagulopathy, hepatic failure, and death. *Yersinia enterocolitica* sepsis may occur.

    D. If the victim survives, scarring from the initial corrosive injury may result in pyloric stricture or other intestinal obstructions.

IV. **Diagnosis** is based on a history of exposure and the presence of vomiting, diarrhea, hypotension, and other clinical signs. Elevation of the white blood count (> 15,000) or blood glucose (> 150 mg/dL) or visible radiopaque pills on abdominal x-ray also suggests significant ingestion. Serious toxicity is very unlikely if the white count, glucose, and x-ray are normal and there is no spontaneous vomiting or diarrhea.

    A. **Specific levels.** If the total serum iron level is higher than 450–500 µg/dL, toxicity is likely to develop. Serum levels higher than 800–1000 µg/dL are associated with severe poisoning. Determine the serum iron level at 4–6 hours after ingestion, and repeat determinations after 8–12 hours to rule out delayed absorption (eg, from a sustained-release tablet or a tablet bezoar). The total iron-binding capacity (TIBC) is unreliable in iron overdose and should not be used to estimate free iron levels.

    B. **Other useful laboratory studies** include CBC, electrolytes, glucose, BUN, creatinine, liver function tests, coagulation studies, and abdominal x-ray.

V. **Treatment.** Patients who have self-limited mild gastrointestinal symptoms or who remain asymptomatic for 6 hours are unlikely to develop serious intoxication. On the other hand, those few with serious ingestion must be promptly and aggressively managed.

    A. **Emergency and supportive measures**

        1. Maintain an open airway and assist ventilation if necessary (see pp 1–7).

        2. Treat shock caused by hemorrhagic gastroenteritis aggressively with intravenous crystalloid fluids (p 5), and replace blood if needed. Patients are often markedly hypovolemic owing to gastrointestinal losses and third-spacing of fluids into the intestinal wall and intestinal space.

        3. Treat coma (p 18), seizures (p 21), and metabolic acidosis (p 31) if they occur.

    B. **Specific treatment.** For seriously intoxicated victims (eg, shock, severe acidosis, and/or serum iron > 500–600 µg/dL), administer **deferoxamine** (see p 355). Monitor the urine for the characteristic orange or pink-red ("vin rose") color of the chelated deferoxamine-iron complex. Therapy may be stopped when the urine color returns to normal or when the serum iron level decreases to the normal range. Prolonged deferoxamine therapy (longer than 36–72 hours) has been associated with adult respiratory distress syndrome (ARDS) and *Yersinia* sepsis.

1. The intravenous route is preferred: give 10–15 mg/kg/h by constant infusion; faster rates (up to 45 mg/kg/h) have been reportedly well tolerated in single cases, but rapid boluses usually cause hypotension. The recommended maximum daily dose is 6 g, but larger amounts have been safely given in massive iron overdoses.

2. Deferoxamine has also been given intramuscularly (eg, as a test dose in suspected poisonings while awaiting laboratory confirmation); the usual dose is 50 mg/kg, with a maximum of 1 g. However, hypotension can also occur with the intramuscular route, and this route is not recommended.

C. **Decontamination** (see p 43)

1. **Prehospital.** Activated charcoal is not effective. Ipecac-induced vomiting may be considered if it can be given within a few minutes of exposure, but keep in mind that it can aggravate iron-induced gastrointestinal irritation and interfere with whole bowel irrigation (see below).

2. **Hospital**

  a. Consider gastric lavage if the product was a liquid formulation or tablets were chewed (intact tablets are not likely to pass through a lavage tube). Do *not* use phosphate-containing solutions for lavage; these may result in life-threatening hypernatremia, hyperphosphatemia, and hypocalcemia. Bicarbonate and deferoxamine lavage are of doubtful efficacy. Deferoxamine lavage is not effective and may enhance iron absorption.

  b. **Whole bowel irrigation** (see p 50) is very effective for ingested tablets and may be considered first-line treatment, especially if large numbers of tablets are visible on plain abdominal x-ray.

  c. **Activated charcoal does not adsorb iron** and is not recommended unless other drugs have been ingested.

  d. Massive ingestions may result in tablet concretions or bezoars. Repeated or prolonged whole bowel irrigation (44.3 L over 5 days in one reported case) may remove the tablets. Endoscopy or surgical gastrotomy is rarely required.

D. **Enhanced elimination**

1. Hemodialysis and hemoperfusion are not effective at removing iron but may be necessary to remove deferoxamine-iron complex in patients with renal failure.

2. **Exchange transfusion** is occasionally used for massive pediatric ingestion but is of questionable efficacy.

▶ ISOCYANATES

Paul D. Blanc, MD, MSPH

Toluene diisocyanate (TDI), methylene diisocyante (MDI), and related chemicals are industrial components in the polymerization of urethane coatings and insulation materials. Most two-part urethane products contain some amount of one of these chemicals, and lesser amounts may contaminate one-part systems. **Methyl isocyanate** (the toxin released in the Bhopal, India, tragedy) is a carbamate insecticide precursor; it is not used in urethanes, has actions different from those of the TDI group of chemicals, and is not discussed here (see Table IV–4, p 495).

I. **Mechanism of toxicity.** Toluene diisocyanate and related isocyanates act as irritants and sensitizers at very low concentrations. The mechanism is poorly understood, but it is thought that they act as haptens. Once a person is sensitized to one isocyanate, cross-reactivity to others may occur.

II. **Toxic dose.** The ACGIH-recommended workplace short-term exposure limit (STEL) for TDI is 0.02 ppm (0.14 mg/m^3), with a threshold limit value (TLV) of 0.005 ppm (0.036 mg/m^3) as an 8-hour time-weighted average. This exposure limit seeks to prevent acute irritant effects. However, in individuals with prior TDI sensitivity, even this level may be hazardous. The level considered immediately dangerous to life or health (IDLH) is 2.5 ppm. Other isocyanates are less volatile but overexposure can occur from spray aerosols.

III. **Clinical presentation.**
   A. **Acute exposure** to irritant levels causes skin and upper respiratory tract toxicity. Burning eyes and skin, cough, and wheezing are common. Noncardiogenic pulmonary edema may occur with severe exposure. Symptoms may occur immediately with exposure or may occasionally be delayed several hours.
   B. **Low-level chronic exposure** may produce dyspnea, wheezing, and other signs and symptoms consistent with asthma. Interstitial lung injury, with radiographic infiltrates and hypoxemia, may occur less commonly.

IV. **Diagnosis** requires a careful occupational history. Pulmonary function testing may document an obstructive deficit or may be normal. Variable airflow or changing measures of airway reactivity (methacholine or histamine challenge) temporally linked to exposure strongly support the diagnosis of isocyanate-induced asthma.
   A. **Specific levels.** There are no specific blood or urine tests for isocyanates.
      1. Test inhalation challenge to isocyanate is not advised except in experienced laboratories owing to the danger of severe asthma attack.
      2. Isocyanate antibody testing, although useful epidemiologically, is difficult to interpret in an individual patient.
   B. **Other useful laboratory studies** include arterial blood gases or oximetry, chest x-ray, and pulmonary function tests.

V. **Treatment.**
   A. **Emergency and supportive measures**
      1. After acute inhalational exposure, maintain an open airway (see p 1), give bronchodilators as needed for wheezing (p 8), and observe for 8–12 hours for pulmonary edema (p 7).
      2. When airway hyperreactivity has been documented, further exposure to isocyanate is contraindicated. Involve public health or OSHA agencies to determine whether other workers are at risk.
   B. **Specific drugs and antidotes.** There is no specific antidote.
   C. **Decontamination** after high-level exposure (see p 43).
      1. **Inhalation.** Remove the victim from exposure, and give supplemental oxygen if available.
      2. **Skin and eyes.** Remove contaminated clothing (liquid or heavy vapor exposure), and wash exposed skin with copious soap and water. Irrigate exposed eyes with copious saline or tepid water.
   D. **Enhanced elimination.** There is no role for these procedures.

▶ **ISONIAZID (INH)**

Christopher R. Brown, MD

Isoniazid (INH), a hydrazide derivative of isonicotinic acid, is the bactericidal drug of choice for tuberculosis. INH is well known for its propensity to cause hepatitis with chronic use. Acute isoniazid overdose is a common cause of drug-induced seizures and metabolic acidosis.

I. **Mechanism of toxicity.**
   A. **Acute overdose.** Isoniazid produces acute toxic effects by competing with brain pyridoxal 5-phosphate, the active form of vitamin B$_6$, for the enzyme glu-

tamic acid decarboxylase. This results in lower levels of γ-aminobutyric acid (GABA), an inhibitory neurotransmitter in the brain, which leads to uninhibited electrical activity manifested as seizures. INH also inhibits the hepatic conversion of lactate to pyruvate, resulting in lactic acidosis.

B. Chronic toxicity. Peripheral neuritis with chronic use is thought to be related to competition with pyridoxine. The mechanism of chronic hepatic injury and INH-induced systemic lupus erythematosus (SLE) is not discussed here.

C. Pharmacokinetics. Peak absorption occurs in 1–2 hours. The volume of distribution is 0.6–0.7 L/kg. Elimination is by hepatic metabolism; the half-life is 0.5–1.6 hours in fast acetylators,and 2–5 hours in slow acetylators. See also Table II–55.

II. Toxic dose.

A. Acute ingestion of as little as 1.5 g can produce toxicity. Severe toxicity is common after ingestion of 80–150 mg/kg.

B. With **chronic use,** 10–20% of patients will develop hepatic toxicity when the dose is 10 mg/kg/d, but less than 2% will develop this toxicity if the dose is 3–5 mg/kg/d. Older persons are more susceptible to chronic toxicity.

III. Clinical presentation.

A. After **acute overdose,** slurred speech, ataxia, coma, and seizures may occur rapidly (usually within 30–60 minutes). Profound anion gap metabolic acidosis (pH 6.8–6.9) often occurs after only one or two seizures, probably owing to muscle release of lactic acid. This usually clears slowly even after the seizure activity is controlled. Hemolysis may occur in patients with glucose-6-phosphate dehydrogenase (G6PD) deficiency.

B. Chronic therapeutic INH use may cause peripheral neuritis, hepatitis, hypersensitivity reactions including drug-induced lupus erythematosus, and pyridoxine deficiency.

IV. Diagnosis is usually made by history and clinical presentation. INH should be considered in any patient with acute onset seizures, especially when accompanied by profound metabolic acidosis.

A. Specific levels. Isoniazid is not usually detected in routine toxicology screening. A 5-mg/kg dose produces a peak INH concentration of 3 mg/L at 1 hour (1–7 mg/L is considered anti-tubercular). Serum levels higher than 30 mg/L are associated with acute toxicity.

B. Other useful laboratory studies include electrolytes, glucose, BUN, creatinine, liver function tests (chronic toxicity), and arterial blood gases.

V. Treatment.

A. Emergency and supportive measures

1. Maintain an open airway and assist ventilation if necessary (see pp 1–7).

2. Treat coma (p 18), seizures (p 21), and metabolic acidosis (p 31) if they occur. Diazepam, 0.1–0.2 mg/kg IV, is usually effective for treatment of seizures.

B. Specific drugs and antidotes. Pyridoxine (vitamin B_6) is a specific antidote and usually terminates diazepam-resistant seizures. Administer at least 5 g IV (see p 407) if the amount of INH ingested is not known; if the amount is known, give an equivalent amount in grams of pyridoxine to grams of ingested INH. If no pyridoxine is available, high-dose diazepam (0.3–0.4 mg/kg) may be effective for status epilepticus. Pyridoxine treatment may also hasten the resolution of metabolic acidosis.

C. Decontamination (see p 43)

1. **Prehospital.** Administer activated charcoal if available. Do **not** induce vomiting because of the risk of rapid onset of coma and seizures.

2. **Hospital.** Administer activated charcoal. Consider gastric lavage for massive ingestions.

D. Enhanced elimination. Although forced diuresis and dialysis have been reported to be successful, there is probably no role for enhanced elimination because the half-life of INH is relatively short (1–5 hours, depending on acetylator status), and toxicity can usually be easily managed with pyridoxine or diazepam.

► ISOPROPYL ALCOHOL

Brett Roth, MD

Isopropyl alcohol is widely used as a solvent, an antiseptic, and a disinfectant and is commonly available in the home as a 70% solution (rubbing alcohol). It is often ingested by alcoholics as a cheap substitute for liquor. Unlike the other common alcohol substitutes methanol and ethylene glycol, isopropyl alcohol is not metabolized to highly toxic organic acids and therefore does not produce a profound anion gap acidosis. Hospitals sometimes color isopropyl alcohol with blue dye to distinguish it from other clear liquids; this has led abusers to refer to it as "blue heaven."

I. **Mechanism of toxicity.**
   A. Isopropyl alcohol is a potent depressant of the CNS, and intoxication by ingestion or inhalation may result in coma and respiratory arrest. It is metabolized to acetone (dimethyl ketone), which may contribute to and prolong CNS depression.
   B. Very large doses of isopropyl alcohol may cause hypotension secondary to vasodilation and possibly myocardial depression.
   C. Isopropyl alcohol is irritating to the gastrointestinal tract and commonly causes gastritis.
   D. **Pharmacokinetics.** Isopropyl alcohol is well absorbed and quickly distributes into body water (volume of distribution 0.6 L/kg). It is metabolized (half-life 2.5–3 hours) by alcohol dehydrogenase to acetone.
II. **Toxic dose.** Isopropyl alcohol is an approximately two- to threefold more potent CNS depressant than ethanol.
   A. **Ingestion.** The toxic oral dose is about 0.5–1 mL/kg of rubbing alcohol (70% isopropyl alcohol) but varies depending on individual tolerance and whether any other depressants were ingested. Fatalities have occurred after adult ingestion of 240 mL, but patients with up to 1-L ingestions have recovered with supportive care.
   B. **Inhalation.** The odor of isopropyl alcohol can be detected at an air level of 40–200 ppm. The recommended workplace limit (ACGIH TLV-TWA) is 400 ppm (983 mg/m^3) as an 8-hour time-weighted average. The air level considered immediately dangerous to life or health (IDLH) is 2000 ppm. Toxicity has been reported in children after isopropyl alcohol sponge baths, probably owing mainly to inhalation as well as skin absorption.
III. **Clinical presentation.** Intoxication mimics drunkenness from ethanol, with slurred speech, ataxia, and stupor followed in large ingestions by coma, hypotension, and respiratory arrest.
   A. Because of the gastric irritant properties of isopropyl alcohol, abdominal pain and vomiting are common, and hematemesis occasionally occurs.
   B. Metabolic acidosis may occur but is usually mild. The osmolar gap is usually elevated (see p 30).
   C. Isopropyl alcohol is metabolized to **acetone**, which contributes to CNS depression and gives a distinct odor to the breath (in contrast, methanol and ethylene glycol and their toxic metabolites are odorless). Acetone is also found in nail polish remover and is widely used as a solvent in industry and chemical laboratories.
IV. **Diagnosis** is usually based on a history of ingestion and the presence of an elevated osmolar gap, the absence of severe acidosis, and the characteristic smell of isopropyl alcohol or its metabolite, acetone. Ketonemia and ketonuria may be present within 1–3 hours of ingestion.
   A. **Specific levels.** Serum isopropyl alcohol and acetone levels are usually available through commercial toxicology laboratories. The serum level may also be estimated by calculating the osmolar gap (see Table I–22, p 31). Isopropyl alcohol levels higher than 150 mg/dL usually cause coma, but patients with levels up to 560 mg/dL have survived with supportive care and dialysis. Serum acetone concentrations may be elevated.

    B. Other useful laboratory studies include electrolytes, glucose, BUN, creatinine, serum osmolality and osmolar gap, and arterial blood gases or oximetry.

V. Treatment.

  A. Emergency and supportive measures

    1. Maintain an open airway and assist ventilation if necessary (see pp 1–7). Administer supplemental oxygen.

    2. Treat coma (p 18), hypotension (p 15), and hypoglycemia (p 33) if they occur.

    3. Admit and observe symptomatic patients for at least 6–12 hours.

  B. Specific drugs and antidotes. There is no specific antidote. Ethanol therapy is *not* indicated because isopropyl alcohol does not produce a toxic organic acid metabolite.

  C. Decontamination (see p 43). Because isopropyl alcohol is rapidly absorbed after ingestion, gastric emptying procedures are not likely to be useful if the ingestion is small (a swallow or two) or if more than 30 minutes has passed. For large ingestions:

    1. Prehospital. Administer activated charcoal if available. Do *not* induce vomiting because of the risk of rapidly developing coma.

    2. Hospital. Administer activated charcoal. Although isopropyl alcohol adsorbs poorly to charcoal, approximately 1 g of charcoal will bind 1 mL of 70% alcohol. Consider gastric lavage for very large recent ingestions.

  D. Enhanced elimination

    1. Hemodialysis effectively removes isopropyl alcohol and acetone but is rarely indicated because the majority of patients can be managed with supportive care alone. Dialysis is indicated when levels are extremely high (eg, > 500–600 mg/dL) or if hypotension does not respond to fluids and vasopressors.

    2. Hemoperfusion, repeat-dose charcoal, and forced diuresis are not effective.

▶ JELLYFISH AND OTHER CNIDARIA

Gerald Joe, PharmD

The large phylum Cnidaria (coelenterates), numbering about 5000 species, includes **fire coral, Portuguese man-of-war, box jellyfish, sea wasps, sea nettle, and anemones**. Despite considerable morphologic variation, all of these organisms have venom contained in microscopic structures like water balloons, called nematocysts.

  I. Mechanism of toxicity. Each nematocyst contains a small ejectable thread soaking in viscous venom. The thread has a barb on the tip and is fired from the nematocyst with enough velocity to pierce human skin. The nematocysts are contained in outer sacs (cnidoblasts) arranged along the tentacles stretched out in the water beneath the body of the jellyfish or along the surface of fire coral and the fingerlike projections of sea anemones. When the cnidoblasts are opened by hydrostatic pressure, physical contact, changes in osmolarity, or chemical stimulants as yet unidentified, they release their nematocysts, which eject the thread and spread venom along and into the skin of the victim. The venom contains numerous chemical components, including neuromuscular toxins, cardiotoxins, hemolysins, dermonecrotoxins, and histaminelike compounds.

  II. Toxic dose. Each time a nematocyst is opened, all of the contained venom is released. The degree of effect will depend on the particular species, the number of nematocysts that successfully discharge venom, the envenomation site, contact time, and individual patient sensitivity (especially in children). Hundreds of thousands of nematocysts may be discharged with a single exposure.

  III. Clinical presentation.

    A. Acute effects. Immediately upon nematocyst discharge, there is stinging, burning pain and a pruritic rash. Depending on the degree of envenomation, there may follow paresthesias, anaphylactoid symptoms, hypotension, muscle spasm, local edema and hemolysis, local and even distal erythematous papular lesions proceeding to pustules and desquamation, chills, fever, nausea, vomiting, abdominal pain, diarrhea, transient elevated liver transaminases, myalgias, arthralgias, headache, anxiety, diaphoresis, pallor, cyanosis, dysphonia, ataxia, paralysis, coma, seizures, pulmonary edema, and cardiac arrhythmias. Lethal outcomes from box jellyfish envenomation are associated with rapid onset of cardiovascular collapse.

B. Potential sequelae include erythema multiforme, keloids, infections, cosmetic tissue damage (fat atrophy and hyperpigmentation), contractures, paresthesias, neuritis, recurrent cutaneous eruptions, paralysis, and regional vasospasm with vascular insufficiency.

C. Corneal stings from the sea nettle are usually painful but resolve within 1–2 days. However, there are reports of prolonged iritis, elevated intraocular pressure, mydriasis, and decreased visual acuity lasting months to years.

IV. Diagnosis is based on the history and observation of characteristic lines of inflammation along the sites of exposure ("tentacle tracks").

A. Specific levels. Specific toxin levels are not available.

B. Other useful laboratory studies include CBC, electrolytes, glucose, BUN, creatinine, CPK, liver transaminases, and urinalysis for hemoglobin.

V. Treatment. Symptomatic care is sufficient for the majority of envenomations, even that of the box jellyfish.

A. Emergency and supportive measures
1. Maintain an open airway and assist ventilation if necessary (see pp 1–7). Administer supplemental oxygen.
2. Treat hypotension (p 15), arrhythmias (pp 10–14), coma (p 18), and seizures (p 21) if they occur.

B. Specific drugs and antidotes. Box jellyfish *(Chironex fleckeri)* antivenin from Australia terminates acute pain and cardiovascular symptoms, prevents tissue effects, and may be located by a regional poison control center (see Table I–42, p 54) for use in severe cases. Local marine biologists can help identify indigenous species for planning of specific therapy.

C. Decontamination. Avoid thrashing about, scratching, scraping, or other mechanical maneuvers that may break open the nematocysts. With double-gloved hands, attempt to wash the affected areas with cold sea or salt water. **Do** *not* use fresh water to wash affected areas because it may cause nematocysts to be discharged. Use vinegar or baking soda as described below.

The above procedures will not relieve symptoms, but they will allow careful removal of tentacles with double-gloved hands or forceps followed by shaving of the area to remove the undischarged nematocysts.

1. For most cnidarian envenomations, spray, soak, or flood the affected area with **vinegar** for 30 minutes to disarm nematocysts.
2. However, for *Chrysaora quinquecirrha* (American sea nettle), *Pelagia noctiluca* (little mauve stinger jellyfish), and *Cyanea captillata* (hair or "lion's mane" jellyfish), *do not* apply vinegar because it may precipitate firing in these species; instead, apply a slurry of **baking soda** for 10 minutes.

D. Enhanced elimination. These procedures are not applicable.

▶ LEAD

Delia A. Dempsey, MD, MS

Lead, a soft metal with no biologic value, is obtained from mining and recycled scrap lead. Lead storage batteries are the major commercial use. Lead is used in the production of pipes, cable sheathing, brass, bronze, steel, ammunition, solder, ceramics, glass, and corrosive-resistant industrial paints. It has been removed from gasoline, house paints, and most food containers. Over the past two decades, blood lead levels have decreased by 80% in adults and children. The fetus, infants, and young children are at the greatest risk from low-dose exposure. The most common source of exposure is from lead-containing paint dust and chips in poorly maintained older houses or during renovation of houses, especially those built before 1950. Other sources include folk remedies (eg, *azarcon* and *greta*), food in contact with lead-glazed ceramics, and other lead-containing food containers. Lead is minimally excreted in breast milk.

Primary prevention of exposure is the paramount goal of lead abatement programs, and universal screening of 1-year-old children is recommended by the CDC (unless the community meets criteria associated with low risk of exposure, in which case only infants and children living in older homes and those from low-income families are screened). Contact your local department of health for local programs and criteria for screening and management of lead exposure in infants and children. Contact OSHA for standards and screening criteria for workers in specific lead industries.

I. **Mechanism of toxicity.** Lead causes enzyme inhibition via sulfhydryl group binding and interacts with essential cations (calcium, zinc, and iron). Pathologic alterations may occur in heme synthesis, cellular and mitochondrial membranes, neurotransmitter release, and nucleotide metabolism. The primary target organs affected are the hematopoietic system, the nervous system, the kidneys, and the reproductive system.

   Pharmacokinetics. Lead is found in three body compartments: blood and soft tissue (the predominant compartment from which lead may be chelated); a shallow bone compartment with an elimination half-life of weeks; and a deep bone compartment with a half-life of decades. In adults, 95% of body lead is in bones, while in children the proportion is 73%. Liberation from bones can occur during prolonged immobilization, pregnancy, and demineralizing bone diseases.

II. **Toxic dose.**
   A. **Dermal** absorption is minimal with inorganic lead, but may occur with organic lead, which may also cause skin irritation.
   B. **Ingestion.** Chronic ingestion is the predominant route of exposure, and daily ingestion of a few paint chips can cause poisoning. Children absorb about 50% of dietary lead while adults absorb only 10%. Absorption is enhanced in children with iron deficiency anemia.
      1. The oral dose associated with the lowest observable effect level (LOEL) in humans is uncertain, but in a 21-day chronic ingestion study, 20 mg/kg/d increased the blood lead level from 15 µg/dL to 40 µg/dL with a concomitant increase in erythrocyte protoporphyrin.
      2. The United States Environmental Protection Agency (EPA) recommended maximum contaminant level (MCL) for lead in drinking water is 20 ppb (parts per billion).
      3. **Acute ingestion** of a single fishing weight or curtain weight has caused encephalopathy and death. Acute ingestion of 15 g of lead acetate caused death.
   C. **Inhalation.** Sanding or torching of lead-containing paint during home remodeling can result in significant inhalation. The OSHA workplace permissible exposure limit (PEL) for inorganic lead dusts and fumes is 0.05 mg/m^3 as an 8-hour time-weighted average. The level considered immediately dangerous to life or health (IDLH) is 700 mg/m^3. The PEL for tetraethyl lead is 0.075 mg/m^3, and the IDLH is 40 mg/m^3.

III. **Clinical presentation.** The multisystem toxicity of lead can produce a spectrum of clinical manifestations.
   A. **Acute ingestion** of large amounts of lead (gram quantities) may cause abdominal pain, hemolytic anemia, and toxic hepatitis and encephalopathy.
   B. **Subacute or chronic exposure**
      1. **Constitutional** effects include fatigue, malaise, irritability, anorexia, insomnia, weight loss, loss of libido, arthralgias, myalgias, and hypertension.
      2. **Gastrointestinal** effects include crampy abdominal pain (lead colic), nausea, constipation, or diarrhea.

3. **CNS** manifestations range from impaired concentration, headache, and diminished visual-motor coordination to overt encephalopathy (a life-threatening emergency characterized by hyperirritability, ataxia, delirium, convulsions, and coma). Chronic low-level exposure in infants and children may lead to decreased intelligence and impaired neurobehavioral development, decreased growth, and diminished auditory acuity.

4. **Peripheral motor neuropathy**, affecting mainly the upper extremities, can cause severe extensor muscle weakness ("wrist drop").

5. **Hematologic** effects include normochromic or microcytic anemia, which may be accompanied by basophilic stippling. Hemolysis may occur.

6. **Nephrotoxic** effects include reversible acute tubular dysfunction (including Fanconilike aminoaciduria in children), and chronic interstitial fibrosis. Hyperuricemia and gout may occur.

7. **Adverse reproductive outcomes** include diminished or aberrant sperm production, increased rate of miscarriage, preterm delivery, decreased gestational age, low birth weight, and impaired neurologic development.

C. **Repeated, intentional inhalation of leaded gasoline** has resulted in ataxia, myoclonic jerking, hyperreflexia, delirium, and convulsions.

IV. **Diagnosis.** Although overt encephalopathy and abdominal colic associated with a suspect activity may readily suggest the diagnosis of severe lead poisoning, the nonspecific symptoms and multisystem signs associated with mild or moderate intoxication may be mistaken for a viral illness or other disorder. Consider lead poisoning in any patient with multisystem findings including abdominal pain, headache, and anemia, and less commonly, motor neuropathy, gout, and renal insufficiency. Consider lead encephalopathy in any child with delirium or convulsions and chronic lead poisoning in any child with neurobehavioral deficits or developmental delays.

A. **Specific levels.** The **whole blood lead** level is the most useful indicator of lead exposure. Relationships between blood lead levels and clinical findings have generally been based on subacute or chronic exposure and not on transiently high values that may result immediately after acute exposure. In addition, there may be considerable interindividual variability. *Note: blood lead samples must be drawn and stored in lead-free syringes and tubes* ("trace metals" tube or royal blue stopper tube containing heparin or EDTA).

1. Blood lead levels are less than 10 µg/dL in populations without occupational or specific environmental exposure. Levels between 10 and 25 µg/dL have been associated with subtle decreases in intelligence and impaired neurobehavioral development in children exposed *in utero* or in early childhood, but these levels are generally without demonstrable toxic effects in adults.

2. Blood lead levels of 25–60 µg/dL may be associated with headache, irritability, difficulty concentrating, slowed reaction time, and other neuropsychiatric effects. Anemia may occur, and subclinical slowing of motor nerve conduction may be detectable.

3. Blood levels of 60–80 µg/dL may be associated with gastrointestinal symptoms and subclinical renal effects.

4. With blood levels in excess of 80 µg/dL, serious overt intoxication may occur, including abdominal pain (lead colic) and nephropathy. Encephalopathy and neuropathy are usually associated with levels over 100 µg/dL.

B. Elevations in **free erythrocyte protoporphyrin (FEP) or zinc protoporphyrin (ZPP)** (> 35 µg/dL) reflect lead-induced inhibition of heme synthesis. Because only actively forming and not mature erythrocytes are affected, elevations will typically lag lead exposure by a few weeks. A high blood lead in the presence of a normal FEP or ZPP therefore suggests very recent exposure. Protoporphyrin elevation is not specific for lead, and may also occur with iron deficiency. Protoporphyrin levels are not sensitive for low-level exposure (blood lead < 300 µg/dL).

202   POISONING & DRUG OVERDOSE

C. **Urinary lead excretion** increases and decreases more rapidly than blood lead. Normal urinary lead excretion is less than 50 µg/d. Several empiric protocols that measure 6- or 24-hour urinary lead excretion after EDTA challenge have been developed to identify persons with elevated body lead burdens; however, many physicians do not use the EDTA challenge test and rely on the blood lead level.

D. Noninvasive in vivo **x-ray fluorescence measurement of lead in bone** is an emerging research method that may provide the best index of long-term cumulative lead exposure and total body lead burden.

E. **Other tests.** Nonspecific laboratory findings that support the diagnosis of lead poisoning include anemia (normocytic or microcytic), basophilic stippling of erythrocytes, and increased urinary coproporphyrin and aminolevulinic acid (ALA). Recently ingested lead paint, glazes, chips, or lead weights may be visible on abdominal x-rays.

V. **Treatment.**

A. **Emergency and supportive measures**

1. Treat seizures (see p 21) and coma (see p 18) if they occur. Provide adequate fluids to maintain urine flow but avoid overhydration, which may aggravate cerebral edema.

2. Patients with increased intracranial pressure may benefit from corticosteroids (eg, dexamethasone, 10 mg IV) and mannitol (1–2 g/kg IV).

B. **Specific drugs and antidotes.** Treatment with chelating agents decreases blood lead concentrations and increases urinary excretion. Although chelation has been associated with improvement in symptoms and decreased mortality, controlled clinical trials demonstrating efficacy are lacking, and *treatment recommendations have been largely empiric.*

1. **Encephalopathy.** Administer **calcium EDTA** (see p 363). Some clinicians initiate treatment with a single dose of **BAL** (see p 341), followed 4 hours later by concomitant administration of calcium EDTA and BAL.

2. **Symptomatic without encephalopathy.** Administer oral **DMSA** (see p 360) or parenteral **calcium EDTA** (see p 363). EDTA is preferred as initial treatment if the patient has severe gastrointestinal toxicity (eg, lead colic).

3. **Asymptomatic children with elevated blood lead levels.** The Centers for Disease Control recommends treatment of children with levels of 45 µg/dL or higher. Use oral **DMSA** (see p 360). There is not yet a consensus on use of chelation for levels less than 45 µg/dL.

4. **Asymptomatic adults.** The usual treatment is removal from exposure and observation. Consider oral DMSA (see p 360) for patients with markedly elevated levels (eg, > 80–100 µg/dL).

5. Although d-penicillamine (see p 397) is an alternative oral treatment, it may be associated with more side effects and less efficient lead diuresis.

C. **Decontamination** (see p 43)

1. **Acute ingestion.** Because even small items (eg, a paint chip or a sip of lead-containing glaze) may contain several hundred milligrams of lead, gut decontamination is indicated after acute ingestion of virtually any lead-containing substance.

   a. Induce vomiting with syrup of ipecac, or perform gastric lavage.

   b. Administer activated charcoal (although efficacy is unknown).

   c. After ingestion of a metallic lead object (fishing or curtain weight), administer activated charcoal.

   d. If lead-containing material is still visible on abdominal x-ray after initial treatment, consider whole bowel irrigation (see p 50), repeated cathartics, or enemas.

2. **Lead-containing buckshot, shrapnel, or bullets** in or adjacent to synovial spaces should be surgically removed if possible, particularly if associated with evidence of systemic lead absorption.

D. **Enhanced elimination.** There is no role for dialysis, hemoperfusion, or repeat-dose charcoal.

E. **Other required measures.** Remove the patient from the source of exposure, and institute control measures to prevent repeated intoxication; in addition, other possibly exposed persons should be promptly evaluated.

  1. **Infants and children.** Action is determined by the blood lead level:
     a. Less than 10 μg/dL: considered nontoxic; no action required.
     b. 10–14 μg/dL: repeat screening; educate parents.
     c. 15–19 μg/dL: repeat screening, and if elevated, identify and abate the source.
     d. 20–44 μg/dL: identify and abate source; perform complete medical evaluation; consider DMSA chelation.
     e. 45–69 μg/dL: identify and abate source; perform medical evaluation; chelate with oral DMSA.
     f. 70 μg/dL or higher: immediately perform medical evaluation.
  2. **Adults with occupational exposure.** Federal OSHA standards for workers exposed to lead provide specific guidelines for periodic blood lead monitoring and medical surveillance. Under the general industry standard, workers must be removed from exposure if a single blood lead level exceeds 60 μg/dL or if the average of three successive monthly levels exceeds 50 μg/dL. In construction workers, removal is required if a single blood lead level exceeds 50 μg/dL. Workers may not return to work until the blood lead level is below 40 μg/dL and any clinical manifestations of toxicity have resolved. *Prophylactic chelation of workers in lead industries is illegal.*

▶ LIONFISH AND OTHER SCORPAENIDAE

Richard F. Clark, MD

The family Scorpaenidae are saltwater fish that are mostly bottom dwellers, noted for their ability to camouflage themselves and disappear into the environment. There are 30 genera and about 300 species, some 30 of which have envenomated humans. Although they were once considered to be an occupational hazard only of commercial fishing, increasing contact with these fish by scuba divers and home aquarists has increased the frequency of envenomations.

I. **Mechanism of toxicity.** Envenomation usually occurs when the fish is being handled or stepped on or when the aquarist has hands in the tank. The dorsal, anal, and pectoral fins are supported by spines that are connected to venom glands. The fish will erect its spines and jab the victim, causing release of venom (and often sloughing of the integumentary sheath of the spine into the wound). The venom of all these organisms is a heat-labile mixture that is not completely characterized.

II. **Toxic dose.** The dose of venom involved in any sting is variable. Interspecies variation in the severity of envenomation is generally the result of the relation between the venom gland and the spines.

  A. *Synanceja* (Australian stonefish) have short, strong spines with the venom gland located near the tip; therefore, large doses of venom are delivered and severe envenomation results.

  B. **Pterois** (lionfish, turkeyfish) have long delicate spines with poorly developed venom glands near the base of the spine and therefore are usually capable of delivering only small doses of venom.

III. **Clinical presentation.** Envenomation typically produces immediate onset of excruciating, sharp, throbbing, intense pain. In untreated cases, the intensity of pain peaks at 60–90 minutes and may last for 1–2 days.

  A. **Systemic intoxication** associated with stonefish envenomation can include the rapid onset of hypotension, tachycardia, cardiac arrhythmias, myocardial ischemia, syncope, diaphoresis, nausea, vomiting, abdominal cramping, dyspnea, pulmonary edema, cyanosis, headache, muscular weakness, and spasticity.

    B. Local tissue effects include erythema, ecchymosis, and swelling. Infection may occur owing to retained portions of integumentary sheath. Hyperalgesia, anesthesia, or paresthesias of the affected extremity may occur, and persistent neuropathy has been reported.

IV. Diagnosis is usually based on a history of exposure, and the severity of envenomation is usually readily apparent.

    A. Specific levels. There are no specific toxin levels available.

    B. Other useful laboratory studies for severe intoxication include electrolytes, glucose, BUN, creatinine, CPK, urinalysis, ECG monitoring, and chest x-ray.

V. Treatment.

    A. Emergency and supportive measures

        1. After severe stonefish envenomation:

            a. Maintain an open airway and assist ventilation if needed (see pp 1–7). Administer supplemental oxygen.

            b. Treat hypotension (p 15) and arrhythmias (pp 10–14) if they occur.

        2. General wound care:

            a. Clean the wound carefully and remove any visible integumentary sheath. Monitor wounds for development of infection.

            b. Give tetanus prophylaxis if needed.

    B. Specific drugs and antidotes. Immediately immerse the extremity in **hot water** (45 °C or 113 °F) for 30–60 minutes. This should result in prompt relief of pain within several minutes. For stonefish envenomations, a specific antivenin can be located by a regional poison control center (see Table I–42, p 54), but most of these cases can be successfully managed with hot water immersion and supportive symptomatic care.

    C. Decontamination procedures are not applicable.

    D. Enhanced elimination. There is no role for these procedures.

▶ LITHIUM

Neal L. Benowitz, MD

Lithium is used for the treatment of bipolar depression and other psychiatric disorders and occasionally to boost the white blood cell count in patients with leukopenia. Serious toxicity is most commonly caused by chronic overmedication in patients with renal impairment. Acute overdose, in contrast, is generally less severe.

I. Mechanism of toxicity. Lithium is a cation that enters cells and substitutes for sodium or potassium. Lithium is thought to stabilize cell membranes. With excessive levels, it depresses neural excitation and synaptic transmission.

    Pharmacokinetics. Lithium is completely absorbed within 6–8 hours of ingestion. The initial volume of distribution (Vd) is about 0.5 L/kg, with slow entry into tissues and a final Vd of 0.7–0.9 L/kg. Entry into the brain is slow, which explains the delay between peak blood levels and central nervous system (CNS) effects after an acute overdose. Elimination is virtually entirely by the kidney, with a half-life of 14–30 hours.

II. Toxic dose. The usual daily dose of lithium ranges from 300 to 2400 mg/d (8–64 meq/d), and the therapeutic serum lithium level is 0.6–1.2 mEq/L. The toxicity of lithium depends on whether the overdose is acute or chronic.

    A. Acute ingestion of 1 meq/kg (40 mg/kg) will produce a blood level after tissue equilibration of approximately 1.2 mEq/L. Acute ingestion of more than 20–30 tablets by an adult would potentially cause serious toxicity.

    B. Chronic intoxication may occur in patients on stable therapeutic doses. Lithium is excreted by the kidney, where it is handled like sodium; any state that causes dehydration, sodium depletion, or excessive sodium reabsorption may lead to increased lithium reabsorption, accumulation, and possibly intoxication. Common states causing lithium retention include acute gastroenteritis, diuretic use, use of nonsteroidal anti-inflammatory drugs, and lithium-induced nephrogenic diabetes insipidus.

III. **Clinical presentation.** Mild to moderate intoxication results in lethargy, muscular weakness, slurred speech, ataxia, tremor, and myoclonic jerks. Rigidity and extrapyramidal effects may be seen. Severe intoxication may result in agitated delirium, coma, convulsions, and hyperthermia. Recovery is often very slow, and patients may remain confused or obtunded for several days to weeks. Cases of rapidly progressive dementia, similar to Jacob-Creutzfeld disease, have occurred and are usually reversible. The ECG commonly shows T-wave inversions; less commonly, bradycardia and sinus node arrest may occur. The white cell count is often elevated (15–20,000/mm^3).

A. **Acute ingestion** may cause initial mild nausea and vomiting, but systemic signs of intoxication are minimal and usually are delayed for several hours while lithium distributes into tissues. Initially high serum levels fall by 50–70% or more with tissue equilibration.

B. In contrast, patients with **chronic intoxication** usually already have systemic manifestations on admission, and toxicity may be severe with levels only slightly above therapeutic. Typically, patients with chronic intoxication have elevated BUN and creatinine levels and other evidence of dehydration or renal insufficiency.

C. **Nephrogenic diabetes insipidus** (see p 34) is a recognized complication of chronic lithium therapy and may lead to dehydration and hypernatremia.

IV. **Diagnosis.** Lithium intoxication should be suspected in any patient with a known psychiatric history who is confused, ataxic, or tremulous.

A. **Specific levels.** The diagnosis is supported by an elevated **lithium** level.

1. Most hospital clinical laboratories can perform a stat serum lithium concentration. However, the serum lithium level is not an accurate predictor of toxicity.

a. With chronic poisoning, toxicity may be associated with levels only slightly above the therapeutic range.

b. On the other hand, peak levels as high as 9.3 mEq/L have been reported early after acute ingestion without signs of intoxication, owing to measurement before final tissue distribution.

c. *Note:* Specimens obtained in a green-top tube (lithium heparin) will give a markedly false elevation of the serum lithium level.

2. Cerebrospinal fluid lithium levels higher than 0.4 mEq/L were associated in one case report with CNS toxicity.

B. **Other useful laboratory studies** include electrolytes (the anion gap may be narrowed owing to elevated chloride or bicarbonate), glucose, BUN, creatinine, and ECG monitoring.

V. **Treatment.**

A. **Emergency and supportive measures**

1. In obtunded patients, maintain an open airway and assist ventilation if necessary (see pp 1–7). Administer supplemental oxygen.

2. Treat coma (p 18), seizures (p 21), and hyperthermia (p 20) if they occur.

3. In dehydrated patients, replace fluid deficits with intravenous crystalloid solutions. Initial treatment should include repletion of sodium and water with 1–2 L of normal saline (children: 10–20 mL/kg). Once fluid deficits are replaced, give hypotonic (eg, half-normal saline) solutions because continued administration of normal saline often leads to hypernatremia, especially in patients with lithium-induced nephrogenic diabetes insipidus.

B. **Specific drugs and antidotes.** There is no specific antidote. Thiazides and indomethacin have been used for treatment of nephrogenic diabetes insipidus (see p 34).

C. **Decontamination** (see p 43) measures are appropriate after acute ingestion but not chronic intoxication.

1. **Prehospital.** Ipecac-induced vomiting may be useful for initial treatment at the scene (eg, children at home) if it can be given within a few minutes of exposure.

2. **Hospital.** Induce vomiting or perform gastric lavage. Activated charcoal does not adsorb lithium but may be useful if other drug ingestion is suspected.

3. Whole bowel irrigation (p 50) may enhance gut decontamination, especially in cases involving sustained-release preparations that do not dissolve readily during the lavage procedure.

   D. **Enhanced elimination** (see p 51). Lithium is excreted exclusively by the kidneys. The clearance is about 25% of the glomerular filtration rate and is reduced by sodium depletion or dehydration.

1. **Hemodialysis** removes lithium effectively and is indicated for intoxicated patients with seizures or severely abnormal mental status and for patients unable to excrete lithium renally (ie, anephric or anuric patients). Repeated and prolonged dialysis may be necessary because of slow movement of lithium out of the CNS.

2. Forced diuresis only slightly increases lithium excretion compared with normal hydration and is not recommended. However, establishing normal urine output may bring the urinary lithium clearance to 25–30 mL/min.

3. Hemoperfusion and repeat-dose charcoal are not effective.

► LOMOTIL AND OTHER ANTIDIARRHEALS

Ilene B. Anderson, PharmD

Lomotil is a combination product containing diphenoxylate and atropine that is commonly prescribed for symptomatic treatment of diarrhea. Children are especially sensitive to small doses of Lomotil and may develop delayed toxicity after accidental ingestion. **Motofen** is a similar drug which contains difenoxin and atropine. **Loperamide** (Imodium) is a nonprescription drug with similar properties.

 I. **Mechanism of toxicity.**
   A. **Diphenoxylate** is an opioid analogue of meperidine. It is metabolized to **difenoxin**, which has fivefold the antidiarrheal activity of diphenoxylate. Both agents have opioid effects (see p 242) in overdose.
   B. **Atropine** is an anticholinergic agent (see p 78) that may contribute to lethargy and coma. It also slows drug absorption and may delay the onset of symptoms.
   C. **Loperamide** is a synthetic piperidine derivative structurally similar to diphenoxylate and haloperidol. It may produce opioidlike toxicity in overdose.
 II. **Toxic dose.**
   A. **Lomotil.** The toxic dose is difficult to predict because of wide individual variability in response to drug effects and promptness of treatment. The lethal dose is unknown, but death in children has been reported after ingestion of **fewer than five tablets**.
   B. **Loperamide.** A single acute ingestion of less than 0.4 mg/kg is not likely to cause serious toxicity in children over 1 year of age. Fatalities, abdominal distension, and paralytic ileus have been reported in children under 1 year of age after ingestion of 0.6–3 mg per day.
III. **Clinical presentation.** Depending on the individual and the time since ingestion, manifestations may be of primarily anticholinergic or opioid intoxication.
   A. **Atropine** intoxication may occur before, during, or after opioid effects. Anticholinergic effects include lethargy or agitation, flushed face, dry mucous membranes, mydriasis (dilated pupils), ileus, hyperpyrexia, and tachycardia.
   B. **Opioid intoxication** produces small pupils, coma, and respiratory arrest, and the onset of these effects is often delayed for several hours after ingestion.
   C. All the antidiarrheals may cause vomiting, abdominal distention, and paralytic ileus.
IV. **Diagnosis** is based on the history and signs of anticholinergic or opioid intoxication.

A. **Specific levels.** Specific serum levels are not available.
B. **Other useful laboratory studies** include electrolytes, glucose, and arterial blood gases (if respiratory insufficiency is suspected).
V. **Treatment.**
  A. **Emergency and supportive measures**
    1. Maintain an open airway and assist ventilation if necessary (see pp 1–7).
    2. Treat coma (p 18) and hypotension (p 15) if they occur.
    3. Because of the danger of abrupt respiratory arrest, observe all children with Lomotil or Motofen ingestion in an intensive care unit for 18–24 hours. Similar precautions should be taken for patients with very large ingestions of loperamide.
  B. **Specific drugs and antidotes**
    1. Administer **naloxone**, 1–2 mg IV (see p 384), to patients with lethargy, apnea, or coma. Repeated doses of naloxone may be required, because its duration of effect (1–2 hours or less) is much shorter than that of the opioids in these products.
    2. There is no evidence that **physostigmine** (see p 402) is beneficial for this overdose, although theoretically it may reverse signs of anticholinergic poisoning.
  C. **Decontamination** (see p 43)
    1. **Prehospital.** Administer activated charcoal, if available. Do *not* induce vomiting because of the risk for unpredictable onset of coma.
    2. **Hospital.** Administer activated charcoal. Gastric emptying is not necessary after a small ingestion if activated charcoal can be given promptly.
  D. **Enhanced elimination.** There is no role for these procedures.

▶ LYSERGIC ACID DIETHYLAMIDE (LSD) AND OTHER HALLUCINOGENS

Karl A. Sporer, MD

Patients seeking medical care after self-administering mind-altering substances may have used any of a large variety of chemicals. Several of these agents are discussed elsewhere in this manual (eg, amphetamines [p 68], cocaine [p 142], marijuana [p 212], phencyclidine [p 254], and toluene [p 307]). The drugs discussed in this section, LSD and other hallucinogens, have become known in some circles as *entactogens* ("to touch within"), and several have been widely used for personal experimentation as well as clinically to facilitate psychotherapeutic interviews. Table II–28 lists some of the more common hallucinogens.
  I. **Mechanism of toxicity.** Despite many intriguing theories and much current research, the biochemical mechanism of hallucinations is not known. LSD stimulates $5\text{-}HT_2$ receptors, and many other agents are thought to alter the activity of serotonin and dopamine in the brain. Central and peripheral sympathetic stimulation may account for some of the side effects such as anxiety, psychosis, dilated pupils, and hyperthermia. Some agents (eg, MDMA) are directly neurotoxic.
  II. **Toxic dose.** The toxic dose is highly variable depending on the agent and the circumstances (Table II–28). In general, entactogenic effects do not appear to be dose-related; therefore, increasing the dose does not intensify the desired effects. Likewise, paranoia or panic attacks may occur with any dose and depend on the surroundings and the patient's current emotional state. On the other hand, hallucinations, visual illusions, and sympathomimetic side effects are dose-related. The toxic dose may be only slightly greater than the therapeutic dose.
  III. **Clinical presentation.**
  A. **Mild to moderate intoxication**
    1. The person experiencing a "bad trip" is conscious, coherent, and oriented but is anxious and fearful and may display paranoid or bizarre reasoning.

TABLE II–28. EXAMPLES OF HALLUCINOGENS

Drug or Compound	Common Name	Comments
5-Hydroxy-N,N-dimethyltryptamine	Bufotenine	From skin secretions of the toad *Bufo vulgaris*.
N, N-dimethyltryptamine	DMT	"Businessman's trip": short duration (30–60 minutes).
2,5-Dimethoxy-4-bromo-amphetamine[a]	DOB	Potent ergotlike vascular spasm may result in ischemia, gangrene.
2,5-Dimethoxy-4-methyl-amphetamine[a]	DOM, STP	Potent sympathomimetic.
4,9-Dihydro-7-methoxy-1-methyl-3-pyrido(3,4)-indole	Harmaline	South American religious and cultural drink called yage or ayahuasca.
Lysergic acid diethylamide	LSD, acid	Potent hallucinogen. Average dose 50–150 µg in tablets, papers.
n-Methyl-1-(1,3-benzodioxol-5-yl)-2-butanamine	MBDB	Nearly pure entactogen without hallucinosis or sympathomimetic stimulation.
3,4-Methylenedioxy-amphetamine[a]	MDA	Potent sympathomimetic. Several hyperthermic deaths reported.
3,4-Methylenedioxy-methamphetamine[a]	MDMA, ecstasy, Adam	Sympathomimetic; hyperthermia reported.
3,4-Methylenedioxy-n-ethylamphetamine[a]	MDE, Eve	
3,4,5-Trimethoxyphenethylamine	Mescaline	Derived from peyote cactus.
3-Methoxy-4,5-methylene-dioxyallylbenzene	Myristicin, nutmeg	
p-Methoxyamphetamine[a]	PMA	
4-Phosphoryloxy-N-N-dimethyltryptamine	Psilocybin	From *Psilocybe* mushrooms.

[a]Amphetamine derivatives. See also p 68.

The patient may also be tearful, combative, or self-destructive. Delayed intermittent "flashbacks" may occur after the acute effects have worn off and are usually precipitated by use of another mind-altering drug.

2. The person with dose-related sympathomimetic side effects may also exhibit tachycardia, mydriasis (dilated pupils), diaphoresis, bruxism, short attention span, tremor, hyperreflexia, hypertension, and fever.

B. **Life-threatening toxicity**
  1. This results from intense sympathomimetic stimulation and includes seizures, severe hyperthermia, hypertension, and cardiac arrhythmias. Hyperthermic patients are usually obtunded, agitated or thrashing about, diaphoretic, and hyperreflexic. Untreated, hyperthermia may result in hypotension, coagulopathy, rhabdomyolysis, and multiple organ failure (see p 20). Hyperthermia has been associated with LSD, methyl-D-aspartate (MDA), MDMA, and phenylmercapturic acid (PMA).
  2. Use of 2,5-dimethoxy-4-bromoamphetamine (DOB) has resulted in ergot-like vascular spasm, circulatory insufficiency, and gangrene (see pp 160 and 68).

IV. **Diagnosis** is based on a history of use and the presence of signs of sympathetic stimulation. Diagnosis of hyperthermia requires a high level of suspicion and use of a thermometer that accurately measures core temperature (rectal, tympanic membrane, or esophageal probe).
  A. **Specific levels.** Serum drug levels are neither widely available nor clinically useful in emergency management. The amphetamine derivatives (DOB, STP, MDA, MDMA, etc) cross-react in many of the available screening procedures for amphetamine class drugs. However, LSD and the other nonamphetamine hallucinogens listed in Table II–28 are not identified on routine toxicology screening. Recently, several LSD screening immunoassays have become available, although they are of limited use because of false-positive and false-negative results and a short window of detection (4–12 hours).
  B. **Other useful laboratory studies** include electrolytes, glucose, BUN, and creatinine. In hyperthermic patients, obtain prothrombin time, CPK, and urinalysis dipstick for occult blood (myoglobinuria will be positive).

V. **Treatment.**
  A. For the patient with a "bad trip" or panic reaction, provide gentle reassurance and relaxation techniques in a quiet environment. Treat agitation (see p 23) or severe anxiety states with diazepam or midazolam (p 342). Butyrophenones such as haloperidol (p 373) or droperidol are useful despite a small theoretic risk of lowering the seizure threshold.
    2. Treat seizures (p 21), hyperthermia (p 20), rhabdomyolysis (p 25), hypertension (p 16), and cardiac arrhythmias (pp 10–14) if they occur.
  B. **Specific drugs and antidotes.** There is no specific antidote. Sedating doses of diazepam (2–10 mg) may alleviate anxiety, and hypnotic doses (10–20 mg) can induce sleep for the duration of the "trip" (usually 4–10 hours).
  C. **Decontamination** (see p 43). Most of these drugs are taken orally in small doses.
    1. **Prehospital.** Administer activated charcoal if available. In general, do **not** induce vomiting, because it is relatively ineffective and is likely to aggravate psychologic distress. Emesis might be considered after a recent massive ingestion if there is no charcoal available and hospital transport will take more than 30 minutes.
    2. **Hospital.** Administer activated charcoal. There is no need for gastric lavage, unless massive ingestion is suspected or the person is unable or unwilling to ingest the charcoal.
  D. **Enhanced elimination.** These procedures are not useful. Although urinary acidification may increase the urine concentration of some agents, it does not significantly enhance total body elimination and may aggravate myoglobinuric renal failure.

▶ MAGNESIUM

Kathryn H. Meier, PharmD

Magnesium (Mg) is a divalent cation required for a variety of enzymatic reactions involving protein synthesis and carbohydrate metabolism. It is also an essential ion for proper neuromuscular functioning. Oral magnesium is widely available in over-the-counter antacids (eg, Maalox and Mylanta) and cathartics (milk of magnesia, magnesium citrate). Intravenous magnesium is used to treat toxemia of pregnancy, polymorphous ventricular tachycardia, refractory ventricular arrhythmias, and rarely, bronchospasm.

I. Mechanism of toxicity.

A. Elevated serum magnesium concentrations act as a CNS depressant and block neuromuscular transmission, perhaps by inhibiting acetylcholine release at the motor endplate.

B. Hypermagnesemia amplifies the response to neuromuscular blockers.

C. Large doses of orally administered magnesium cause diarrhea, usually within 3 hours. Repeated or excessive doses of cathartics can cause serious fluid and electrolyte abnormalities.

II. Toxic dose. Only about 30% of orally administered magnesium is absorbed from the gastrointestinal tract, and excess magnesium is usually rapidly excreted by the kidneys. Hypermagnesemia rarely occurs after acute or chronic overexposure except in patients with renal insufficiency or massive overdose.

A. Commonly available antacids (eg, Maalox, Mylanta, and others) contain 12.5–37.5 mEq of magnesium per 15 mL (one tablespoon), milk of magnesia contains about 40 meq per 15 mL, and magnesium sulfate contains 8 mEq per g.

B. Ingestion of 200 g of magnesium sulfate (1600 meq magnesium) caused coma in a young woman with normal renal function.

III. Clinical presentation. Moderate toxicity may cause nausea, vomiting, weakness, and cutaneous flushing. Larger doses can cause cardiac conduction abnormalities, hypotension, severe muscle weakness, and lethargy. Very high levels can cause coma, respiratory arrest, and asystole (see Table II–29).

IV. Diagnosis should be suspected in a patient with renal insufficiency who presents with weakness or hypotonia, especially if there is a history of using magnesium-containing antacids or cathartics.

A. Specific levels. Determination of serum magnesium concentration is usually rapidly available. The normal range is 1.5–2.2 mEq/L. Therapeutic levels for treatment of toxemia of pregnancy (eclampsia) are 2.5–5 mEq/L.

B. Other useful laboratory studies include electrolytes, BUN, creatinine, serum osmolality and osmolar gap (magnesium may elevate the osmolar gap), calcium, and ECG.

V. Treatment.

A. Emergency and supportive measures

1. Maintain an open airway and assist ventilation if necessary (see pp 1–7).

TABLE II–29. MAGNESIUM POISONING

Magnesium Serum Levels (mEq/L)	Symptoms
> 3	Nausia, vomiting, weakness, cutaneous flushing
> 5	ECG changes—prolonged PR, QRS, QT intervals
7–10	Hypotension, loss of deep tendon reflexes, sedation
> 10	Muscle paralysis, respiratory arrest , hypotension, arrrhythmias
> 14	Death from respiratory arrest or asystole

2. Replace fluid and electrolyte losses caused by excessive catharsis.
3. Treat hypotension with intravenous fluids and dopamine (see p 15).
  B. Specific drugs and antidotes. There is no specific antidote. Administration of intravenous **calcium** (see p 350) may temporarily alleviate respiratory depression.
  C. Decontamination (see p 43)
   1. Prehospital. Ipecac-induced vomiting may be useful for initial treatment at the scene (eg, children at home) if it can be given within a few minutes of exposure.
   2. Hospital. Consider gastric lavage for large recent ingestions. Do **not** administer a cathartic. Activated charcoal is not effective.
  D. Enhanced elimination
   1. Hemodialysis rapidly removes magnesium and is the only route of elimination in anuric patients.
   2. Hemoperfusion and repeat-dose charcoal are not effective.

▶ MANGANESE

Paul D. Blanc, MD, MSPH

Manganese intoxication is generally caused by chronic rather than acute exposure. Sources of exposure are almost universally industrial–mining, metal working, smelting, foundries, and welding. Recent studies also suggest a possible link between an organic manganese fungicide (Maneb) and chronic neurologic toxicity. A gasoline additive, methylcyclopentadienyl manganese tricarbonyl (MMT), has been promoted for combustion efficiency but has potential health concerns.
  I. Mechanism of toxicity. The precise mechanism is not known. The central nervous system is the target organ.
 II. Toxic dose. The primary route of exposure is inhalation; inorganic manganese is poorly absorbed from the gastrointestinal tract. The OSHA workplace permissible exposure limit (PEL) for manganese dust is 5 mg/m^3. The air level considered to be immediately dangerous to life or health (IDLH) is 10,000 ppm.
III. Clinical presentation. Acute high-level manganese inhalation can produce an irritant-type pneumonitis (see p 181). More typically, toxicity occurs after chronic exposure to low levels over months or years. The patient usually presents with an effective psychiatric disorder, frequently misdiagnosed as schizophrenia or atypical psychosis. Organic signs of neurologic toxicity, such as parkinsonism or other extrapyramidal movement disorders, usually appear later, some time after a primarily psychiatric presentation.
IV. Diagnosis depends on a thorough occupational and psychiatric history.
  A. Specific levels. Testing of whole blood, serum, or urine may be performed, but the results should be interpreted with caution, as they may not correlate with clinical effects.
   1. Normal serum manganese concentrations are usually less than 1.2 μg/L.
   2. Elevated urine manganese concentrations (> 2 μg/L) may confirm recent acute exposure. Exposures at the OSHA PEL usually do not raise urinary levels above 8 μg/L. Chelation challenge does not have a role in diagnosis.
   3. Hair and nail levels are not useful.
  B. Other useful laboratory studies include arterial blood gases or oximetry, chest x-ray (after acute, heavy, symptomatic inhalation exposure), and magnetic resonance imaging (MRI) of the brain.
 V. Treatment.
  A. Emergency and supportive measures
   1. Acute inhalation. Administer supplemental oxygen. Treat bronchospasm (see p 8) and noncardiogenic pulmonary edema (see p 7) if they occur.
   2. Chronic intoxication. Psychiatric and neurologic effects are treated with the usual psychiatric and antiparkinsonian drugs, but often respond poorly.

B. **Specific drugs and antidotes.** EDTA and other chelators have **not** been
proved effective after chronic neurologic damage has occurred. The efficacy
of chelators early after acute exposure has not been studied.
C. **Decontamination** (see p 43)
1. **Acute inhalation.** Remove the victim from exposure and give supplemental oxygen if available.
2. **Ingestion.** Because inorganic manganese is so poorly absorbed from the
gastrointestinal tract, gut decontamination is probably not necessary. For
massive ingestions, particularly of organic compounds (eg, Maneb and
MMT), gastric lavage and activated charcoal may be appropriate but have
not been studied.
D. **Enhanced elimination.** There is no known role for dialysis or hemoperfusion.

▶ MARIJUANA

Neil L. Benowitz, MD

Marijuana consists of the leaves and flowering parts of the plant *Cannabis sativa* and is
usually smoked in cigarettes ("joints" or "reefers") or pipes or added to food (usually
cookies or brownies). Resin from the plant may be dried and compressed into blocks
called hashish. Marijuana contains a number of cannabinoids; the primary psychoactive one is delta-9-tetrahydrocannabinol (THC). THC is also available in capsule form
(dronabinol or Marinol) as an appetite stimulant, used primarily for AIDS-related
anorexia, and as treatment for vomiting associated with cancer chemotherapy.
I. **Mechanism of toxicity.** THC, which binds to anandamide receptors in the brain,
may have stimulant, sedative, or hallucinogenic actions depending on the dose
and time after consumption. Both catecholamine release (resulting in tachycardia) and inhibition of sympathetic reflexes (resulting in orthostatic hypotension)
may be observed.
Pharmacokinetics. Only about 10–20% of ingested dronabinol is absorbed,
with onset of effects within 30–60 minutes and peak absorption at 2–4 hours. Metabolized by hydroxylation to active and inactive metabolites. Elimination half-life
is 20–30 hours, but may be longer in chronic users.
II. **Toxic dose.** Typical marijuana cigarettes contain 1–3% THC, but more potent
varieties may contain up to 15% THC. Hashish contains 3–6% and hashish oil
30–50% THC. Dronabinol is available in 2.5-, 5-, and 10-mg capsules. Toxicity is
dose-related, but there is much individual variability, influenced in part by prior
experience and degree of tolerance.
III. **Clinical presentation.**
A. **Subjective effects** after smoking a marijuana cigarette include euphoria, palpitations, heightened sensory awareness, and altered time perception followed after about 30 minutes by sedation. More severe intoxication may result in impaired short-term memory, depersonalization, visual hallucinations,
and acute paranoid psychosis. Occasionally, even with low doses of THC,
subjective effects may precipitate a panic reaction.
B. **Physical findings** may include tachycardia, orthostatic hypotension, conjunctival injection, incoordination, slurred speech, and ataxia. Stupor with pallor,
conjunctival injection, fine tremor, and ataxia have been observed in children
after they have eaten marijuana cookies.
C. **Other health problems** include salmonellosis and pulmonary aspergillosis
from use of contaminated marijuana. Marijuana may be contaminated by
paraquat, but the latter is destroyed by pyrolysis and there have been no reports of paraquat toxicity from smoking marijuana.
D. **Intravenous use** of marijuana extract or hash oil may cause dyspnea, abdominal pain, fever, shock, disseminated intravascular coagulation, acute
renal failure, and death.

IV. **Diagnosis** is usually based on the history and typical findings such as tachycardia and conjunctival injection combined with evidence of altered mood or cognitive function.
  A. **Specific levels.** Blood levels are not commonly available. Cannabinoid metabolites may be detected in the urine by enzyme immunoassay for up to several days after single acute exposure or weeks after chronic THC exposure. Urine levels do not correlate with degree of intoxication or functional impairment. Hemp and hemp seed products (eg, hemp seed nutrition bars) may provide alternative explanations for positive urine testing. While barely capable of causing a true positive for THC metabolite, they have no pharmacologic effect.
  B. **Other useful laboratory studies** include electrolytes and glucose.
V. **Treatment.**
  A. **Emergency and supportive measures**
    1. Most psychologic disturbances may be managed by simple reassurance, possibly with adjunctive use of diazepam or midazolam (p 342).
    2. Sinus tachycardia usually does not require treatment but if necessary may be controlled with beta blockers such as propranolol (p 405).
    3. Orthostatic hypotension responds to head-down position and intravenous fluids.
  B. **Specific drugs and antidotes.** There is no specific antidote.
  C. **Decontamination** after ingestion (see p 45)
    1. **Prehospital.** Administer activated charcoal if available. Ipecac-induced vomiting may be useful for initial treatment at the scene (eg, children at home) if it can be given within a few minutes of exposure.
    2. **Hospital.** Administer activated charcoal. Gastric emptying is not necessary if activated charcoal can be given promptly.
  D. **Enhanced elimination.** These procedures are not effective owing to the large volume of distribution of cannabinoids.

▶ MERCURY

Saralyn Williams, MD

Mercury (Hg) is a naturally occurring metal that is mined chiefly as HgS in cinnabar ore. It is converted to three primary forms, each with a distinct toxicology: elemental (metallic) mercury (Hg^0), inorganic mercury salts (eg, mercuric chloride [$HgCl_2$]), and organic (alkyl) mercury (eg, methylmercury). Approximately one-third of commercial mercury use is in the manufacture of chlorine and caustic soda; other major uses include electrical equipment, thermometers and other measuring and control instruments, dental amalgam, paints and pigments, and gold mining and extracting. Previous use in pharmaceuticals and biocides has sharply declined, although mercuric chloride is still commonly used as a stool fixative, and mercurochrome and thimerosal are still used as topical antiseptics. Aquatic organisms can convert inorganic mercury into methylmercury, with resulting bioaccumulation in large carnivorous fish such as swordfish.
  I. **Mechanism of toxicity.** Mercury reacts with sulfhydryl (SH) groups, resulting in enzyme inhibition and pathologic alteration of cellular membranes.
    A. Elemental and methylmercury are particularly toxic to the CNS. Metallic mercury vapor is also a pulmonary irritant. Methylmercury is teratogenic.
    B. Inorganic mercuric salts are corrosive to the skin, eyes, and gastrointestinal tract, and are nephrotoxic.
  II. **Toxic dose.** The pattern and severity of toxicity are highly dependent on the form of mercury and the route of exposure, mostly because of different pharmacokinetic profiles. Chronic exposure to any form may result in toxicity. See Table II–30 for a summary of absorption and toxicity.
    A. **Elemental (metallic) mercury** is a highly volatile liquid at room temperature.

1. Hg^0 vapor is rapidly absorbed by the lungs and distributed to the CNS. Airborne exposure to 10 mg/m^3 is considered immediately dangerous to life or health (IDLH), and chemical pneumonitis may occur at levels in excess of 1 mg/m^3. The recommended workplace limit (ACGIH TLV-TWA) is 0.025 mg/m^3 as an 8-hour time-weighted average; however, recent data suggest that subclinical effects on the CNS and kidneys may occur below this level.
2. Liquid metallic mercury is poorly absorbed from the gastrointestinal tract, and acute ingestion has been associated with poisoning only in the presence of abnormal gut motility that markedly delays normal fecal elimination, or after peritoneal contamination.
B. **Inorganic mercuric salts.** The acute lethal oral dose of mercuric chloride is approximately 1–4 g. Severe toxicity and death have been reported after use of peritoneal lavage solutions containing mercuric chloride concentrations of 0.2–0.8%.
C. **Organic mercury** antiseptics undergo limited skin penetration; however, in rare cases, such as topical application to an infected omphalocele, intoxication has resulted. Oral absorption is significant and may also pose a hazard. Methylmercury is well absorbed after inhalation, ingestion, and probably dermal exposure. Ingestion of 10–60 mg/kg may be lethal, and chronic daily ingestion of 10 µg/kg may be associated with adverse neurologic and reproductive effects. The United States Environmental Protection Agency (EPA) reference dose (RfD), the daily lifetime dose believed to be without potential hazard, is 0.3 µg/kg/d.
III. **Clinical presentation.**
A. **Acute inhalation of high concentrations of metallic mercury vapor** may cause severe chemical pneumonitis and noncardiogenic pulmonary edema. Acute gingivostomatitis may also occur.
B. **Chronic intoxication from inhalation of mercury vapor** produces a classic triad of tremor, neuropsychiatric disturbances, and gingivostomatitis.
1. Early stages feature a fine intention tremor of the fingers, but involvement of the face and progression to choreiform movements of the limbs may occur.
2. Neuropsychiatric manifestations include fatigue, insomnia, anorexia, and memory loss. There may be an insidous change in mood to shyness, withdrawal, and depression, combined with explosive irritability and frequent blushing ("erethism").
3. Subclinical changes in peripheral nerve function and renal function have been reported, but frank neuropathy and nephropathy are rare.
4. Acrodynia, a rare idiosyncratic reaction to chronic mercury exposure, occurs mainly in children and has the following features: pain in the extremities, often accompanied by pinkish discoloration and desquamation ("pink disease"); hypertension; profuse sweating; anorexia, insomnia, irritability, and/or apathy; and a miliarial rash.

TABLE II–30. SUMMARY OF ABSORPTION AND TOXICITY OF MERCURY COMPOUNDS

| | Absorption | | Toxicity | |
Form	Oral	Inhalation	Neurologic	Renal
Elemental (metallic) mercury				
Hg^0 liquid	Poor	NA*	Rare	Rare
Hg^0 vapor	NA*	Good	Likely	Possible
Inorganic mercuric salts				
Hg^{2+}	Good	Rare but possible	Rare	Likely
Organic (alkyl) mercury				
RHg^+	Good	Rare but possible	Likely	Possible

*NA = Not applicable.

C. **Acute ingestion of inorganic mercuric salts**, particularly mercuric chloride, causes an abrupt onset of hemorrhagic gastroenteritis and abdominal pain. Intestinal necrosis, shock, and death may ensue. Acute oliguric renal failure from acute tubular necrosis may occur within days. Chronic exposure may result in CNS toxicity.

D. **Organic mercury compounds**, particularly short-chain alkyl compounds such as methylmercury, primarily affect the CNS, causing paresthesias, ataxia, dysarthria, hearing impairment, and progressive constriction of the visual fields. Symptoms first become apparent after several weeks or months.

1. Ethylmercury compounds may also cause gastroenteritis.
2. Phenylmercury compounds produce a pattern of toxicity intermediate between alkyl and inorganic mercury.
3. Methylmercury is a potent teratogen, and perinatal exposure has caused mental retardation and a cerebral palsy-type syndrome in offspring.

IV. **Diagnosis** depends on integration of characteristic findings with a history of known or potential exposure and presence of elevated mercury blood levels or urinary excretion.

A. **Specific levels.** Elemental and inorganic mercury follow a biphasic elimination rate (initially rapid, then slow), and both urinary and fecal excretion occur. The urinary elimination half-time is approximately 40 days.

1. **Metallic and inorganic mercury.** Whole blood, and preferably urine mercury, levels are useful in confirming exposure. In most people without occupational exposure, whole blood Hg is less than 2 μg/dL and urine Hg is less than 10 μg/L. Overt neurologic effects have occurred in persons with chronic urine Hg levels greater than 100–200 μg/L. In patients with acute inorganic mercury poisoning resulting in gastroenteritis and acute tubular necrosis, blood Hg levels are often greater than 50 μg/dL.
2. **Organic mercury.** Methylmercury undergoes biliary excretion and enterohepatic recirculation, with 90% eventually excreted in the feces; as a result, urine levels are not useful. Whole blood Hg levels greater than 20 μg/dL have been associated with symptoms. The blood mercury half-life is 50–70 days. Hair levels have been used to document remote exposure.

B. **Other useful laboratory studies** include electrolytes, glucose, BUN, creatinine, liver transaminases, urinalysis, chest x-ray, and arterial blood gases (if pneumonitis is suspected). Urinary markers of early nephrotoxicity (microalbuminuria, retinol binding protein, β_2-microglobulin, and N-acetylglucosaminidase) may aid detection of early adverse effects. Formal visual field examination may be useful for organic mercury exposure.

V. **Treatment.**

A. **Emergency and supportive measures**

1. **Inhalation.** Observe closely for several hours for development of acute pneumonitis and pulmonary edema (see p 7), and give supplemental oxygen if indicated.
2. **Mercuric salt ingestion.** Anticipate severe gastroenteritis and treat shock aggressively with intravenous fluid replacement (see p 15). Vigorous hydration may also help maintain urine output. Acute renal failure is usually reversible, but hemodialysis may be required for 1–2 weeks.
3. **Organic mercury ingestion.** Provide symptomatic supportive care.

B. **Specific drugs and antidotes**

1. **Metallic (elemental) mercury.** In acute or chronic poisoning, oral **DMSA** (see p 360) may enhance urinary Hg excretion (although its effect on clinical outcome has not been fully studied). Although penicillamine (see p 397) is an alternative oral treatment, it may be associated with more side effects and less efficient Hg excretion.
2. **Inorganic mercury salts.** Treatment with intramuscular **BAL** (see p 341), if begun within minutes to a few hours after ingestion, may reduce or avert severe renal injury. Because prompt intervention is necessary, do not

delay treatment while waiting for specific laboratory confirmation. Oral **DMSA** (see p 360) is also effective, but its absorption may be limited by gastroenteritis and shock, and it is more appropriately used as a follow-up to BAL treatment.

3. **Organic mercury.** In methylmercury intoxication, limited data suggest that oral **DMSA** (see p 360) may be effective in decreasing Hg levels in tissues, including the brain.

4. Because BAL may redistribute mercury to the brain from other tissue sites, it should not be used in poisoning by metallic or organic mercury, because the brain is a key target organ.

C. **Decontamination** (see p 43)
   1. **Inhalation**
      a. Immediately remove the victim from exposure and give supplemental oxygen if needed.
      b. Even minute indoor spills (eg, 1 mL) of metallic mercury can result in hazardous chronic airborne levels. Cover the spill with powdered sulfur, and carefully clean up and discard all residue and contaminated carpeting, porous furniture, and permeable floor covering. Do **not** use a home vacuum cleaner, as this may disperse the liquid mercury, increasing its airborne concentration. For large spills, professional cleanup with self-contained vacuum systems is recommended.
   2. **Ingestion of metallic mercury.** In healthy persons, metallic mercury passes through the intestinal tract with minimal absorption, and there is no need for gut decontamination. With extremely large ingestions, or in patients with abnormally diminished bowel motility or intestinal perforation, there is a risk of chronic intoxication. Multiple-dose cathartics, whole bowel irrigation (see p 50), or even surgical removal may be necessary, depending on x-ray evidence of mercury retention or elevated blood or urine Hg levels.
   3. **Ingestion of inorganic mercuric salts**
      a. **Prehospital.** Administer activated charcoal if available. Do **not** induce vomiting because of the risk of serious corrosive injury.
      b. **Hospital.** Perform gastric lavage. Administer activated charcoal, although it is of uncertain benefit.
      c. Arrange for endoscopic examination if corrosive injury is suspected.
   4. **Ingestion** of organic mercury. After acute ingestion, perform gastric lavage and administer activated charcoal. Immediately stop breast feeding, but continue to express and discard milk, as some data suggest this may accelerate reduction of blood Hg levels.

D. **Enhanced elimination**
   1. There is no role for dialysis, hemoperfusion, or repeat-dose charcoal in removing metallic or inorganic mercury. However, dialysis may be required for supportive treatment of renal failure, and it may slightly enhance removal of the mercury-chelator complex in patients with renal failure (hemodialysis clearance of the mercury-BAL complex is about 5 mL/min).
   2. In patients with chronic methylmercury intoxication, repeated oral administration of an experimental polythiol resin was effective in enhancing Hg elimination by interrupting enterohepatic recirculation.

▶ METALDEHYDE

Gerald Joe, PharmD

Metaldehyde is widely used in the United States as a snail and slug poison. In Europe, it is also used as a solid fuel for small heaters. The pellets are often mistaken for cereal or candy. Common commercial products containing metaldehyde (2–4%)

include Cory's Slug and Snail Death, Deadline for Slugs and Snails, and Bug-Geta Snail and Slug Pellets.

I. **Mechanism of toxicity.** The mechanism of toxicity is not well understood. Metaldehyde, like paraldehyde, is a polymer of acetaldehyde, and depolymerization to form acetaldehyde may account for some of its toxic effects. Further metabolism to acetone bodies may contribute to metabolic acidosis.

Pharmacokinetics. Readily absorbed with onset of effects in 1–3 hours. Volume of distribution and protein binding are not known. The elimination half-life is approximately 27 hours.

II. **Toxic dose.** Ingestion of 100–150 mg/kg may cause myoclonus and convulsions, and ingestion of more than 400 mg/kg is potentially lethal. Death occurred in a child after ingestion of 3 g.

III. **Clinical presentation.** Symptoms usually begin within 1–3 hours after ingestion.
   A. Small ingestions (5–10 mg/kg) cause salivation, facial flushing, vomiting, abdominal cramps, diarrhea, and fever.
   B. Larger doses may produce irritability, ataxia, drowsiness, myoclonus, opisthotonus, convulsions, and coma. Rhabdomyolysis and hyperthermia may result from seizures or excessive muscle activity. Liver and kidney damage has been reported.
   C. Metabolic acidosis and elevated osmolar gap have been reported.

IV. **Diagnosis** is based on a history of ingestion and clinical presentation. Ask about containers in the garage or planting shed; metaldehyde is frequently packaged in brightly colored cardboard boxes similar to cereal containers.
   A. **Specific levels.** Serum levels are not generally available.
   B. **Other useful laboratory studies** include electrolytes, glucose, BUN, creatinine, osmolar gap (may be elevated), and liver enzymes. If rhabdomyolysis is suspected, also perform a urine dipstick for occult blood (myoglobin is positive) and obtain a serum CPK.

V. **Treatment.**
   A. **Emergency and supportive measures**
      1. Maintain an open airway and assist ventilation if necessary (see pp 1–7).
      2. Treat coma (p 18) and seizures (p 21) if they occur. Paraldehyde should **not** be used to treat seizures because of its chemical similarity to metaldehyde.
      3. Treat fluid loss from vomiting or diarrhea with intravenous crystalloid fluids (p 15).
      4. Monitor asymptomatic patients for at least 4–6 hours after ingestion.
   B. **Specific drugs and antidotes.** There is no specific antidote.
   C. **Decontamination** (see p 43)
      1. **Prehospital.** Administer activated charcoal, if available. Do **not** induce vomiting, because of the risk of abrupt onset of seziures.
      2. **Hospital.** Administer activated charcoal. Gastric emptying is not necessary if activated charcoal can be given promptly.
   D. **Enhanced elimination.** There is no apparent benefit from dialysis, hemoperfusion, or forced diuresis. Repeat-dose charcoal has not been studied.

▶ METAL FUME FEVER

Paul D. Blanc, MD, MSPH

Metal fume fever is an acute febrile illness associated with the inhalation of respirable particles of zinc oxide. Although metal fume fever has also been invoked as a generic effect of exposure to numerous metal oxides (copper, cadmium, iron, magnesium, and manganese), there is little evidence to support this. Metal fume fever usually occurs in workplace settings involving welding, melting, or flame-cutting galvanized metal or in brass foundry operations. Zinc chloride exposure may occur from smoke bombs; while it is a severe lung irritant, it does not cause metal fume fever.

I. **Mechanism of toxicity.** Metal fume fever results from inhalation of zinc oxide (neither ingestion nor parenteral administration induces the illness). The mechanism is uncertain, but may be cytokine-mediated. It does not involve sensitization and can occur with the first exposure.

II. **Toxic dose.** The toxic dose is variable. Resistance to the condition develops after repeated days of exposure but wears off rapidly when exposure ceases. The ACGIH recommended workplace exposure limit (TLV-TWA) for zinc oxide fumes is 5 mg/m^3 as an 8-hour time-weighted average, which is intended to prevent metal fume fever in most exposed workers. The air level considered immediately dangerous to life or health (IDLH) is 500 mg/m^3.

III. **Clinical Presentation.**
   A. Symptoms begin 4–8 hours after exposure, when the victim develops fever, malaise, myalgias, and headache. The white blood cell count may be elevated (12,000–16,000). The chest x-ray is usually normal. Typically, all symptoms resolve spontaneously within 24–36 hours.
   B. Rare asthmatic responses to zinc oxide fumes have been reported but are not part of the metal fume fever syndrome.
   C. Pulmonary infiltrates and hypoxemia are not consistent with pure metal fume fever and if present suggest possible heavy metal pneumonitis resulting from cadmium or other toxic inhalations (eg, phosgene and nitrogen oxides) associated with metal-working, foundry operations, or welding.

IV. **Diagnosis.** A history of welding, especially with galvanized metal, and typical symptoms and signs are sufficient to make the diagnosis.
   A. **Specific levels.** There are no specific tests to diagnose or exclude metal fume fever. Blood or urine zinc determinations do not have a role in clinical diagnosis of the syndrome.
   B. **Other useful laboratory studies** include CBC, arterial blood gases or oximetry, and chest x-ray (to exclude other disorders).

V. **Treatment.**
   A. **Emergency and supportive measures**
      1. Administer supplemental oxygen, and give bronchodilators if there is wheezing (see pp 7–8). If hypoxemia or wheezing is present, consider other toxic inhalations (see p 181).
      2. Provide symptomatic care (eg, acetaminophen or other antipyretic) as needed; symptoms are self-limited.
   B. **Specific drugs and antidotes.** There is no specific antidote.
   C. **Decontamination** is not necessary; by the time symptoms develop, the exposure has usually been over for several hours.
   D. **Enhanced elimination.** There is no role for these procedures.

▶ **METHANOL**

Ilene B. Anderson, PharmD

Methanol (wood alcohol) is a common ingredient in many solvents, windshield-washing solutions, duplicating fluids, and paint removers. It is sometimes used as an ethanol substitute by alcoholics. Although methanol itself produces mainly inebriation, its metabolic products may cause metabolic acidosis, blindness, and death after a characteristic latent period of 6–30 hours.

I. **Mechanism of toxicity.** Methanol is slowly metabolized by alcohol dehydrogenase to formaldehyde and subsequently by aldehyde dehydrogenase to formic acid (formate). Systemic acidosis is caused by the formic acid as well as by lactic acid, while blindness is caused primarily by formate. Both ethanol and methanol compete for the enzyme alcohol dehydrogenase; the preference of this enzyme for metabolizing ethanol forms the basis for ethanol therapy in methanol poisonings.

Pharmacokinetics. Methanol is readily absorbed and quickly distributed to the body water (Vd = 0.6 L/kg). It is not protein bound. It is metabolized slowly by alcohol dehydrogenase via zero-order kinetics, at a rate about one-tenth that of ethanol. The reported "half-life" ranges from 2–24 hours, depending on whether metabolism is blocked (eg, by ethanol or fomepizole). Only about 3% is excreted unchanged by the kidneys and less than 10% through the breath.

II. **Toxic dose.** The fatal oral dose of methanol is estimated to be 30–240 mL (20–150 g). The minimum toxic dose is approximately 100 mg/kg. Elevated serum methanol levels have been reported after extensive dermal exposure and concentrated inhalation. The ACGIH recommended workplace exposure limit (TLV-TWA) for inhalation is 200 ppm as an 8-hour time-weighted average, and the level considered immediately dangerous to life or health (IDLH) is 6000 ppm.

III. **Clinical presentation.**
   A. **In the first few hours** after ingestion, methanol-intoxicated patients present with inebriation and gastritis. Acidosis is not usually present because metabolism to toxic products has not yet occurred. There may be a noticeable elevation in the osmolar gap (see p 30); an osmolar gap of as little as 10 mOsm/L is consistent with toxic concentrations of methanol.
   B. **After a latent period** of up to 30 hours, severe anion gap metabolic acidosis, visual disturbances, blindness, seizures, coma, and death may occur. Patients describe the visual disturbance as haziness or "like standing in a snow-field." Fundoscopic examination may reveal optic disc hyperemia, venous engorgement, or papilledema. The latent period is longer when ethanol has been ingested concurrently with methanol.

IV. **Diagnosis** is usually based on the history, symptoms, and laboratory findings because stat methanol levels are rarely available. Calculation of the osmolar and anion gaps (see p 30) can be used to estimate the methanol level and to predict the severity of the ingestion. A large anion gap not accounted for by elevated lactate suggests possible methanol (or ethylene glycol) poisoning, because the anion gap in these cases is mostly nonlactate.
   A. **Specific levels**
      1. **Serum methanol** levels higher than 20 mg/dL should be considered toxic, and levels higher than 40 mg/dL should be considered very serious. After the latent period, a low or nondetectable methanol level does not rule out serious intoxication in a symptomatic patient because all the methanol may already have been metabolized to formate.
      2. Elevated **serum formate** concentrations may confirm the diagnosis and are a better measure of toxicity, but formate levels are not yet widely available.
   B. **Other useful laboratory studies** include electrolytes, glucose, BUN, creatinine, serum osmolality and osmolar gap, arterial blood gases, ethanol level, and lactate level.

V. **Treatment.**
   A. **Emergency and supportive measures**
      1. Maintain an open airway and assist ventilation if necessary (see pp 1–7).
      2. Treat coma (p 18) and seizures (p 21) if they occur.
      3. Treat metabolic acidosis with intravenous sodium bicarbonate (p 345). Correction of acidosis should be guided by arterial blood gases.
   B. **Specific drugs and antidotes**
      1. Administer **fomepizole** (see p 370) or **ethanol** (see p 367) to saturate the enzyme alcohol dehydrogenase and prevent the formation of methanol's toxic metabolites. Therapy is indicated in patients with the following:
         a. A history of significant methanol ingestion, when methanol serum levels are not immediately available and the osmolar gap is greater than 5 mOsm/L.
         b. Metabolic acidosis and an osmolar gap greater than 5–10 mOsm/L not accounted for by ethanol.
         c. A methanol blood concentration greater than 20 mg/dL.

2. **Folic acid** (see p 370) may enhance the conversion of formate to carbon dioxide and water. A reasonable dose is 50 mg IV every 4 hours.
   C. **Decontamination** (see p 43)
      1. **Prehospital.** Do *not* induce vomiting.
      2. **Hospital.** Perform gastric lavage. Activated charcoal has not been shown to efficiently adsorb methanol in vivo.
   D. **Enhanced elimination.** Hemodialysis rapidly removes both methanol (half-life reduced to 3–6 hours) and formate. The indications for dialysis are suspected methanol poisoning with significant metabolic acidosis, an osmolar gap greater than 10 mOsm/L, or a measured serum methanol concentration greater than 40 mg/dL. Dialysis should be continued until the methanol concentration is less than 20 mg/dL. *Note:* The ethanol infusion must be increased during dialysis (see Ethanol, p 367).

▶ METHEMOGLOBINEMIA

Paul D. Blanc, MD, MSPH

Methemoglobin is an oxidized form of hemoglobin. Many oxidant chemicals and drugs are capable of inducing methemoglobinemia: nitrites and nitrates, bromates and chlorates, aniline derivatives, antimalarial agents, dapsone, sulfonamides, local anesthetics, and numerous others (Table II–31). Occupational risk groups include chemical and munitions workers. An important environmental source for methemoglobinemia in infants is nitrate-contaminated well water. Amyl and butyl nitrite are abused for their alleged sexual enhancement properties. Oxides of nitrogen and other oxidant combustion products make smoke inhalation an important potential cause of methemoglobinemia.

I. **Mechanism of toxicity.**
   A. Methemoglobin inducers act by oxidizing ferrous (Fe^{2+}) to ferric (Fe^{3+}) hemoglobin. This abnormal hemoglobin is incapable of carrying oxygen, inducing a functional anemia. In addition, the shape of the oxygen-hemoglobin dissociation curve is altered, aggravating cellular hypoxia.
   B. Methemoglobinemia does not directly cause hemolysis; however, many oxidizing agents that induce methemoglobinemia may also cause hemolysis through either hemoglobin (Heinz body) or cell membrane effects, particularly in patients with low tolerance for oxidative stress (eg, those with glucose-6–phosphate dehydrogenase [G6PD] deficiency).
II. **Toxic dose.** The ingested dose or inhaled air level of toxin required to induce methemoglobinemia is highly variable. Neonates and persons with congenital methemoglobin reductase deficiency or G6PD deficiency have an impaired ability to regenerate normal hemoglobin and are therefore more likely to accumulate

TABLE II–31. SELECTED AGENTS CAPABLE OF INDUCING METHOMOGLOBINEMIA

Local anesthetics	Analgesics	Miscellaneous
Benzocaine	Phenazopyridine	Aminophenol
Lidocaine	Phenacetin	Aniline dyes
Antimicrobials	**Nitrites and nitrates**	Bromates
Chloroquine	Ammonium nitrate	Chlorates
Dapsone	Amyl nitrite	Metoclopramide
Primaquine	Butyl nitrite	Nitrobenzene
Sulfonamides	Isobutyl nitrite	Nitroethane
Trimethoprim	Sodium nitrate	Nitrogen oxides
	Sodium nitrite	Nitroglycerin

methemoglobin after oxidant exposure. Concomitant hemolysis suggests either heavy oxidant exposure or increased cell vulnerability.

III. **Clinical presentation.** The severity of symptoms usually correlates with measured methemoglobin levels (Table II–32).

    A. Symptoms and signs are caused by decreased blood oxygen content and cellular hypoxia and include headache, dizziness, and nausea, progressing to dyspnea, confusion, seizures, and coma. Even at low levels, skin discoloration ("chocolate cyanosis"), especially of the nails, lips, and ears, is striking.

    B. Usually, mild methemoglobinemia (< 15 – 20%) is well-tolerated and will resolve spontaneously. Continued metabolism of oxidant compounds from a long-acting parent compound (eg, dapsone) may lead to prolonged effects (2–3 days).

IV. **Diagnosis.** The patient with mild to moderate methemoglobinemia appears markedly cyanotic, yet may be relatively asymptomatic. The arterial oxygen partial pressure (pO_2) is normal. The diagnosis is suggested by the finding of "chocolate brown" blood (dry a drop of blood on filter paper and compare with normal blood), which is usually apparent when the methemoglobin level exceeds 15%. Differential diagnosis includes other causes of cellular hypoxia (eg, carbon monoxide, cyanide, and hydrogen sulfide) and sulfhemoglobinemia.

    A. Specific levels. The co-oximeter type of arterial blood gas analyzer will directly measure oxygen saturation and methemoglobin percentages (measure as soon as possible, because levels fall rapidly in vitro).

        1. *Note:* Sulfhemoglobin and the antidote methylene blue both produce erroneously high levels on the co-oximeter: a dose of 2 mL/kg methylene blue gives a false-positive methemoglobin of approximately 15%.

        2. The routine arterial blood gas machine measures the serum pO_2 (which is normal) and calculates a falsely normal oxygen saturation.

        3. Pulse oximetry is *not* reliable; it will appear deceptively near-normal in a patient with severe methemoglobinemia, and falsely desaturated in a patient who has been given methylene blue.

    B. Other useful laboratory studies include electrolytes and glucose. If hemolysis is suspected, add CBC, haptoglobin, peripheral smear, and urinalysis dipstick for occult blood (free hemoglobin is positive).

V. **Treatment.**

    A. Emergency and supportive measures

        1. Maintain an open airway and assist ventilation if necessary (see pp 1–7). Administer supplemental oxygen.

        2. Usually, mild methemoglobinemia (<15 – 20%) will resolve spontaneously and requires no intervention.

    B. Specific drugs and antidotes

        1. Methylene blue (see p 381) is indicated in the symptomatic patient with methemoglobin levels higher than 20% or when even minimal compromise of oxygen-carrying capacity is potentially harmful (eg, pre-existing anemia,

TABLE II–32. CORRELATION OF SYMPTOMS WITH METHEMOGLOBIN LEVELS

Methemoglobin Level[a]	Typical Symptoms
< 15%	Usually asymptomatic
15–20%	Cyanosis, mild symptoms
20–45%	Marked cyanosis, moderate symptoms
45–70%	Severe cyanosis, severe symptoms
> 70%	Usually lethal

[a]These percentages assume normal range total hemoglobin concentrations. Concomitant anemia may lead to more severe symptoms at lower proportional methemoglobinemia.

congestive heart failure, pneumocystis pneumonia, angina pectoris, etc). Give methylene blue, 1–2 mg/kg (0.1–0.2 mL/kg of 1% solution) over several minutes. *Caution:* methylene blue can slightly worsen methemoglobinemia when given in excessive amounts; in patients with G6PD deficiency, it may aggravate methemoglobinemia and cause hemolysis.

2. **Ascorbic acid**, which can reverse methemoglobin by an alternate metabolic pathway, is of minimal use acutely because of its slow action.

C. **Decontamination** (see p 43) depends on the specific agent involved.

D. **Enhanced elimination** (see p 51)
   1. If methylene blue is contraindicated (eg, G6PD deficiency) or has not been effective, **exchange transfusion** may rarely be necessary in patients with severe methemoglobinemia.
   2. **Hyperbaric oxygen** is theoretically capable of supplying sufficient oxygen independent of hemoglobin, and may be useful in extremely serious cases that do not respond rapidly to antidotal treatment.

▶ METHYL BROMIDE

Delia A. Dempsey, MS, MD

Methyl bromide is an odorless, colorless extremely toxic gas used as a fumigant (against fungi, nematodes, insects, weeds, and rodents) on soil, perishable foods, and in buildings. It is a potent alkylating agent and is used in the chemical industry. Before World War II, liquid methyl bromide was used as a refrigerant and in some fire extinguishers. Although its predominant present use is agricultural, urban use for structural pest control has been steadily increasing. For its use as a fumigant, fields or buildings are evacuated and covered with a giant tarp, and the gas is introduced. After 12–24 hours, the tarp is removed, and the area is ventilated and then tested for residual methyl bromide before reoccupation.

Methyl bromide is threefold heavier than air and may accumulate in low-lying areas (including basements and underground connecting tunnels). It may condense to a liquid at cold temperatures (38.5 °F or 3.6 °C), then vaporize when temperatures rise. Methyl bromide gas has poor warning properties, so the lacrimator chloropicrin (2%) is usually added. However, chlorpicrin has a different vapor pressure and may dissipate at a different rate, limiting its warning properties.

I. **Mechanism of toxicity.** Methyl bromide is a potent nonspecific alkylating agent with a special affinity for sulfhydryl and amino groups. Limited data indicate that toxicity is either the result of direct alkylation of cellular components (eg, glutathione, proteins, or DNA) or formation of toxic metabolites from methylated glutathione. Animal data clearly indicate that its toxicity does not result from dissociation into methyl alcohol and bromide ion.

   Pharmacokinetics. Inhaled methyl bromide is rapidly distributed to all tissues and metabolized. In sublethal animal studies, approximately 50% is eliminated as exhaled carbon dioxide, 25% is excreted in urine and feces, and 25% is bound to tissues as a methyl group. The elimination half-life of the bromide ion is 9–15 days.

II. **Toxic dose.**

A. **Inhalation** is the most important route of exposure. The ACGIH recommended workplace exposure limit (TLV-TWA) in air is 1 ppm ($3.9 mg/m^3$) as an 8-hour time-weighted average. Toxic effects are generally seen at levels of 200 ppm, and the air level considered immediately dangerous to life or health (IDLH) is 250 ppm. NIOSH considers methyl bromide a potential occupational carcinogen.

B. **Skin** irritation and absorption may occur, causing burns and systemic toxicity. Methyl bromide may penetrate clothing and some protective gear. Retention of the gas in clothing and rubber boots can be a source of prolonged percutaneous exposure.

III. **Clinical presentation.**
  A. **Acute irritant effects** are limited, and lethal exposures can occur without warning if chlorpicrin has not been added. Chloropicrin is probably responsible for most reports of eye, mucous membrane, and upper respiratory irritation after low-level exposures. Moderate skin exposure can result in dermatitis and, in severe cases, chemical burns.
  B. **Acute systemic effects** are usually delayed several hours and may include malaise, visual disturbances, headache, nausea, vomiting, tremor, seizures, and coma. In some cases there is a 6- to 48-hour prodrome of nausea, vomiting, and other symptoms before the onset of intractable seizures and coma. Death may be caused by fulminant respiratory failure with noncardiogenic pulmonary edema or complications of status epilepticus. Sublethal exposure may result in flulike symptoms, respiratory complaints, or chronic effects.
  C. **Chronic neurologic sequelae** can result from chronic exposure or a sublethal acute exposure. A wide spectrum of neurologic and psychiatric problems may occur that may take months or years to resolve, or may be irreversible. Reported problems include agitation, delirium, dementia, psychoneurotic symptoms, psychosis, visual disturbances, vertigo, aphasia, ataxia, peripheral neuropathies, myoclonic jerking, tremors, and seizures.

IV. **Diagnosis** is based on a history of exposure to the compound and on clinical presentation.
  A. **Specific levels.** Methylation of tissues releases free bromide ions. Endogenous serum bromide does not usually exceed 5 mg/L (0.06 mEq/L). Although elevated bromide concentrations may indicate exposure, they do not correlate with clinical severity after acute methyl bromide poisoning, and levels of 40–400 mg/L (0.5–5 mEq/L) have been reported with both lethal and nonlethal exposures. Moreover, commonly used assays (eg, the gold chloride spectrophotometric method) are not sensitive enough to accurately determine bromide levels lower than 50 mg/L (0.6 mEq/L), which means that methyl bromide poisoning is not necessarily ruled out by negative test results.
  B. **Other useful laboratory studies** include electrolytes (falsely elevated chloride is seen with some methods: 1 mEq bromide = 1.5 mEq chloride), glucose, BUN, and creatinine. If there is respiratory distress, also perform arterial blood gases or oximetry and chest x-ray.

V. **Treatment.**
  A. **Emergency and supportive measures**
    1. Administer supplemental oxygen, and treat bronchospasm (p 8), pulmonary edema (p 7), seizures (p 21), and coma (p 18) if they occur. Seizures are often intractable and may require induction of barbiturate coma with a short-acting agent such as pentobarbital (p 398); consult a neurologist as soon as possible.
    2. Monitor patients for a minimum of 6–12 hours to detect development of delayed symptoms, including seizures and noncardiogenic pulmonary edema.
  B. **Specific drugs and antidotes.** Theoretically, N-acetylcysteine (NAC, p 334) or dimercaprol (BAL, p 341) can offer a reactive sulfhydryl group to bind free methyl bromide, although neither agent has been critically tested. Some data suggest that toxicity may be due to toxic metabolites formed from methylated glutathione; if this is true then N-acetylcysteine (NAC) could possibly exacerbate toxicity. Neither agent can be recommended at this time.
  C. **Decontamination** (see p 43). Properly trained personnel should use self-contained breathing apparatus and chemical-protective clothing before entering contaminated areas. The absence of irritant effects from chloropicrin does not guarantee that it is safe to enter without protection.
    1. Remove victims from exposure and administer supplemental oxygen if available.

2. If exposure is to liquid methyl bromide, remove contaminated clothing and wash affected skin with soap and water. Irrigate exposed eyes with copious water or saline.
D. **Enhanced elimination.** There is no role for these procedures.

▶ METHYLENE CHLORIDE

Paul D. Pearigen, MD

Methylene chloride (dichloromethane) is widely used in paint and varnish removers and as a solvent in degreasing operations; it is found in some Christmas tree lights and magic trick sets. It is also used as a fumigant for fruits and grains. Methylene chloride is metabolized to carbon monoxide in vivo and may produce phosgene, chlorine, or hydrogen chloride upon combustion. It was considered to be the least toxic of all the chlorinated hydrocarbon solvents before its implication as a suspected human carcinogen.

I. **Mechanism of toxicity.** Methylene chloride, like other chlorinated hydrocarbon solvents, is an irritant to mucous membranes, defats the skin epithelium, is a direct CNS depressant, and may sensitize the myocardium to arrhythmogenic effects of catecholamines.
   A. *Carbon monoxide* (CO) is generated in vivo during metabolism by the mixed-function oxidases in the liver. The contribution of CO to methylene chloride intoxication is minor.
   B. Methylene chloride is a **suspected human carcinogen**.
II. **Toxic dose.** Toxicity may occur after inhalation or ingestion.
   A. **Inhalation.** OSHA considers methylene chloride a potential human carcinogen. The ACGIH workplace exposure threshold limit value (TLV-TWA) is 50 ppm (174 mg/m^3) for an 8-hour shift, which may result in a carboxyhemoglobin level of 3–4%. The air level considered immediately dangerous to life or health (IDLH) is 2300 ppm.
   B. **Ingestion.** The acute oral toxic dose is approximately 0.5–5 mL/kg.
III. **Clinical presentation.**
   A. **Inhalation** is the most common route of exposure and results in mucous membrane and skin irritation, nausea, vomiting, and headache. Severe exposures may lead to pulmonary edema, cardiac arrhythmias, and CNS depression with respiratory arrest.
   B. **Ingestion** can cause corrosive gastrointestinal injury and systemic intoxication.
   C. Extensive **skin exposure** can cause significant burns and systemic symptoms owing to skin absorption.
   D. **Chronic exposure** can cause bone marrow, hepatic, and renal toxicity.
IV. **Diagnosis** is based on a history of exposure and clinical presentation.
   A. **Specific levels**
      1. **Carboxyhemoglobin** levels should be obtained, although they may not correlate with the severity of the intoxication.
      2. Expired air and blood or urine levels of **methylene chloride** may be obtained to assess workplace exposure but are not useful in clinical management.
   B. **Other useful laboratory studies** include CBC, electrolytes, glucose, BUN, creatinine, liver transaminases, and ECG monitoring.
V. **Treatment.**
   A. **Emergency and supportive measures**
      1. Maintain an open airway and assist ventilation if necessary (see pp 1–7).
      2. Administer supplemental oxygen, and treat coma (p 18) and pulmonary edema (p 7) if they occur.

3. Monitor the ECG for at least 4–6 hours, and treat arrhythmias (p 13) if they occur. Avoid the use of epinephrine, which may aggravate cardiac arrhythmias. Tachyarrhythmias caused by myocardial sensitization may be treated with **propranolol** (see p 405), 1–2 mg IV, or **esmolol** (see p 366), 25–100 μg/kg/min IV.

4. If corrosive injury is suspected after ingestion, consult a gastroenterologist regarding possible endoscopy.

B. **Specific drugs and antidotes.** Administer 100% **oxygen** by tight-fitting mask or endotracheal tube if the carboxyhemoglobin level is elevated.

C. **Decontamination** (see p 43)
   1. **Inhalation.** Remove the victim from exposure and give supplemental oxygen, if available.
   2. **Skin and eyes.** Remove contaminated clothing, and wash exposed skin with soap and water. Irrigate exposed eyes with copious saline or tap water.
   3. **Ingestion** (see p 45)
      a. **Prehospital.** Administer activated charcoal if available. Do **not** induce vomiting because of the risk of rapid CNS depression.
      b. **Hospital.** Perform gastric lavage (if there has been a large, recent ingestion), and administer activated charcoal. The effectiveness of charcoal is not known.

D. **Enhanced elimination.** There is no documented efficacy for repeat-dose activated charcoal, hemodialysis, hemoperfusion, or hyperbaric oxygen.

▶ MONOAMINE OXIDASE INHIBITORS

Neal L. Benowitz, MD

Most monoamine oxidase (MAO) inhibitors are used in treating severe depression; **procarbazine** is a cancer chemotherapeutic drug. Available drugs in this class include **furazolidone** (Furoxone), **isocarboxazid** (Marplan), **pargyline** (Eutonyl), **phenelzine** (Nardil), **procarbazine** (Matulane), and **tranylcypromine** (Parnate). **Moclobemide** (Aurorix) is available in many countries but not in the United States. Serious toxicity from MAO inhibitors occurs either with overdose or owing to interactions with certain other drugs or foods (Table II–33). **Selegiline** (Eldepryl), a MAO type B inhibitor, is not generally associated with the same toxicity or drug interactions with the other MAO inhibitors (which act on MAO type A), although there have been reports of adverse interactions with meperidine. The popular herbal product for de-

TABLE II–33. INTERACTIONS WITH MONOAMINE OXIDASE INHIBITORS[a]

Drugs		Foods
Amphetamines	Metaraminol	Beer
Buspirone	Methyldopa	Broad bean pods and Fava beans
Clomipramine	Methylphenidate	Cheese (natural or aged)
Cocaine	Paroxetine	Chicken liver
Dextromethorphan	Phenylephrine	Pickled herring
Ephedrine	Phenylpropanolamine	Smoked, pickled, or aged meats
Fluoxetine	Reserpine	Snails
Fluoxetine	Sertraline	Spoiled or bacterially contaminated foods
Guanethidine	Tramadol	Summer sausage
L-Dopa	Trazodone	Wine (red)
LSD (lysergic acid diethylamide)	Tryptophan	Yeast (dietary supplement and Marmite)
MDMA	Venlafaxine	
Meperidine (Demerol)		

[a]Possible interactions, based on case reports or pharmacologic considerations.

pression, **St. John's Wort** (*Hypericum perforatum*), appears to act as a monoamine oxidase inhibitor.

I. **Mechanism of toxicity.** MAO inhibitors irreversibly inactivate MAO, an enzyme responsible for degradation of catecholamines within neurons in the CNS. MAO is also found in the liver and the intestinal wall, where it metabolizes tyramine and therefore limits its entry into the systemic circulation. Moclobemide is a reversible MAO inhibitor and is less hazardous than the other agents.

   A. Toxicity results from release of excessive neuronal stores of vasoactive amines, inhibition of metabolism of catecholamines or interacting drugs, or absorption of large amounts of dietary tyramine (which in turn releases catecholamines from neurons).

   B. In addition, severe rigidity and hyperthermia may occur when patients receiving MAO inhibitors use therapeutic doses of meperidine (Demerol), dextromethorphan, fluoxetine (Prozac), paroxetine (Paxil), sertraline (Zoloft), venlafaxine (Effexor), or tryptophan; the mechanism is unknown but may be related to inhibition of serotonin metabolism in the CNS, resulting in "serotonin syndrome" (see p 21).

II. **Toxic dose.** MAO inhibitors have a low therapeutic index. Acute ingestion of 2–3 mg/kg or more should be considered potentially life-threatening. Serious drug or food interactions may occur in patients receiving therapeutic doses of MAO inhibitors. *Note:* Because of irreversible MAO inhibition, adverse drug interactions may occur for up to 2 weeks after discontinuing MAO inhibitors. Interactions may also occur when MAO inhibitors are started within 10 days of stopping fluoxetine, owing to the long half-life of fluoxetine.

III. **Clinical presentation.** Symptoms may be delayed 6–24 hours after acute overdose, but occur rapidly after ingestion of interacting drugs or foods in a patient on chronic MAO inhibitor therapy. Because of irreversible inactivation of MAO, toxic effects (and the potential for drug or food interactions) may persist for several days.

   A. Anxiety, restlessness, flushing, headache, tremor, myoclonus, hyperreflexia, sweating, shivering, tachypnea, tachycardia, and moderate hypertension are common with mild intoxication.

   B. Severe intoxication may result in severe hypertension (which may be complicated by intracranial hemorrhage), delirium, hyperthermia, and eventually cardiovascular collapse and multisystem failure.

   C. Hypotension, particularly when upright (orthostatic hypotension), is seen with therapeutic dosing and also may occur with overdose.

IV. **Diagnosis** is based on clinical features of sympathomimetic drug intoxication with a history of MAO inhibitor use, particularly with use of drugs or foods known to interact. Serotonin syndrome (see p 21) is suspected when the patient has myoclonic jerking, hyperreflexia, diaphoresis, and hyperthermia.

   A. **Specific levels.** Specific drug levels are not available. Most agents are not detectable on comprehensive urine toxicology screening.

   B. **Other useful laboratory studies** include electrolytes, glucose, BUN, creatinine, CPK, 12-lead ECG and ECG monitoring. If intracranial hemorrhage is suspected, perform a CT head scan.

V. **Treatment.**

   A. **Emergency and supportive measures**
      1. Maintain an open airway and assist ventilation if necessary (see p 1–7). Administer supplemental oxygen.
      2. Treat hypertension (p 16), hypotension (p 15), coma (p 18), seizures (p 21), and hyperthermia (p 20) if they occur.
      3. Continuously monitor temperature, other vital signs, and ECG for a minimum of 6 hours in asymptomatic patients, and admit all symptomatic patients for continuous monitoring for 24 hours.

   B. **Specific drugs and antidotes**
      1. Since the hypertension is catecholamine-mediated, alpha-adrenergic blockers (eg, phentolamine, p 400) or combined alpha- and beta-adrenergic blockers (eg, labetalol, p 377) are particularly useful.

2. **Serotonin syndrome** should be treated with sedation and cooling. Anecdotal reports suggest possible benefit with methysergide (Sansert), 2 mg PO every 6 hours for 3 doses, or cyproheptadine (Periactin), 4 mg PO every hour for 3 doses, presumably because of their serotonin-antagonist activity.

C. **Decontamination** (see p 43)

1. **Prehospital.** Administer activated charcoal if available. Ipecac-induced vomiting may be useful for initial treatment at the scene (eg, children at home) if it can be given within a few minutes of an acute overdose. However, it should not be used for patients with suspected food or drug interaction because of the risk of aggravating hypertension.

2. **Hospital.** Administer activated charcoal. Perform gastric lavage for a suspected large overdose.

D. **Enhanced elimination.** Dialysis and hemoperfusion are not effective. Repeat-dose activated charcoal has not been studied.

▶ MUSHROOMS

Kent R. Olson, MD

There are more than 5000 varieties of mushrooms in the United States, about 100 of which are potentially toxic. The majority of toxic mushrooms cause mild to moderate self-limited gastroenteritis. A few species may cause severe or even fatal reactions. The major categories of poisonous mushrooms are described in Table II–34. *Amanita phalloides* and other amatoxin-containing mushrooms are discussed on p 228.

TABLE II–34. CLASSIFICATION OF MUSHROOM TOXICITY[a]

Toxins	Mushrooms	Onset	Symptoms and Signs
Amatoxins (See p 228)	*Amanita phalloides, A ocreata, A verna, A virosa,* some *Lepiota* and *Galerina* species.	6–12 h	Vomiting, diarrhea, abdominal cramps, hepatic failure.
Monomethylhydrazine	*Gyrometra (Helvella) esculenta,* others.	6–12 h	Vomiting, diarrhea, weakness, seizures, hemolysis, hepatitis, methemoglobinemia.
Muscarine	*Clitocybe dealbata, C cerusata, Inocybe, Omphalotus olearius.*	0.5–2 h	Salivation, sweating, vomiting, diarrhea, miosis.
Coprine	*Coprinus armamentarius, Clitocybe clavipes.*	30 min	Disulfiramlike reaction with alcohol may occur up to 5 days after ingesting fungi.
Ibotenic acid, muscimol	*Amanita muscaria, A pantherina,* others.	0.5–2 h	Muscular jerking, anticholinergic syndrome, hallucinations.
Allenic norleucine	*Amanita smithiana.*	1–6 days	Acute renal failure.
Orellanine	*Cortinarius orellanus,* other *Cortinarius* spp.	1–12 days	Acute renal failure (tubulointerstitial nephritis).
Psilocybin	*Psilocybe cubensis,* others.	0.5–1 h	Hallucinations.
Gastrointestinal irritants	Many species.	0.5–2 h	Vomiting, diarrhea.

[a]Modified and reproduced, with permission, from Becker CE et al: Diagnosis and treatment of *Amanita phalloides*-type mushroom poisoning: Use of thioctic acid. *West J Med* 1976;**125**:100.

I. **Mechanism of toxicity.** The various mechanisms thought responsible for poisoning are listed in Table II–34. The majority of toxic incidents are caused by gastrointestinal irritants that produce vomiting and diarrhea shortly after ingestion.

II. **Toxic dose.** This is not known. The amount of toxin varies considerably among members of the same species, depending on local geography and weather conditions. In most cases, the exact amount of toxic mushroom ingested is unknown because the victim has unwittingly added a toxic species to a meal of edible fungi.

III. **Clinical presentation.** The various clinical presentations are described in Table II–34. In most cases, the onset of vomiting and diarrhea is rapid. A delay in onset of more than 6–12 hours suggests amatoxin, monomethylhydrazine, or orellanine poisoning.

IV. **Diagnosis** may be difficult because the victim may not realize that the illness has been caused by mushrooms, especially if symptoms are delayed 12 or more hours after ingestion. If leftover mushrooms are available, obtain assistance from a mycologist through a local university or mycologic society. However, note that the mushrooms brought for identification may not be the same ones that were eaten.

   A. **Specific levels.** Specific toxin levels are not available.

   B. **Other useful laboratory studies** include electrolytes, glucose, BUN, creatinine, liver transaminases, and prothrombin time (PT).

V. **Treatment.**

   A. **Emergency and supportive measures**

      1. Treat hypotension from gastroenteritis with intravenous crystalloid solutions (see p 15) and supine positioning.

      2. Monitor patients for 12–24 hours for delayed-onset gastroenteritis associated with amatoxin or monomethylhydrazine poisoning.

      3. For suspected *Cortinarius* spp. ingestion, monitor renal function for 1–2 weeks.

   B. **Specific drugs and antidotes**

      1. For **monomethylhydrazine** poisoning, give pyridoxine, 20–30 mg/kg IV (see p 407) for seizures; treat methemoglobinemia with methylene blue, 1 mg/kg IV (p 381).

      2. For **muscarine** intoxication, atropine, 0.01–0.03 mg/kg IV (p 340), may alleviate cholinergic symptoms.

      3. **Ibotenic acid-induced** or **muscimol-induced** anticholinergic symptoms may improve with physostigmine (p 402).

      4. Treat **amatoxin-type** poisoning as described below.

   C. **Decontamination** (see p 43)

      1. **Prehospital.** Administer activated charcoal if available. Ipecac-induced vomiting may be useful for initial treatment at the scene (eg, children at home) if it can be given within a few minutes of exposure.

      2. **Hospital.** Administer activated charcoal. Gastric emptying is not necessary if activated charcoal can be given promptly.

   D. **Enhanced elimination.** There is no accepted role for enhanced removal procedures.

▶ MUSHROOMS, AMATOXIN-TYPE

Shoshana Zevin, MD

Amatoxins (α-amanitin, μ-amanitin, and others) are a group of highly toxic peptides found in several species of mushrooms, including *Amanita phalloides, Amanita virosa, Amanita ocreata, Amanita verna, Galerina autumnalis, Galerina marginata,* and some species of *Lepiota.* These mushrooms are often picked and eaten by amateur foragers who have misidentified them as an edible species.

I. **Mechanism of toxicity.** Amatoxins are highly stable and resistant to heat and are not removed by any form of cooking. They are thought to act by inhibiting cellular protein synthesis by interfering with RNA polymerase.

    A. Absorption of amatoxins (and phalloidins) by intestinal cells causes cell death and sloughing after a delay of 8–12 hours.

    B. Absorption by the liver and kidneys results in severe hepatic necrosis and renal failure.

    C. **Pharmacokinetics.** Amanitin is rapidly absorbed. The volume of distribution is not known. In dogs, 85% of the dose is excreted within the first 6 hours. Enterohepatic recirculation may contribute to sustained toxicity.

II. **Toxic dose.** Amatoxins are among the most potent toxins known; the minimum lethal dose is about 0.1 mg/kg. One *Amanita* cap may contain 10–15 mg. In contrast, *Galerina* species contain far less toxin; 15–20 caps would be a fatal dose for an adult.

III. **Clinical presentation.** The onset of symptoms is characteristically delayed 8–12 hours or more after ingestion. Death occurring within the first 1–2 days usually results from massive fluid loss owing to gastroenteritis, while death occurring later usually results from hepatic failure.

    A. **Gastroenteritis.** Initially, vomiting is accompanied by severe abdominal cramps and explosive watery diarrhea. Severe fluid losses and electrolyte imbalance can occur rapidly, and some patients die of shock within 24 hours.

    B. **Hepatic failure.** Liver injury may be apparent within 24–36 hours, with rapidly rising transaminase levels. Fulminant hepatic failure may follow, with jaundice, encephalopathy, and death. Encephalopathy, metabolic acidosis, severe coagulopathy, and hypoglycemia are grave prognostic signs and usually predict a fatal outcome.

IV. **Diagnosis** is usually based on a history of wild-mushroom ingestion and the characteristic delay of 8–12 hours before onset of severe gastroenteritis (see also monomethylhydrazine-type mushrooms, p 227). However, if a variety of mushrooms has been eaten, stomach upset may occur much earlier owing to a different toxic species, making diagnosis of amatoxin poisoning more difficult.

    Any available mushroom specimens that may have been ingested should be examined by a mycologist. Pieces of mushroom retrieved from the emesis or even mushroom spores found on microscopic examination may provide clues to the ingested species.

    A. **Specific levels**

        1. A radioimmunoassay has been developed for amatoxins but is not widely available. The toxin is rapidly bound in the body within the first several hours after ingestion, and amatoxins are generally not detectable in the serum or urine more than 24 hours after exposure.

        2. A qualitative test (the Meixner test) may determine the presence of amatoxins in mushroom specimens. A single drop of concentrated hydrochloric acid is added to dried juice from the mushroom cap that has been dripped onto newspaper or other unrefined paper; a blue color suggests the presence of amatoxins. *Caution:* This test has unknown reliability and can be misinterpreted or poorly performed; it should not be used to determine the edibility of mushroom specimens!

    B. **Other useful laboratory studies** include electrolytes, glucose, BUN, creatinine, liver transaminases, bilirubin, and prothrombin time (PT).

V. **Treatment.** The mortality rate may be higher than 60% if the patient is not treated for severe fluid losses, but is probably less than 10–20% with intensive supportive care.

    A. **Emergency and supportive measures**

        1. Maintain an open airway and assist ventilation if necessary (see pp 1–7). Administer supplemental oxygen.

        2. Treat fluid and electrolyte losses aggressively, because massive fluid losses may cause circulatory collapse. Administer normal saline or another crystalloid solution, 10- to 20-mL/kg boluses, with monitoring of central ve-

nous pressure or even pulmonary artery pressure (p 15) to guide fluid therapy.
3. Provide vigorous supportive care for hepatic failure (p 38); orthotopic **liver transplantation** may be lifesaving in patients who develop fulminant hepatic failure. Contact a liver transplantation service for assistance.
B. **Specific drugs and antidotes.** There is no proved effective antidote for amatoxin poisoning, although over the years many therapies have been promoted. Animal studies suggest that early treatment with silibinin (an extract of the milk thistle) or high doses of penicillin may partially protect against hepatic injury, but human studies are lacking. There are no data to support the use of cimetidine or *N*-acetylcysteine. Consult a medical toxicologist or a regional poison control center (see Table I–42, p 54) for further information.
C. **Decontamination** (see p 45)
   1. **Prehospital.** Administer activated charcoal if available. Ipecac-induced vomiting may be useful for initial treatment at the scene (eg, children at home) if it can be given within a few minutes of exposure.
   2. **Hospital.** Administer activated charcoal. Gastric lavage may not remove mushroom pieces.
D. **Enhanced elimination.** There is no proved role for forced diuresis, hemoperfusion, or hemodialysis in the removal of amatoxins.
   1. Repeat-dose activated charcoal may trap small quantities of amatoxin undergoing enterohepatic recirculation.
   2. Cannulation of the bile duct and removal of bile have been effective in dog studies.

▶ NAPHTHALENE AND PARADICHLOROBENZENE

Mark J. Galbo, MS

Naphthalene and paradichlorobenzene are common ingredients in diaper pail and toilet bowl deodorizers and moth repellants. Both compounds have a similar pungent odor and clear to white crystalline substances, and they are therefore difficult to distinguish visually. Naphthalene 10% in oil has been used as a scabicide in the past. Naphthalene is no longer commonly used because it has been largely replaced by the far less toxic paradichlorobenzene.
I. **Mechanism of toxicity.** Both compounds cause gastrointestinal upset, and both may cause CNS stimulation. In addition, naphthalene may produce hemolysis, especially in patients with glucose-6-phosphate dehydrogenase (G6PD) deficiency.
II. **Toxic dose.**
   A. **Naphthalene.** As little as one mothball containing naphthalene (250–500 mg) may produce hemolysis in a patient with G6PD deficiency. The amount necessary to produce lethargy or seizures is not known but may be as little as 1–2 g (4–8 mothballs). Several infants developed serious poisoning from clothes and bedding that had been stored in naphthalene mothballs.
   B. **Paradichlorobenzene** is much less toxic than naphthalene; up to 20-g ingestions have been well-tolerated in adults. The oral LD_{50} for paradichlorobenzene in rats is 2.5–3.2 g/kg.
   C. **Pharmacokinetics.** Both compounds are rapidly absorbed orally or by inhalation.
III. **Clinical presentation.** Acute ingestion usually causes prompt nausea and vomiting. Both compounds are volatile, and inhalation of vapors may cause eye, nose, and throat irritation.
   A. **Naphthalene.** Agitation, lethargy, and seizures may occur with naphthalene ingestion. In patients with G6PD deficiency, naphthalene ingestion may cause acute hemolysis.

B. Paradichlorobenzene ingestions are virtually always innocuous. Serious poisoning in animals is reported to cause tremors and hepatic necrosis. Paradichlorobenzene decomposes to hydrochloric acid, which may explain some of its irritant effects.

IV. Diagnosis is usually based on a history of ingestion and the characteristic "mothball" smell around the mouth and in the vomitus. Differentiation between naphthalene and paradichlorobenzene by odor or color is difficult. Paradichlorobenzene is reportedly more rapidly soluble in turpentine. In an in-vitro x-ray study, paradichlorobenzene was radiopaque, but naphthalene was not visible.

A. Specific levels. Serum levels are not available.

B. Other useful laboratory studies include CBC and, if hemolysis is suspected, haptoglobin, free hemoglobin, and urine dipstick for occult blood (positive with hemoglobinuria).

V. Treatment.

A. Emergency and supportive measures

1. Maintain an open airway and assist ventilation if necessary (see pp 1–7).
2. Treat coma (p 18) and seizures (p 21) if they occur.
3. Treat hemolysis and resulting hemoglobinuria if they occur, by intravenous hydration and urinary alkalinization (see Rhabdomyolysis, p 25).

B. Specific drugs and antidotes. There is no specific antidote.

C. Decontamination (see p 43)

1. **Naphthalene**
   a. **Prehospital.** Administer activated charcoal if available. Do **not** induce vomiting, because of the risk of lethargy and seizures. Do not administer milk, fats, or oils, which may enhance absorption.
   b. **Hospital.** Administer activated charcoal. Gastric emptying is not necessary if activated charcoal can be given promptly.
2. **Paradichlorobenzene.** Gut emptying and charcoal are not necessary unless a massive dose has been ingested. Do not administer milk, fats, or oils, which may enhance absorption.
3. **Inhalation.** Either agent: remove the victim from exposure; fresh air is all that is required.

D. Enhanced elimination. There is no role for these procedures.

▶ NICOTINE

Neal L. Benowitz, MD

Nicotine poisoning may occur in children after they ingest tobacco or drink saliva expectorated by a tobacco chewer (which is often collected in a can or other containers); in children or adults after accidental or suicidal ingestion of nicotine-containing pesticides (such as Black Leaf 40, which contains 40% nicotine sulfate); and occasionally after cutaneous exposure to nicotine, such as among tobacco harvesters. Nicotine chewing gum (Nicorette), transdermal delivery formulations (Habitrol, Nicoderm, Nicotrol, and Prostep), and nicotine nasal spray are widely available as adjunctive therapy for smoking cessation.

I. Mechanism of toxicity. Nicotine binds to nicotinic cholinergic receptors, resulting initially, via actions on ganglia, in predominantly sympathetic nervous stimulation. With higher doses, parasympathetic stimulation and then ganglionic and neuromuscular blockage may occur. Direct effects on the brain may also result in vomiting and seizures.

Pharmacokinetics. Nicotine is rapidly absorbed by all routes. The apparent volume of distribution (Vd) is 1 L/kg. It is rapidly metabolized and excreted in the urine with a half-life of 30–80 min (the rate of elimination is pH-dependent and faster in an acidic urine).

II. **Toxic dose.** Owing to presystemic metabolism and spontaneous vomiting, which limit absorption, the bioavailability of nicotine that is swallowed is about 30–40%. Rapid absorption of 2–5 mg can cause nausea and vomiting, particularly in a person who does not habitually use tobacco. Absorption of 40–60 mg in an adult is said to be lethal, although this dose spread throughout the day is not unusual in a cigarette smoker.

A. **Tobacco.** Cigarette tobacco contains about 1.5% nicotine, or 10–15 mg of nicotine per cigarette. Moist snuff is also about 1.5% nicotine; most containers hold 30 g of tobacco. Chewing tobacco contains 2.5–8% nicotine. In a child, ingestion of one cigarette or three cigarette butts should be considered potentially toxic, although serious poisoning from ingestion of cigarettes is very uncommon.

B. **Nicotine gum** contains 2 or 4 mg per piece, but owing to its slow absorption and high degree of presystemic metabolism, nicotine intoxication from these products is uncommon.

C. **Transdermal nicotine patches** deliver an average of 5–22 mg of nicotine over the 16–24 hours of intended application, depending on the brand and size. Transdermal patches may produce intoxication in light smokers or in nonsmokers, particularly children to whom a used patch inadvertently sticks. Ingestion of a discarded patch may also potentially produce poisoning.

D. **Nicotine nasal spray** delivers about 1 mg (a single dose is one spray in each nostril).

III. **Clinical presentation.** Nicotine intoxication commonly causes dizziness, nausea, vomiting, pallor, and diaphoresis. Abdominal pain, salivation, lacrimation, and diarrhea may be noted. Pupils may be dilated or constricted. Confusion, agitation, lethargy, and convulsions are seen with severe poisonings. Initial tachycardia and hypertension may be followed by bradycardia and hypotension. Respiratory muscle weakness with respiratory arrest is the most likely cause of death.

Symptoms usually begin within 15 minutes after acute liquid nicotine exposure and resolve in 1 or 2 hours, although more prolonged symptoms may be seen with higher doses or cutaneous exposure, the latter owing to continued absorption from the skin. Delayed onset and prolonged symptoms may also be seen with nicotine gum or transdermal patches.

IV. **Diagnosis** is suggested by vomiting, pallor, and diaphoresis, although these symptoms are nonspecific. The diagnosis is usually made by a history of tobacco, insecticide, or therapeutic nicotine product exposure. Nicotine poisoning should be considered in a small child with unexplained vomiting whose parents consume tobacco.

A. **Specific levels.** Nicotine or its metabolite cotinine are detected in comprehensive urine toxicology screens, but because these are so commonly present, they will not usually be reported unless specifically requested. Serum levels can be performed but are not useful in acute management.

B. **Other useful laboratory studies** include electrolytes, glucose, and arterial blood gases or oximetry.

V. **Treatment.**

A. **Emergency and supportive measures**

1. Maintain an open airway and assist ventilation if necessary (see pp 1–7). Administer supplemental oxygen.

2. Treat seizures (p 21), coma (p 18), hypotension (p 15), hypertension (p 16), and arrhythmias (pp 10–14) if they occur.

3. Observe for at least 4–6 hours to rule out delayed toxicity, especially after skin exposure. For ingestion of intact gum tablets or transdermal patches, observe for a longer period (up to 12–24 hours).

B. **Specific drugs and antidotes**

1. **Mecamylamine** (Inversine) is a specific antagonist of nicotine actions; however, it is available only in tablets, a form not suitable for a patient who is vomiting, convulsing, or hypotensive.

2. Signs of muscarinic stimulation (bradycardia, salivation, wheezing, etc), if they occur, may respond to **atropine** (see p 340).

C. Decontamination (see p 43). *Caution:* Rescuers should wear appropriate skin-protective gear when treating patients with oral or skin exposure to liquid nicotine.

    1. Skin and eyes. Remove all contaminated clothing and wash exposed skin with copious soap and water. Irrigate exposed eyes with copious saline or water.

    2. Ingestion (see p 45). For asymptomatic small-quantity cigarette ingestions, no gut decontamination is necessary.

        a. Prehospital. Administer activated charcoal if available. Do *not* induce vomiting because of the risk of abrupt onset of seizures.

        b. Hospital. Administer activated charcoal. Consider gastric lavage for large recent ingestions of liquid nicotine.

        c. For ingestion by transdermal patches or large amounts of gum, consider repeated doses of charcoal and whole bowel irrigation (see p 50).

D. Enhanced elimination. These procedures are not likely to be useful because the endogenous clearance of nicotine is high, its half-life is relatively short (2 hours), and the volume of distribution is large.

▶ NITRATES AND NITRITES

Neal L. Benowitz, MD

Organic nitrates (eg, nitroglycerin, isosorbide dinitrate, and isosorbide mononitrate) are widely used as vasodilators for the treatment of ischemic heart disease and heart failure. Organic nitrates such as nitroglycerin are also used in explosives. Bismuth subnitrate, ammonium nitrate, and silver nitrate are used in antidiarrheal, diuretic, and topical burn medications, respectively. Sodium and potassium nitrate and nitrite are used in preserving cured foods and may also occur in high concentrations in some well water. Butyl, amyl, ethyl, and isobutyl nitrites are often sold as "room deodorizers" or "liquid incense" and are sometimes inhaled for abuse purposes.

I. Mechanism of toxicity. Nitrates and nitrites both cause vasodilation, which can result in hypotension.

    A. Nitrates relax veins at lower doses and arteries at higher doses. Nitrates may be converted into nitrites in the gastrointestinal tract, especially in infants.

    B. Nitrites are potent oxidizing agents. Oxidation of hemoglobin by nitrites may result in methemoglobinemia (see p 220), which hinders oxygen-carrying capacity and oxygen delivery. Many organic nitrites (eg, amyl nitrite and butyl nitrite) are volatile and may be inhaled.

II. Toxic dose. In the quantities found in food, nitrates and nitrites are generally not toxic; however, infants may develop methemoglobinemia after ingestion of sausages or well water because they readily convert nitrate to nitrite and because their hemoglobin is more susceptible to oxidation compared with that of adults.

    A. Nitrates. The estimated adult lethal oral dose of nitroglycerin is 200–1200 mg. Hypotension occurs at low doses, but massive doses are required to produce methemoglobinemia.

    B. Nitrites. Ingestion of as little as 15 mL of butyl nitrite produced 40% methemoglobinemia in an adult. The estimated adult lethal oral dose of sodium nitrite is 1 g.

III. Clinical presentation. Headache, skin flushing, and orthostatic hypotension with reflex tachycardia are the most common adverse effects of nitrates and nitrites and occur commonly even with therapeutic doses of organic nitrates.

A. **Hypotension** may aggravate or produce symptoms of cardiac ischemia or cerebrovascular disease and may even cause seizures. However, fatalities from hypotension are rare.

B. Workers or patients regularly exposed to nitrates may develop tolerance and may suffer **angina** or **myocardial infarction** owing to rebound coronary vasoconstriction upon sudden withdrawal of the drug.

C. Methemoglobinemia (see p 220) is most common after nitrite exposure; the skin is cyanotic, even at levels low enough to be otherwise asymptomatic (eg, 15%).

IV. **Diagnosis** is suggested by hypotension with reflex tachycardia and headache. Methemoglobinemia of 15% or more may be diagnosed by noting a chocolate brown coloration of the blood when it is dried on filter paper.

A. **Specific levels.** Blood levels are not commercially available. With the use of a nitrite dipstick (normally used to detect bacteria in urine), nitrite can be detected in the serum of patients intoxicated by alkyl nitrites.

B. **Other useful laboratory studies** include electrolytes, glucose, arterial blood gases or oximetry, methemoglobin concentration, and ECG and ECG monitoring.

V. **Treatment.**

A. **Emergency and supportive measures**

1. Maintain an open airway and assist ventilation if necessary (see pp 1–7). Administer supplemental oxygen.

2. Treat hypotension with supine positioning, intravenous crystalloid fluids, and low-dose pressors if needed (see p 15).

3. Monitor vital signs and ECG for 4–6 hours.

B. **Specific drugs and antidotes.** Symptomatic methemoglobinemia may be treated with **methylene blue** (see p 381).

C. **Decontamination** (see p 43)

1. **Inhalation.** Remove victims from exposure and administer supplemental oxygen if available.

2. **Skin and eyes.** Remove contaminated clothing and wash with copious soap and water. Irrigate exposed eyes with water or saline.

3. **Ingestion** (see p 45)

   a. **Prehospital.** Administer activated charcoal if available.

   b. **Hospital.** Administer activated charcoal. Gastric emptying is not necessary for small ingestions if activated charcoal can be given promptly.

D. **Enhanced elimination.** Hemodialysis and hemoperfusion are not effective. Severe methemoglobinemia in infants not responsive to methylene blue therapy may require **exchange transfusion**.

▶ NITROGEN OXIDES

Kent R. Olson, MD

Nitrogen oxides (nitric oxide or nitrogen dioxide; *not* nitrous oxide [p 236]) are dangerous chemical gases commonly released from nitrous or nitric acid, from reactions between nitric acid and organic materials, and from burning of nitrocellulose and many other products. Exposure to nitrogen oxides occurs in electric arc welding, electroplating, and engraving. Nitrogen oxides are found in engine exhaust, and they are produced when stored grain with a high nitrite content ferments in storage silos.

I. **Mechanism of toxicity.** Nitrogen oxides are irritant gases with relatively low water solubility. Slow accumulation and hydration to nitric acid in the alveoli results in delayed onset of chemical pneumonitis. In addition, nitrogen oxides can oxidize hemoglobin to methemoglobin.

II. **Toxic dose.** The ACGIH-recommended workplace exposure limit (threshold limit value; TLV-TWA) for nitric oxide is 25 ppm (31 mg/m^3), and for nitrogen dioxide it is 3 ppm (5.6 mg/m^3) as an 8-hour time-weighted average. The air levels considered immediately dangerous to life or health (IDLH) are 100 and 20 ppm, respectively.

III. **Clinical presentation.** Because of the poor water solubility of nitrogen oxides, there is very little upper respiratory irritation at low levels (< 10 ppm nitrogen dioxide) and allowing prolonged exposure with no warning symptoms other than mild cough or nausea. With more concentrated exposures, upper respiratory symptoms such as burning eyes, sore throat, and painful brassy cough may occur.

   A. After a delay of up to 24 hours, chemical pneumonia may develop, with progressive cough, tachypnea, hypoxemia, and pulmonary edema. The onset may be more rapid after exposure to higher concentrations.
   B. After recovery from acute chemical pneumonia and after chronic low-level exposure to nitrogen oxides, permanent restrictive and obstructive lung disease from bronchiolar damage may become evident.
   C. Methemoglobinemia has (see p 220) been described in victims exposed to nitrogen oxides in smoke during major structural fires.

IV. **Diagnosis** is based on a history of exposure, if known. Because of the potential for delayed effects, all patients with significant smoke inhalation should be observed for several hours.
   A. **Specific levels.** There are no specific blood levels.
   B. **Other useful laboratory studies** include arterial blood gases or oximetry, methemoglobin level, chest x-ray, and pulmonary function tests.

V. **Treatment.**
   A. **Emergency and supportive measures**
      1. Observe closely for signs of upper-airway obstruction, and intubate the trachea and assist ventilation if necessary (see pp 1–7). Administer humidified supplemental oxygen.
      2. Observe symptomatic victims for a minimum of 24 hours after exposure and treat chemical pneumonia and noncardiogenic pulmonary edema (see p 7) if they occur.
   B. **Specific drugs and antidotes**
      1. Administration of corticosteroids has been recommended, but there is no convincing evidence that they can improve nitrogen oxide-induced chemical pneumonia or pulmonary edema or prevent chronic bronchitis.
      2. Treat methemoglobinemia with **methylene blue** (see p 381).
   C. **Decontamination** (see p 43). Rescuers should wear self-contained breathing apparatus, and if there is the potential for high-level gas exposure or exposure to liquid nitric acid, chemical-protective clothing.
      1. **Inhalation.** Remove victims from exposure immediately and give supplemental oxygen, if available.
      2. **Skin and eyes.** Remove any wet clothing, and flush exposed skin with water. Irrigate exposed eyes with copious water or saline.
   D. **Enhanced elimination.** There is no role for enhanced elimination procedures.

▶ NITROPRUSSIDE

Neal L. Benowitz, MD

Sodium nitroprusside is a short-acting parenterally administered vasodilator used to treat severe hypertension and cardiac failure. It is also used to induce hypotension for certain surgical procedures. Toxicity may occur with acute high-dose nitroprusside treatment or with prolonged infusions.

I. **Mechanism of toxicity.** Nitroprusside is rapidly hydrolyzed (half-life 11 min) and releases free cyanide, which is normally quickly converted to thiocyanate by rhodanase enzymes in the liver and blood vessels.
   A. **Acute cyanide poisoning** (see p 150) may occur with short-term high-dose nitroprusside infusions (eg, > 10–15 µg/kg/min for 1 hour or longer).
   B. **Thiocyanate** is eliminated by the kidney and may accumulate in patients with renal insufficiency, especially after prolonged infusions.

II. **Toxic dose.** The toxic dose depends on renal function and the rate of infusion.
   A. **Cyanide** poisoning is uncommon at nitroprusside infusion rates of less than 8–10 µg/kg/min, but has been reported after infusion of 4 µg/kg/min for 3 hours.
   B. **Thiocyanate** toxicity does not occur with acute brief use in persons with normal renal function, but may result from prolonged infusions (eg, > 3 µg/kg/min for 48 hours or longer), especially in persons with renal insufficiency (with rates as low as 1 µg/kg/min).

III. **Clinical presentation.** The most common adverse effect of nitroprusside is hypotension, which is often accompanied by reflex tachycardia. Peripheral and cerebral hypoperfusion can lead to lactic acidosis and altered mental status.
   A. **Cyanide** poisoning is accompanied by headache, hyperventilation, anxiety, agitation, seizures, and metabolic acidosis. The ECG may reveal ischemic patterns.
   B. **Thiocyanate** accumulation causes somnolence, confusion, delirium, tremor, and hyperreflexia. Seizures and coma may rarely occur with severe toxicity.
   C. Methemoglobinemia occurs rarely and is usually mild.

IV. **Diagnosis.** Lactic acidosis, coma, or seizures after short-term high-dose nitroprusside infusion should suggest cyanide poisoning, while confusion or delirium developing gradually after several days of continuous use should suggest thiocyanate poisoning.
   A. **Specific levels.** Cyanide levels may be obtained but are not usually available rapidly enough to guide treatment when cyanide poisoning is suspected. Cyanide levels may not accurately reflect toxicity because of simultaneous production of methemoglobin, which binds some of the cyanide. Cyanide levels greater than 1 mg/L usually produce a demonstrable lactic acidosis. **Thiocyanate** levels higher than 50–100 mg/L may cause delirium and somnolence.
   B. **Other useful laboratory studies** include electrolytes, glucose, BUN, creatinine, serum lactate, ECG, arterial blood gases and measured arterial and venous oxygen saturation (see Cyanide, p 150), and methemoglobin level.

V. **Treatment.**
   A. **Emergency and supportive measures**
      1. Maintain an open airway and assist ventilation if necessary (see pp 1–7). Administer supplemental oxygen.
      2. For hypotension, stop the infusion immediately and administer intravenous fluids or even pressors if necessary (p 15).
   B. **Specific drugs and antidotes.** If cyanide poisoning is suspected, administer **sodium thiosulfate** (see p 408). Sodium nitrite treatment may aggravate hypotension and should not be used. **Hydroxocobalamin** (see p 374), 25 mg/h IV infusion, is sometimes coadministered with high-dose nitroprusside as prophylaxis against cyanide toxicity.
   C. **Decontamination.** These procedures are not relevant because the drug is administered only parenterally.
   D. **Enhanced elimination.** Nitroprusside and cyanide are both metabolized rapidly, so there is no need to consider enhanced elimination for these. Hemodialysis may accelerate **thiocyanate** elimination and is especially useful in patients with renal failure.

▶ **NITROUS OXIDE**

Kent R. Olson, MD

Nitrous oxide, or laughing gas, is used as a general anesthetic agent and as a propellant in many commercial products such as whipped cream or cooking oil spray. Nitrous oxide is used by many U.S. dentists, in some cases without adequate scavenging equipment. Abuse of nitrous oxide is not uncommon in the medical and dental professions.

I. **Mechanism of toxicity.**
   A. **Acute toxicity** after exposure to nitrous oxide is mainly caused by asphyxia if adequate oxygen is not supplied with the gas.
   B. **Chronic toxicity** to the hematologic and nervous systems is believed to be secondary to the selective inactivation of vitamin B_{12}. Adverse reproductive outcomes have been reported in workers chronically exposed to nitrous oxide.
II. **Toxic dose.** The toxic dose is not established. Chronic occupational exposure to 2000 ppm nitrous oxide produced asymptomatic but measurable depression of vitamin B_{12} in dentists. The ACGIH-recommended workplace exposure limit (TLV-TWA) is 50 ppm (90 mg/m^3) as an 8-hour time-weighted average.
III. **Clinical presentation.**
   A. Signs of **acute toxicity** are related to **asphyxia**. These include headache, dizziness, confusion, syncope, seizures, and cardiac arrhythmias. Interstitial emphysema and pneumomediastinum have been reported after forceful inhalation from a pressurized whipped cream dispenser.
   B. **Chronic nitrous oxide abuse** may produce megaloblastic anemia, thrombocytopenia, leukopenia, peripheral neuropathy, and myelopathy, similar to effects of vitamin B_{12} deficiency.
IV. **Diagnosis** is based on a history of exposure and clinical presentation (eg, evidence of asphyxia and an empty can or tank). It should also be considered in a patient with manifestations suggesting chronic vitamin B_{12} deficiency but with normal vitamin B_{12} levels.
   A. **Specific levels.** Specific levels are not generally available and are unreliable owing to off-gassing.
   B. **Other useful laboratory studies** include CBC, platelet count, and vitamin B_{12}.
V. **Treatment.**
   A. **Emergency and supportive measures**
      1. Maintain an open airway and assist ventilation if necessary (see pp 1–7). Administer high-flow supplemental oxygen.
      2. After significant asphyxia, anticipate and treat coma (p 18), seizures (p 21), and cardiac arrhythmias (pp 10–14).
   B. **Specific drugs and antidotes.** There is no specific antidote. Chronic effects may resolve over 2–3 months after discontinuing exposure.
   C. **Decontamination.** Remove victims from exposure and give supplemental oxygen if available.
   D. **Enhanced elimination.** These procedures are not effective.

▶ NONSTEROIDAL ANTI-INFLAMMATORY DRUGS

Kathryn H. Keller, PharmD

The nonsteroidal anti-inflammatory drugs (NSAIDs) are a chemically diverse group of agents that share similar pharmacologic properties and are widely used for control of pain and inflammation (Table II–35). Overdose by most of the agents in this group usually produces only mild gastrointestinal upset. However, toxicity may be severe after overdose with **oxyphenbutazone, phenylbutazone, mefenamic acid, piroxicam,** or **diflunisal**.

I. **Mechanism of toxicity.** NSAIDs produce their pharmacologic and most toxicologic effects by inhibiting the enzyme cyclo-oxygenase; this results in decreased production of prostaglandins and decreased pain and inflammation. CNS, hemodynamic, pulmonary, and hepatic dysfunction also occur with some agents, but the relationship to prostaglandin production remains uncertain. Prostaglandins are also involved in maintaining the integrity of the gastric mucosa and regulating renal blood flow; thus, acute or chronic intoxication may affect these organs.

TABLE II–35. COMMON NSAIDs

Drug	Maximum Daily Adult Dose (mg)	Half-Life (h)	Comments
Carboxylic acids			
Bromfenac sodium	150	1–2	Chronic use associated with severe liver injury
Diclofenac	200	2	
Diflunisal	1500	8–12	
Etodolac	1000	7	
Fenoprofen	3200	3	Acute renal failure
Ibuprofen[a]	3200	2–4	Massive overdose may cause coma, renal failure, metabolic acidosis, and cardiorespiratory depression.
Indomethacin	200	3–11	
Ketoprofen[a]	300	2–4	
Ketorolac	40 (PO) 60–120 (IV)	4–6	High risk of renal failure
Meclofenamate	400	1–3	
Mefenamic acid	1000	2	Seizures, twitching
Naproxen[a]	1500	10–20	Seizures, acidosis
Oxaprozin	1800	42–50	
Sulindac	400	7–16	Extensive enterohepatic recirculation
Tolmetin	1800	1	
Enolic acids			
Nabumetone	2000	24	
Oxyphenbutazone	600	27–64	Seizures, acidosis
Phenylbutazone	600	50–100	Seizures, acidosis
Piroxicam	20	45–50	Seizures, coma

[a]Currently available in the US as nonprescription formulations.

Pharmacokinetics. NSAIDs are generally well-absorbed, and volumes of distribution (Vd) are relatively small (eg, 0.15 L/kg for ibuprofen). Most agents are highly protein bound, and most are eliminated through hepatic metabolism and renal excretion with variable half-lives (eg, 1.5–2.5 hours for ibuprofen and 13–15 hours for naproxen). (See also Table II–55.)

II. **Toxic dose.** Human data are insufficient to establish a reliable correlation between amount ingested, plasma concentrations, and clinical toxic effects. Generally, significant symptoms occur after ingestion of more than 5–10 times the usual therapeutic dose.

III. **Clinical presentation.** In general, patients with NSAID overdose are asymptomatic or have mild gastrointestinal upset (nausea, vomiting, abdominal pain, sometimes hematemesis). Occasionally patients exhibit drowsiness, lethargy, ataxia, nystagmus, tinnitus, and disorientation.

   A. With the more toxic agents **oxyphenbutazone, phenylbutazone, mefenamic acid,** or **piroxicam** and with massive **ibuprofen** overdose, seizures, coma, renal failure, and cardiorespiratory arrest may occur. Hepatic dysfunction, hypoprothrombinemia, and metabolic acidosis are also commonly reported.

B. **Diflunisal** overdose produces toxicity resembling salicylate poisoning (see p 284).

C. Chronic use of **bromfenac** for more than 10 days has resulted in fatal hepatotoxicity.

D. **Phenylbutazone** and **antipyrine** use has been associated with agranulocytosis and other blood dyscrasias.

IV. **Diagnosis** is usually based primarily on a history of ingestion of NSAIDs, because symptoms are mild and nonspecific and quantitative levels are not usually available.

A. **Specific levels** are not usually readily available and do not contribute to clinical management.

B. **Other useful laboratory studies** include CBC, electrolytes, glucose, BUN, creatinine, liver transaminases, prothrombin time (PT), and urinalysis.

V. **Treatment.**

A. **Emergency and supportive measures**

1. Maintain an open airway and assist ventilation if necessary (see pp 1–7). Administer supplemental oxygen.

2. Treat seizures (p 21), coma (p 18), and hypotension (p 15) if they occur.

3. Antacids may be used for mild gastrointestinal upset. Replace fluid losses with intravenous crystalloid solutions.

B. **Specific drugs and antidotes.** There is no antidote. Vitamin K (see p 409) may be used for patients with elevated prothrombin time (PT) caused by hypoprothrombinemia.

C. **Decontamination** (see p 43)

1. **Prehospital.** Administer activated charcoal if available. Ipecac-induced vomiting may be useful for initial treatment at the scene (eg, children at home) if it can be given within a few minutes of exposure.

2. **Hospital.** Administer activated charcoal. Gastric emptying is not necessary for most ingestions if activated charcoal can be given promptly. Consider gastric lavage for massive overdoses.

D. **Enhanced elimination.** NSAIDs are highly protein bound and extensively metabolized. Thus, hemodialysis, peritoneal dialysis, and forced diuresis are not likely to be effective.

1. **Charcoal hemoperfusion** may be effective for **phenylbutazone** overdose, although there are limited clinical data to support its use.

2. There are no data on the use of repeat-dose activated charcoal therapy.

▶ **NONTOXIC OR MINIMALLY TOXIC HOUSEHOLD PRODUCTS**

Ilene B. Anderson, PharmD

There are a variety of products commonly found around the home that are either completely nontoxic or have little or no toxicity after typical accidental exposures. Treatment is rarely required because the ingredients are not toxic, the concentrations of potentially toxic ingredients are minimal, or the construction or packaging of the product is such that a significant dose of a harmful ingredient is extremely unlikely.

Table II-36 lists a number of products considered nontoxic. However, the taste or texture of the product may be disagreeable or cause mild stomach upset. Also, some of the products listed can create a foreign body effect or a choking hazard depending on the formulation and the age of the child. Table II-37 provides examples of products that may cause mild gastrointestinal upset but are generally not considered toxic after small ingestions. Stomach cramps, vomiting, or diarrhea may occur but is usually mild and self-limited. Table II-38 lists several other products that are often ingested by small children with minimal effect. While they may contain potentially toxic ingredients, the concentrations or packaging make it very unlikely that symptoms will occur after a small exposure.

TABLE II–36. NONTOXIC PRODUCTS[a]

Air fresheners	Eye makeup	Playdoh
Aluminum foil	Felt-tip markers and pens	Putty
Antiperspirants	Fingernail polish (dry)	Rouge
Ashes, wood/fireplace	Glitter	Rust
Baby lotion	Glow stick/jewelry	Saccharin
Baby wipes	Gum	Shellac (dry)
Ball-point pen ink	Gypsum	Sheetrock
Calamine lotion	Incense	Shoe polish
Candles	Indelible markers	Silica gel
Caulk	Ink (w/out aniline dyes)	Silly putty
Charcoal	Kitty litter	Soil
Charcoal briquettes	Lip balm	Stamp pad ink
Cigarette ashes	Lipstick	Starch
Cigarette filter tips (unsmoked)	Magic markers	Styrofoam
Clay	Makeup	Sunscreen products
Cold packs (for large ingestions,	Mascara	Suntan lotions
see Nitrates, p 233)	Matches (< 3 paper books)	Superglue
Crayons	Mylar balloons	Teething rings
Crazy Glue	Newspaper	Thermometers (<0.5 mL elemental
Cyanoacrylate glues	Paraffin	mercury or phthalates/alcohol)
Deodorants	Pencils (contain graphite, not lead)	Wall board
Desiccants	Photographs	Watercolor paints
Diapers, disposable	Plaster	Wax
Erasers	Plastic	Zinc oxide ointment

[a]These items are virtually nontoxic in small to moderate exposures. However, the taste or texture of the product may result in mild stomach upset. In addition, some of the products may cause a foreign body effect or choking hazard depending on the size of the product and the age of the child.

In all cases involving exposures to these substances, attempt to confirm the identity and/or ingredients of the product and assure that no other more toxic products were involved. Determine whether there are any unexpected symptoms or evidence of choking or foreign body effect. Advise the parent that mild gastrointestinal upset may occur. Water or other liquid may be given to reduce the taste or texture of the product. For symptomatic eye exposures, follow the instructions for ocular decontamination (see p 44).

TABLE II–37. MILD GASTROINTESTINAL IRRITANTS[a]

A & D Ointment	Clotrimazole cream	Kaolin
Antacids	Corticosteroids	Lactase
Antibiotic ointments	Dishwashing liquid soaps (not	Lanolin
Baby bath	electric dishwashing type)	Latex paint
Baby shampoo	Fabric softeners	Liquid soaps
Bar soap	Fertilizers (nitrogen, phosphoric	Miconazole
Bath oil beads	acid, and potash)	Petroleum jelly
Bleach (household, less than 6%	Glycerin	Plant food
hypochlorite)	Guaifenesin	Prednisone
Body lotions and creams	Hair conditioners	Shaving cream
Bubble bath	Hair shampoos	Simethicone
Bubbles	Hand soaps	Spermicides (nonoxynol-9 < 10%)
Carbamide peroxide 6.5%	Hydrocortisone cream	Steroid creams
Chalk (calcium carbonate)	Hydrogen peroxide 3%	Toothpaste (without fluoride)

[a]The items in this list usually have little or no effect in small ingestions. In moderate to large ingestions, gastrointestinal effects such as diarrhea, constipation, stomach cramps, or vomiting may occur. The effects are usually mild and rarely require medical intervention.

TABLE II–38. OTHER LOW-TOXICITY PRODUCTS[a]

Products	Comments
Holiday hazards	
Angel hair	Finely spun glass. Dermal or ocular irritation or corneal abrasion is possible.
Bubble lights	May contain a tiny amount of methylene chloride.
Christmas tree ornaments	Can cause foreign body effect or choking hazard. Antique or foreign-made ornaments may be decorated with lead-based paint.
Christmas tree preservatives	Homemade solutions may contain aspirin, bleach, or sugar. Commercial products usually contain only concentrated sugar solution.
Easter egg dyes	Most of these contain nontoxic dyes and sodium bicarbonate. Older formulations may contain sodium chloride, which can cause hypernatremia if a large amount is ingested (see p 34).
Fireplace crystals	May contain salts of copper, selenium, arsenic, and antimony. Small amounts can cause irritation to the mouth or stomach. (Larger ingestions could conceivably result in heavy metal poisoning; see specific heavy metal).
Halloween candy	Tampering rarely occurs. X-ray of candy provides a false sense of security; although it may reveal radiopaque glass or metallic objects, most poisons are radiolucent. Prudent approach is to discard candy or food items that are not commercially packaged or if the package is damaged.
Snow scenes	The "snow" is comprised of insoluble particles of calcium carbonate that are not toxic. The fluid may have bacterial growth.
Snow sprays	Sprays may contain hydrocarbon solvent or methylene chloride (see pp 183 and 224) vehicle. Inhalation may cause headache and nausea. Once dried, the snow is not toxic.
Miscellaneous	
Capsaicin sprays	These self-defense sprays contain capsaicin, the main ingredient in chili peppers. Exposure causes intense mucous membrane irritation and burning sensation.
Cyanoacrylate glues	Ingestion of the polymerized glue is harmless. Cyanide is not released. Corneal abrasions may occur following ocular exposure. Adhesion of skin and eyelids is possible following dermal exposure.
Fire extinguishers	The 2 common types contain sodium bicarbonate (white powder) or monoammonium phosphate (yellow powder). Small ingestions result in little to no effect. Mucous membrane irritation is common. Major risk is pneumonitis after extensive inhalation.
Fluorescent light bulbs	Contain inert gases and nontoxic powder that may be irritating to mucous membranes.
Oral contraceptives	Birth control pills contain varying amounts of estrogens and progesterones. In excessive amounts these may cause stomach upset, and in females (even prepubertal) may cause transient vaginal spotting. Some formulations may contain iron.
Household pesticides	Numerous formulations, some contain hydrocarbon solvents, others are water-based. Pesticides used may include pyrethrins, organophosphates, or carbamates, but generally low potency and in concentrations less than 1.5%. The risk of pesticide poisoning is very low unless intentional misuse results in massive exposure. Major potential toxicity is related to inhalation of the hydrocarbon solvent.
Respiratory irritants	
Baby powders Spray starch	These products have little or no toxicity when injested. However, if aspirated into the lungs, they can cause an inflammatory pneumonitis.

[a]These products may contain small amounts of potentially toxic ingredients, but rarely cause problems because of the small concentrations or conditions of exposure

TABLE II–39. COMMON OPIATES AND OPOIDS[a]

Drug	Type of Activity	Usual Adult Dose[a] (mg)	Elimination Half-Life (h)	Duration of Analgesia (h)
Butorphanol	Mixed	2	3–4	3–4
Codeine	Agonist	60	2–4	4–6
Fentanyl	Agonist	0.2	1–5	0.5–2
Heroin[b]	Agonist	4	(b)	3–4
Hydrocodone	Agonist	5	3–4	4–8
Hydromorphone	Agonist	1.5	1–4	4–5
Meperidine	Agonist	100	2–5	2–4
Methadone	Agonist	10	20–30	4–8[c]
Morphine	Agonist	10	2–4	3–6
Nalbuphine	Mixed	10	5	3–6
Oxycodone	Agonist	4.5	2–5	4–6
Pentazocine	Mixed	50	2–3	2–3
Propoxyphene	Agonist	100	6–12	4–6

[a]Usual dose: Dose equivalent to 10 mg of morphine.
[b]Rapidly hydrolyzed to morphine.
[c]Sedation and coma may last 2–3 days

▶ OPIATES AND OPIOIDS

Timothy E. Albertson, MD, PhD

Opiates are a group of naturally occurring compounds derived from the juice of the poppy *Papaver somniferum*. Morphine is the classic opiate derivative used widely in medicine; heroin (diacetylmorphine) is a well-known, highly addictive street narcotic. The term *opioids* refers to these and other derivatives of naturally occurring opium (eg, morphine, heroin, codeine, and hydrocodone) as well as new, totally synthetic opiate analogues (eg, fentanyl, butorphanol, meperidine, and methadone Table II–39). A wide variety of prescription medications contain opioids, often in combination with aspirin or acetaminophen. **Dextromethorphan** (see p 155) is an opioid derivative with potent antitussive but no analgesic or addictive properties. **Tramadol** (Ultram) is a newer analgesic that is unrelated chemically to the opiates but acts on mu (μ) opioid receptors.

I. **Mechanism of toxicity.** In general, opioids share the ability to stimulate a number of specific opiate receptors in the CNS, causing sedation and respiratory depression. Death results from respiratory failure, usually as a result of apnea or pulmonary aspiration of gastric contents. In addition, acute noncardiogenic pulmonary edema may occur by unknown mechanisms.

  Pharmacokinetics. Usually, peak effects occur within 2–3 hours, but absorption may be slowed by their pharmacologic effects on gastrointestinal motility. Most drugs have large volumes of distribution (3–5 L/kg). The rate of elimination is highly variable, from 1–2 hours for fentanyl derivatives versus 15–30 hours for methadone. See also Tables II–39 and II–55.

II. **Toxic dose.** The toxic dose varies widely depending on the specific compound, the route and rate of administration, and tolerance to the effects of the drug as a result of chronic use. Some newer fentanyl derivatives have a potency up to 2000 times that of morphine.

III. **Clinical presentation.**

A. **With mild or moderate overdose**, lethargy is common. The pupils are usually small, often "pinpoint" size. Blood pressure and pulse rate are decreased, bowel sounds are diminished, and the muscles are usually flaccid.
B. **With higher doses**, coma is accompanied by respiratory depression, and apnea often results in sudden death. Noncardiogenic pulmonary edema may occur, often after resuscitation and administration of the opiate antagonist naloxone.
C. **Seizures** are not common after opioid overdose but occur occasionally with certain compounds (eg, dextromethorphan, meperidine, propoxyphene, and tramadol). Seizures may occur in patients with renal compromise who receive repeated doses of meperidine, owing to accumulation of the metabolite normeperidine.
D. **Cardiotoxicity** similar to that seen with tricyclic antidepressants (p 310) and quinidine (p 277) can occur in patients with severe **propoxyphene** intoxication.
E. Some newer synthetic opioids have mixed agonist and antagonist effects with unpredictable results in overdose.
F. Opioid **withdrawal syndrome** can cause anxiety, piloerection (goosebumps), abdominal cramps and diarrhea, and insomnia.
IV. **Diagnosis** is simple when typical manifestations of opiate intoxication are present (pinpoint pupils and respiratory and CNS depression), and the patient quickly awakens after administration of naloxone. Signs of intravenous drug abuse (eg, needle track marks) may be present.
A. **Specific levels** are not usually performed because of poor correlation with clinical effects. Qualitative screening of the urine is an effective way to confirm recent use. Fentanyl derivatives, tramadol, and some other synthetic opioids may not be detected by routine toxicologic screens.
B. **Other useful laboratory studies** include electrolytes, glucose, arterial blood gases or oximetry, chest x-ray, and stat serum acetaminophen or salicylate levels (if the ingested overdose was of a combination product).
V. **Treatment.**
A. **Emergency and supportive measures**
   1. Maintain an open airway and assist ventilation if necessary (see pp 1–7). Administer supplemental oxygen.
   2. Treat coma (p 18), seizures (p 21), hypotension (p 15), and noncardiogenic pulmonary edema (p 7) if they occur.
B. **Specific drugs and antidotes.**
   1. **Naloxone** (p 384) is a specific opioid antagonist with no agonist properties of its own; large doses may be given safely.
      a. Administer naloxone, 0.4–2 mg IV. As little as 0.2–0.4 mg is usually effective for heroin overdose. Repeat doses every 2–3 minutes if there is no response, up to a total dose of 10–20 mg if an opioid overdose is strongly suspected.
      b. *Caution:* The duration of effect of naloxone (1–2 hours) is shorter than that of many opioids. Therefore, do not release the patient who has awakened after naloxone treatment until at least 3–4 hours have passed since the last dose of naloxone. In general, if naloxone was required to reverse opioid-induced coma, it is safer to admit the patient for at least 6–12 hours of observation.
   2. **Nalmefene** (p 384) is an opioid antagonist with a longer duration of effect (3–5 hours).
      a. Nalmefene may be given in doses of 0.1–2 mg IV, with repeated doses up to 10–20 mg if an opioid overdose is strongly suspected.
      b. *Caution:* While nalmefene's duration of effect is longer than that of naloxone, it is still much shorter than the duration of effect of methadone. If a methadone overdose is suspected, the patient should be observed for at least 8–12 hours after the last dose of nalmefene.
   3. **Sodium bicarbonate** (p 345) may be effective for QRS interval prolongation or hypotension associated with propoxyphene poisoning.
C. **Decontamination** (see p 43)

1. **Prehospital.** Administer activated charcoal if available. Do *not* induce vomiting, because of the potential for developing lethargy and coma.
2. **Hospital.** Administer activated charcoal. Gastric emptying is not necessary if activated charcoal can be given promptly.
   D. **Enhanced elimination.** Because of the very large volumes of distribution of the opioids and the availability of an effective antidotal treatment, there is no role for enhanced elimination procedures.

▶ ORGANOPHOSPHATES AND CARBAMATES

Olga F. Woo, PharmD

Organophosphates and carbamates, also known generally as cholinesterase inhibitors, are widely used pesticides that may cause poisonings after accidental or suicidal exposure. Poisonings are particularly common in rural areas and third-world countries where more potent agents are widely available. Several **chemical warfare agents** (eg, GA [Tabun], GB [Sarin], GD [Soman], GF, and VX) contain extremely potent organophosphates (see Table II–40). Household insect sprays often contain low-potency organophosphates or carbamates. Many commercial products contain solvents such as toluene or xylene that can themselves produce toxic effects in an overdose.

I. **Mechanism of toxicity.**

A. **Organophosphates** and their potent sulfoxidation ("-oxon") derivatives inhibit the enzyme acetylcholinesterase, allowing the accumulation of excessive acetylcholine at muscarinic receptors (cholinergic effector cells), at nicotinic receptors (skeletal neuromuscular junctions and autonomic ganglia), and in the central nervous system. Permanent damage to the acetylcholinesterase enzyme ("aging") may occur after a variable delay unless antidotal treatment with an enzyme reactivator is given.

B. **Carbamates** also inhibit acetylcholintesterase and produce similar clinical effects. However, binding to the enzyme is reversible and toxicity is usually brief and self-limited.

C. Organophosphates and carbamates are well absorbed by inhalation and ingestion and through the skin (with the exception of aldicarb, most carbamates are poorly absorbed across the skin compared with organophosphates). Some organophosphates (eg, disulfoton, fenthion, and others) are highly lipophilic and are stored in fat tissue, which may lead to delayed and persistent toxicity for several days after exposure.

D. **Aldicarb** is an important carbamate because it is relatively more potent and is translocated systemically by certain plants (eg, melons) and concentrated in their fruit. An acute outbreak of aldicarb poisoning occurred in California in 1985 after ingestion of watermelons that had been grown in a field previously sprayed with aldicarb. A similar outbreak after ingestion of contaminated cucumbers occurred in Dublin, Ireland in 1992.

II. **Toxic dose.** There is a wide spectrum of relative potency of the organophosphates and carbamates (Table II–41). The degree of intoxication is also affected by the rate of exposure (acute versus chronic), the ongoing metabolic degradation and elimination of the agent, and for organophosphates, the rate of metabolism to their more toxic "-oxon" derivatives. Some agents, including the highly toxic "nerve gases" developed for chemical warfare, are direct and powerful inhibitors of cholinesterase.

III. **Clinical presentation.** Signs and symptoms of acute organophosphate poisoning usually occur within 1–2 hours of exposure but may be delayed up to several hours, especially after skin exposure. Clinical manifestations may be classified into muscarinic, nicotinic, and CNS effects. In addition, chemical pneumonitis

TABLE II–40. EXAMPLES OF CHEMICAL AND BIOLOGICAL WEAPONS[a]

Type of Agent	Toxicity
Nerve agents GA (tabun) GB (sarin) GD (soman) GF VX	Cholinesterase inhibition. Estimated lethal dose in adult human 10–1000 mg (applied to skin), depending on the agent.
Vesicants mustard (sulfur mustard; H; HD) Lewisite (L) phosgene oxime (CX)	Erythema, blisters, eye irritation, and corneal injury; airway irritation and bronchoalveolar damage. Onset after mustard exposure delayed 2–24 h.
Cyanides cyanide salts (CN) hydrogen cyanide (HCN, AC) cyanogen chloride (CK)	See also Cyanide, p 150. Anxiety, agitation, dyspnea, weakness, nausea, syncope, convulsions. CK also causes irritation to the eyes, nose, and throat.
Pulmonary irritants phosgene (CG) perflurorisobutylene (PFIB) HC; chlorine	See also Phosgene, p 262, and Irritant Gases, p 181. Phosgene causes delayed onset pulmonary edema; latency period (1–24 h) depends on concentration and duration of exposure. Chlorine is more rapid-acting.
Botulin toxin	See Botulism, p 112. With an oral LD$_{50}$ of 0.001 μg/kg, it is the most potent toxin known. May be delivered as an aerosol or added to food or water.
Staphylococcal enterotoxin B	An exotoxin of *Staphylococcus aureus*. After a latent period of 3–12 h, victim develops fever, headache, and myalgias; vomiting and diarrhea are more likely with oral exposure. In severe cases pulmonary edema and ARDS can develop. LD$_{50}$ in animals, 27 μg/kg.
Ricin	Toxin derived from beans of *Ricinus communis*. More potent by aerosol than other routes of exposure. Inhalation can cause severe irritation and pulmonary edema. Ingestion causes vomiting and diarrhea, and systemic absorption can lead to multiple organ injury.
Trichothecene (T2) mycotoxins	"Yellow rain." Heat-stable toxins produced by various filamentous fungi. Skin or eye contact causes rapid onset of burning pain, redness, blisters, and necrosis. Inhalation can cause nasal irritation, sneezing, and cough. Vomiting and diarrhea, weakness, ataxia, syncope, hypotension, and tachycardia can occur with systemic toxicity.

[a]References: *Medical Management of Chemical Casualties.* U.S. Army Medical Research Institute of Infectious. Diseases. Fort Detrick, MD, 1996; and *Medical Management of Biological Casualties.* Medical Research Institute of Chemical Defense, Aberdeen Proving Ground, MD, 1995.

(see p 183) may occur if a product containing a hydrocarbon solvent is aspirated into the lungs.

   A. **Muscarinic** manifestations include vomiting, diarrhea, abdominal cramping, bronchospasm, miosis, bradycardia, and excessive salivation and sweating. Severe diaphoresis can actually lead to dehydration with systemic hypovolemia, resulting in shock.
   B. **Nicotinic** effects include muscle fasciculations, tremor, and weakness. Death is usually caused by respiratory muscle paralysis. Blood pressure and pulse rate may be increased because of nicotinic effects or decreased because of muscarinic effects.
   C. **Central nervous system** poisoning may cause agitation, seizures, and coma.

D. Some organophosphates may cause a delayed, often permanent peripheral neuropathy. An **"intermediate syndrome"** has also been described, characterized by recurrent muscle weakness occurring within several days of the exposure. It may be associated with inadequate pralidoxime therapy.

IV. Diagnosis is based on the history of exposure and the presence of characteristic muscarinic, nicotinic, and CNS manifestations of acetylcholine excess. There may be a solvent odor, and some organophosphates have a strong garlicky odor.

    A. Specific levels

        1. Laboratory evidence of **organophosphate** poisoning may be obtained by measuring decreases in the plasma pseudocholinesterase (PChE) and red blood cell acetylcholinesterase (AChE) activities. However, because of

TABLE II–41. RELATIVE TOXICITIES OF ORGANOPHOSPHATES AND CARBAMATES[a]

ORGANOPHOSPHATES		
Low toxicity (LD$_{50}$ > 1000 mg/kg)	**Moderate toxicity** (LD$_{50}$ 50–1000 mg/kg)	**High toxicity** (LD$_{50}$ < 50 mg/kg)
Bromophos mg/kg)	Acephate	Azinphos-methyl
Etrimfos	Bensulide	Bomyl
Iodofenphos (jodfenphos)	Chlorpyrifos	Carbophenothion
Malathion	Crotoxyphos	Chlorfenvinphos
Phoxim	Cyanophos	Chlormephos
Primiphos-methyl	Cythioate	Coumaphos
Propylthiopyrophosphate	DEF	Cyanofenphos
Temephos	Demeton-S-methyl	Demeton
Tetrachlorvinphos	Diazinon	Dialifor
	Dichlofenthion	Dicrotophos
	Dichlorvos (DDVP)	Disulfoton
	Dimethoate	EPN
	Edifenphos	Famphur
	EPBP	Fenamiphos
	Ethion	Fenophosphon
	Ethoprop	Fensulfothion
	Fenthion	Fonofos
	Fenitrothion	Isofenphos
	Formothion	Isofluorphate
	Heptenophos	Mephosfolan
	IBP (Kitacin)	Methamidophos
	Isoxathion	Methidathion
	Leptophos	Mevinphos
	Methyl trithion	Monocrotophos
	Naled	Parathion
	Oxydemeton-methyl	Phorate
	Oxydeprofos	Phosfolan
	Phencapton	Phosphamidon
	Phenthoate	Prothoate
	Phosalone	Schradan
	Phosmet	Sulfotep
	Pirimiphos-ethyl	Terbufos
	Profenofos	Tetraethylpyrophosphate
	Propetamphos	Triorthocresylphosphate
	Pyrazophos	
	Pyridaphenthion	
	Quinalphos	
	Sulprofos	
	Thiometon	
	Triazophos	
	Tribufos	
	Trichlorfon	

TABLE II–41. RELATIVE TOXICITIES OF ORGANOPHOSPHATES AND CARBAMATES (CONTINUED)

CARBAMATES

Low toxicity (LD$_{50}$ > 200 mg/kg)	Moderate toxicity (LD$_{50}$ 50–200 mg/kg)	High toxicity (LC$_{50}$ < 50 mg/kg)
BPMC (Fenocarb)	Benfuracarb	Aldicarb
Carbaryl	Bufencarb	Aldoxycarb
Ethiofencarb	Carbosulfan	Aminocarb
Isoprocarb	Dioxacarb	Bendiocarb
MPMC (Meobal)	Propoxur	Carbofuran
MTMC (Metacrate)	Pirimicarb	Dimetilan
XMC (Cosban)	Promecarb	Formetanate
	Thiodicarb	Isolan
	Trimethacarb	Mecarbam
		Methiocarb
		Methomyl
		Mexacarbate
		Oxamyl

^{a}Based on oral LD$_{50}$ values in the rat.

wide inter-individual variability, significant depression of enzyme activity may occur but still fall within the "normal" range. It is most helpful if the patient had a pre-exposure baseline measurement for comparison (eg, as part of a workplace health surveillance program).

   a. The AChE activity provides a more reliable measure of the toxic effect; a 25% or greater depression in activity from baseline generally indicates a true exposure effect.

   b. PChE activity is a sensitive indicator of exposure but is not as specific as AChE activity (PChE may be depressed owing to genetic deficiency, medical illness, or chronic organophosphate exposure). PChE activity usually recovers within weeks after exposure, whereas AChE recovery may take several months.

  2. Carbamate poisoning produces reversible acetylcholinesterase inhibition, and spontaneous recovery of enzyme activity may occur within several hours, making these tests less useful.

  3. Assay of blood and urine for specific agents and their metabolites may also provide evidence of exposure, but these tests are not widely available.

 B. Other useful laboratory studies include electrolytes, glucose, BUN, creatinine, liver transaminases, arterial blood gases or oximetry, ECG monitoring, and chest x-ray (if pulmonary edema or aspiration of hydrocarbon solvent is suspected).

V. Treatment.

 A. Emergency and supportive measures. *Caution:* rescuers and health care providers must take measures to prevent direct contact with the skin or clothing of contaminated victims, because secondary contamination and serious illness may result, especially with potent pesticides and nerve agents. (see Section IV, pp 415 and 416)

  1. Maintain an open airway and assist ventilation if necessary (see pp 1–7). Pay careful attention to respiratory muscle weakness; sudden respiratory arrest may occur. If intubation is required, note potential interactions between neuromuscular blockers and cholinesterase inhibitors (see p 386). Administer supplemental oxygen.

  2. Treat hydrocarbon pneumonitis (p 7), seizures (p 21), and coma (p 18) if they occur.

3. Observe patients for at least 6–8 hours to rule out delayed-onset symptoms resulting from skin absorption.
B. **Specific drugs and antidotes.** Specific treatment includes the antimuscarinic agent **atropine** and the enzyme reactivator **pralidoxime.**
 1. Give **atropine**, 0.5–2 mg IV initially (see p 340), repeated frequently as needed. Large cumulative doses of atropine (up to 100 mg or more) may occasionally be required in severe cases. The most clinically important indication for continued atropine administration is persistent wheezing or bronchorrhea. **Note:** Atropine will reverse muscarinic but not nicotinic effects.
 2. **Pralidoxime** (2-PAM, Protopam; see p 403) is a specific antidote for organophosphate toxicity, that acts to regenerate the enzyme activity at all affected sites (muscarinic, nicotinic, and probably CNS; however, it does *not* reactivate plasma cholinesterase).
   a. Pralidoxime should be given immediately to reverse muscular weakness and fasciculations: 1–2 g initial bolus dose (20–40 mg/kg in children) IV over 5–10 minutes, followed by a continuous infusion (see p 403). It is most effective if started within the first 24 hours of the exposure before irreversible phosphorylation of the enzyme, but may still be effective if given late, particularly after exposure to highly lipid soluble compounds.
   b. Pralidoxime is not generally recommended for carbamate intoxication, because in such cases the cholinesterase inhibition is spontaneously reversible and short-lived. However, if the exact agent is not identified and the patient has significant toxicity, pralidoxime should be given empirically.
C. **Decontamination** (see p 43). **Note:** Rescuers must wear chemical-protective clothing and gloves when handling a grossly contaminated victim. If there is heavy liquid contamination with a solvent such as xylene or toluene, clothing removal and victim decontamination should be carried out outdoors or in a room with high-flow ventilation.
 1. **Skin.** Remove all contaminated clothing and wash exposed areas with soap and water, including the hair and under the nails. Irrigate exposed eyes with copious tepid water or saline.
 2. **Ingestion** (see p 45)
   a. **Prehospital.** Administer activated charcoal, if available. Do *not* induce vomiting because of the risk of abrupt onset of toxicity.
   b. **Hospital.** Administer activated charcoal (cathartics are not necessary if the patient already has diarrhea). Perform gastric lavage for large recent ingestions.
D. **Enhanced elimination.** Dialysis and hemoperfusion are not generally indicated because of the large volume of distribution of organophosphates and the effectiveness of the specific therapy described above. Repeat-dose activated charcoal (see p 54) is theoretically applicable to **aldicarb** poisoning, because the agent undergoes significant enterohepatic recirculation.

▶ **OXALIC ACID**

Kent R. Olson, MD

Oxalic acid and oxalates are used as bleaches, metal cleaners, and rust removers and in chemical synthesis and leather tanning. Soluble and insoluble oxalate salts are found in several species of plants.
I. **Mechanism of toxicity.**
 A. **Oxalic acid solutions** are highly irritating and corrosive. Ingestion and absorption of oxalate cause acute hypocalcemia resulting from precipitation of the insoluble calcium oxalate salt. Calcium oxalate crystals may then deposit in the brain, heart, kidneys, and other sites, causing serious systemic damage.

B. Insoluble calcium oxalate salt found in dieffenbachia and similar plants is not absorbed but causes local mucous membrane irritation.

II. **Toxic dose.** Ingestion of 5–15 g of oxalic acid has caused death. The recommended workplace limit (ACGIH TLV-TWA) for oxalic acid vapor is 1 mg/m^3 as an 8-hour time-weighted average. The level considered immediately dangerous to life or health (IDLH) is 500 mg/m^3.

III. **Clinical presentation.** Toxicity may occur as a result of skin or eye contact, inhalation, or ingestion.

    A. Acute skin or eye contact causes irritation and burning, which may lead to serious corrosive injury if the exposure and concentration are high.

    B. Inhalation may cause sore throat, cough, and wheezing. Large exposures may lead to chemical pneumonitis or pulmonary edema.

    C. Ingestion of soluble oxalates may result in weakness, tetany, convulsions, and cardiac arrest owing to profound hypocalcemia. The QT interval may be prolonged, and variable conduction defects may occur. Oxalate crystals may be found on urinalysis. Insoluble oxalate crystals are not absorbed but can cause irritation and swelling in the oropharynx and esophagus.

IV. **Diagnosis** is based on a history of exposure and evidence of local or systemic effects or oxalate crystalluria.

    A. Specific levels. Serum oxalate levels are not available.

    B. Other useful laboratory studies include electrolytes, glucose, BUN, creatinine, calcium, ECG monitoring, and urinalysis.

V. **Treatment.**

    A. Emergency and supportive measures

        1. Protect the airway (see p 1), which may become acutely swollen and obstructed after significant ingestion or inhalation. Administer supplemental oxygen, and assist ventilation if necessary (pp 2–7).

        2. Treat coma (p 18), seizures (p 21), and arrhythmias (pp 10–14) if they occur.

        3. Monitor the ECG and vital signs for at least 6 hours after significant exposure, and admit symptomatic patients to an intensive care unit.

    B. Specific drugs and antidotes. Administer 10% **calcium solution** (chloride or gluconate) to counteract symptomatic hypocalcemia.

    C. Decontamination (see p 43)

        1. **Insoluble oxalates** in plants: Flush exposed areas. For ingestions, dilute with plain water; do not induce vomiting or give charcoal.

        2. **Oxalic acid or strong commercial oxalate solutions.** Immediately flush with copious water. Do *not* induce vomiting because of the risk of aggravating corrosive injury; instead, give water to dilute, and on arrival in the hospital perform gastric lavage.

        3. **Plants containing soluble oxalates.** Induce vomiting with syrup of ipecac if it can be administered within a few minutes of the ingestion. In the hospital, consider gastric lavage. Alternately, attempt to precipitate ingested oxalate in the stomach by administering calcium (calcium chloride or gluconate, 1–2 g; or calcium carbonate [Tums], several tablets) orally or via gastric tube. The effectiveness of activated charcoal is unknown.

    D. Enhanced elimination. Maintain high-volume urine flow (3–5 mL/kg/h) to help prevent calcium oxalate precipitation in the tubules. Oxalate is removed by hemodialysis, but the indications for this treatment are not established.

▶ **PARALDEHYDE**

Timothy McCarthy, PharmD

Paraldehyde is a cyclic trimer of acetaldehyde. Although it has been largely replaced by newer agents, paraldehyde was widely used in the past as an anticonvulsant, a sedative-hypnotic, and an anesthetic. It has a characteristic penetrating odor and a disagreeable taste. It is incompatible with plastic and must be stored and administered in glass containers only. It rapidly decomposes to acetaldehyde and acetic acid upon exposure to light and air.

I. **Mechanism of toxicity.** Paraldehyde is a potent CNS depressant. It is a strong irritant to intestinal mucosa, especially if it has partially decomposed to acetic acid. If the produce has developed a brown discoloration or the pungent smell of acetic acid, it should not be used.

II. **Toxic dose.** The typical therapeutic dose of paraldehyde for control of seizures or alcohol withdrawal is 5–10 mL IM or PO or 0.1–0.2 mL/kg IV every 4–6 hours. Deaths have been reported after a rectal dose of only 12 mL (undecomposed paraldehyde) and an oral dose of 25 mL. However, survival has been reported after ingestion of 125 mL. Co-ingestion of alcohol or other depressant drugs increases the risk of serious toxicity.

III. **Clinical presentation.** Peak effects are usually seen within 30–60 minutes after ingestion but may be delayed up to 2–3 hours after rectal administration. Lethargy, stupor, and coma are common. Gastritis, often hemorrhagic, may occur. Metabolic acidosis with an elevated anion gap may be a result of acetic acid or may be a manifestation of starvation-type ketoacidosis in a patient with paraldehyde-induced gastritis. Severe leukocytosis (> 30,000), hypercoagulability, tachycardia, hypotension, tachypnea, right ventricular failure, and pulmonary edema have been reported.

IV. **Diagnosis** is based on a history of exposure and is suggested by the typical pungent odor on the breath, metabolic acidosis, and altered mental status.
  A. **Specific levels.** Serum levels are not routinely available. The anticonvulsant therapeutic level is approximately 200 mg/L; serum levels higher than 500 mg/L are often associated with death.
  B. **Other useful laboratory studies** include electrolytes, glucose, and arterial blood gases or oximetry.

V. **Treatment.**
  A. **Emergency and supportive measures**
    1. Maintain the airway and assist ventilation if necessary (see pp 1–7). Administer supplemental oxygen.
    2. Treat coma (p 18), hypotension (p 15), metabolic acidosis (p 31), and pulmonary edema (p 8) if they occur.
  B. **Specific drugs and antidotes.** There is no specific antidote.
  C. **Decontamination** (see p 43)
    1. **Prehospital.** Administer activated charcoal, if available. Do **not** induce emesis because paraldehyde is mildly corrosive and because of the risk of abrupt decline in mental status.
    2. **Hospital.** Administer activated charcoal. Consider gastric lavage for large recent ingestion.
  D. **Enhanced elimination.** The volume of distribution is 0.9 L/kg, making paraldehyde accessible to enhanced elimination procedures. However, there are few data to support use of extracorporeal methods of enhanced elimination.

▶ **PARAQUAT AND DIQUAT**

Rick Geller, MD

Paraquat and diquat are dipyridyl herbicides used for weed control and as defoliants. Paraquat has been used for large-scale control of illegal marijuana growing. Dipyridyl product formulations differ by country. In the United States, paraquat is encountered most commonly as a concentrated (20–37%) liquid. Diquat is sold in aqueous concentrates containing 8–36% of the herbicide. Granular formulations containing a 2.5% mixture of paraquat and diquat salts are also widely available.

I. **Mechanism of toxicity.**

A. **Paraquat and diquat** are strong cations in aqueous solution, and concentrated solutions (eg, >20%) may cause severe corrosive injury when ingested or applied to the skin, eyes, or mucous membranes. The dipyridil herbicides are extremely potent systemic toxins when absorbed and can cause multiple system organ damage. Reaction of these dicationic compounds with NADPH produces highly reactive free radicals, leading to tissue destruction through lipid peroxidation.

  1. **Paraquat** is selectively taken up and concentrated by pulmonary alveolar cells, leading to cell necrosis followed by connective tissue proliferation and pulmonary fibrosis.

  2. **Diquat** does not cause pulmonary fibrosis, but is associated with gastrointestinal fluid sequestration, renal failure, and cerebral and brain stem hemorrhagic infarctions.

B. **Pharmacokinetics**

  1. **Absorption.** Paraquat and diquat are rapidly absorbed from the gastrointestinal tract, and peak serum levels are reached within 2 hours of ingestion. The presence of food may significantly reduce absorption. Although absorption is poor through intact skin, the dipyridil herbicides can be taken up through abraded skin or after prolonged contact with concentrated solutions. Fatalities usually result from ingestion, but have been reported after intramuscular injection, vaginal and percutaneous exposure, and rarely after inhalation.

  2. **Distribution.** Paraquat has an apparent volume of distribution (Vd) of 1.2–1.6 L/kg. It is distributed most avidly to lung, kidney, liver, and muscle tissue; in the lungs, paraquat is actively taken up against a concentration gradient.

  3. **Elimination.** Paraquat is eliminated renally, with more than 90% excreted unchanged within 12–24 hours if renal function is normal. Diquat is eliminated renally and via the gastrointestinal tract.

II. **Toxic dose.** Diquat is less toxic than paraquat. However, this distinction may be of little comfort, as both compounds are extremely toxic.

A. **Paraquat.** Ingestion of as little as 2–4 g, or 10–20 mL, of concentrated 20% paraquat solution has resulted in death. The estimated lethal dose of 20% paraquat is 10–20 mL for adults and 4–5 mL for children.

  1. If food is present in the stomach, it may bind paraquat, preventing its absorption and reducing its toxicity.

  2. Once applied to plants or soil, paraquat is rapidly bound and is not likely to be toxic. When burned, it is combusted and does not produce poisoning.

B. **Diquat.** The animal LD_{50} is approximately 400 mg/kg. The estimated lethal dose for adults is 30–60 mL of 20% diquat.

III. **Clinical presentation.**

A. **Paraquat.** After ingestion of concentrated solutions, there is pain and swelling in the mouth and throat and oral ulcerations may be visible. Nausea, vomiting, and abdominal pain are common. The severity and tempo of illness depend on the dose. Ingestion of more than 40 mg/kg (about 14 mL of a 20% solution in an adult) leads to corrosive gastrointestinal injury, rapid onset of renal failure, myonecrosis, shock, and death within hours to a few days. Ingestion of 20–40 mg/kg causes a more indolent course evolving over several days, with most patients dying from pulmonary fibrosis after days to weeks.

B. **Diquat** causes similar initial symptoms. Severe gastroenteritis and gastrointestinal fluid sequestration may cause massive fluid and electrolyte loss contributing to renal failure. Pulmonary fibrosis has not been reported, but cerebral and brain stem hemorrhagic infarctions may occur.

IV. **Diagnosis** is based on a history of ingestion and the presence of gastroenteritis and oral burns. The oral mucosal burns may have the appearance of a pseudomembrane on the soft palate, sometimes confused with diphtheria.

A. **Specific levels.** The prognosis may be correlated with specific serum levels, but these levels are not likely to be available in a timeframe useful for emer-

gency management. Assistance in obtaining and interpreting paraquat and diquat levels can be obtained through Zeneca (1-800-327-8633). Paraquat levels associated with a high likelihood of death are 2 mg/L at 4 hours, 0.9 mg/L
at 6 hours, and 0.1 mg/L at 24 hours after ingestion.
  B. **Other useful laboratory studies** include electrolytes, glucose, BUN, creati-
     nine, liver transaminases, urinalysis, arterial blood gases or oximetry, and
     chest x-ray.
V. **Treatment.**
  A. **Emergency and supportive measures.** Expert assistance for managing
     paraquat and diquat exposure can be obtained 24 hours a day by contacting
     the **Zeneca Agricultural Products Emergency Information Network (1-
     800-327-8633).**
     1. Maintain an open airway and assist ventilation if necessary (see pp 1–7).
     2. Treat fluid and electrolyte imbalance caused by gastroenteritis with intra-
        venous crystalloid solutions.
     3. Avoid excessive oxygen administration in patients with **paraquat** poison-
        ing, as this may aggravate lipid peroxidation reactions in the lungs. Treat
        significant hypoxemia with supplemental oxygen, but use only the lowest
        oxygen concentration necessary to achieve a pO_2 of about 60 mm.
  B. **Specific drugs and antidotes.** There is no specific antidote.
  C. **Decontamination** (see p 43)
     1. **Skin and eyes.** Remove all contaminated clothing, and wash exposed
        skin with soap and water. Irrigate exposed eyes with copious saline or
        water.
     2. **Ingestion** (see p 45). Immediate and aggressive gastrointestinal decon-
        tamination is probably the only treatment that may significantly affect out-
        come after paraquat or diquat ingestion.
        a. **Prehospital.** Administer activated charcoal if available. Ingestion of any
           food—*or even plain dirt*—may afford some protection if charcoal is not
           immediately available. Ipecac-induced vomiting may be useful for initial
           treatment at the scene (eg, children at home) if it can be given within a
           few minutes of exposure. Note that many commercial solutions contain
           an added emetic agent.
        b. **Hospital.** Immediately administer 100 g of activated charcoal and re-
           peat the dose in 1–2 hours. Gastric lavage may be helpful if performed
           within an hour of the ingestion. Various clays, such as bentonite and
           Fuller's earth, adsorb paraquat and diquat but are probably no more ef-
           fective than charcoal.
  D. **Enhanced elimination** (see p 51). Although charcoal hemoperfusion has
     been advocated, and early animal studies and human case reports suggested
     benefits, no controlled study has demonstrated improved outcome, and the
     current consensus is that the procedure is not indicated. Hemodialysis and
     forced diuresis are not effective.

▶ PENTACHLOROPHENOL AND DINITROPHENOL

Delia A. Dempsey, MS, MD

Pentachlorophenol (Penchlor, Chlorophen, Pentachlorofenol, Penta, Pentanol,
Pentachlorophenate, PCP, and others) is a chlorinated aromatic hydrocarbon widely
used as a fungicide, as well as a herbicide and defoliant. It is applied to wood,
leather, burlap, twine, and rope to prevent fungal rot and decay. It is used predominantly in wood preservation and in the paper industry. Sodium pentachlorophenol is
an ingredient in some paints. It has a pungent mothball-like odor.
  Dinitrophenols (Dinoseb, DNP, Dinitrobutylphenol, and analogs Disophenol and
Dinitrocresol) are insecticides, herbicides, fungicides, and chemical intermediaries

and are used in some explosives, dyes, and photographic chemicals. Dinitrophenol has also been taken orally for weight reduction but is banned for this use.

I. **Mechanism of toxicity.**
   A. Pentachlorophenol and dinitrophenols uncouple oxidative phosphorylation in the mitochondria. Substrates are metabolized but the energy produced is dissipated as heat instead of producing adenosine triphosphate (ATP). The basal metabolic rate increases, placing increased demands on the cardiorespiratory system. Excess lactic acid results from anaerobic glycolysis.
   B. Dinitrophenols may oxidize hemoglobin to methemoglobin (see p 220).
   C. In animal studies, pentachlorophenol is mutagenic, teratogenic, and carcinogenic. DNP is teratogenic and may be weakly carcinogenic.

II. **Toxic dose.** These agents are readily absorbed through the skin, lungs, and gastrointestinal tract.
   A. **Inhalation.** The air level of pentachlorophenol considered immediately dangerous to life or health (IDLH) is 2.5 mg/m^3. The ACGIH recommended workplace air exposure limit (TLV-TWA) is 0.5 mg/m^3 as an 8-hour time-weighted average.
   B. **Skin.** This is the main route associated with accidental poisoning. An epidemic of moderate intoxication occurred in a neonatal nursery after diapers were inadvertently washed in 23% sodium pentachlorophenate.
   C. **Ingestion.** The minimum lethal oral dose of pentachlorophenol for humans is not known, but death occurred after ingestion of 2 g. Ingestion of 1–3 g of dinitrophenol is considered lethal.

III. **Clinical presentation.** The toxic manifestations of pentachlorophenol and dinitrophenol are nearly identical. Profuse sweating, fever, tachypnea, and tachycardia are universally reported in serious poisonings.
   A. **Acute exposure** causes irritation of the skin, eyes, and upper respiratory tract. Systemic absorption may cause headache, vomiting, weakness, and lethargy. Profound sweating, hyperthermia, tachycardia, tachypnea, convulsions, and coma are associated with severe or fatal poisonings. Pulmonary edema may occur. Death is usually caused by cardiovascular collapse or hyperthermia. After death an extremely rapid onset of rigor mortis is frequently reported. Dinitrophenol may also induce methemoglobinemia, liver and kidney failure, and yellow-stained skin.
   B. **Chronic exposure** may present in a similar manner and in addition may cause weight loss, gastrointestinal disturbances, fevers and night sweats, weakness, flulike symptoms, contact dermatitis, and aplastic anemia (rare). Cataracts and glaucoma have been associated with DNP.

IV. **Diagnosis** is based on history of exposure and clinical findings, and should be suspected in patients with fever, metabolic acidosis, diaphoresis, and tachypnea.
   A. **Specific levels.** Blood levels are not readily available or useful for emergency management.
   B. **Other useful laboratory studies** include CBC, electrolytes, glucose, BUN, creatinine, CPK, liver transaminases, amylase, urine dipstick for occult blood (positive with hemolysis or rhabdomyolysis), arterial blood gases, methemoglobin level, and chest x-ray.

V. **Treatment.**
   A. **Emergency and supportive measures**
      1. Maintain an open airway and assist ventilation if necessary (see pp 1–7).
      2. Treat coma (p 18), seizures (p 21), hypotension (p 15), or hyperthermia (p 20) if they occur. Dehydration from tachypnea, fever, and sweating is common and may require large-volume fluid replacement.
      3. Monitor asymptomatic patients for at least 6 hours after exposure.
      4. Do **not** use salicylates or anticholinergic agents, as these may worsen hyperthermia. Paralysis with neuromuscular blockers may not be helpful given the intracellular mechanism for hyperthermia. Barbiturates (p 101) may be of some value.
   B. **Specific drugs and antidotes.** There is no specific antidote. Treat **methemoglobinemia** with methylene blue (see p 381).

C. Decontamination (see p 43)
   1. **Inhalation.** Remove the victim from exposure and administer supplemental oxygen if available.
   2. **Skin and eyes.** Remove contaminated clothing and store in a plastic bag; wash exposed areas thoroughly with soap and copious water. Irrigate exposed eyes with copious saline or tepid water. Rescuers should wear appropriate protective clothing and respirators to avoid exposure.
   3. **Ingestion** (see p 45)
      a. **Prehospital.** Administer activated charcoal if available. Do *not* induce vomiting, because of the risk of seizures.
      b. **Hospital.** Place a gastric tube, immediately administer a dose of activated charcoal, and then perform gastric lavage. After lavage, administer activated charcoal. For small ingestions, charcoal may be given without gut emptying.
D. Enhanced elimination. There is no evidence that enhanced elimination procedures are effective.

▶ PHENCYCLIDINE (PCP)

Kent R. Olson, MD

Phencyclidine (PCP) is a dissociative anesthetic agent with properties similar to those of ketamine. It was previously marketed for veterinary use, and it became popular as an inexpensive street drug in the late 1960s. PCP is commonly smoked, but may also be snorted, ingested, or injected, and it is frequently substituted for or added to other illicit psychoactive drugs such as THC (tetrahydrocannabinol or marijuana), mescaline, or LSD. PCP is known by a variety of street names, including "peace pill," "angel dust," "hog," "goon," "animal tranquilizer," and "krystal."

I. **Mechanism of toxicity.** PCP is a dissociative anesthetic that produces generalized loss of pain perception with little or no depression of airway reflexes or ventilation. Psychotropic effects are mediated through several mechanisms, including stimulation of sigma opioid receptors; inhibition of reuptake of dopamine, norepinephrine, and serotonin; and blocking of potassium conductance.

   Pharmacokinetics. PCP is rapidly absorbed by inhalation or ingestion. The volume of distribution (Vd) is about 6 L/kg. The duration of clinical effects after an overdose is highly variable and ranges from 11–14 hours in one report to 1–4 days in another. PCP is eliminated mainly by hepatic metabolism, although renal and gastric excretion account for a small fraction and are pH dependent. (See also Table II–55.)

II. **Toxic dose.** In tablet form the usual street dose is 1–6 mg, which results in hallucinations, euphoria, and disinhibition. Ingestion of 6–10 mg causes toxic psychosis and signs of sympathomimetic stimulation. Acute ingestion of 150–200 mg has resulted in death. Smoking PCP produces rapid onset of effects and thus may be an easier route for users to titrate to the desired level of intoxication.

III. **Clinical presentation.** Clinical effects may be seen within minutes of smoking PCP and can last 24 hours or longer depending on the dose.
   A. **Mild intoxication** causes lethargy, euphoria, hallucinations, and occasionally bizarre or violent behavior. Patients may abruptly swing between quiet catatonia and loud or agitated behavior. Vertical and horizontal nystagmus are prominent.
   B. **Severe intoxication** produces signs of adrenergic hyperactivity, including hypertension, rigidity, localized dystonic reactions, hyperthermia, tachycardia, diaphoresis, convulsions, and coma. The pupils are sometimes paradoxically small. **Death** may occur as a result of self-destructive behavior or as a complication of hyperthermia (eg, rhabdomyolysis, renal failure, coagulopathy, or brain damage).

IV. **Diagnosis** is suggested by the presence of rapidly fluctuating behavior, vertical nystagmus, and signs of sympathomimetic excess.
  A. **Specific levels**
    1. Specific serum PCP levels are not readily available, nor do they correlate reliably with the degree of intoxication. Levels of 30–100 ng/mL have been associated with toxic psychosis.
    2. Qualitative urine screening for PCP is widely available. PCP analogues may not appear on routine screening, although they can cross-react in some immunologic assays.
  B. **Other useful laboratory studies** include electrolytes, glucose, BUN, creatinine, CPK, and urinalysis dipstick for occult blood (positive with myoglobinuria).
V. **Treatment.**
  A. **Emergency and supportive measures**
    1. Maintain an open airway and assist ventilation if necessary (see pp 1–7).
    2. Treat coma (p 21), seizures (p 18), hypertension (p 16), hyperthermia (p 20), and rhabdomyolysis (p 25) if they occur.
    3. Agitated behavior (p 23) may respond to limiting sensory stimulation but may require sedation with haloperidol (see p 373), midazolam or diazepam (see p 342). Do *not* use physostigmine.
    4. Monitor temperature and other vital signs for a minimum of 6 hours, and admit all patients with hyperthermia or other evidence of significant intoxication.
  B. **Specific drugs and antidotes.** There is no specific antidote.
  C. **Decontamination.** No decontamination measures are necessary after smoking or injecting PCP. For ingestion (see p 45):
    1. **Prehospital.** Administer activated charcoal, if available. Do *not* induce vomiting.
    2. **Hospital.** Administer activated charcoal. Gastric emptying is not necessary if activated charcoal can be given promptly.
  D. **Enhanced elimination.** Because of its large volume of distribution, PCP is not effectively removed by dialysis, hemoperfusion, or other enhanced removal procedures.
    1. Repeat-dose activated charcoal has not been studied but might marginally increase elimination by adsorbing PCP partitioned into the acidic stomach fluid. Continuous nasogastric suction has also been proposed for removal of gastric-partitioned PCP.
    2. Although urinary acidification increases the urinary concentration of PCP, there is no evidence that this significantly enhances systemic elimination; and it may be dangerous because urinary acidification can aggravate myoglobinuric renal failure.

▶ **PHENOL AND RELATED COMPOUNDS**

Olga F. Woo, PharmD

Phenol (carbolic acid) was introduced into household use as a potent germicidal agent but has limited use today because less toxic compounds have replaced it. Now phenol is most commonly found in topical skin products (eg, Campho-phenique contains 9.7% phenol) and is also used cosmetically as a skin-peeling agent. **Hexachlorophene** is a chlorinated biphenol that was widely used as a topical antiseptic and preoperative scrub until its adverse neurologic effects were recognized. Other phenolic compounds include **creosote, creosol, hydroquinone, eugenol,** and **phenylphenol** (bisphenol, the active ingredient in Lysol). **Pentachlorophenol** and **dinitrophenols** are discussed on p 252.

I. **Mechanism of toxicity.** Phenol denatures protein, disrupts the cell wall, and produces coagulative necrosis. It may cause corrosive injury to the eyes, skin, and respiratory tract. Systemic absorption causes CNS stimulation. The mechanism of CNS intoxication is not known. Some phenolic compounds (eg, dinitrophenol and hydroquinone) may induce **methemoglobinemia** (see p 220).

II. **Toxic dose.** The minimum toxic and lethal doses have not been well established. Phenol is well absorbed by inhalation, skin application, and ingestion.

   A. **Inhalation.** The ACGIH-recommended workplace exposure limit (TLV-TWA) is 5 ppm (19 mg/m^3) as an 8-hour time-weighted average. The level considered immediately dangerous to life or health (IDLH) is 250 ppm.

   B. **Skin application.** Death has occurred in infants from repeated dermal applications of small doses (one infant died after a 2% solution of phenol was applied for 11 hours on the umbilicus under a closed bandage). Solutions >5% are corrosive.

   C. **Ingestion.** Deaths have occurred after adult ingestions of 1–32 g of phenol; however, survival after ingestion of 45–65 g has been reported. As little as 50–500 mg has been reported as fatal in infants.

   D. **Pharmacokinetics.** Phenol is rapidly absorbed by all routes. Its elimination half-life is 0.5–4.5 hours.

III. **Clinical presentation.** Toxicity may result from inhalation, skin or eye exposure, or ingestion.

   A. **Inhalation.** Vapors of phenol may cause respiratory tract irritation and chemical pneumonia. Smoking of clove cigarettes (clove oil contains the phenol derivative eugenol) may cause severe tracheobronchitis.

   B. **Skin and eyes.** Topical exposure to the skin may produce a deep white patch that turns red, then stains the skin brown. This lesion is often relatively painless. Eye irritation and severe corneal damage may occur if concentrated liquids are spilled into the eye.

   C. **Ingestion** usually causes vomiting and diarrhea, and diffuse corrosive gastrointestinal tract injury may occur. Systemic absorption may cause agitation, confusion, seizures, coma, hypotension, arrhythmias, and respiratory arrest.

IV. **Diagnosis** is based on a history of exposure, the presence of a characteristic odor, and painless white skin burns.

   A. **Specific levels.** Normal urine phenol levels are less than 20 mg/L. Urine phenol levels may be elevated in workers exposed to benzene and after use of phenol-containing throat lozenges and mouthwashes.

   B. **Other useful laboratory studies** include CBC, electrolytes, glucose, BUN, creatinine, and ECG. After hydroquinone exposure, obtain a methemoglobin level.

V. **Treatment.**

   A. **Emergency and supportive measures**

      1. Maintain an open airway and assist ventilation if necessary (see pp 1–7).

      2. Treat coma (p 18), seizures (p 21), hypotension (p 15), and arrhythmias (pp 10–14) if they occur.

      3. If corrosive injury to the gastrointestinal tract is suspected, consult a gastroenterologist for possible endoscopy.

   B. **Specific drugs and antidotes.** No specific antidote is available. If **methemoglobinemia** occurs, administer methylene blue (see p 381).

   C. **Decontamination** (see p 43)

      1. **Inhalation.** Remove victims from exposure and administer supplemental oxygen if available.

      2. **Skin and eyes.** Remove contaminated clothing and wash exposed skin with soapy water or, if available, mineral oil, olive oil, or petroleum jelly. Immediately flush exposed eyes with copious tepid water or saline.

      3. **Ingestion** (see p 45)

         a. **Prehospital.** Administer activated charcoal if available. Do **not** induce vomiting, because phenol is corrosive and may cause seizures.

         b. **Hospital.** Administer activated charcoal, orally or by gastric tube. Consider gastric lavage for large recent ingestions.

D. Enhanced elimination. Enhanced removal methods are generally not effective because of the large volume of distribution of these lipid-soluble compounds. Hexachlorophene is excreted in the bile, and repeat-dose activated charcoal (see p 54) may possibly be effective in increasing its clearance from the gut.

▶ PHENOTHIAZINES AND OTHER ANTIPSYCHOTIC DRUGS

Karl A. Sporer, MD

Phenothiazines, butyrophenones, and other related drugs are widely used to treat psychosis and agitated depression. In addition, some of these drugs (eg, prochlorperazine, promethazine, and droperidol) are used as antiemetic agents. Suicidal overdoses are common, but because of the high toxic-therapeutic ratio, acute overdose seldom results in death. A large number of newer agents have been developed; overdose experience with these agents is limited. Table II–42 describes available antipsychotic agents.

I. **Mechanism of toxicity.** A variety of pharmacologic effects are responsible for toxicity involving primarily the cardiovascular and central nervous systems.

A. **Cardiovascular.** Anticholinergic effects produce tachycardia. Alpha-adrenergic blockade causes orthostatic hypotension. With very large overdoses of some agents, quinidinelike membrane-depressant effects on the heart may occur.

TABLE II–42. COMMON PHENOTHIAZINES AND OTHER ANTIPSYCHOTIC DRUGS

Drug	Type[a]	Usual Adult Daily Dose (mg)	Toxicity[b]
Chlorpromazine	P	200–2000	E, A, H
Chlorprothixene	T	75–200	E
Clozapine	D	100–900	A, H
Ethopropazine	P	50–400	A, H
Fluphenazine	P	2.5–20	E, A
Haloperidol	B	1–100	E
Loxapine	D	60–100	E
Mesoridazine	P	150–400	A, H
Molindone	O	50–225	E
Olanzapine	D	5–10	E, A, H
Perphenazine	P	10–30	E
Prochlorperazine[c]	P	15–40	E
Promethazine[c]	P	25–200	A, E
Risperidone	O	4–16	E, H
Thioridazine	P	150–300	A, H
Thiothixene	T	5–60	E
Trifluoperazine	P	1–40	E
Trimethobenzamide[c]	O	600–1000	A, E

[a]P = Phenothiazine; T = Thiothixine; B = Butyrophenone; D = Dibenzodiazepine; O = Other.
[b]E = Extrapyramidal reactions; A = Anticholinergic effects; H = Hypotension.
[c]Used primarily as an antiemetic.

B. **Central nervous system.** Centrally mediated sedation and anticholinergic effects contribute to CNS depression. Alpha-adrenergic blockade causes small pupils, despite anticholinergic effects on other systems. Extrapyramidal dystonic reactions are relatively common with therapeutic doses and are probably caused by central dopamine receptor blockade. The seizure threshold may be lowered by unknown mechanisms. Temperature regulation is also disturbed, resulting in poikilothermia

C. **Pharmacokinetics.** These drugs have large volumes of distribution (Vd = 10–30 L/kg), and most have long elimination half-lives (eg, chlorpromazine, = 18–30 hours). Elimination is largely by hepatic metabolism. See Table II–55, p 319.

II. **Toxic dose.** Extrapyramidal reactions, anticholinergic side effects, and orthostatic hypotension are often seen with therapeutic doses. Tolerance to the sedating effects of the antipsychotics is well-described, and patients on chronic therapy may tolerate much larger doses than other persons.

A. Typical daily doses are given in Table II–42.

B. The toxic dose after acute ingestion is highly variable. Serious CNS depression and hypotension may occur after ingestion of 200–1000 mg of chlorpromazine in children or 3–5 g in adults.

III. **Clinical presentation.** Major toxicity is manifested in the cardiovascular and central nervous systems. Also, anticholinergic intoxication (see p 78) may occur as a result of ingestion of benztropine (Cogentin) or other co-administered drugs.

A. **Mild intoxication** causes sedation, small pupils, and orthostatic hypotension. Anticholinergic manifestations include dry mouth, absence of sweating, tachycardia, and urinary retention. Paradoxically, clozapine causes hypersalivation through an unknown mechanism.

B. **Severe intoxication** may cause coma, seizures, and respiratory arrest. The ECG usually shows QT interval prolongation and occasionally QRS prolongation (particularly with thioridazine [Mellaril]). Hypothermia or hyperthermia may occur. Clozapine can cause a prolonged confusional state and rarely cardiac toxicity. Risperidone can cause QT interval prolongation, but delirium is less severe.

C. **Extrapyramidal** dystonic side effects of therapeutic doses include torticollis, jaw muscle spasm, oculogyric crisis, rigidity, bradykinesia, and pill-rolling tremor.

D. Patients on chronic antipsychotic medication may develop the **neuroleptic malignant syndrome** (see p 20) characterized by rigidity, hyperthermia, sweating, lactic acidosis, and rhabdomyolysis.

E. Clozapine use has been associated with agranulocytosis.

IV. **Diagnosis** is based on a history of ingestion and findings of sedation, small pupils, hypotension, and QT interval prolongation. Dystonias in children should always suggest the possibility of antipsychotic exposure, often as a result of intentional administration by parents. Phenothiazines are occasionally visible on plain abdominal x-rays (see Table I–35).

A. **Specific levels.** Quantitative blood levels are not routinely available and do not help in diagnosis or treatment. Qualitative screening may easily detect phenothiazines in urine or gastric juice, but butyrophenones such as haloperidol are usually not included in toxicologic screens (see Table I–30, p 39).

B. **Other useful laboratory studies** include electrolytes, glucose, BUN, creatinine, CPK, arterial blood gases or oximetry, abdominal x-ray (to look for radiopaque pills), and chest x-ray.

V. **Treatment.**

A. **Emergency and supportive measures**

1. Maintain an open airway and assist ventilation if necessary (see pp 1–7). Administer supplemental oxygen.

2. Treat coma (p 18), seizures (p 21), hypotension (p 15), and hyperthermia (p 20) if they occur.

3. Monitor vital signs and ECG for at least 6 hours, and admit the patient for at least 24 hours if there are signs of significant intoxication. Children with

antipsychotic intoxication should be evaluated for possible intentional abuse.

B. Specific drugs and antidotes. There is no specific antidote.

    1. Dystonic reactions. Give **diphenhydramine**, 0.5–1 mg/kg IM or IV (see p 359) or benztropine (see p 344).

    2. QRS interval prolongation. Treat quinidinelike cardiotoxic effects with **bicarbonate**, 1–2 mEq/kg IV (see p 345).

C. Decontamination (see p 43)

    1. Prehospital. Administer activated charcoal if available. Do **not** induce vomiting.

    2. Hospital. Administer activated charcoal. Gastric emptying is not necessary if activated charcoal can be given promptly.

D. Enhanced elimination. Owing to extensive tissue distribution, these drugs are not effectively removed by dialysis or hemoperfusion. Repeat-dose activated charcoal has not been evaluated.

▶ PHENYLPROPANOLAMINE AND OTHER DECONGESTANTS

Neal L. Benowitz, MD

Phenylpropanolamine (PPA), phenylephrine, ephedrine, and pseudoephedrine are sympathomimetic drugs widely available in nonprescription nasal decongestants and cold preparations. These remedies usually also contain antihistamines and cough suppressants. PPA is also widely used as an appetite suppressant. Combinations of nonprescription sympathomimetics and caffeine are sometimes sold on the underground market as amphetamine or cocaine substitutes. Ephedrine and ephedra-containing herbal preparations (eg, "Ma Huang" or "Herbal Ecstasy") are often used as alternatives to the amphetamine derivative ecstasy (see p 208) or as adjuncts to body building or weight loss programs.

I. Mechanism of toxicity. All these agents stimulate the adrenergic system, with variable effects on alpha- and beta-adrenergic receptors depending on the compound. Generally, these agents stimulate the central nervous system much less than other phenylethylamines (see amphetamines, p 68).

    A. PPA and phenylephrine are direct alpha-adrenergic agonists. In addition, PPA produces mild beta-1-adrenergic stimulation and acts in part indirectly by enhancing norepinephrine release.

    B. Ephedrine and pseudoephedrine have both direct and indirect alpha- and beta-adrenergic activity but clinically produce more beta-adrenergic stimulation than PPA or phenylephrine.

    C. Pharmacokinetics. Peak effects occur within 1–3 hours although absorption may be delayed with sustained-release products. The drugs have large volumes of distribution (eg, the Vd for PPA is 2.5–5 L/kg). Elimination half-lives are 3–7 hours. See also Table II–55, p 319.

II. Toxic dose. Table II–43 lists the usual therapeutic doses of each agent. Patients developing autonomic insufficiency and those taking monoamine oxidase (MAO) inhibitors (see p 225) may be extraordinarily sensitive to these and other sympathomimetic drugs, developing severe hypertension after ingestion of even subtherapeutic doses.

    A. PPA, phenylephrine, and ephedrine have low toxic:therapeutic ratios, with toxicity often occurring after ingestion of just 2–3 times the therapeutic dose.

    B. Pseudoephedrine is slightly less toxic, with symptoms occurring after four- to fivefold the usual therapeutic dose.

III. Clinical presentation. The time course of intoxication by these drugs is usually brief, with resolution within 4–6 hours (unless sustained-release preparations are involved). The major toxic effect of these drugs is **hypertension**, which may lead to headache, confusion, seizures, and intracranial hemorrhage.

TABLE II–43. COMMON OVER-THE-COUNTER SYMPATHOMIMETIC DRUGS

Drug	Major Effects[a]	Usual Daily Adult Dose (mg)	Usual Daily Pediatric Dose (mg/kg)
Ephedrine	β, α	100–200	2–3
Phenylephrine	α	40–60	0.5–1
Phenylpropanolamine	α	100–150	1–2
Pseudoephedrine	β, α	180–360	3–5

[a]α = alpha-adrenergic; β = beta-adrenergic.

- **A. Intracranial hemorrhage** may occur in normal, healthy young persons after what might appear to be only modest elevation of the blood pressure (ie, 170/110 mm Hg) and is often associated with focal neurologic deficits, coma, or seizures.
- **B. Bradycardia or atrioventricular block** is common in patients with moderate to severe hypertension associated with PPA and phenylephrine, owing to the baroreceptor reflex response to hypertension. The presence of drugs such as antihistamines or caffeine prevents reflex bradycardia and may enhance the hypertensive effects of PPA and phenylephrine.
- **C. Myocardial infarction** and diffuse myocardial necrosis have been associated with PPA intoxication.

IV. **Diagnosis** is usually based on a history of excessive ingestion of diet pills or decongestant medications and the presence of hypertension. Bradycardia or AV block suggests PPA or phenylephrine. Severe headache, focal neurologic deficits, or coma should raise the possibility of intracerebral hemorrhage.
- **A. Specific levels.** Serum drug levels are not generally available and do not alter treatment. These agents may produce positive results for amphetamines on urine testing (see Table I–33, p 41), but can be distinguished on confirmatory testing.
- **B. Other useful laboratory studies** include electrolytes, glucose, BUN, creatinine, CPK with MB isoenzymes, 12-lead ECG and ECG monitoring, and CT head scan if intracranial hemorrhage is suspected.

V. **Treatment.**
- **A. Emergency and supportive measures**
  1. Maintain an open airway and assist ventilation if necessary (see pp 1–7). Administer supplemental oxygen.
  2. Treat hypertension aggressively (p 16 and **B**, below). Treat seizures (p 21) and ventricular tachyarrhythmias (p 13) if they occur. Do **not** treat reflex bradycardia, except indirectly by lowering blood pressure.
  3. Monitor the vital signs and ECG for a minimum of 4–6 hours after exposure, and longer if a sustained-release preparation has been ingested.
- **B. Specific drugs and antidotes**
  1. **Hypertension.** Treat hypertension if the diastolic pressure is higher than 100–105 mm Hg, especially in a patient with no prior history of hypertension. If there is computed tomographic or obvious clinical evidence of intracranial hemorrhage, lower the diastolic pressure cautiously, to no lower than 90 mm Hg, and consult a neurosurgeon immediately.
     - a. Use a vasodilator such as **phentolamine** (p 400) or **nitroprusside** (p 392).
     - b. *Caution:* Do *not* use beta blockers alone to treat hypertension without first giving a vasodilator; paradoxic worsening of the hypertension may result.
     - c. Many patients have moderate orthostatic variation in the blood pressure; therefore, for immediate partial relief of severe hypertension, try placing the patient in an upright position.

2. Arrhythmias
  a. Tachyarrhythmias usually respond to low-dose **propranolol** (p 405) or **esmolol** (p 366).
  b. *Caution:* Do *not* treat AV block or sinus bradycardia associated with hypertension; increasing the heart rate with atropine may abolish this reflex response that serves to limit hypertension, resulting in worsening elevation of the blood pressure.
C. Decontamination (see p 43)
  1. Prehospital. Administer activated charcoal if available. Do *not* induce vomiting.
  2. Hospital. Administer activated charcoal. Gastric emptying is not necessary if activated charcoal can be given promptly.
D. Enhanced elimination. Dialysis and hemoperfusion are not effective. Urinary acidification may enhance elimination of PPA, ephedrine, and pseudo-ephedrine, but may also aggravate myoglobin deposition in the kidney if the patient has rhabdomyolysis.

▶ PHENYTOIN

Kathryn H. Keller, PharmD

Phenytoin is used orally for the prevention of generalized (grand mal) and psychomotor seizures. Intravenous phenytoin is used to treat status epilepticus and occasionally as an antiarrhythmic agent. Oral formulations include suspensions, capsules, and tablet preparations. The brand Dilantin Kapseals exhibits delayed absorption characteristics not usually shared by generic products.

I. Mechanism of toxicity. Toxicity may be caused by the phenytoin itself or by the propylene glycol diluent used in parenteral preparations.
  A. Phenytoin alters neuronal ion fluxes, increasing refractory periods and decreasing repetitive neuronal firing. It is also known to increase brain concentrations of γ-aminobutyric acid (GABA). Toxic levels usually cause central nervous system depression.
  B. The **propylene glycol** diluent in parenteral preparations may cause myocardial depression and cardiac arrest when infused rapidly (> 40–50 mg/min [0.5–1 mg/kg/min]). The mechanism is not known.
  C. Pharmacokinetics. Absorption may be slow and unpredictable. The time to peak plasma levels varies with the dosage. The volume of distribution (Vd) is about 0.5–0.8 L/kg. Protein binding is about 90% at therapeutic levels. Hepatic elimination is saturable (zero-order kinetics) at levels near the therapeutic range, so the apparent "half-life" increases as levels rise (26 hours at 10 mg/L, 40 hours at 20 mg/L, and 60 hours at 40 mg/L). See also Table II–55 (p 319).
II. Toxic dose. The minimum acute toxic oral overdose is approximately 20 mg/kg. Because phenytoin exhibits dose-dependent elimination kinetics, accidental intoxication can easily occur in patients on chronic therapy owing to drug interactions or slight dosage adjustments.
III. Clinical presentation. Toxicity caused by phenytoin may be associated with acute oral overdose or chronic accidental overmedication. In acute oral overdose, absorption and peak effects may be delayed.
  A. Mild to moderate intoxication commonly causes nystagmus, ataxia, and dysarthria. Nausea, vomiting, diplopia, hyperglycemia, agitation, and irritability have also been reported.
  B. Severe intoxication can cause stupor, coma, and respiratory arrest. Although seizures have been reported, literature reports are unconvincing; seizures in a phenytoin-intoxicated patient should prompt a search for other causes (eg, anoxia, hyperthermia, or an overdose of another drug).

   C. Rapid intravenous injection, usually at rates exceeding 50 mg/min, can cause profound hypotension, bradycardia, or cardiac arrest. Cardiac toxicity does not occur with oral overdose.

IV. Diagnosis is based on a history of ingestion or is suspected in any epileptic patient with altered mental status or ataxia.

   A. Specific levels. Serum phenytoin concentrations are generally available in all hospital clinical laboratories. Obtain repeated blood samples because slow absorption may result in delayed peak levels. The therapeutic concentration range is 10–20 mg/L.

     1. Above 20 mg/L, nystagmus is common. Above 30 mg/L, ataxia, slurred speech, and tremor are common. With levels higher than 40 mg/L, lethargy, confusion, and stupor ensue. Survival has been reported in three patients with levels above 100 mg/L.

     2. Because phenytoin is protein bound, patients with renal failure or hypoalbuminemia may experience toxicity at lower serum levels. Free (unbound) serum phenytoin levels are not routinely available.

   B. Other useful laboratory studies include electrolytes, glucose, BUN, creatinine, serum albumin, and ECG monitoring (during intravenous infusion).

V. Treatment.

   A. Emergency and supportive measures

     1. Maintain an open airway and assist ventilation if necessary (see pp 1–7). Administer supplemental oxygen.

     2. Treat stupor and coma (p 18) if they occur. Protect the patient from self injury caused by ataxia.

     3. If seizures occur, consider an alternative diagnosis and treat with other usual anticonvulsants (p 22).

     4. If hypotension occurs with intravenous phenytoin administration, immediately stop the infusion and administer intravenous fluids and pressors (p 15) if necessary.

   B. Specific drugs and antidotes. There is no specific antidote.

   C. Decontamination (see p 43)

     1. Prehospital. Administer activated charcoal if available. Ipecac-induced vomiting may be useful for initial treatment at the scene (eg, children at home) if it can be given within a few minutes of exposure.

     2. Hospital. Administer activated charcoal. Gastric emptying is not necessary if activated charcoal can be given promptly.

   D. Enhanced elimination. Repeat-dose activated charcoal (see p 54) may enhance phenytoin elimination. There is no role for diuresis, dialysis, or hemoperfusion.

▶ PHOSGENE

John Balmes, MD

Phosgene was originally manufactured as a war gas. It is now used in the manufacture of dyes, resins, and pesticides. It is also commonly produced when chlorinated compounds are burned, such as in a fire, or in the process of welding metal that has been cleaned with chlorinated solvents.

I. Mechanism of toxicity. Phosgene is an irritant. However, because it is poorly water-soluble, in lower concentrations it does not cause immediate upper-airway or skin irritation. Thus, an exposed individual may inhale phosgene deeply into the lungs for prolonged periods, where it is slowly hydrolyzed to hydrochloric acid. This results in necrosis and inflammation of the small airways and alveoli, which may lead to noncardiogenic pulmonary edema.

II. Toxic dose. The ACGIH-recommended workplace exposure limit (TLV-TWA) is 0.1 ppm (0.4 mg/m^3) as an 8-hour time-weighted average. The level considered immediately dangerous to life or health (IDLH) is 2 ppm. Exposure to 50 ppm may be rapidly fatal.

III. Clinical presentation. Exposure to moderate concentrations of phosgene causes mild cough and minimal mucous membrane irritation. After an asymptomatic interval of 30 minutes to 8 hours (depending on the duration and concentration of exposure), the victim develops dyspnea and hypoxemia. Pulmonary edema may be delayed up to 24 hours. Permanent pulmonary impairment may be a sequela of serious exposure.

IV. Diagnosis is based on a history of exposure and the clinical presentation. Many other toxic gases may cause delayed-onset pulmonary edema (see p 7).
  A. Specific levels. There are no specific blood or urine levels.
  B. Other useful laboratory studies include chest x-ray and arterial blood gases or oximetry.

V. Treatment.
  A. Emergency and supportive measures
    1. Maintain an open airway and assist ventilation if necessary (see pp 1–7). Administer supplemental oxygen, and treat noncardiogenic pulmonary edema (see p 7) if it occurs.
    2. Monitor the patient for at least 12–24 hours after exposure because of the potential for delayed-onset pulmonary edema.
  B. Specific drugs and antidotes. There is no specific antidote.
  C. Decontamination. Remove the victim from exposure and give supplemental oxygen if available. Rescuers should wear self-contained breathing apparatus.
  D. Enhanced elimination. These procedures are not effective.

▶ PHOSPHINE AND PHOSPHIDES

Peter Wald, MD, MPH

Phosphine is a colorless gas that is heavier than air. It has a characteristic fishy or garliclike odor. It has been used for fumigation, and it is a serious potential hazard in operations producing metal phosphides, where phosphine can be released in the chemical reaction of water and metal alloys. Workers at risk include metal refiners, acetylene workers, fire fighters, pest-control operators, and those in the semiconductor industry. **Zinc phosphide** and **aluminum phosphide** are used as fumigants and rodenticides.

I. Mechanism of toxicity. Phosphine is a highly toxic gas, especially to organs of high oxygen flow and demand such as the lungs, brain, kidneys, heart, and liver. The pathophysiologic action of phosphine is not clearly understood, but may be related to inhibition of electron transport in mitochondria. Zinc and aluminum phosphides liberate phosphine gas upon contact with moisture.

II. Toxic dose.
  A. Phosphine gas. The ACGIH-recommended workplace exposure limit (TLV-TWA) is 0.3 ppm (0.42 mg/m^3), much lower than the minimal detectable (fishy odor) concentration of 1–3 ppm. Hence, the odor threshold does not provide sufficient warning of dangerous concentrations. An air level of 50 ppm is considered immediately dangerous to life or health (IDLH). Chronic exposure to sublethal concentrations for extended periods may produce toxic symptoms.
  B. Phosphides. Ingestion of as little as 500 mg *aluminum phosphide* has caused death in an adult. In a recent case series, survivors ingested about 1.5 g (range 1.5–18) while fatal cases had ingested an average of 2.3 g (range 1.5–36). The LD$_{50}$ for *zinc phosphide* in rats is 40 mg/kg; the lowest reported lethal dose in humans is 4 g. A 36-year-old man who ingested 6 mg/kg zinc phosphide and was treated with ipecac and activated charcoal remained asymptomatic.

III. **Clinical presentation.** Inhalation of phosphine gas is associated with cough, dyspnea, headache, dizziness, and vomiting. Phosphide ingestion may cause nausea, vomiting, diarrhea, hypotension unresponsive to pressors, and a rotten fish or garlicky odor. In both exposures, pulmonary edema, myocardial necrosis, convulsions, and coma may occur. Renal and hepatic toxicity are also reported. The onset of symptoms is usually rapid, although delayed onset of pulmonary edema has been described.

IV. **Diagnosis** is based on a history of exposure to the agent. *Caution:* Pulmonary edema may have a delayed onset, and initial respiratory symptoms may be mild or absent.

   A. **Specific levels.** Body fluid phosphine levels are not clinically useful.

   B. **Other useful laboratory studies** include BUN, creatinine, electrolytes, liver transaminases, arterial blood gases or oximetry, and chest x-ray.

V. **Treatment.**

   A. **Emergency and supportive measures**

      1. Maintain an open airway and assist ventilation if necessary (see pp 1–7). Administer supplemental oxygen, and treat noncardiogenic pulmonary edema (p 7) if it occurs.

      2. Treat seizures (p 21) and hypotension (p 15) if they occur.

      3. Patients with a history of significant phosphine inhalation or phosphide ingestion should be admitted and observed for 48–72 hours for delayed onset of pulmonary edema.

   B. **Specific drugs and antidotes.** There is no specific antidote.

   C. **Decontamination**

      1. **Prehospital.** Administer activated charcoal if available. Ipecac-induced vomiting may be useful for initial treatment at the scene (eg, children at home) if it can be given within a few minutes of exposure.

      2. **Hospital.** Administer activated charcoal, although studies have not determined its binding affinity for phosphides. Consider gastric lavage for large recent ingestion. Use of 3–5% sodium bicarbonate in the lavage has been proposed (to reduce stomach acid and resulting production of phosphine) but is not of proven benefit.

   D. **Enhanced elimination.** Dialysis and hemoperfusion have not been shown to be useful in hastening elimination of phosphine.

▶ **PHOSPHORUS**

Peter Wald, MD, MPH

There are two naturally occurring types of elemental phosphorus: red and white-yellow. **Red phosphorus** is not absorbed and is essentially nontoxic. In contrast, **white** or **yellow phosphorus** is a highly toxic cellular poison. Although no longer a component of matches, white phosphorus is still used in the manufacture of fireworks and fertilizer and as a rodenticide.

I. **Mechanism of toxicity.**

   A. Phosphorus is highly corrosive and is also a general cellular poison. Cardiovascular collapse occurring after ingestion probably results not only from fluid loss owing to vomiting and diarrhea but also from direct toxicity on the heart and vascular tone.

   B. White-yellow phosphorus spontaneously combusts in air to yield phosphorus oxide, a highly irritating fume.

II. **Toxic dose.**

   A. **Ingestion.** The fatal oral dose of white-yellow phosphorus is approximately 1 mg/kg. Deaths have been reported after ingestion of as little as 15 mg.

   B. **Inhalation.** The recommended workplace limit (ACGIH TLV-TWA) for white-yellow phosphorus is 0.1 mg/m^3 (0.02 ppm) as an 8-hour time-weighted average. The air level considered immediately dangerous to life or health is 5 mg/m^3.

III. Clinical presentation.

A. Acute inhalation may cause conjunctivitis, mucous membrane irritation, cough, wheezing, chemical pneumonitis, and noncardiogenic pulmonary edema. **Chronic inhalation** of phosphorus (over at least 10 months) may result in mandibular necrosis ("phossy jaw").

B. Skin or eye contact may cause severe dermal or ocular burns.

C. Acute ingestion may cause gastrointestinal burns, severe vomiting, and diarrhea with "smoking" stools. Systemic effects include headache, confusion, seizures, coma, arrhythmias, and shock. Metabolic derangements may occur, including hypocalcemia and hyperphosphatemia (or hypophosphatemia). If the victim survives, hepatic or renal failure may occur after 4–8 days.

IV. Diagnosis is based on a history of exposure and the clinical presentation. Smoking stools caused by spontaneous combustion of elemental phosphorus suggest phosphorus ingestion.

A. Specific levels. Because serum phosphorus may be elevated, depressed, or normal, it is not a useful test for diagnosis or estimation of severity.

B. Other useful laboratory studies include BUN, creatinine, liver transaminases, urinalysis, arterial blood gases or oximetry, and chest x-ray (acute inhalation).

V. Treatment.

A. Emergency and supportive measures
1. Observe the victim of inhalation closely for signs of upper-airway injury and perform endotracheal intubation and assist ventilation if necessary (see p 4). Administer supplemental oxygen. Treat bronchospasm (p 8) and pulmonary edema (p 7) if they occur.
2. Treat fluid losses from gastroenteritis with aggressive intravenous crystalloid fluid replacement.
3. Consider endoscopy if oral, esophageal, or gastric burns are suspected (p 129).

B. Specific drugs and antidotes. There is no specific antidote.

C. Decontamination (see p 43). Rescuers should wear appropriate protective gear to prevent accidental exposure. If solid phosphorus is brought into the emergency department, immediately cover it with water or wet sand.
1. **Inhalation.** Remove the victim from exposure and give supplemental oxygen, if available.
2. **Skin and eyes.** Remove contaminated clothing and wash exposed areas with soap and water. Irrigate exposed eyes with copious tepid water or saline. Covering exposed areas may help prevent spontaneous combustion of white-yellow phosphorus.
3. **Ingestion** (see p 45)
   a. **Prehospital.** Administer activated charcoal if available (although there is no evidence that it adsorbs phosphorus). Do **not** induce vomiting because of the potential for corrosive injury.
   b. **Hospital.** Perform careful gastric lavage. Administer activated charcoal (although there is no evidence that it adsorbs phosphorus).

D. Enhanced elimination. There is no effective method of enhanced elimination.

▶ PLANTS AND HERBAL MEDICINES

Olga F. Woo, PharmD

Plant ingestions are second only to drugs as the most common poisoning exposure in children. Fortunately, serious poisoning or death is extremely rare because the quantity of toxin ingested is small. During the past 2 decades, public interest in natural foods and traditional medical remedies and in "herbal highs" has resulted in increasing use of herbal products. Unfortunately, there is little consumer awareness of the potential harm from some herbal preparations. Besides toxicity from natural products contained in some medicinal plants, "herbal" or "traditional" preparations may

sometimes actually contain allopathic drugs such as phenylbutazone, corticosteroids, salicylates, ephedrine, or toxic metal salts such as mercury or lead.
  I. **Mechanism of toxicity.** Table II–44 is a list of potentially toxic plants and herbs,
     categorized in Groups 1, 2a, 2b, and 3.
     A. **Group 1** plants contain systemically active poisons that may cause serious
        intoxication.
     B. **Group 2a** plants contain insoluble calcium oxalate crystals that cause burning
        pain and swelling of mucous membranes.
     C. **Group 2b** plants contain soluble oxalate salts (sodium or potassium) that can
        produce acute hypocalcemia, renal injury, and other organ damage sec-
        ondary to precipitation of calcium oxalate crystals in various organs (see
        p 248). Mucous membrane irritation and gastroenteritis may also occur.
     D. **Group 3** plants contain various chemical agents that generally produce only
        mild to moderate gastrointestinal irritation after ingestion or dermatitis after
        skin contact.

TABLE II–44. POISONOUS PLANTS AND HERBS

Common Name	Botanical Name	Toxic Group	Remarks
Acorn	*Quercus* spp	3	Tannin; irritant
Akee	*Blighia sapida*	1	Hypoglycemia and hepatotoxicity
Almond, bitter	*Prunus* spp	1	Cyanogenic glycosides (see p 150)
Aloe vera	*Aloe vera*	3	Hypersensitivity; skin irritant
Amaryllis	*Hippeastrum equestre*	3	
American bittersweet	*Celastrus scandens*	3	
American ivy	*Parthenocissus* spp	2b	Soluble oxalates (see p 248)
Angel's trumpet	*Brugmansia arborea*	1, 3	Anticholinergic alkaloids (see p 78)
Anthurium	*Anthurium* spp	2a	Calcium oxalate crystals
Apple (seeds)	*Malus domestica*	1	Cyanogenic glycosides (see p 150)
Apricot (chewed pits)	*Prunus* spp	1	Cyanogenic glycosides (see p 150)
Arrowhead vine	*Syngonium podophyllum*	2a	Calcium oxalate crystals (see text)
Asparagus fern	*Asparagus plumosus*	3	
Autumn crocus	*Colchicum autumnale*	1	Colchicine (see p 145)
Avocado (leaves)	*Avocado*	1	Unknown toxin
Azalea	*Rhododendron* genus	1	Andromedotoxin; hypotension, brady-cardia, AV block; lethargy
Bahia	*Bahia oppositifolia*	1	Cyanogenic glycosides (see p 150)
Baneberry	*Actaea* spp	3	Irritant oil protoanemonin: severe gastroenteritis
Barbados nut; purging nut	*Jatropha* spp	1	Phytotoxins: severe gastroenteritis
Barberry	*Berberis* spp	3	
Beech	*Fagus sylvatica*	3	Saponins
Begonia	*Begonia rex*	2a	Calcium oxalate crystals
Belladonna	*Atropa belladonna*	1	Atropine (see p 78)
Bellyache bush	*Jatropha* spp	1	Phytotoxins: severe gastroenteritis
Be-still tree	*Thevetia peruviana*	1	Cardiac glycosides (see p 128)
Birch (bark, leaves)	*Betula* spp	1, 3	Methyl salicylate (see p 284), irritant oils
Bird of paradise	*Poinciana gillesi*	3	
Black cohosh	*Cimicifuga* spp	3	
Black locust	*Robinia pseudoacacia*	1	Phytotoxins: severe gastroenteritis
Black nightshade	*Hyoscyamus* spp	1	Anticholinergic alkaloids (see p 78)
Black snakeroot	*Zigadenus* spp	1	Similar to veratramine: hypotension, bradycardia, lethargy
Bleeding heart	*Dicentra*	3	
Bloodroot	*Sanguinaria canadensis*	3	
Blue cohosh	*Caulophyllum thalictroides*	1, 3	Cytisine: similar to nicotine (see p 231)

(continued)

TABLE II–44. POISONOUS PLANTS AND HERBS (CONTINUED)

Common Name	Botanical Name	Toxic Group	Remarks
Boston ivy	*Parthenocissus* spp	2b	Soluble oxalates (see p 248)
Boxwood; box plant	*Buxus* spp	3	
Broom; scotch broom	*Cytisus* spp	1, 3	Cytisine: similar to nicotine (see p 231); sparteine: cardiotoxic; sparteione: diuretic, oxytoxic
Buckeye	*Aesculus* spp	1, 3	Coumarin glycosides (see p 148)
Buckthorn; tullidora	*Karwinskia humboltiana*	1	Chronic ingestion may cause ascending paralysis
Buckthorn	*Rhamnus* spp	3	Anthraquinone cathartic
Bunchberry	*Cornus canadensis*	3	
Burdock root	*Arctium minus*	1,3	Anticholinergic alkaloids (see p 78)
Burning bush	*Euonymus* spp	3	
Buttercups	*Ranunculus* spp	3	Irritant oil protoanemonin
Cactus (thorn)	*Cactus*	3	Cellulitis, abscess may result
Caladium	*Caladium* spp; *Xanthosoma* spp	2a	Calcium oxalate crystals (see text)
California geranium	*Senecio* spp	1	Hepatotoxic pyrrolizidine alkaloids
California privet	*Ligustrum* spp	3	
Calla lily	*Zantedeschia* spp	2a	Calcium oxalate crystals (see text)
Cannabis	*Cannabis sativa*	1	Mild hallucinogen
Caraway	*Carum carvi*	3	When used as herbal medication
Cardinal flower	*Lobelia* spp	1	Lobeline: nicotinelike alkaloid (see p 231)
Carnation	*Dianthus caryophyllus*	3	
Carolina allspice	*Calycanthus* spp	1	Strychninelike alkaloid (see p 298)
Cascara	*Rhamnus* spp	3	Anthraquinone cathartic
Cassava	*Manihot esculenta*	1	Cyanogenic glycosides (see p 150)
Castor bean	*Ricinus communis*	1	Ricin: severe gastroenteritis
Catnip	*Nepeta cataria*	1, 3	Mild hallucinogen
Century plant	*Agave americana*	3	Thorns can cause cellulitis
Chamomile	*Chamomilla recucita*	3	Potentially antigenic
Cherry (chewed pits)	*Prunus* spp	1	Cyanogenic glycosides (see p 150)
Chili pepper	*Capsicum* spp	3	Irritant to skin, eyes, mucous membranes
Chinaberry	*Melia azedarach*	1, 3	Severe fatal gastroenteritis reported; contains convulsant
Christmas rose	*Helleborus niger*	1, 3	Similar to cardiac glycosides (see p 128)
Chrysanthemum; mum	*Chrysanthemum* spp	3	Pyrethrins (see p 276)
Coffeeberry	*Rhamnus* spp	3	Anthraquinone cathartic
Cola nut; gotu kola	*Cola* spp	1	Caffeine (see p 118), theobromine
Comfrey	*Symphytum officinale*	1, 3	Irritant tannin and hepatotoxic pyrrolizidine alkaloids
Conquer root	*Exogonium purga*	3	
Coral bean	*Sophora secundiflora*	1	Cytisine: similar to nicotine (see p 231)
Coral berry	*Symphoricarpos* spp	3	
Coriaria	*Coriaria myrtifolia*	1	Contains convulsant agent
Cotoneaster	*Cotoneaster*	1,3	Cyanogenic glycosides (see p 150)
Coyotillo	*Karwinskia humboldtiana*	1	Chronic ingestion may cause ascending paralysis
Creeping charlie	*Glecoma hederacea*	1, 3	Volatile oils; mild stimulant
Crown of thorns	*Euphorbia* spp	3	
Cyclamen	*Cyclamen*	3	
Daffodil (bulb)	*Narcissus* spp	3	
Daphne	*Daphne* spp	1, 3	Bark: coumarin glycosides (see p 148) berries: blisters
Deadly nightshade	*Atropa belladonna*	1	Atropine (see p 78)
Death camas	*Zigadenus* spp	1	Similar to veratramine: hypotension, bradycardia, lethargy
Devils ivy	*Scindapsus aureus*	2a	Calcium oxalate crystals (see text)

(continued)

TABLE II–44. POISONOUS PLANTS AND HERBS (CONTINUED)

Common Name	Botanical Name	Toxic Group	Remarks
Dogbane	Apocynum spp	1	Cardiac glycosides (see p 128)
Dolls-eyes	Actaea spp	3	Irritant oil protoanemonin: severe gastroenteritis
Dragon root	Arisaema spp	2a	Calcium oxalate crystals (see text)
Dumbcane	Dieffenbachia spp	2a	Calcium oxalate crystals (see text)
Dusty miller	Senecio spp	1	Hepatotoxic pyrrolizidine alkaloids
Elderberry	Sambucus	1	Unripe berries contain cyanogenic glycosides (see p 150)
Elephant's ear; taro	Alacasia spp; Colocasia spp; Philodendron spp	2a	Calcium oxalate crystals (see text)
English ivy; heart ivy	Hedera helix	3	Saponins
English laurel	Prunus laurocerasus	1	Cyanogenic glycosides (see p 150)
Ergot	Claviceps spp	1	Ergot alkaloids (see p 160)
Eucalyptus	Eucalyptus	3	Irritant oils
False hellebore	Veratrum spp	1, 3	Veratramine: hypotension, AV block, arrhythmias; seizures
Fava bean	Vicia faba	1	Hemolytic anemia in G6PD-deficient persons
Ficus (sap)	Ficus benjamina	3	
Firethorn	Pyracantha	3	
Fool's parsley	Conium maculatum	1	Coniine: nicotinelike alkaloid (see p 231)
Four o'clock	Mirabilis jalapa	3	Seeds have hallucinogenic effects
Foxglove	Digitalis purpurea	1	Cardiac glycosides (see p 128)
Glacier ivy	Hedera glacier	3	Saponins
Glory pea	Sesbania spp	3	Saponins
Goldenrod; rayless	Haplopappus heterophyllus	1	Higher alcohol tremetol: CNS depression
Golden chain	Labumum anagyroides	1	Cytisine: similar to nicotine (see p 231)
Golden seal	Hydrastis spp	1, 3	Fatalities reported after use as herbal tea
Gordolobo	Senecio spp	1	Hepatotoxic pyrrolizidine alkaloids
Grindelia	Grindelia spp	1	Balsamic resin: renal, cardiac toxicity
Groundsel	Senecio spp	1	Hepatotoxic pyrrolizidine alkaloids
Guaiac	Guaiacum officinale	3	
Harmaline	Banisteriopsis spp	1	Harmaline: hallucinogen (see p 208)
Harmel; Syrian rue	Peganum harmala	1	Harmaline: hallucinogen (see p 208)
Heart leaf	Philodendron spp	2a	Calcium oxalate crystals (see text)
Heath	Ericaceae family	1, 3	Andromedotoxin: hypotension, AV block, arrhythmias: lethargy
Heliotrope	Heliotropium spp	1	Pyrrolizidine alkaloids: hepatotoxicity
Hemlock; poison hemlock	Conium maculatum	1	Coniine: nicotinelike alkaloid (see p 231)
Henbane; black henbane	Hyoscyamus spp	1	Anticholinergic alkaloids (see p 78)
Holly (berry)	Ilex aquifolium	3	
Honeysuckle	Caprifoliaceae family	3	Red berries contain toxin
Hops	Humulus lupulus	1	Sedative
Horse chestnut	Aesculus spp	1, 3	Coumarin glycosides (see p 148)
Hyacinth	Hyacinthus	3	
Hydrangea	Hydrangea spp	1, 3	Cyanogenic glycosides (see p 150)
Indian currant	Symphoricarpos spp	3	
Indian tobacco	Lobelia spp	1	Lobeline: nicotinelike alkaloid (see p 231)
Inkberry	Phytolacca americana	3	If absorbed may cause hemolysis; cooked berries edible
Iris	Iris	3	
Ivy bush; sheepkill	Kalmia spp	1	Andromedotoxin: hypotension, AV block, arrhythmias; lethargy

(continued)

TABLE II–44. POISONOUS PLANTS AND HERBS (CONTINUED)

Common Name	Botanical Name	Toxic Group	Remarks
Jack-in-the-pulpit	*Arisaema* spp	2a	Calcium oxalate crystals (see text)
Jalap	*Exogonium purga*	3	
Jequirity bean	*Abrus precatorius*	1	Phytotoxin abrin: severe fatal gastroenteritis reported
Jerusalem cherry	*Solanum pseudocapsicum*	1, 3	Unripe berry contains solanine and anticholinergic alkaloids (see p 78)
Jessamine, Carolina or Yellow	*Gelsemium sempervirens*	1	Alkaloids similar to strychnine (see p 298)
Jessamine, day or night	*Cestrum* spp	1, 3	Solanine and anticholinergic alkaloids (see p 78)
Jetberry bush, Jetbead	*Rhodotypos scandens*	1	Cyanogenic glycosides (see p 150)
Jimmyweed	*Haplopappus heterophyllus*	1	High alcohol tremetol: CNS depression
Jimsonweed	*Brugmansia arborea*	1, 3	Anticholinergic alkaloids (see p 78)
Jimsonweed; thornapple	*Datura stramonium*	1	Anticholinergic alkaloids (see p 78)
Juniper	*Juniperus macropoda*	1,3	Hallucinogen
Kava-kava	*Piper methysticum*	1	Mild hallucinogen
Kentucky coffee tree	*Gymaocladus dioica*	1	Cytisine: similar to nicotine (see p 231)
Khat; chat	*Catha edulis*	1	Mild hallucinogen and stimulant
Labrador tea	*Ledum* spp	1	Andromedotoxin: hypotension, AV block, arrhythmias; lethargy
Lantana	*Lantana camara*	1	Hepatotoxic in animals; ingestion of unripe berries may cause cardiovascular collapse and death
Larkspur	*Delphinium*	1	Delphinine: arrhythmias, AV block
Licorice root	*Glycyrrhiza lepidata*	1, 3	Hypokalemia after chronic use
Lily of the Nile	*Agapanthus*	3	Burning sensation when ingested
Lily-of-the-valley	*Convallaria majalis*	1	Cardiac glycosides (see p 128)
Lily-of-the-valley shrub	*Pieris japonica*	1	Andromedotoxin: hypotension, AV block, arrhythmias; lethargy
Mandrake	*Mandragora officinarum*	1	Anticholinergic alkaloids (see p 78)
Mandrake	*Podophyllum peltatum*	1, 3	Oil is keratolytic, irritant; hypotension, seizures reported after ingestion of resin; ripe fruit nontoxic
Marble queen	*Scindapsus aureus*	2a	Calcium oxalate crystals (see text)
Marijuana	*Cannabis sativa*	1	Mild hallucinogen
Marsh marigold	*Caltha palustris*	3	Irritant oil protoanemonin
Mate	*Ilex paraguayensis*	1, 3	Irritant tannins; caffeine
Mayapple	*Podophyllum peltatum*	1, 3	Oil is keratolytic, irritant; hypotension, seizures reported
Meadow crocus	*Colchicum autumnale*	1	Colchicine (see p 145)
Mescal bean	*Sophora secundiflora*	1	Cytisine: similar to nicotine (see p 231)
Mescal button	*Lophophora williamsii*	1	Mescaline: hallucinogen (see p 208)
Milkweed	*Asclepias* spp	3	Galitoxin: fatal poisonings in livestock
Mistletoe, American	*Phoradendron flavescens*	1, 3	Cardiotoxic phoratoxin: potential pressor effects
Mistletoe, European	*Viscum album*	1	Cardiotoxic viscotoxin: vasoconstrictor
Mock azalea	*Menziesia ferruginea*	1	Andromedotoxin: hypotension, AV block, arrhythmias; lethargy
Monkshood	*Aconitum napellus*	1	Aconite: hypotension, AV block, arrhythmias; seizures
Moonseed	*Menispermaceae*	1	Contains convulsant agent
Mormon tea	*Ephedra viridis*	1	Sympathomimetic (see p 259)
Morning glory	*Ipomoea violacea*	1	Seeds are hallucinogenic
Mountain laurel	*Kalmia* spp	1	Andromedotoxin: hypotension, AV block, arrhythmias: lethargy

(continued)

TABLE II–44. POISONOUS PLANTS AND HERBS (CONTINUED)

Common Name	Botanical Name	Toxic Group	Remarks
Nectarine (chewed pits)	*Prunus* spp	1	Cyanogenic glycosides (see p 150)
Nephthytis	*Syngonium podophyllum*	2a	Calcium oxalate crystals (see text)
Nightshade	*Solanum* spp	1, 3	Solanine and anticholinergic alkaloids (see p 78)
Nightshade, black	*Hyoscyamus* spp	1	Anticholinergic alkaloids (see p 78)
Nightshade, deadly	*Atropa belladonna*	1	Atropine (see p 78)
Nutmeg	*Myristica fragrans*	1	Hallucinogen (see p 208)
Oakleaf ivy	*Toxicodendron* spp	3	Urushiol oleoresin: contact dermatitis
Oleander	*Nerium oleander*	1	Cardiac glycosides (see p 128)
Oleander, yellow	*Thevetia peruviana*	1	Cardiac glycosides (see p 128)
Pampas grass	*Cortaderia selloana*	1	Cyanogenic glycosides (see p 150)
Paraguay tea	*Ilex paraguayensis*	1, 3	Irritant tannins; caffeine
Peach (chewed pits)	*Prunus* spp	1	Cyanogenic glycosides (see p 150)
Pear (chewed seeds)	*Prunus* spp	1	Cyanogenic glycosides (see p 150)
Pennyroyal (oil)	*Mentha pulegium*	1	Hepatotoxic (see p 122); seizures
Periwinkle	*Vinca*	1	*Vinca* alkaloids
Periwinkle, rose	*Catharanthus roseus*	1	Hallucinogen
Peyote; mescal	*Lophophora williamsii*	1	Mescaline: hallucinogen (see p 208)
Pheasant's-eye	*Adonis* spp	1	Cardiac glycosides (see p 128)
Pigeonberry	*Duranta repens*	3	Saponins
Pigeonberry	*Phytolacca americana*	3	If absorbed may cause hemolysis; cooked berries edible
Plum (chewed pits)	*Prunus* spp	1	Cyanogenic glycosides (see p 150)
Poinsettia	*Euphorbia* spp	3	
Poison ivy; poison oak; poison sumac; poison vine	*Toxicodendron* spp	3	Urushiol oleoresin contact dermatitis (*Rhus* dermatitis)
Pokeweed (unripe berries)	*Phytolacca americana*	3	If absorbed may cause hemolysis; cooked berries edible
Potato (unripe)	*Solanum* spp	1, 3	Solanine and anticholinergic alkaloids (see p 78)
Pothos; yellow pothos	*Scindapsus aureus*	2a	Calcium oxalate crystals (see text)
Prickly poppy	*Argemone mexicana*	1	Narcotic-analgesic, smoked as euphoriant
Pride-of-Madeira	*Echium* spp	1	Pyrrolizidine alkaloids: hepatotoxicity
Privet; common privet	*Ligustrum* spp	3	
Purslane	*Portulaca oleracea*	2b	Soluble oxalates (see p 248)
Pyracantha	*Pyracantha*	3	
Ragwort, tansy	*Senecio* spp	1	Pyrrolizidine alkaloids: hepatotoxic
Rattlebox	*Sesbania* spp	3	Saponins
Rattlebox, bush tea	*Crotalaria* spp	1	Pyrrolizidine alkaloids: hepatotoxicity
Rattlebox, purple	*Daubentonia* spp	3	
Rhododendron	*Rhododendron* genus	1	Andromedotoxin: hypotension, bradycardia, AV block; lethargy
Rhubarb	*Rheum rhaponticum*	2b	Soluble oxalates (see p 248)
Rosary pea; rosary bean	*Abrus precatorius*	1	Phytotoxin abrin: severe fatal gastroenteritis reported
Rose periwinkle	*Catharanthus roseus*	1	Hallucinogen
Rustyleaf	*Menziesia ferruginea*	1	Andromedotoxin: hypotension, AV block, arrhythmias; lethargy
Sassafras	*Sassafras albidium*	1	Hepatocarcinogenic
Scotch broom	*Cytisus scoparins*	1, 3	Cytisine: gastrointestional nicotinic effects; sparteine; cardiotoxic; sparteione: diuretic, oxytoxic
Shamrock	*Oxalis* spp	2b	Soluble oxalates (see p 248)
Skunk cabbage	*Symplocarpus foetidus*	2a	Calcium oxalate crystals (see text)

(continued)

TABLE II–44. POISONOUS PLANTS AND HERBS (CONTINUED)

Common Name	Botanical Name	Toxic Group	Remarks
Skunk cabbage	*Veratrum* spp	1, 3	Veratramine: hypotension, AV block, arrhythmias; seizures
Sky-flower	*Duranta repens*	3	Saponins
Snakeroot	*Rauwolfia serpentina*	1	Antihypertensive reserpine; tranquilizer
Snowberry	*Symphoricarpos* spp	3	
Sorrel; soursob	*Oxalis* spp	2b	Soluble oxalate (see p 248)
Spathiphyllum	*Spathiphyllum*	2a	Calcium oxalate crystals (see text)
Spindle tree	*Euonymus* spp	3	
Split leaf	*Philodendron* spp	2a	Calcium oxalate crystals (see text)
Sprengeri fern	*Asparagus densiflorus*	3	
Squill	*Scilla; Urginea maritima*	1	Cardiac glycosides (see p 128)
Star-of-Bethlehem	*Ornithogalum* spp	1	Cardiac glycosides (see p 128)
St. John's Wort	*Hypericum perforatum*	1	Mild MAO inhibition (see p 225)
String of pearls/beads	*Senecio* spp	1	Hepatotoxic pyrrolizidine alkaloids
Strychnine	*Strychnos nux-vomica*	1	Strychnine (see p 298)
Sweet clover	*Melilotus* spp	1	Coumarin glycosides (see p 148)
Sweet pea	*Lathyrus odoratus*	1	Neuropathy (lathyrism) after chronic use
Swiss cheese plant	*Monstera friedrichsthali*	2a	Calcium oxalate crystals (see text)
Tobacco	*Nicotiana* spp	1	Nicotine (see p 231)
Tomato (leaves)	*Lycopersicon esculentum*	1	Solanine: sympathomimetic; bradycardia
Tonka bean	*Dipteryx odorata*	1	Coumarin glycosides (see p 148)
Toyon (leaves)	*Heteromeles arbutifolia*	1	Cyanogenic glycosides (see p 150)
Tulip (bulb)	*Tulipa*	3	
Tung tree; candle nut	*Aleurites* spp	1, 3	Phytotoxins, saponins
Turbina	*Turbina corymbosa*	1	Hallucinogen
T'u-san-chi	*Gynura segetum*	1	Hepatotoxic pyrrolizidine alkaloids
Umbrella plant	*Cyperus alternifolius*	1	See essential oils (p 122)
Uva-ursi	*Arctostaphylos uvo-ursi*	1, 3	Hydroquinone: berries edible
Valerian	*Valeriana officinalis*	1	Valerine alkaloids: used as mild tranquilizer
Walnut (green shells)	*Juglans*	1	Moldy parts contain convulsant mycotoxins
Water hemlock	*Cicuta maculata*	1	Cicutoxin: seizures; vomiting; diaphoresis, salivation
Wild calla	*Calla palustris*	2a	Calcium oxalate crystals (see text)
Wild onion	*Zigadenus* spp	1	Similar to veratramine: hypotension, bradycardia, lethargy
Windflower	*Anemone*	3	Irritant oil protoanemonin
Wisteria	*Wisteria*	3	Severe gastroenteritis
Woodruff	*Galium odoratum*	1	Coumarin glycosides (see p 148)
Wood rose	*Ipomoea violacea; Merremia tuberosa*	1	Seeds are hallucinogenic
Wormwood	*Artemesia absinthium*	1	Absinthe
Yarrow	*Achillea millefolium*	3	Prepared as a tea
Yellow oleander	*Thevetia peruviana*	1	Cardiac glycosides (see p 128)
Yew	*Taxus*	1	Taxine; similar to cardiac glycosides (see p 128); seizures
Yohimbine	*Corynanthe yohimbe*	1	Purported aphrodisiac; mild hallucinogen; α_2-blocker

II. **Toxic dose.**
  A. **Plants.** The amount of toxin ingested is usually unknown. Concentrations of the toxic agent may vary depending on the plant part, the season, and soil conditions. In general, childhood ingestion of a single leaf or a few petals from even Group 1 plants results in little or no toxicity because of the small amount of toxin absorbed.
  B. **Herbs.** Herbal teas and medications may contain variable amounts of active or poisonous substances. Homeopathic medicines are usually extremely diluted, and toxicity is rare. On the other hand, naturopathic medicines or steeped teas may be highly concentrated. In addition, commercial packaged products ("patent" medicines or nutritional supplements) may contain multiple different herbal and mineral products in various concentrations. Nutritional supplements may contain toxic plants or herbal medicines (see Table II–45). Contamination or adulteration with unlabelled substances may also be present.
III. **Clinical presentation.**
  A. **Group 1.** The presentation depends upon the active toxic agent (Table II–44). In most cases, vomiting, abdominal pain, and diarrhea occur within 60–90 minutes of a significant ingestion. With some toxins (eg, ricin), severe gastroenteritis may result in massive fluid and electrolyte loss.

TABLE II–45. SELECTED DIETARY SUPPLEMENTS AND ALTERNATIVE REMEDIES[a]

Product	Source or Active Ingredient	Common or Purported Use	Clinical Effects & Potential Toxicity
Aconite	*Aconitum* sp.	Chinese traditional medicine	Nausea, vomiting, arrhythmias, shock
Anabolic steroids	Methandrostenolone, oxandrolone, testolactone, many other steroid derivatives	Body building	Virilization; feminization; cholestatic hepatitis; aggressiveness, mania, or psychosis; hypertension; acne; hyperlipidemia; immune suppression
Azarcon (Greta)	Lead salts	Hispanic folk remedy for abdominal pain, colic	Lead poisoning (see p 199)
Bufotoxin	Bufotenine (toad venom); "love stone"; Chan su	Purported aphrodisiac; hallucinogen	Cardiac glycosides (see Digoxin, p 128)
Chromium	Chromium picolinate	Body building; athletic performance enhancement	Gastrointestinal irritation; niacin-like flushing reaction with picolinate salt (see p 317)
Comfrey	*Symphytum officinale*	Anti-inflammatory; gastritis; diarrhea	Hepatic veno-occlusive disaease; possible teratogen/carcinogen. (Note: many other plants also contain hepatotoxic pyrrolizidine alkaloids–*see* Table II–44)
Creatine	Creatine monohydrate; creatine monophosphate	Athletic performance enhancement	Gastrointestinal irritation.
DHEA	Dihydroepiandrosterone	Anticancer; anti-aging	Androgenic effects in females; possible stimulation of prostate cancer
Echinacea	*Echinacea angustifolia; Echinacea pallida; Echinacea purpurea*	Immune stimulation	CNS stimulant; allergic dermatitis; anaphylaxis
Garlic	*Allium sativum*	Hyperlipidemia; hypertension	Rash; gastrointestinal irritation; asthma

(continued)

TABLE II-45. SELECTED DIETARY SUPPLEMENTS AND ALTERNATIVE REMEDIES[a] (CONTINUED)

Product	Source or Active Ingredient	Common or Purported Use	Clinical Effects & Potential Toxicity
Ginko	Extract of *Ginko biloba*	Alzheimer's disease	Gastrointestinal irritation; allergic dermatitis
Ginseng	*Panex ginseng; Panex quinquefolium*	Fatigue/stress; immune stimulation; many ailments	Decreases serum glucose; increases cortisol. *Ginseng abuse syndrome:* nervousness; insomnia; gastrointestinal distress
Glucosamine	Glucosamine chondroitin	Osteoarthritis	Unknown
Goldenseal	*Hydrastis canadensis*	Dyspepsia; postpartum bleeding; drug test adulterant	Nausea; vomiting; diarrhea; paresthesia; seizures; hypo- or hypertension
Guarana	Caffeine	Athletic performance enhancement; appetite suppressant	Tachycardia, tremor; vomiting (See Caffeine, p 118)
Jin bu huan	l-Tetrahydropalmatine	Chinese traditional medicine	Acute CNS depression and bradycardia; chronic hepatitis
Ma Huang	Ephedrine (various *Ephedra* sp.)	Stimulant; athletic performance enhancement; appetite suppressant	Hypertension; tachycardia (see p 259)
Melatonin	Pineal gland	Sleep aid	Sedation; headache; loss of libido
Pennyroyal oil	Pulegone, menthofuran	Abortifacient	Coma, hepatic necrosis
Rattlesnake powder	*Polvo de vibora; carne de viboro; viboro de cascabel*	Hispanic traditional remedy	*Salmonella* sepsis
Saw Palmetto	Extract of Saw Palmetto berry	Prostatic hypertrophy	Unknown
Senna	*Cassia angustifolia; Cassia acutifolia*	Weight loss; laxative	Watery diarrhea; abdominal cramps; dehydration
Spirulina	Some blue-green algae	Body building	Niacinlike flushing reaction (see p 317)
St. John's Wort	*Hypericum perforatum*	Antidepressant	MAO inhibition (see p 225); photosensitivity
Tea tree oil	*Melaleuca alternifolia*	Topical antifungal; vaginitis; acne	Sedation; ataxia; contact dermatitis
Valerian root	*Valeriana officinalis; Valeriana edulis*	Sleep aid	Sedation; vomiting
Vanadium	Vanadyl sulfate; ammonium vanadyl tartrate	Body building	Intestinal cramps, diarrhea; black stools
Yohimbine	*Corynanthe yohimbe*	Stimulant; purported aphrodisiac	Hallucinations; MAO inhibition; hypertension; irritability; gastrointestinal irritation
Zinc	Zinc gluconate lozenges	Flu/cold symptoms	Nausea; mouth/throat irritation

[a]Most of these products are legally considered neither food nor drugs and, therefore, are not regulated by the FDA (Dietary Supplement Health and Education Act, 1994). Toxicity may be related to the active ingredient(s) or to impurities, contaminants, or adulterants in the product. See also Caffeine (p 118), Essential Oils (p 122), Salicylates (p 284), and Vitamins (p 317). *This table was compiled by Christine A Haller, MD.*

B. **Group 2a.** Insoluble calcium oxalate crystals cause immediate burning, prickly pain upon contact with mucous membranes. Swelling of the lips, tongue, and pharynx may occur, and in rare cases glottic edema may result in airway obstruction. Symptoms usually resolve within a few hours.

C. **Group 2b.** Soluble oxalates may be absorbed into the circulation, where they precipitate with calcium, resulting in acute hypocalcemia and multiple-organ injury, including renal tubular necrosis.

D. **Group 3.** Skin or mucous membrane irritation may occur, although it is less severe than with Group 2 plants. Vomiting and diarrhea are common but are usually mild and self-limited. Fluid and electrolyte imbalances caused by severe gastroenteritis are rare.

IV. **Diagnosis** is usually based on a history of exposure and is suspected when plant material is seen in vomitus. Identification of the plant is essential to proper treatment. Because common names sometimes refer to more than one plant, it is preferable to confirm the botanical name. If in doubt about the plant identification, take the specimen to a local nursery, florist, or college botany department.

A. **Specific levels.** Serum toxin levels are not available for most plant toxins. In selected cases, laboratory analyses for therapeutic drugs may be used (eg, digoxin assay for oleander glycosides).

B. **Other useful laboratory studies** include, for patients with gastroenteritis, CBC, electrolytes, glucose, BUN, creatinine, and urinalysis. If hepatotoxicity is suspected, also obtain liver transaminases and prothrombin time (PT).

V. **Treatment.** Most ingestions cause no symptoms or only mild gastroenteritis, and patients recover quickly with supportive care.

A. **Emergency and supportive measures**
 1. Maintain an open airway and assist ventilation if necessary (see pp 1–7). Administer supplemental oxygen.
 2. Treat coma (p 18), seizures (p 21), arrhythmias (pp 10–14), and hypotension (p 15) if they occur.
 3. Replace fluid losses caused by gastroenteritis with intravenous crystalloid solutions.

B. **Specific drugs and antidotes.** There are few effective antidotes. See the "Remarks" column in Table II–44 for specific information or referral to additional discussion elsewhere in Section II.

C. **Decontamination** (see p 43)
 1. **Group 1 and Group 2b plants**
  a. **Prehospital.** Administer activated charcoal if available. Ipecac-induced vomiting may be useful for initial treatment at the scene (eg, children at home) if it can be given within a few minutes of exposure.
  b. **Hospital.** Administer activated charcoal. Gastric emptying is not necessary if activated charcoal can be given promptly.
 2. **Group 2a and Group 3 plants**
  a. Wash the affected areas with plain water and give water or milk to drink.
  b. Do **not** induce vomiting, because of potential aggravation of irritant effects. Gastric lavage and activated charcoal are not necessary.

D. **Enhanced elimination.** These procedures are not generally effective.

▶ **POLYCHLORINATED BIPHENYLS (PCBs)**

Diane Liu, MD, MPH

Polychlorinated biphenyls (PCBs) are a group of chlorinated hydrocarbon compounds that were once widely used as high-temperature insulators for transformers and other electrical equipment and were also found in carbonless copy papers and some inks and paints. Since 1974, all uses in the United States are confined to closed systems. Most PCB poisonings are chronic occupational exposures, with delayed-onset symptoms being the first indication that an exposure has occurred. In 1977, the U.S. Environmental Protection Agency (EPA) banned further manufacturing of PCBs because they are suspected carcinogens and are highly persistent.

I. **Mechanism of toxicity.** PCBs are irritating to mucous membranes. When burned, PCBs may produce the more highly toxic polychlorinated dibenzodioxins (PCDDs) and polychlorinated dibenzofurans (PCDFs; see p 156). It is difficult to establish the specific effects of PCB intoxication because PCBs are nearly always contaminated with small amounts of these compounds. PCBs, and particularly the PCDD and PCDF contaminants, are mutagenic and teratogenic and are considered potential human carcinogens.

II. **Toxic dose.** PCBs are well absorbed by all routes (skin, inhalation, and ingestion) and are widely distributed in fat; bioaccumulation occurs even with low-level exposure.

   A. **Inhalation.** PCBs are mildly irritating to the skin at airborne levels of 0.1 mg/m^3 and very irritating at 10 mg/m^3. The recommended workplace limits (ACGIH TLV-TWA) are 0.5 mg/m^3 (for PCBs with 54% chlorine) and 1 mg/m^3 (for PCBs with 42% chlorine) as 8-hour time-weighted averages. The air level considered immediately dangerous to life or health (IDLH) for either type is 5 mg/m^3.

   B. **Ingestion.** Acute toxicity after ingestion is unlikely; the oral LD_{50} is 1–10 g/kg.

III. **Clinical presentation.**

   A. **Acute PCB exposure** may cause skin, eye, nose, and throat irritation.

   B. **Chronic exposure** may cause **chloracne** (cystic acneiform lesions predominantly found on the posterior neck, axillas, and upper back); the onset is usually 6 weeks or longer after exposure. Skin pigmentation and porphyria may occur. Elevation of hepatic transaminases may occur.

IV. **Diagnosis** is usually based on a history of exposure and the presence of chloracne or elevated hepatic transaminases.

   A. **Specific levels.** PCB serum and fat levels are poorly correlated with health effects. Serum PCB concentrations are usually less than 20 μg/L; higher levels may indicate exposure but not necessarily toxicity.

   B. **Other useful laboratory studies** include BUN, creatinine, and liver enzymes.

V. **Treatment.**

   A. **Emergency and supportive measures**

      1. Treat bronchospasm (see p 8) if it occurs.

      2. Monitor for elevated hepatic enzymes; chloracne; and nonspecific eye, gastrointestinal, and neurologic symptoms.

   B. **Specific drugs and antidotes.** There is no specific antidote.

   C. **Decontamination** (see p 43)

      1. **Inhalation.** Remove the victim from exposure and give supplemental oxygen if available.

      2. **Skin and eyes.** Remove contaminated clothing and wash exposed skin with soap and water. Irrigate exposed eyes with copious tepid water or saline.

      3. **Ingestion** (see p 45)

         a. **Prehospital.** Administer activated charcoal if available. Ipecac-induced vomiting may be useful for initial treatment if it can be given within a few minutes of exposure.

         b. **Hospital.** Administer activated charcoal. Gastric emptying is not necessary if activated charcoal can be given promptly.

   D. **Enhanced elimination.** There is no role for dialysis, hemoperfusion, or repeat-dose charcoal. Lipid-clearing drugs (eg, clofibrate and resins) have been suggested, but insufficient data exist to recommend them.

▶ PYRETHRINS AND PYRETHROIDS

Brent R. Ekins, PharmD

Pyrethrins are naturally occurring insecticides derived from the chrysanthemum plant. Pyrethroids (Table II–46) are synthetically derived compounds. Acute human poisoning from exposure to these insecticides is rare; however, they can cause skin and upper-airway irritation and hypersensitivity reactions. Piperonyl butoxide is added to these compounds to prolong their activity by inhibiting mixed oxidase enzymes in the liver that metabolize the pyrethrins. Common pyrethrin-containing pediculides include A-200, Triple-X, and RID.

I. **Mechanism of toxicity.** In insects, pyrethrins and pyrethroids rapidly cause death by paralyzing the nervous system through disruption of the membrane ion transport system in nerve axons, and pyrethroids prolong sodium influx and also may block inhibitory pathways. Mammals are generally able to metabolize these compounds rapidly and thereby render them harmless.

II. **Toxic dose.** The toxic oral dose in mammals is greater than 100–1000 mg/kg, and the potentially lethal acute oral dose is 10–100 g. Pyrethrins are not well absorbed across the skin or from the gastrointestinal tract. They have been used for many years as oral anthelmintic agents with minimum adverse effects other than mild gastrointestinal upset.

    A. **Deltamethrin.** There is one report of seizures in a young woman who ingested 30 mL of 2.5% deltamethrin (750 mg). **Chinese chalk** (sold under a variety of names, including Miraculous Insecticide Chalk and Cockroach Wipeout Chalk) contains up to 37.6 mg of deltamethrin per stick of chalk. Ingestion of a single chalk is generally considered nontoxic.

    B. A 45-year-old man died after ingesting beans cooked in 10% **cypermethrin.**

III. **Clinical presentation.** Toxicity to humans is primarily associated with hypersensitivity reactions and direct irritant effects rather than any pharmacologic property.

    A. **Anaphylactic** reactions including bronchospasm, oropharyngeal edema, and shock may occur in hypersensitive individuals.

    B. **Inhalation** of these compounds may precipitate wheezing in asthmatics. Inhalation or pulmonary aspiration may also cause a hypersensitivity pneumonitis.

    C. **Skin** exposure may cause burning, tingling, numbness, and erythema.

    D. **Eyes.** Accidental eye exposure during scalp application of A-200 Pyrinate has caused corneal injury including keratitis and denudation. The cause is uncertain, but may be related to the surfactant (Triton-X) contained in the product.

    E. **Ingestion.** With large ingestions (200–500 mL of concentrated solution), the central nervous system (CNS) may be affected, resulting in seizures, coma, or respiratory arrest.

IV. **Diagnosis** is based on a history of exposure. There are no characteristic clinical symptoms or laboratory tests that are specific for identifying these compounds.

    A. **Specific levels.** These compounds are rapidly metabolized in the body, and methods for determining the parent compound are not routinely available.

    B. **Other useful laboratory studies** include electrolytes, glucose, and arterial blood gases or oximetry.

TABLE II–46. PYRETHROIDS

Allethrin	Cypermethrin	Furamethrin
Barthrin	Decamethrin	Permethrin
Bioallethrin	Deltamethrin	Phthalthrin
Bioresmethrin	Dimethrin	Resmethrin
Cismethrin	Fenothrin	Supermethrin
Cymethrin	Fenvalerate	Tetramethrin

V. Treatment.
A. Emergency and supportive measures
1. Treat bronchospasm (see p 8) or anaphylaxis (see p 26) if they occur.
2. Observe patients with a history of large ingestions for at least 4–6 hours for any signs of CNS depression or seizures.
B. Specific drugs and antidotes. There is no specific antidote.
C. Decontamination (see p 43)
1. **Inhalation.** Remove victims from exposure and give supplemental oxygen if needed.
2. **Skin.** Wash with copious soap and water. Topical application of vitamin E in vegetable oil was reported anecdotally to relieve paresthesias.
3. **Eyes.** Irrigate with copious water. After irrigation, perform a fluorescein examination and refer the victim to an ophthalmologist if there is evidence of corneal injury.
4. **Ingestion** (see p 45). In the majority of cases, a subtoxic dose has been ingested and no decontamination is necessary. However, after a large ingestion of Chinese chalk or a concentrated solution:
   a. **Prehospital.** Administer activated charcoal if available. Do *not* induce vomiting, because of the risk of lethargy and seizures.
   b. **Hospital.** Administer activated charcoal. Gastric lavage is not necessary if activated charcoal can be given promptly.
D. Enhanced elimination. These compounds are rapidly metabolized by the body, and extracorporeal methods of elimination would not be expected to enhance their elimination.

▶ QUINIDINE AND OTHER TYPE Ia ANTIARRHYTHMIC DRUGS

Neal L. Benowitz, MD

Quinidine, procainamide (Pronestyl), and disopyramide (Norpace) are type Ia antiarrhythmic agents. Quinidine and procainamide are commonly used for suppression of acute and chronic supraventricular and ventricular arrhythmias. Disopyramide is used for ventricular arrhythmias. All three agents have a low toxic:therapeutic ratio and may produce fatal intoxication (Table II–47). See description of other antiarrhythmic agents, p 72.

I. Mechanism of toxicity.
A. Type Ia agents depress the fast sodium-dependent channel, slowing phase zero of the cardiac action potential. At high concentrations, this results in reduced myocardial contractility and excitability, and severe depression of cardiac conduction velocity. Repolarization is also delayed, resulting in a pro-

TABLE II–47. TYPE Ia ANTIARRHYTHMIC DRUGS

Drug	Serum High-Life (h)	Usual Adult Daily Dose (mg)	Therapeutic Serum Levels (mg/L)	Major Toxicity[a]
Quinidine	6–8	1000–2000	2–4	S, B, V, H
Disopyramide	4–10	400–800	2–4	B, V, H
Procainamide	4	1000–4000	4–10	B, V, H
NAPA[b]	5–7	N/A	15–25	H

[a]S = seizures; B = bradycardia; V = ventricular tachycardia; H = hypotension.
[b]NAPA = N-acetylprocainamide, an active metabolite of procainamide.

longed QT interval that may be associated with polymorphic ventricular tachy-cardia (torsades de pointes; see Figure I–7, p 14).

B. Quinidine and disopyramide also have anticholinergic activity; quinidine has alpha-adrenergic receptor-blocking activity, and procainamide has ganglionic- and neuromuscular-blocking activity.

C. Pharmacokinetics. See Table II–55, p 319.

II. Toxic dose. Acute adult ingestion of 1 g of quinidine, 5 g of procainamide, or 1 g of disopyramide, and any ingestion in children, should be considered potentially lethal.

III. Clinical presentation. The primary manifestations of toxicity involve the cardio-vascular and central nervous systems.

A. Cardiotoxic effects of the type Ia agents include sinus bradycardia; sinus node arrest or asystole; PR, QRS, or QT interval prolongation; sinus tachy-cardia (caused by anticholinergic effects); polymorphous ventricular tachycar-dia (torsades des pointes); and depressed myocardial contractility, which, along with alpha-adrenergic or ganglionic blockade, may result in hypotension and occasionally pulmonary edema.

B. Central nervous system toxicity. Quinidine and disopyramide can cause anticholinergic effects such as dry mouth, dilated pupils, and delirium. All type Ia agents can produce seizures, coma, and respiratory arrest.

C. Other effects. Quinidine commonly causes nausea, vomiting, and diarrhea after acute ingestion and, especially with chronic doses, cinchonism (tinnitus, vertigo, deafness, or visual disturbances). Procainamide may cause gastroin-testinal upset and, with chronic therapy, a lupuslike syndrome.

IV. Diagnosis is based on a history of exposure and typical cardiotoxic features such as QRS and QT interval prolongation, AV block, or polymorphous ventricu-lar tachycardia.

A. Specific levels. Rapid serum levels are generally available for each agent. Serious toxicity with these drugs usually occurs only with levels above the therapeutic range; however, some complications, such as QT prolongation and polymorphous ventricular tachycardia, may occur at therapeutic levels.

1. Methods for detecting quinidine may vary in specificity, with some also measuring metabolites and contaminants.

2. Procainamide has an active metabolite, N-acetylprocainamide (NAPA); with therapeutic procainamide dosing, NAPA levels can range up to 15 mg/L.

B. Other useful laboratory studies include electrolytes, glucose, BUN, creati-nine, arterial blood gases or oximetry, and ECG monitoring.

V. Treatment.

A. Emergency and supportive measures

1. Maintain an open airway and assist ventilation if necessary (see pp 1–7).

2. Treat hypotension (p 15), arrhythmias (pp 10–14), coma (p 18), and seizures (p 21) if they occur.

3. Treat recurrent ventricular tachycardia with lidocaine, phenytoin, or over-drive pacing (p 14). Do *not* use other type Ia or Ic agents, because they may worsen cardiac toxicity.

4. Continuously monitor vital signs and ECG for a minimum of 6 hours, and admit symptomatic patients until the ECG returns to normal.

B. Specific drugs and antidotes. Treat cardiotoxic effects such as wide QRS intervals or hypotension with **sodium bicarbonate** (see p 345), 1–2 meq/kg rapid IV bolus, repeated every 5–10 minutes and as needed. Markedly impaired conduction or high-degree atrioventricular (AV) block un-responsive to bicarbonate therapy is an indication for insertion of a cardiac pacemaker.

C. Decontamination (see p 43)

1. Prehospital. Administer activated charcoal if available. Do *not* induce vomiting because of the risk of abrupt onset of seizures and coma.

2. Hospital. Administer activated charcoal. Consider gastric lavage for large ingestions.

D. Enhanced elimination (see p 51)

1. **Quinidine** has a very large volume of distribution, and therefore it is not effectively removed by dialysis. Acidification of the urine may enhance excretion, but this is not recommended because it may aggravate cardiac toxicity.

2. **Disopyramide, procainamide,** and **N-acetylprocainamide (NAPA)** have smaller volumes of distribution and are effectively removed by hemoperfusion or dialysis.

3. The efficacy of repeat-dose activated charcoal has not been studied for the type Ia agents.

► **QUININE**

Neal L. Benowitz, MD

Quinine is an optical isomer of quinidine. Quinine was once widely used for treatment of malaria and is still occasionally used for chloroquine-resistant cases, but it is now prescribed primarily for the treatment of nocturnal muscle cramps. Quinine is found in tonic water and has been used to cut street heroin. It has also been used as an abortifacient.

I. **Mechanism of toxicity.** The mechanism of quinine toxicity is believed to be similar to that of quinidine (see p 277); however, quinine is a much less potent cardiotoxin. Quinine also has toxic effects on the retina that can result in blindness. At one time, vasoconstriction of retinal arterioles resulting in retinal ischemia was thought to be the cause of blindness; however, recent evidence indicates a direct toxic effect on photoreceptor and ganglion cells.

II. **Toxic dose.** Quinine sulfate is available in capsules and tablets containing 130–325 mg. The minimum toxic dose is approximately 3–4 g in adults; 1 g has been fatal in a child.

III. **Clinical presentation.** Toxic effects involve the cardiovascular and central nervous systems, the eyes, and other organ systems.

A. **Mild intoxication** produces nausea, vomiting, and cinchonism (tinnitus, deafness, vertigo, headache, and visual disturbances).

B. **Severe intoxication** may cause ataxia, obtundation, convulsions, coma, and respiratory arrest. With massive intoxication, quinidinelike cardiotoxicity (hypotension, QRS and QT interval prolongation, AV block, and ventricular arrhythmias) may be fatal.

C. **Retinal toxicity** occurs 9–10 hours after ingestion and includes blurred vision, impaired color perception, constriction of visual fields, and blindness. The pupils are often fixed and dilated. Funduscopy may reveal retinal artery spasm, disk pallor, and macular edema. Although gradual recovery occurs, many patients are left with permanent visual impairment.

D. **Other toxic effects** of quinine include hypokalemia, hypoglycemia, hemolysis (in patients with glucose-6-phosphate dehydrogenase [G6PD] deficiency), and congenital malformations when used in pregnancy.

IV. **Diagnosis** is based on a history of ingestion and the presence of cinchonism and visual disturbances. Quinidinelike cardiotoxic effects may or may not be present.

A. **Specific levels.** Serum quinine levels can be measured by the same assay as for quinidine, as long as quinidine is not present. Plasma quinine levels above 10 mg/L have been associated with visual impairment; 87% of patients with levels above 20 mg/L reported blindness. Levels above 16 mg/L have been associated with cardiac toxicity.

B. **Other useful laboratory studies** include CBC, electrolytes, glucose, BUN, creatinine, arterial blood gases or oximetry, and ECG monitoring.

V. **Treatment.**

A. **Emergency and supportive measures**

1. Maintain an open airway and assist ventilation if necessary (see pp 1–7).

2. Treat coma (p 18), seizures (p 21), hypotension (p 15), and arrhythmias (pp 10–14) if they occur.
3. Avoid types Ia and Ic antiarrhythmic drugs; they may worsen cardiotoxicity.
4. Continuously monitor vital signs and the ECG for at least 6 hours after ingestion, and admit symptomatic patients to an intensive care unit.

B. Specific drugs and antidotes
1. Treat cardiotoxicity with **sodium bicarbonate** (see p 345), 1–2 meq/kg rapid IV bolus.
2. Stellate ganglion block has previously been recommended for quinine-induced blindness, the rationale being to increase retinal blood flow. However, recent evidence indicates that this treatment is not effective, and the procedure may have serious complications.

C. Decontamination (see p 43)
1. **Prehospital.** Administer activated charcoal if available. Do **not** induce vomiting because of the risk of abrupt onset of seizures or coma.
2. **Hospital.** Administer activated charcoal. Consider gastric lavage for large ingestions.

D. Enhanced elimination. Because of extensive tissue distribution (volume of distribution is 3 L/kg), dialysis and hemoperfusion procedures are ineffective. Acidification of the urine may slightly increase renal excretion but does not significantly alter the overall elimination rate and may aggravate cardiotoxicity.

▶ RADIATION (IONIZING)

Evan T. Wythe, MD

Radiation poisoning is a rare but potentially challenging complication of the nuclear age. Dependence on nuclear energy, and the expanded use of radioactive isotopes in industry and medicine, increase the possibility of accidental exposures. Ionizing radiation may be generated from a variety of sources. **Particle-emitting** sources may produce beta and alpha particles and neutrons. Ionizing **electromagnetic** radiation includes gamma rays and x-rays. In contrast, magnetic fields, microwaves, radio waves, and ultrasound are examples of *nonionizing* electromagnetic radiation.

Management of a radiation accident depends on whether the victim has been contaminated or only irradiated. **Irradiated** victims pose no threat to health care providers and may be managed with no special precautions. On the other hand, **contaminated** victims must be decontaminated to prevent spread of radioactive materials to others and the environment.

I. Mechanism of toxicity.
A. Radiation impairs biologic function by ionizing atoms and breaking chemical bonds, leading to the formation of highly reactive free radicals that can damage cell walls, organelles, and DNA. Affected cells are either killed or inhibited in division. Cells with a high turnover rate (eg, bone marrow, epithelial coverings such as skin, gastrointestinal tract, and pulmonary system) are more sensitive to radiation. Lymphocytes are particularly sensitive.
B. Radiation also causes a poorly understood inflammatory response and microvascular effects after moderately high doses (eg, 600 rads).
C. Radiation effects may be deterministic or stochastic. Deterministic effects are associated with a threshold dose and usually occur within an acute time frame (within a year). Stochastic effects have no known threshold and may occur after a latency period of years (eg, cancer).

II. Toxic dose. Various terms are used to describe radiation exposure and dose: **R** (roentgen) is a measure of exposure, whereas **rad** (radiation absorbed dose) and **rem** (radiation equivalent, man) are measures of dose. Rad is the unit of radiation dose commonly referred to in exposures, whereas rem is useful in describing dose-equivalent biologic damage. For most exposures, these units can be considered interchangeable. The exception is alpha particle exposure (eg, plutonium), which causes greater double-stranded DNA damage and a higher rem compared with rad.

A. Toxicity thresholds

1. **Acute effects.** Exposure to more than 75 rad causes nausea and vomiting. Exposure to more than 400 rad is potentially lethal without medical intervention. Vomiting within 1–5 hours of exposure suggests an exposure of at least 600 rad. Brief exposure to 5000 rad or more usually causes death within minutes to hours.

2. **Carcinogenesis.** Radiation protection organizations have not agreed on a threshold dose for stochastic effects such as cancer.

B. Recommended exposure limits

1. **Exposure to the general population.** The National Council on Radiation Protection (NCRP) recommends a maximum of 0.5 rem per person per year. The background radiation level at sea level is about 35 millirem (0.035 rem) per year.

2. **Occupational exposure to x-rays.** The federal government has set standards for such exposures: 5 rem/year to the total body, gonads, or blood-forming organs; 75 rem/year to the hands or feet. A single chest x-ray results in a radiation exposure of about 15 millirem (mrem) to the patient, and about 0.006 mrem to nearby health care personnel (at a distance of 160 cm). A head CT scan gives about 1 rad to the head; an abdominal CT scan may give as much as 2–5 rad to the area of concern.

3. **Radiation during pregnancy.** Established guidelines vary but generally recommend a maximum exposure of no more than 50 mrem per month (NCRP). Exposure to the ovaries and fetus from a routine abdominal (KUB) film may be as high as 146 mrem; from a chest x-ray, the dose is about 15 mrem.

4. **Exposure guidelines for emergency health care personnel.** To save a life, the NCRP-recommended maximum exposure for a rescuer is 50 rem whole body exposure.

III. Clinical presentation.

A. Acute radiation syndrome (ARS) consists of a constellation of symptoms and signs indicative of systemic radiation injury. It is often described in four stages (prodrome, latency, manifest illness, and recovery). The onset and severity of each stage of radiation poisoning are determined largely by the dose.

1. The *prodromal* stage, from 0–48 hours, may include nausea, vomiting, abdominal cramps, and diarrhea. Severe exposures are associated with diaphoresis, disorientation, fever, ataxia, coma, shock, and death.

2. During the *latent* stage, there may be an improvement in symptoms. The duration of this stage is usually hours to days, but may be shorter or absent with massive exposures.

3. The *manifest illness* stage, from 1–60 days, is characterized by multiple organ system involvement, particularly bone marrow suppression, which may lead to sepsis and death.

4. The *recovery* phase may be accompanied by hair loss, disfiguring burns, and scars.

B. Gastrointestinal system. Exposure to 100 R or more usually produces nausea, vomiting, abdominal cramps, and diarrhea within a few hours. After exposure to 600 rad or more, loss of integrity of the GI mucosal layer results in denudation and severe necrotic gastroenteritis, which may lead to marked dehydration, gastrointestinal bleeding, and death within a few days. Doses of 1500 rad are thought to completely destroy gastrointestinal stem cells.

C. Central nervous system. With acute exposures of several thousand rads, confusion and stupor may occur, followed within minutes to hours by ataxia, convulsions, coma, and death. In animal models of massive exposure, a phenomenon known as "early transient incapacitation" occurs.

D. **Bone marrow depression** may be subclinical but apparent on a CBC after exposure to as little as 25 rad. Immunocompromise usually follows exposure to more than 100 rad.

1. Early neutropenia is caused by margination; the true nadir occurs at about 30 days or as soon as 14 days after severe exposure. Neutropenia is the most significant factor in septicemia.

2. Thrombocytopenia is usually not evident for 2 weeks or more after exposure.

3. The lymphocyte count is of great prognostic importance and usually reaches a nadir within 48 hours of serious exposure; a count of less than 300–500 lymphocytes/mm^3 during this period indicates a poor prognosis, while 1200/mm^3 or more suggests likely survival.

E. **Other complications** of high-dose acute radiation syndrome include multisystem organ failure, veno-occlusive disease of the liver, interstitial pneumonitis, renal failure, tissue fibrosis, skin burns, and hair loss.

IV. **Diagnosis** depends on the history of exposure. The potential for contamination should be assessed by determining the type of radionuclide involved and the potential route(s) of exposure.

A. **Specific levels**

1. **Detection.** Depending on the circumstances, the presence of radionuclides may be verified by one or more of the following devices: survey meters with either pancake or alpha probes; whole body counts; chest counts; or nuclear medicine cameras.

2. **Biologic specimens.** Nasopharyngeal and wound swabs, sputum, vomitus, skin wipes, wound bandages, and clothing articles (particularly shoes) may be collected for radionuclide analysis and counts. Collection of urine and feces for 24–72 hours may assist in estimation of an internal dose. Serum levels of radioactive materials are not generally available or clinically useful.

3. **Other methods.** Chromosomal changes in lymphocytes are the most sensitive indication of exposures to as little as 10 rad; DNA fragments, dicentric rings, and deletions may be present. Exposure to 15 rad may cause oligospermia first seen about 45 days after the exposure.

B. **Other useful laboratory studies** include CBC (repeat every 6 hours), electrolytes, glucose, BUN, creatinine, and urinalysis. Immediately draw lymphocytes for human leukocyte antigen (HLA) typing in case bone marrow transplant is required later.

V. **Treatment.** For expert assistance in evaluation and treatment of victims and in on-scene management, immediately contact the **Radiation Emergency Assistance Center & Training Site (REAC/TS): telephone (615) 576-3131 or (615) 481-1000.** REAC/TS is operated for the U.S. Department of Energy (DOE) by the Oak Ridge Associated Universities, and assistance is available 24 hours a day. Also contact the local state agency responsible for radiation safety.

A. **Emergency and supportive measures.** Depending on the risk to rescuers, treatment of serious medical problems takes precedence over radiologic concerns. If there is a potential for contamination of rescuers and equipment, appropriate radiation response protocols should be implemented, and rescuers should wear protective clothing and respirators. *Note:* If the exposure was to electromagnetic radiation only, the victim is not contaminating and does not pose a risk to downstream personnel.

1. Maintain an open airway and assist ventilation if necessary (see pp 1–7).

2. Treat coma (p 18) and seizures (p 21) if they occur.

3. Replace fluid losses from gastroenteritis with intravenous crystalloid solutions (see p 15).

4. Treat leukopenia and resulting infections as needed. Immunosuppressed patients require reverse isolation and appropriate broad-spectrum antibiotic therapy. Bone marrow stimulants may help selected patients.

B. **Specific drugs and antidotes.** Chelating agents or pharmacologic blocking drugs may be useful in some cases of ingestion or inhalation of certain biologically active radioactive materials, if they are given before or shortly after exposure (Table II–48). Contact REAC/TS (see above) for specific advice on use of these agents.

C. **Decontamination** (p 43)
  1. **Exposure to particle-emitting solids or liquids.** *The victim is potentially highly contaminating to rescuers, transport vehicles, and attending health personnel.*
      a. Remove victims from exposure, and if their conditions permit, remove all contaminated clothing and wash the victims with soap and water.
      b. All clothing and cleansing water must be saved, evaluated for radioactivity, and properly disposed of.
      c. Rescuers should wear protective clothing and respiratory gear to avoid contamination. At the hospital, measures must be taken to prevent contamination of facilities and personnel (see Section IV, pp 415 and 416).
      d. Induce vomiting or perform gastric lavage (see p 45) if radioactive material has been ingested. Administer activated charcoal (see p 48), although its effectiveness is unknown. Certain other adsorbent materials may also be effective (see Table II–48).
      e. Contact REAC/TS (see above) and the state radiologic health department for further advice. In some exposures, unusually aggressive steps may be needed (eg, lung lavage for significant inhalation of plutonium).
  2. **Electromagnetic radiation exposure.** *The patient is not radioactive and does not pose a contamination threat.* There is no need for decontamination once the patient has been removed from the source of exposure, unless electromagnetic radiation emitter fragments are embedded in body tissues.

TABLE II–48. CHELATING AND BLOCKING AGENTS FOR SOME RADIATION EXPOSURES[a]

Radionuclide	Chelating or Blocking Agents
Cesium-137	Prussian blue (ferric hexacyanoferrate) adsorbs cesium in the GI tract, and may also enhance elimination. Dose: 500 mg PO 6 times daily in 100–200 mL of water.
Iodine-131	Potassium iodide dilutes radioactive iodine and blocks thyroid iodine uptake. Dose: 300 mg PO immediately, then 130 mg PO daily. Perchlorate, 200 mg PO, then 100 mg every 5 h, has also been recommended.
Plutonium-239	DTPA (diethylenetriamine pentaacetic acid): chelator. Dose: 1 g in 250 mL D5W IV over 30–60 min daily. Wounds: Irrigate with 1 g DTPA in 250 mL water. EDTA (see p 363) may also be effective if DTPA is not immediately available. Aluminum-containing antacids may bind plutonium in GI tract.
Strontium-90	Alginate or aluminum hydroxide-containing antacids may reduce intestinal absorption of strontium. Dose: 10 g, then 1 g 4 times daily. Barium sulfate may also reduce Sr absorption. Dose: 100 g in 250 mL water PO. Calcium gluconate may dilute the effect of strontium. Dose: 2 g in 500 mL PO or IV. Ammonium chloride is a demineralizing agent. Dose: 3 g PO 3 times daily.
Tritium	Forced fluids, diuretics, (?) hemodialysis. Water dilutes tritium, enhances urinary excretion.
Uranium-233, -235, -238	Sodium bicarbonate forms a carbonate complex with uranyl ion, which is then eliminated in the urine. Dose: 100 mEq in 500 mL D5W by slow constant IV infusion. Aluminum-containing antacids may help prevent uranium absorption.

[a]References: Bhattacharyya ANL et al: Methods of treatment. Pages 27–36 in: *Radiation Protection Dosimetry.* Gerber GB, Thomas RG (editors). Vol. 41, No. 1 (1992); and Ricks RC; *Hospital Emergency Department Management of Radiation Accidents.* Oak Ridge Associated Universities, 1984.

D. Enhanced elimination. Chelating agents and forced diuresis may be useful for certain exposures (Table II–48).

▶ SALICYLATES

Susan Kim, PharmD

Salicylates are widely used for their analgesic and anti-inflammatory properties. They are found in a variety of prescription and over-the-counter analgesics, cold preparations, and topical keratolytic products (methyl salicylate), and even Pepto-Bismol (bismuth subsalicylate). Before the introduction of child-resistant containers, aspirin overdose was one of the leading causes of accidental death in children. Two distinct syndromes of intoxication may occur, depending on whether the exposure is **acute** or **chronic**.

I. **Mechanism of toxicity.** Salicylates have a variety of toxic effects.
   A. Central stimulation of the respiratory center results in hyperventilation, leading to respiratory alkalosis. Secondary effects from hyperventilation include dehydration and compensatory metabolic acidosis.
   B. Intracellular effects include uncoupling of oxidative phosphorylation and interruption of glucose and fatty acid metabolism, which contribute to metabolic acidosis.
   C. The mechanism by which cerebral and pulmonary edema occurs is not known but may be related to an alteration in capillary integrity.
   D. Salicylates alter platelet function and may also prolong the prothrombin time.
   E. **Pharmacokinetics.** Acetylsalicylic acid is well absorbed from the stomach and small intestine. Large tablet masses and enteric coated products may dramatically delay absorption (hours to days). The volume of distribution of salicylate is about 0.1–0.3 L/kg, but this can be increased by acidemia, which enhances movement of the drug into cells. Elimination is mostly by hepatic metabolism at therapeutic doses, but renal excretion becomes important with overdose. The elimination half-life is normally 2–4.5 hours but as long as 18–36 hours after overdose. Renal elimination is dependent on urine pH. See also Table II–55 (p 320).

II. **Toxic dose.** The average therapeutic single dose is 10 mg/kg, and the usual daily therapeutic dose is 40–60 mg/kg/d. Each tablet of aspirin contains 325–650 mg of acetylsalicylic acid. One teaspoon of concentrated **oil of wintergreen** contains 5 g of methyl salicylate, equivalent to about 7.5 g of aspirin.
   A. **Acute ingestion** of 150–200 mg/kg will produce mild intoxication; severe intoxication is likely after acute ingestion of 300–500 mg/kg.
   B. **Chronic intoxication** may occur with ingestion of more than 100 mg/kg/d for 2 or more days.

III. **Clinical presentation.** Patients may become intoxicated after an acute accidental or suicidal overdose or as a result of chronic repeated overmedication for several days.
   A. **Acute ingestion.** Vomiting occurs shortly after ingestion, followed by hyperpnea, tinnitus, and lethargy. Mixed respiratory alkalemia and metabolic acidosis are apparent when arterial blood gases are determined. With severe intoxication, coma, seizures, hypoglycemia, hyperthermia, and pulmonary edema may occur. Death is caused by central nervous system failure and cardiovascular collapse.
   B. **Chronic intoxication.** Victims are usually young children or confused elderly. The diagnosis is often overlooked because the presentation is nonspecific; confusion, dehydration, and metabolic acidosis are often attributed to sepsis, pneumonia, or gastroenteritis. However, morbidity and mortality rates are much higher than after acute overdose. Cerebral and pulmonary edema are more common than with acute intoxication, and severe poisoning occurs at lower salicylate levels.

IV. Diagnosis is not difficult if there is a history of acute ingestion, accompanied by typical signs and symptoms. In the absence of a history of overdose, diagnosis is suggested by the characteristic arterial blood gases, which reveal a mixed respiratory alkalemia and metabolic acidosis.

    A. Specific levels. Obtain stat and serial serum salicylate concentrations. Systemic acidemia increases brain salicylate concentrations, worsening toxicity.

        1. Acute ingestion. Serum levels greater than 900–1000 mg/L (90–100 mg/dL) are usually associated with severe toxicity. Single determinations are **not** sufficient because of the possibility of prolonged or delayed absorption from sustained-release tablets or a tablet mass or bezoar (especially after massive ingestion). Most toxicologists no longer use the Done Nomogram to estimate toxicity.

        2. Chronic intoxication. Symptoms correlate poorly with serum levels, and the Done Nomogram cannot be used to predict toxicity. Chronic therapeutic concentrations in arthritis patients range from 100 to 300 mg/L (10–30 mg/dL). A level greater than 600 mg/L (60 mg/dL) accompanied by acidosis and altered mental status is considered very serious.

    B. Other useful laboratory studies include electrolytes (anion gap calculation), glucose, BUN, creatinine, prothrombin time (PT), arterial blood gases, and chest x-ray.

V. Treatment.

    A. Emergency and supportive measures

        1. Maintain an open airway and assist ventilation if necessary (see pp 1–7). **Warning:** ensure adequate ventilation to prevent respiratory acidosis, and do not allow controlled mechanical ventilation to interfere with the patient's need for compensatory efforts to maintain the serum pH. Administer supplemental oxygen. Obtain serial arterial blood gases and chest x-rays to observe for pulmonary edema (more common with chronic or severe intoxication).

        2. Treat coma (p 18), seizures (p 21), pulmonary edema (p 7), and hyperthermia (p 20) if they occur.

        3. Treat metabolic acidosis with intravenous sodium bicarbonate (p 345). Do **not** allow the serum pH to fall below 7.4.

        4. Replace fluid and electrolyte deficits caused by vomiting and hyperventilation with intravenous crystalloid solutions. Be cautious with fluid therapy, because excessive fluid administration may contribute to pulmonary edema.

        5. Monitor asymptomatic patients for a minimum of 6 hours (longer if an enteric-coated preparation or a massive overdose has been ingested and there is suspicion of a tablet bezoar). Admit symptomatic patients to an intensive care unit.

    B. Specific drugs and antidotes. There is no specific antidote for salicylate intoxication. **Sodium bicarbonate** is frequently given both to prevent acidemia and to promote salicylate elimination by the kidneys (see **D**, below).

    C. Decontamination (see p 43). Decontamination is not necessary for patients with *chronic* intoxication.

        1. Prehospital. Administer activated charcoal if available. Ipecac-induced vomiting may be useful for initial treatment of children at home if it can be given within 30 minutes of exposure.

        2. Hospital. Administer activated charcoal orally or by gastric tube. Gastric lavage is not necessary after small ingestions (ie, <300 mg/kg) if activated charcoal is given promptly.

        3. Note: With very large ingestions of salicylate (eg, 30–60 g), very large doses of activated charcoal (300–600 g) are theoretically necessary to adsorb all the salicylate and prevent desorption. In such cases, the charcoal may be given in several 25- to 50-g doses at 3- to 5-hour intervals. Charcoal should be continued until the serum salicylate levels are clearly falling.

D. Enhanced elimination (see p 51)

1. **Urinary alkalinization** is effective in enhancing urinary excretion of salicylate, although often difficult to achieve in dehydrated or critically ill patients.

    a. Add 100 mEq of sodium bicarbonate to 1 L of 5% dextrose in quarter normal saline, and infuse intravenously at 200 mL/h (3–4 mL/kg/h). If the patient is dehydrated, start with a bolus of 10–20 mL/kg. Fluid and bicarbonate administration is potentially dangerous in patients at high risk for pulmonary edema (eg, chronic intoxication).

    b. Unless renal failure is present, also add potassium, 30–40 mEq, to each liter of intravenous fluids (potassium depletion inhibits alkalinization).

    c. Alkalemia is not a contraindication to bicarbonate therapy, considering that patients often have a significant base deficit in spite of the elevated serum pH.

2. **Hemodialysis** is very effective in rapidly removing salicylate and correcting acid-base and fluid abnormalities. Indications for urgent hemodialysis are as follows:

    a. Patients with acute ingestion and serum levels higher than 1200 mg/L (120 mg/dL), or with severe acidosis and other manifestations of intoxication.

    b. Patients with chronic intoxication with serum levels higher than 600 mg/L (60 mg/dL) accompanied by acidosis, confusion, or lethargy, especially if the patient is elderly or debilitated.

    c. Any patient with severe manifestations of intoxication.

3. **Hemoperfusion** is also very effective but does not correct acid-base or fluid disturbances.

4. **Repeat-dose activated charcoal** therapy effectively reduces the serum salicylate half-life, but it is not as rapidly effective as dialysis, and frequent stooling may contribute to dehydration and electrolyte disturbances.

▶ SCORPIONS

Richard F. Clark, MD

The order Scorpionida contains several families, genera, and species of scorpions. All have paired venom glands in a bulbous segment called the telson, located just anterior to a stinger on the end of the 6 terminal segments of the abdomen (often called a tail).The only dangerous species in the United States is the *Centruroides exilicauda* (formerly *C sculpturatus*), also known as the bark scorpion. The most serious envenomations are usually reported in children under age 10 years. This scorpion is found primarily in the arid southwestern United States but has been found as a stowaway in cargo as far north as Michigan. Other dangerous scorpions are found in Mexico (*Centruroides* species), Brazil (*Tityus* species), India (*Buthus* species), the Middle East, and north Africa and the eastern Mediterranean (*Leiurus* and *Androctonus* species).

I. **Mechanism of toxicity.** The scorpion grasps its prey with its anterior pincers, arches its pseudoabdomen, and stabs with the stinger. Stings also result from stepping on the stinger. The venom of *C exilicauda* contains numerous digestive enzymes (eg, hyaluronidase and phospholipase) and also several neurotoxins. Alteration in sodium channel flow results in excessive stimulation at neuromuscular junctions and the autonomic nervous system.

II. **Toxic dose.** Variable amounts of venom from none to the complete contents of the telson may be ejected through the stinger.

III. **Clinical presentation.**

    A. **Common scorpion stings.** Most stings result only in local, immediate, burning pain. Some local tissue inflammation and occasionally local paresthesias may occur. Symptoms usually resolve within several hours. This represents the typical scorpion sting seen in the United States.

B. Dangerous scorpion stings. In some victims, especially children under age 10 years, systemic symptoms occur, including weakness, restlessness, diaphoresis, diplopia, nystagmus, roving eye movements, hyperexcitability, muscle fasciculations, opisthotonos, priapism, salivation, slurred speech, hypertension, tachycardia, and, rarely, convulsions, paralysis, and respiratory arrest. Envenomations by *Tityus, Buthus, Androctonus,* and *Leiurus* species have caused pulmonary edema, cardiovascular collapse, and death, as well as coagulopathies, disseminated intravascular coagulation, pancreatitis, and renal failure with hemoglobinuria and jaundice. In nonfatal cases, recovery usually occurs within 12–36 hours.

IV. Diagnosis. Either the patient saw the scorpion, or the clinician must recognize the symptoms. In the case of *Centruroides* stings, tapping on the sting site usually produces severe pain ("tap test").

A. Specific levels. Body fluid toxin levels are not available.

B. No other useful laboratory studies are needed for minor envenomations. For severe envenomations, obtain CBC, electrolytes, glucose, BUN, creatinine, coagulation profile, and arterial blood gases.

V. Treatment. The majority of scorpion stings in the United States, including those by *Centruroides*, can be managed with symptomatic care at home, consisting of oral analgesics and cool compresses or intermittent ice packs.

A. Emergency and supportive measures

1. For severe envenomations, maintain an open airway and assist ventilation if necessary (see pp 1–7). Administer supplemental oxygen.
2. Treat hypertension (p 16), tachycardia (p 12), and convulsions (p 21) if they occur.
3. Do *not* overtreat with excessive sedation.
4. Clean the wound and provide tetanus prophylaxis if indicated.
5. Do *not* immerse the injured extremity in ice or perform local incision or suction.

B. Specific drugs and antidotes. An antivenin effective against severe *Centruroides* envenomations is available only in Arizona. Specific antivenins against other species may be available in other parts of the world, but are not approved in the USA.

C. Decontamination. These procedures are not applicable.

D. Enhanced elimination. These procedures are not applicable.

▶ SEDATIVE-HYPNOTIC AGENTS

Paul D. Pearigen, MD

Sedative-hypnotic agents are widely used for the treatment of anxiety and insomnia. As a group they are one of the most frequently prescribed medications. Barbiturates (see p 101), benzodiazepines (p 106), antihistamines (p 84), skeletal muscle relaxants (p 291), antidepressants (pp 79 and 310), and anticholinergic agents (p 78) are discussed elsewhere in this book. In this section (and Table II–49) are listed some of the less commonly used hypnotic agents.

I. Mechanism of toxicity. The exact mechanism of action and the pharmacokinetics (see Table II–55, p 319) vary for each agent. The major toxic effect that causes serious poisoning or death is central nervous system depression resulting in coma, respiratory arrest, and pulmonary aspiration of gastric contents.

II. Toxic dose. The toxic dose varies considerably between drugs and also depends largely on individual tolerance and the presence of other drugs such as alcohol. For most of these drugs, ingestion of 3–5 times the usual hypnotic dose results in coma. However, co-ingestion of alcohol or other drugs may cause

TABLE II-49. COMMON SEDATIVE-HYPNOTIC AGENTS[a]

Drug	Usual Adult Oral Hypnotic Dose (mg)	Approximate Lethal Dose (g)	Toxic Concentration (mg/L)	Usual Half-Life[b] (h)
Buspirone	5–20	Unknown	—	2–4
Chloral hydrate[c]	500–1000	5–10	> 20	8–10
Ethchlorvynol	500–1000	5–10	> 10	10–30
Glutethimide	250–500	10–20	> 10	10–15
Meprobamate	600–1200	10–20	> 60	8–17
Methaqualone	150–250	3–8	> 5	20–40
Methyprylon	200–400	5–10	> 10	3–11

[a]See also anticholinergic agents (p 78), antihistamines (p 84), barbiturates (p 101), benzodiazepines (p 106), paraldehyde (p 249), and skeletal muscle relaxants (p 291).
[b]Half-life in overdose may be considerably longer.
[c]Toxic concentration is measured as trichloroethanol.

coma after smaller ingestions, while individuals chronically using large doses of these drugs may tolerate much higher acute doses.
III. **Clinical presentation.** Overdose with any of these drugs may cause drowsiness, ataxia, nystagmus, stupor, coma, and respiratory arrest. Deep coma may result in absent reflexes, fixed pupils, and depressed or absent electroencephalographic (EEG) activity. Hypothermia is common. Most agents also slow gastric motility and decrease muscle tone. Hypotension with a large overdose is caused primarily by depression of cardiac contractility and, to a lesser extent, loss of venous tone.
   A. **Chloral hydrate** is metabolized to trichloroethanol, which also has CNS-depressant activity. Trichloroethanol may also sensitize the myocardium to the effects of catecholamines, resulting in cardiac arrhythmias.
   B. **Buspirone** may cause nausea, vomiting, drowsiness, and miosis. There are no reported deaths.
   C. **Ethchlorvynol** has a pungent odor sometimes described as pearlike, and gastric fluid often has a pink or green color depending on the capsule form (200- and 500-mg are red; 750-mg is green).
   D. **Glutethimide** often produces mydriasis (dilated pupils) and other anticholinergic side effects, and patients may exhibit prolonged and cyclic or fluctuating coma. It is sometimes taken in combination with codeine ("loads"), which may produce opioid effects.
   E. **Meprobamate** has been reported to form tablet concretions in large overdoses, occasionally requiring surgical removal. Hypotension is more common with this agent than with other sedative-hypnotics.
   F. **Methaqualone** is unusual among sedative-hypnotic agents in frequently causing muscular hypertonicity, clonus, and hyperreflexia.
   G. **Chlorzoxazone** may cause hepatitis.
IV. **Diagnosis** is usually based on a history of ingestion, because clinical manifestations are fairly nonspecific. Hypothermia and deep coma may cause the patient to appear dead; thus, careful evaluation should precede the diagnosis of brain death. Chloral hydrate is radiopaque and may be visible on plain abdominal x-rays.
   A. **Specific levels** and qualitative urine screening are usually available through commercial toxicology laboratories.
      1. Drug levels do not always correlate with severity of intoxication, especially in patients who have tolerance to the drug or who have also ingested other

drugs or alcohol. In addition, early after ingestion blood levels may not reflect brain concentrations.

   2. Some agents (chloral hydrate and glutethimide) have active metabolites,
   levels of which may correlate better with the state of intoxication.

B. Other useful laboratory studies include electrolytes, glucose, serum
ethanol, BUN, creatinine, arterial blood gases, ECG, and chest x-ray.

V. Treatment.

A. Emergency and supportive measures

   1. Maintain an open airway and assist ventilation if necessary (see pp 1–7).
   Administer supplemental oxygen.

   2. Treat coma (p 18), hypothermia (p 19), hypotension (p 15), and pulmonary
   edema (p 8) if they occur.

   3. Monitor patients for at least 6 hours after ingestion, because delayed absorption may occur. Patients with **chloral hydrate** ingestion should be
   monitored at least 18–24 hours because of the risk of cardiac arrhythmias.
   Tachyarrhythmias caused by myocardial sensitization may be treated with
   propranolol (see p 405), 1–2 mg IV, or **esmolol** (see p 366), 25–100
   μg/kg/min IV.

B. Specific drugs and antidotes.
Flumazenil (see p 369) is a specific antago-
nist of benzodiazepine receptors. It does not appear to cross-react with other
sedative agents.

C. Decontamination (see p 43)

   1. Prehospital. Administer activated charcoal if available. Do **not** induce
   vomiting, because of the risk of lethargy and coma.

   2. Hospital. Administer activated charcoal. Gastric emptying is not necessary if activated charcoal can be given promptly; however, consider gastric
   lavage for massive ingestions.

D. Enhanced elimination.
Because of extensive tissue distribution, dialysis and
hemoperfusion are not very effective for most of the drugs in this group.

   1. Repeat-dose charcoal may enhance elimination of glutethimide (which undergoes enterohepatic recirculation) and meprobamate, although no studies have been performed to document clinical effectiveness.

   2. Meprobamate has a relatively small volume of distribution (0.75 L/kg), and
   hemoperfusion is indicated for deep coma complicated by intractable hypotension.

   3. Resin hemoperfusion has been reported to be partially effective for
   ethchlorvynol overdose.

▶ SELENIUM

Janet Weiss, MD

Selenium is a trace metal considered an essential element in the human diet, with
multiple roles in metabolic chemistry. It is present as selenocysteine at the active site
of glutathione peroxidase and has an important antioxidant function. Excessive selenium absorption can cause acute and chronic toxicity. Selenium is used in the electronics industry in rectifiers, photoelectric cells, and solar batteries; in glass, rubber,
steel, and ceramic manufacturing; and in some paints, inks, varnishes, fungicides,
and insecticides. **Selenious acid** is used in gun blueing solutions. Food sources of
selenium include seafood (especially shrimp), meat, and milk products. Geographic
concentration of selenium resulting from environmental factors has been reported.
Self-medication with selenium-containing supplements and excessive use of selenium-containing shampoos have caused toxicity.

   I. Mechanism of toxicity. Elemental selenium is not well absorbed and poses no
   significant risk. Other forms of selenium are better absorbed by the skin, lungs,
   and gastrointestinal tract. Organic selenium compounds (selenomethionine) are

more bioavailable, while inorganic selenite and selenate are less well absorbed. Once absorbed, selenium may have a variety of toxic effects, including inhibition of sulfhydryl enzymes and displacement of sulfur in certain tissues.

  A. **Hydrogen selenide** (selenium hydride) is a highly irritating gas produced by acid reaction with metal selenides.
  B. **Selenious acid** is a corrosive agent with systemic toxic effects. Selenium oxide is converted to selenious acid on contact with water and is highly toxic.

II. **Toxic dose.**

  A. **Ingestion.** Little is known about the oral toxic dose because there are few reports of poisoning. Co-ingestion of vitamin C may reduce selenite to elemental selenium and decrease its absorption.
  1. **Acute overdose.** The oral mean lethal dose of selenite salts in the dog is about 4 mg/kg. Ingestion of 1–5 mg/kg sodium selenite in five adults caused moderate reversible toxicity. Ingestion of as little as 20 mL of gun blueing solution (2% selenious acid) has been fatal.
  2. **Chronic ingestion.** The recommended nutritional daily intake is 50–200 µg/d. The drinking water maximum contaminant level (MCL) is 10 µg/L. Chronic ingestion of 850 µg/day has been associated with toxicity.
  B. **Inhalation.** The recommended workplace exposure levels considered immediately dangerous to life or health (IDLH) are listed in Table II–50.

III. **Clinical presentation.**

  A. **Acute inhalation** of hydrogen selenide may cause burning eyes and throat, metallic taste, coughing, wheezing, chemical pneumonitis, and noncardiogenic pulmonary edema.
  B. **Skin** irritation is common after direct exposure.
  C. **Acute ingestion** may cause vomiting, hypersalivation, garlicky odor on the breath, esophageal burns, abdominal pain, restlessness, and muscle spasms. Cardiovascular effects include hypotension, hemoconcentration, peripheral vasodilation, myocardial depression, and prolonged QT intervals and T-wave changes. Neurologic dysfunction including coma and convulsions may occur. Hepatic dysfunction has been reported. **Death** has occurred after small ingestions of selenious acid in gun blueing solutions.
  D. **Chronic ingestion** of large quantities of selenium has been associated with reddish discoloration and loss of hair and nails, polyneuritis, fatigue, irritability, decreased cognitive function, garlicky breath, elevation of hepatic transaminases, dermatitis, nausea, and vomiting. Animal studies suggest that chronic excessive selenium exposure is embryotoxic and teratogenic, causes hepatic cirrhosis, and may be carcinogenic.
  E. **Chronic inhalation** of hydrogen selenide may cause nausea, vomiting, chronic diarrhea, abdominal pain, bitter taste, garlicky breath, dizziness, fatigue, conjunctivitis, dental caries, and impaired pulmonary function.

IV. **Diagnosis** is difficult without a history of exposure but should be suspected in a patient with hair and nail loss or discoloration and other characteristic symptoms.

TABLE II–50. TOXIC LEVELS OF SELENIUM COMPOUNDS

Selenium Compound	TLV[a]	Level Immediately Dangerous to Life or Health (IDLH)
Hydrogen selenide (selenium hydride)	0.16 mg/m³ (0.05 ppm)	1 ppm
Selenium compounds, general	0.2 mg/m³ (as Se)	1 mg/m³
Selenium hexafluoride	0.16 mg/m³ (0.05 ppm)	2 ppm

[a]TLV = ACGIH recommended exposure limit (threshold limit value) as an 8-hour time-weighted average (TLV-TWA).

A. Specific levels. Selenium can be measured in the blood, hair, and urine. Whole blood levels are most reliable and remain elevated longer than serum levels, which are typically 40–60% lower.

    1. On a normal diet, whole blood selenium levels range from 0.1 to 0.2 mg/L. One patient with chronic intoxication after ingestion of 31 mg/d had a whole blood selenium of 0.53 mg/L.

    2. Average hair levels are up to 0.5 ppm. The relationship between hair and tissue concentrations is not well understood.

    3. Both whole blood and urinary concentrations reflect dietary intake. Overexposure should be considered when blood selenium levels exceed 0.4 mg/L or urinary excretion exceeds 600–1000 µg/d.

B. Other useful laboratory studies include electrolytes, glucose, BUN, creatinine, liver transaminases, and ECG. After inhalation exposure, obtain arterial blood gases or oximetry and chest x-ray.

V. Treatment.

A. Emergency and supportive measures

    1. Maintain an open airway and assist ventilation if necessary (see pp 1–7). Administer supplemental oxygen.

    2. Treat coma (p 18), convulsions (p 21), bronchospasm (p 8), and pulmonary edema (p 7) if they occur.

    3. Observe for at least 6 hours after exposure.

    4. After ingestion of selenious acid, consider endoscopy to rule out esophageal or gastric corrosive injury.

B. Specific drugs and antidotes. There is no established specific antidote. Although chelation with EDTA (p 363) and dimercaprol (BAL, p 341) has been studied in animals, their use is not supported in humans. N-acteylcysteine (NAC) (p 334) may have therapeutic value, but further studies are needed. High-dose vitamin C (several grams daily) has produced equivocal results.

C. Decontamination (see p 43)

    1. Inhalation. Immediately remove the victim from exposure and give supplemental oxygen if available.

    2. Skin and eyes. Remove contaminated clothing and wash exposed skin with soap and copious water. Irrigate exposed eyes with copious tepid water or saline.

    3. Ingestion (see p 45)

        a. Prehospital. Administer activated charcoal if available. Do *not* administer ipecac or induce vomiting because of risk of corrosive injury and potential for abrupt onset of seizures.

        b. Hospital. If tablets, solids, or a large quantity of liquid (more than 1–2 oz) has been ingested, perform gastric lavage, and administer activated charcoal. (Gastric lavage may not be effective after ingestion of small amounts of liquid or delayed presentation.)

        c. In vitro experiments indicate that vitamin C can reduce selenium salts to elemental selenium, which is poorly absorbed. Its use has not been studied in vivo, but oral or nasogastric administration of several grams of ascorbic acid is probably reasonable.

D. Enhanced elimination. There is no known role for any enhanced removal procedure.

► SKELETAL MUSCLE RELAXANTS

Karl A. Sporer, MD

Various drugs have been used to treat muscle spasm. Most compounds in this group act as simple sedative-hypnotic agents and produce skeletal muscle relaxation indirectly. The drugs commonly used as skeletal muscle relaxants are listed in

Table II–51. Meprobamate, a metabolite of carisoprodol, was at one time a popular sedative-hypnotic agent (see p 287).

I. **Mechanism of Toxicity.**
   A. **Central Nervous System.** Most of these drugs cause generalized CNS depression.
      1. **Cyclobenzaprine** and **orphenadrine** have anticholinergic side effects.
      2. **Baclofen** is an agonist at the GABA-B receptor and can produce profound CNS and respiratory depression as well as paradoxical muscle hypertonicity and seizurelike activity.
      3. Spastic encephalopathy is also common with **carisoprodol** overdose.
   B. **Cardiovascular effects.** Hypotension may occur after overdose. **Baclofen** has caused bradycardia in up to 30% of ingestions. Massive **orphenadrine** ingestions have caused supraventricular tachycardia.
   C. **Pharmacokinetics** vary with the drug. Absorption may be delayed because of anticholinergic effects. See also Table II–55, p 319.
II. **Toxic Dose.** The toxic dose varies considerably between drugs and also depends largely on individual tolerance and can be influenced by the presence of other drugs such as ethanol. For most of these drugs, ingestion of more than 3–5 times the usual therapeutic dose may cause stupor or coma.
III. **Clinical presentation.** Onset of CNS depression is usually seen within 30–120 minutes of ingestion. Lethargy, slurred speech, ataxia, coma, and respiratory arrest may occur. Larger ingestions, especially when combined with alcohol, can produce unresponsive coma.
   A. **Carisoprodol** may cause hyperreflexia, opisthotonus, and increased muscle tone.
   B. **Cyclobenzaprine** and **orphenadrine** can produce anticholinergic findings, such as tachycardia, dilated pupils, and delirium. Despite its structural similarity to tricyclic antidepressants, cyclobenzaprine has not been reported to cause quinidinelike cardiotoxicity
   C. **Baclofen** overdose causes coma, respiratory depression, occasional bradycardia, and paradoxical seizurelike activity. Onset is rapid but may last 12–48 hours.
IV. **Diagnosis** is usually based on the history of ingestion and findings of CNS depression, often accompanied by muscle twitching or hyperreflexia. The differential diagnosis should include other sedative-hypnotic agents (see p 287).
   A. **Specific levels.** Many of these drugs can be detected on comprehensive urine toxicology screening. Quantitative drug levels do not always correlate with severity of intoxication, especially in patients who have tolerance to the drug or who have also ingested other drugs or alcohol. In addition, early after ingestion blood levels may not reflect brain concentrations.
   B. **Other useful laboratory studies** include electrolytes, glucose, serum ethanol, BUN, creatinine, arterial blood gases, and chest x-ray.
V. **Treatment.**

TABLE II–51. COMMON SKELETAL MUSCLE RELAXANTS

Drug	Usual Half Life	Usual Daily Adult Dose (mg)
Baclofen	2.5–4	40–80
Carisoprodol[a]	1.5–8	800–1600
Chlorzoxazone	1	1500–3000
Cyclobenzaprine	24–72	30–60
Methocarbamol	1–2	4000–4500
Orphenadrine	14–16	200

[a]Metabolized to methocarbamol

A. **Emergency and supportive measures**
   1. Maintain an open airway and assist ventilation if necessary (see pp 1–7). Administer supplemental oxygen.
   2. Treat coma (p 18), hypothermia (p 19), hypotension (p 15), and pulmonary edema (p 7) if they occur. Hypotension usually responds promptly to supine position and intravenous fluids.
   3. Monitor patients for at least 6 hours after ingestion, because delayed absorption may occur.
B. **Specific drugs and antidotes.** There are no specific antidotes. Flumazenil (see p 369) is a specific antagonist of benzodiazepine receptors, and it does not appear to cross-react with skeletal muscle relaxants or other sedative agents. While physostigmine may reverse anticholinergic symptoms associated with cyclobenzaprine and orphenadrine overdose, it is not generally needed and may cause seizures.
C. **Decontamination** (see p 43)
   1. **Prehospital.** Administer activated charcoal if available. Do *not* induce vomiting because of the risk of lethargy and coma.
   2. **Hospital.** Administer activated charcoal. Gastric emptying is not necessary if activated charcoal can be given promptly; however, consider gastric lavage for massive ingestions.
D. **Enhanced elimination.** Because of extensive tissue distribution, dialysis and hemoperfusion are not very effective for most of the drugs in this group. Repeat-dose charcoal may enhance elimination of meprobamate, although no studies have been performed to document this.

▶ SNAKEBITE

Richard F. Clark, MD

Of the 14 families of snakes, 5 are poisonous (Table II–52). The annual incidence of snakebite in the United States is three to four bites per 100,000 population. Clinically significant morbidity occurs in less than 60%, and only a few deaths are reported each year. Rattlesnake bite is the most common envenomation in the United States, and the victim is often a young, intoxicated male who was teasing or trying to capture the snake. Snakes strike accurately to about one-third their body length, with a maximum striking distance of a few feet.

I. **Mechanism of toxicity.** Snake venoms are complex mixtures of 50 or more components that function to immobilize, kill, and predigest prey. In human victims, these substances produce local "digestive" effects on tissues as well as hemotoxic, neurotoxic, and other systemic effects. The relative predominance of digestive, hemotoxoic, or neurotoxic venom components depends on the species of the snake and geographic variables.

II. **Toxic dose.** The potency of the venom and the amount of venom injected vary considerably. About 20% of all snake strikes are "dry" bites in which there is no envenomation.

III. **Clinical presentation.** The most common snake envenomations in the United States are from rattlesnakes (Crotalidae). Bites from common North American Elapidae (eg, coral snakes) and Colubridae (eg, king snakes) are also discussed here. For information about bites from other exotic snakes, contact a regional poison control center (see Table I–42, p 54) for a specific consultation.
   A. **Crotalidae.** Fang marks may look like puncture wounds or lacerations, the latter resulting from a glancing blow by the snake or sudden movement by the victim. The fangs often penetrate only a few millimeters but occasionally enter deeper tissue spaces or veins.
      1. **Local effects.** Within minutes of envenomation, stinging, burning pain begins. Progressive swelling, erythema, petechiae, ecchymosis, and hemorrhagic blebs develop over the next several hours. The limb may swell to

TABLE II-52. EXAMPLES OF POISONOUS SNAKES

Family and Genera	Common Name	Comments
Colubridae		
Lampropeltis	King snake	Human envenomation difficult because of small mouth
Heterodon	Hognose	and small fixed fangs in the rear of mouth. May cause
Coluber	Racer	severe systemic coagulopathy.
Dispholidus	Boomslang	
Crotalidae		
Crotalus	Rattlesnake	Most common envenomation in USA. Long rotating
Agkistrodon	Copperhead, cottonmouth	fangs in the front of the mouth. Heat-sensing facial pits
Bothrops	Fer-de-lance	(hence the name "pit vipers").
Elapidae		
Micrurus	Coral snake	Human envenomation difficult because of small mouth
Naja	Cobra	and small fixed fangs in rear of mouth. Neurotoxicity
Bungarus	Krait	usually predominates.
Dendroaspis	Mamba	
Hydrophidae	Sea snakes	Also have small rear-located fangs.
Viperidae		
Bitis	Puff adder, gaboon viper	Long rotating fangs in the front of the mouth, but no
Cerastes	Cleopatra's asp	heat-sensing facial pits.
Echis	Saw-scaled viper	

twice its normal size within the first few hours. Hypovolemic shock and local compartment syndrome may occur secondary to fluid and blood sequestration in injured areas.

2. **Systemic effects** may include nausea and vomiting, weakness, muscle fasciculations, diaphoresis, perioral and peripheral parasthesias, a metallic taste, thrombocytopenia, and coagulopathy. Circulating vasodilatory compounds may contribute to hypotension. Pulmonary edema and cardiovascular collapse have been reported.

3. **Mojave rattlesnake** (*Crotalus scutulatus*) bites deserve special consideration and caution, because neurologic signs and symptoms of envenomation may be delayed and there is often little swelling or evidence of tissue damage. The onset of muscle weakness, ptosis, and respiratory arrest may occur several hours after envenomation. Facial and laryngeal edema have also been reported.

B. **Elapidae.** Coral snake envenomation is rare because of the snake's small mouth and fangs. The snake must hold on and "chew" the extremity for several seconds or more to work its rear fangs into the skin.

1. **Local effects.** There is usually minimal swelling and inflammation around the fang marks. Local paresthesias may occur.

2. **Systemic effects.** Systemic symptoms usually occur within a few hours but may be delayed 12 hours or more. Nausea and vomiting, euphoria, confusion, diplopia, dysarthria, muscle fasciculations, generalized muscle weakness, and respiratory arrest may occur.

C. **Colubridae.** These small-mouthed rear-fanged snakes must also hang onto their victims and "chew" the venom into the skin before significant envenomation can occur.

1. **Local effects.** There is usually little local reaction other than mild pain and paresthesias, although swelling of the extremity may occur.

2. **Systemic effects.** The most serious effect of envenomation is systemic coagulopathy, which can be fatal.

IV. Diagnosis. Correct diagnosis and treatment depend on proper identification of the offending snake, especially if more than one indigenous poisonous species or an exotic snake is involved.

A. Determine whether the bite was by an indigenous (wild) species or an exotic zoo animal or illegally imported pet. (The owner of an illegal pet snake may be reluctant to admit this for fear of fines or confiscation.) Envenomation occurring during the fall and winter months (October-March) when snakes usually hibernate is not likely to be caused by a wild species.

B. If the snake is available, attempt to have it identified by a herpetologist. ***Caution:*** Be careful not to handle a "dead" snake; accidental envenomation may still occur up to several hours after death.

C. Specific levels. These tests are not applicable.

D. Other useful laboratory studies include CBC, platelet count, prothrombin time (PT), fibrin split products, fibrinogen, CPK, and urine dipstick for occult blood (positive with free myoglobin or hemoglobin). For severe envenomations with frank bleeding, hemolysis, or anticipated bleeding problems, obtain a blood type and screen early. If compromised respiratory function is suspected, closely monitor oximetry and arterial blood gases.

V. Treatment.

A. Emergency and supportive measures. Regardless of the species, prepare for both local and systemic manifestations. Monitor patients closely for at least 6–8 hours after a typical crotalid bite and for at least 12–24 hours after *C scutulatus* or an elapid bite.

1. Local effects

a. Monitor local swelling at least hourly with measurements of limb girth, the presence and extent of local ecchymosis, and assessment of circulation.

b. When indicated, obtain consultation with an experienced surgeon for management of serious wound complications. Do not perform fasciotomy unless compartment syndrome is documented with tissue compartment pressure monitoring.

c. Provide tetanus prophylaxis if needed.

d. Administer broad-spectrum antibiotics only if there are signs of infection.

2. Systemic effects

a. Monitor the victim for respiratory muscle weakness. Maintain an open airway and assist ventilation if necessary (see p 1–7). Administer supplemental oxygen.

b. Treat bleeding complications with fresh-frozen plasma (and antivenin; see below). Treat hypotension with intravenous crystalloid fluids (p 15), and rhabdomyolysis (p 25) with fluids and sodium bicarbonate.

B. Specific drugs and antidotes. For patients with documented envenomation, be prepared to administer specific **antivenin**. Virtually all local and systemic manifestations of envenomation improve after antivenin administration. ***Caution:*** Life-threatening anaphylactic reactions may occur with antivenin administration, even after a negative skin test.

1. For **rattlesnake** and other **Crotalidae** envenomations, the presence of fang marks, limb swelling, ecchymosis, and severe pain at the bite site are considered minimal indications for **polyvalent Crotalidae antivenin** (see p 336). Progressive systemic manifestations such as generalized fasciculations, coagulopathy, and muscle weakness are indications for prompt and aggressive treatment. For a Mojave rattlesnake bite, the decision to administer antivenin is more difficult because there are few local signs of toxicity.

2. For **coral snake** envenomation, consult a regional poison control center (see Table I–42, p 54) or an experienced medical toxicologist to determine the advisability of ***Micrurus fulvius*** antivenin (see p 338). In general, if there is evidence of coagulopathy or neurologic toxicity, administer antivenin.

3. For **Colubridae** envenomations, there are no antivenins available.
4. For **other exotic snakes**, consult a regional poison control center (see Table I–42, p 54) for assistance in diagnosis, location of specific antivenin, and indications for administration.

C. **Decontamination.** First-aid measures are generally ineffective and may cause additional tissue damage.
   1. Remain calm, remove the victim to at least 20 feet from the snake, wash the area with soap and water, and remove any constricting clothing or jewelry. Apply ice sparingly to the site (excessive ice application or immersion in ice water can lead to frostbite and aggravate tissue damage).
   2. Loosely splint or immobilize the extremity near heart level. *Do not apply a tourniquet.*
   3. Do *not* make cuts over the bite site. If performed within 15 minutes, **suction** over the fang marks (ie, with a Sawyer extractor) may remove some venom but this should not delay transport to a hospital. Mouth suction of the wound is not advised.

D. **Enhanced elimination.** Dialysis, hemoperfusion, and charcoal administration are not applicable.

▶ **SPIDERS**

Richard F. Clark, MD

Most of the more than 50,000 species of spiders in the United States possess poison glands connected to fangs in the large, paired, jawlike structures known as chelicerae. However, only a very few spiders have fangs long and tough enough to pierce human skin. In the United States, these include *Latrodectus* (black widow), *Loxosceles* (brown recluse spider), *Phidippus* (jumping spider), and **tarantulas** (a common name given to many large spiders). Tarantulas rarely cause significant envenomation but can produce a painful bite because of their large size. Spiders not common to North America are not discussed here.

Latrodectus species (black widow) are ubiquitous in the continental United States, and the female can cause serious envenomations with rare fatalities. They are usually encountered in the summer months while gardening or moving firewood, or during house repairs. The spider has a body size of 1–2 cm and is characteristically shiny black with a red hourglass shape on its bulbous abdomen. Other related species may be brown or red, or have irregular red markings on a black body. *Latrodectus* makes coarse, irregular webs in dimly lit locations.

Loxosceles species (brown recluse) are found mainly in the central and southeastern US (Missouri, Kansas, Arkansas, and Tennessee), but have been identified nationwide. The spider's nocturnal hunting habits and reclusive temperament result in infrequent contact with humans; most encounters occur at outdoor woodpiles or in basements. The spider is 1–3 cm in length, light to dark brown in color, with a characteristic violin- or fiddle-shaped marking on its cephalothorax (back).

I. **Mechanism of toxicity.** Spiders use their hollow fangs (chelicerae) to inject their venoms, which contain various protein and polypeptide toxins that are poorly characterized but appear to be designed to induce rapid paralysis of the insect victim and to aid in digestion.
   A. *Latrodectus* (black widow) spider venom contains alpha-latrotoxin. This extremely potent toxin binds to specific synaptic membrane receptor proteins and causes opening of nonspecific cation channels, leading to an increased influx of calcium, indiscriminate release of acetylcholine, and excessive stimulation of the motor endplate.
   B. *Loxosceles* (brown spiders) and *Phidippus* (jumping spiders) toxins contain a variety of digestive enzymes such as collagenases, proteases, and phospholipases. *Loxosceles* venom also contains sphingomyelinase D, which is

cytotoxic and chemotactically attracts white blood cells to the bite site, and also has a role in producing systemic symptoms such as hemolysis.

II. **Toxic dose.** Spider venoms are generally extremely potent toxins (far more potent than most snake venoms), but the delivered dose is extremely small. The size of the victim may be an important variable.

III. **Clinical presentation.** Manifestations of envenomation are quite different depending on the species.

A. *Latrodectus* (black widow) inflicts a bite that can range from mild erythema to a target lesion with a central punctate site with central blanching and an outer erythematous ring.

1. The bite is often initially painful but may go unnoticed. It almost always becomes painful within 30–120 minutes. By 3–4 hours, painful cramping and muscle fasciculations occur in the involved extremity. This cramping progresses toward the chest, back, or abdomen and can produce boardlike rigidity, weakness, dyspnea, headache, and paresthesias. Black widow envenomation may mimic myocardial infarction or an acute surgical abdomen. Symptoms often persist for 1–2 days.

2. Additional common symptoms may include hypertension, regional diaphoresis, restlessness, nausea, vomiting, and tachycardia.

3. Other less common symptoms include leukocytosis, fever, delirium, arrhythmias, and paresthesias. Rarely, hypertensive crisis or respiratory arrest may occur after severe envenomation, mainly in very young or very old victims.

B. *Loxosceles* syndrome is often called "loxoscelism" or "necrotic arachnidism."

1. Envenomation usually produces a painful burning sensation at the bite site within 10 minutes, but can be delayed. Over the next 1–12 hours, a "bull's-eye" lesion forms, consisting of a central vesicle (which may be hemorrhagic) surrounded by a blanched ring enclosed by a ring of ecchymosis. The entire lesion can range from 1 to 5 cm in diameter. Over the next 24–72 hours, an indolent necrotic ulcer develops that may persist for a month or more. However, in most cases necrosis is limited and healing occurs rapidly.

2. Systemic illness may occur in the first 24–48 hours and does not necessarily correlate with the severity of the ulcer. Systemic manifestations include fever, chills, malaise, nausea, and myalgias. Rarely, intravascular hemolysis and disseminated intravascular coagulopathy may occur.

C. *Phidippus.* Many necrotic spider bites in the United States are probably caused by *Phidippus* species, which inflict a painful bite, resulting in localized wheals, rashes, ecchymosis, and pruritus that are occasionally complicated by arthralgias, myalgias, headache, fever, nausea, vomiting, and hypotension. The duration of effects is generally no more than 1–4 days, and death is very rare.

IV. **Diagnosis** is most commonly made based on the characteristic clinical presentation. Bite marks of all spiders but the tarantulas are usually too small to be easily visualized, and victims often do not recall feeling the bite or seeing the spider.

Besides *Loxosceles* and *Phidippus*, many arthropods and insects may also produce small puncture wounds, pain, itching, redness, swelling, and even necrotic ulcers, so the offending animal often cannot be precisely identified unless it was captured or seen by the victim.

A. **Specific levels.** Serum toxin levels are not currently available. In the future, diagnostic serologic tests may be useful in diagnosing the specific responsible spider.

B. **Other useful laboratory studies**

1. *Latrodectus*. Electrolytes, calcium, glucose, CPK, and ECG (for chest pain).

2. *Loxosceles*. CBC, platelets, BUN, and creatinine. If hemolysis is suspected, haptoglobin and urine dipstick for occult blood (positive with free hemoglobin) are useful; repeat daily for 1–2 days.

V. Treatment.
  A. Emergency and supportive measures
    1. General
      a. Cleanse the wound and apply cool compresses or intermittent ice packs. Treat infection if it occurs.
      b. Give tetanus prophylaxis if indicated.
    2. *Latrodectus* envenomation
      a. Monitor victims for at least 6–8 hours.
      b. Maintain an open airway and assist ventilation if necessary (see pp 1–7), and treat severe hypertension (p 16) if it occurs.
    3. *Loxosceles* or *Phidippus* envenomation
      a. Do not excise or debride aggressively on initial evaluation.
      b. Admit patients with systemic symptoms and monitor for hemolysis, renal failure, and other complications.
  B. Specific drugs and antidotes
    1. *Latrodectus*
      a. Muscle cramping may be treated with **intravenous calcium** (p 350) or muscle relaxants such as **methocarbamol** (p 380). However, these therapies are often ineffective when used alone.
      b. Most patients will also require opioids such as **morphine** (p 383) and often are admitted for 24–48 hours for pain control.
      c. Equine-derived antivenin (**antivenin *Latrodectus mactans*; see p 337) is rapidly effective, but rarely used because symptomatic therapy is usually adequate and because of the small risk of anaphylaxis. It may still be indicated for seriously ill, elderly, or pediatric patients who do not respond to conventional therapy for hypertension, muscle cramping, or respiratory distress and for pregnant victims threatening premature labor.
    2. *Loxosceles*. Therapy for necrotic arachnidism has been difficult to evaluate because of the inherent difficulty of accurate diagnosis.
      a. *Dapsone* has shown some promise in reducing the severity of necrotic ulcers in anecdotal case reports, but has not been effective in controlled animal models.
      b. Steroids are not usually recommended.
      c. A goat-derived antivenin has been studied, but is not FDA-approved or commercially available.
      d. Hyperbaric oxygen has been proposed for significant necrotic ulcers, but results from animal studies are equivocal, and insufficient data exist to recommend its use.
  C. Decontamination. These measures are not applicable. There is no proven value in the sometimes popular early excision of *Loxosceles* bites to prevent necrotic ulcer formation.
  D. Enhanced elimination. These procedures are not applicable.

▶ STRYCHNINE

Neal L. Benowitz, MD

Strychnine is an alkaloid derived from the seeds of a tree, *Strychnos nux-vomica*. At one time strychnine was an ingredient in a variety of over-the-counter tonics and laxatives. Today strychnine is no longer used in any pharmaceuticals. Instead it is used primarily as a rodenticide and is sometimes found as an adulterant in illicit drugs such as cocaine or heroin.

  I. Mechanism of toxicity. Strychnine competitively antagonizes glycine, an inhibitory neurotransmitter released by post-synaptic inhibitory neurons in the spinal cord. This causes increased neuronal excitability, which results in generalized seizurelike contraction of skeletal muscles. Simultaneous contraction of opposing flexor and extensor muscles causes severe muscle injury, with rhabdomyolysis, myoglobinuria, and, in some cases, acute renal failure.

  Pharmcokinetics. Strychnine is rapidly absorbed after ingestion. The volume of distribution is very large (Vd = 13 L/kg). Elimination is by hepatic metabolism with a half-life of about 10 hours after overdose.

II. **Toxic dose.** It is difficult to establish a toxic dose, although 16 mg was fatal in an adult in one case. Because life-threatening clinical manifestations can occur rapidly and because management decisions are based on clinical findings rather than on a history of ingested amounts, any dose of strychnine should be considered life-threatening.

III. **Clinical presentation.** Symptoms and signs usually develop within 15–30 minutes of ingestion and may last several hours (the serum elimination half-life of strychnine was 10 hours in one reported overdose).
   A. Muscular stiffness and painful cramps precede generalized muscle contractions and opisthotonos. The face may be drawn into a forced grimace ("sardonic grin," or *risus sardonicus*). Muscle contractions are intermittent and are easily triggered by emotional or physical stimuli. Repeated and prolonged muscle contractions often result in hyperthermia, rhabdomyolysis, myoglobinuria, and renal failure.
   B. Muscle spasms may resemble the tonic phase of a grand mal seizure, but strychnine does not cause true seizures, and the patient is awake and painfully aware of the contractions.
   C. Victims may also experience hyperacusis, hyperalgesia, and increased visual stimulation. Sudden noises or other sensory input may trigger muscle contractions.
   D. Death is usually caused by respiratory arrest owing to intense contraction of the respiratory muscles. Death may also be secondary to hyperthermia or rhabdomyolysis and renal failure.

IV. **Diagnosis** is based on a history of ingestion of a rodenticide or recent intravenous drug abuse and the presence of seizurelike generalized muscle contractions, often accompanied by hyperthermia, lactic acidosis, and rhabdomyolysis (with myoglobinuria and elevated serum creatine phosphokinase [CPK]). In the differential diagnosis (see Table I–15, p 24), one should consider other causes of generalized muscle rigidity such as a black widow spider bite (p 296), neuroleptic malignant syndrome (p 20), or tetanus (see p 301).
   A. **Specific levels.** Strychnine can be measured in the gastric fluid, urine, or blood. The toxic serum concentration is reported to be 1 mg/L, although in general, blood levels do not correlate well with the severity of toxicity.
   B. **Other useful laboratory studies** include electrolytes, BUN, creatinine, CPK, arterial blood gases or oximetry, and urine test for occult blood (positive in the presence of urine myoglobinuria).

V. **Treatment.**
   A. **Emergency and supportive measures**
      1. Maintain an open airway and assist ventilation if necessary (see pp 1–7).
      2. Treat hyperthermia (p 20), metabolic acidosis (p 31), and rhabdomyolysis (p 25) if they occur.
      3. Limit external stimuli such as noise, light, and touch.
      4. **Treat muscle spasms** aggressively.
         a. Administer **diazepam** (see p 342), 0.1–0.2 mg/kg IV or **midazolam** 0.05–0.1 mg/kg IV, to patients with mild muscle contractions. Give **morphine** (p 383) for pain relief. *Note:* These agents may impair the respiratory drive.
         b. In more severe cases, use **pancuronium** 0.06–0.1 mg/kg IV or another neuromuscular blocker (see p 386), to produce complete neuromuscular paralysis. *Caution:* Neuromuscular paralysis will cause respiratory arrest; patients will need endotracheal intubation and assisted ventilation.
   B. **Specific drugs and antidotes.** There is no specific antidote.

C. Decontamination (see p 43)
   1. Prehospital. Administer activated charcoal, if available. Do *not* induce vomiting because of the risk of aggravating muscle spasms.
   2. Hospital. Administer activated charcoal orally or by gastric tube. Gastric lavage is not necessary for small ingestions if activated charcoal can be given promptly.
D. Enhanced elimination. Symptoms usually abate within several hours and can be managed effectively with intensive supportive care, so there is little to be gained from accelerated drug removal by dialysis or hemoperfusion. The use of repeat-dose activated charcoal has not been studied.

▶ SULFUR DIOXIDE

John Balmes, MD

Sulfur dioxide is a colorless, nonflammable gas formed by the burning of materials that contain sulfur. It is a major air pollutant from automobiles, smelters, and plants burning soft coal or oils high in sulfur content. It is soluble in water to form sulfurous acid, which may be oxidized to sulfuric acid; both are components of acid rain. Occupational exposures to sulfur dioxide occur in ore and metal refining, chemical manufacturing, and wood pulp treatment and in its use as a disinfectant, refrigerant, and dried-food preservative.

  I. Mechanism of toxicity. Sulfur dioxide is an irritant because it rapidly forms sulfurous acid on contact with moist mucous membranes. Most effects occur in the upper respiratory tract because 90% of inhaled sulfur dioxide is rapidly deposited there, but with very large exposures sufficient gas reaches the lower airways to cause chemical pneumonitis and pulmonary edema.
 II. Toxic dose. The sharp odor or taste of sulfur dioxide is noticed at 1–5 ppm. Throat and conjunctival irritation begins at 8–12 ppm and is severe at 50 ppm. The ACGIH-recommended workplace permissible limit (TLV-TWA) is 2 ppm (5.2 mg/m^3) as an 8-hour time-weighted average, the short-term exposure limit (STEL) is 5 ppm (13 mg/m^3), and the air level considered immediately dangerous to life or health (IDLH) is 100 ppm. Persons with asthma may experience bronchospasm with brief exposure to 0.5–1 ppm.
III. Clinical presentation.
   A. Acute exposure causes burning of the eyes, nose, and throat; lacrimation; and cough. Laryngospasm may occur. Wheezing may be seen in normal subjects as well as asthmatics. Chemical bronchitis is not uncommon. With a very high-level exposure, chemical pneumonitis and noncardiogenic pulmonary edema may occur.
   B. Asthma and chronic bronchitis may be exacerbated.
   C. Sulfhemoglobinemia due to absorption of sulfur has been reported.
   D. Frostbite injury to the skin may occur from exposure to liquid sulfur dioxide.
 IV. Diagnosis is based on a history of exposure and the presence of airway and mucous membrane irritation. Symptoms usually occur rapidly after exposure.
   A. Specific levels. Blood levels are not available.
   B. Other useful laboratory studies include arterial blood gases or oximetry, chest x-ray, and spirometry or peak expiratory flow rate.
  V. Treatment.
   A. Emergency and supportive measures
     1. Remain alert for progressive upper-airway edema or obstruction, and be prepared to intubate the trachea and assist ventilation if necessary (see p 4).
     2. Administer humidified oxygen, treat wheezing with bronchodilators (p 8), and observe the victim for at least 4–6 hours for development of pulmonary edema (p 7).
   B. Specific drugs and antidotes. There is no specific antidote.

C. Decontamination
1. **Inhalation.** Remove the victim from exposure and give supplemental oxygen if available.
2. **Skin and eyes.** Wash exposed skin and eyes with copious tepid water or saline. Treat frostbite injury as for thermal burns.
D. Enhanced elimination. There is no role for these procedures.

▶ TETANUS

Karl A. Sporer, MD

Tetanus is a rare disease in the United States, with fewer than 50 cases reported annually. It is caused by an exotoxin produced by *Clostridium tetani*, an anaerobic, spore-forming, gram-positive rod found widely in soil and in the gastrointestinal tract. Tetanus is typically seen in older persons (especially older women), recent immigrants, and intravenous drug users who have not maintained adequate tetanus immunization.

I. **Mechanism of toxicity.** The growth of *C tetani* in a wound under anaerobic conditions produces the toxin tetanospasmin. The toxin enters the myoneural junction of alpha motor neurons and travels via retrograde axonal transport to the synapse. There it blocks the release of the presynaptic inhibitory neurotransmitters γ-aminobutyric acid (GABA) and glycine, causing intense muscular spasms.

II. **Toxic dose.** Tetanospasmin is an extremely potent toxin. Fatal tetanus can result from a minor puncture wound in a susceptible individual.

III. **Clinical presentation.** The incubation period between the initial wound and development of symptoms averages 1–2 weeks (range 2–56 days). The wound is not apparent in about 5% of cases. Wound cultures are positive for *C tetani* only about one-third of the time.
   A. The most common initial complaint is pain and stiffness of the jaw, progressing to trismus, *risus sardonicus*, and opisthotonos over several days. Uncontrollable and painful reflex spasms involving all muscle groups are precipitated by minimal stimuli and can result in fractures, rhabdomyolysis, hyperpyrexia, and asphyxia. The patient remains awake during the spasms. In survivors, the spasms may persist for days or weeks.
   B. A syndrome of sympathetic hyperactivity often accompanies the muscular manifestations, with hypertension, tachycardia, arrhythmias, and diaphoresis.
   C. Neonatal tetanus occurs frequently in developing countries, owing to inadequate maternal immunity and poor hygiene, especially around the necrotic umbilical stump. Localized tetanus has been reported, involving rigidity and spasm only in the affected limb. Cephalic tetanus is uncommonly associated with head wounds and involves primarily the cranial nerves.

IV. **Diagnosis** is based on the finding of characteristic muscle spasms in an awake person with a wound and an inadequate immunization history. Strychnine poisoning (p 298) produces identical muscle spasms and should be considered in the differential diagnosis. Other considerations include hypocalcemia and dystonic reactions.
   A. **Specific levels.** There are no specific toxin assays. A serum antibody level of 0.01 IU/mL or greater suggests prior immunity and makes the diagnosis less likely.
   B. **Other useful laboratory studies** include electrolytes, glucose, calcium, BUN, creatinine, CPK, arterial blood gases, and urine dipstick for occult blood (positive with myoglobinuria). A diagnostic electromyographic pattern has been described but is not commonly used.

V. **Treatment.**
   A. **Emergency and supportive measures**
   1. Maintain an open airway and assist ventilation if necessary (see pp 1–7).

2. Treat hyperthermia (p 20), arrhythmias (pp 10–14), metabolic acidosis (p 31), and rhabdomyolysis (p 25) if they occur.
3. Limit external stimuli such as noise, light, and touch.
4. **Treat muscle spasms** aggressively:
    a. Administer **diazepam** (see p 342), 0.1–0.2 mg/kg IV, or **midazolam,** 0.05–0.1 mg/kg IV, to patients with mild muscle contractions. Give **morphine** (see p 383) for pain relief. *Note:* These agents may impair respiratory drive.
    b. In more severe cases, use **pancuronium,** 0.06–0.1 mg/kg IV or another neuromuscular blocker (see p 386), to produce complete neuromuscular paralysis. *Caution:* Neuromuscular paralysis will cause respiratory arrest; patients will need endotracheal intubation and assisted ventilation.
B. **Specific drugs and antidotes**
    1. **Human tetanus immune globulin** (TIG), 3000–5000 IU administered IM, will neutralize circulating toxin but has no effect on toxin already fixed to neurons. TIG should be given as early as possible to a patient with suspected tetanus and to persons with a fresh wound but possibly inadequate prior immunization.
    2. **Prevention** can be ensured by an adequate immunization series with tetanus toxoid in childhood and repeated boosters at 10-year intervals. Survival of tetanus may not protect against future exposures, because the small amount of toxin required to cause disease is inadequate to confer immunity.
C. **Decontamination.** Thoroughly debride and irrigate the wound, and administer appropriate antibiotics (penicillin is adequate for *C tetani*).
D. **Enhanced elimination.** There is no role for these procedures.

▶ THALLIUM

Thomas J. Ferguson, MD, PhD

Thallium is a soft metal that quickly oxidizes upon exposure to air. It is a minor constituent in a variety of ores. Thallium salts are used in the manufacture of jewelry, semiconductors, and optical devices. Thallium is no longer used in the United States as a depilatory or a rodenticide because of its high human toxicity.

I. **Mechanism of toxicity.** The mechanism of thallium toxicity is not known. It appears to affect a variety of enzyme systems, resulting in generalized cellular poisoning. Thallium metabolism has some similarities to that of potassium, and it may inhibit potassium flux across biological membranes by binding to Na-K ATP transport enzymes.

II. **Toxic dose.** The minimum lethal dose of thallium salts is probably 12–15 mg/kg, although toxicity varies widely depending on the compound, and there are reports of death after adult ingestion of as little as 200 mg. The more water-soluble salts (eg, thallous acetate and thallic chloride) are slightly more toxic than the less soluble forms (thallic oxide and thallous iodide). Some thallium salts are well absorbed across intact skin.

III. **Clinical presentation.** Symptoms do not occur immediately but are typically delayed 12–14 hours after ingestion.
A. **Acute effects** include abdominal pain, nausea, vomiting, and diarrhea (sometimes with hemorrhage). Shock may result from massive fluid or blood loss. Within 2–3 days, delirium, seizures, respiratory failure, and death may occur.
B. **Chronic effects** include painful peripheral neuropathy, myopathy, chorea, stomatitis, and ophthalmoplegia. Hair loss and nail dystrophy (Mees' lines) may appear after 2–4 weeks.

IV. Diagnosis. Thallotoxicosis should be considered when gastroenteritis and painful parasthesia are followed by alopecia.
- **A. Specific levels.** Urinary thallium is normally less than 0.8 μg/L. Concentrations greater than 20 μg/L are evidence of excessive exposure and may be associated with subclinical toxicity during workplace exposures. Blood thallium levels are not considered reliable measures of exposure, except after large exposures. Hair levels are of limited value, mainly in documenting past exposure or in forensic cases.
- **B. Other useful laboratory studies** include CBC, electrolytes, glucose, BUN, creatinine, and hepatic transaminases. Since thallium is radiopaque, plain abdominal x-rays may be useful after acute ingestion.

V. Treatment.
- **A. Emergency and supportive measures**
  1. Maintain an open airway and assist ventilation if necessary (see pp 1–7).
  2. Treat seizures (p 21) and coma (p 18) if they occur.
  3. Treat gastroenteritis with aggressive intravenous replacement of fluids (and blood if needed). Use pressors only if shock does not respond to fluid therapy (p 15).
- **B. Specific drugs and antidotes.** There is currently no recommended specific treatment in the United States.
  1. **Prussian blue** (ferric ferrocyanide) is the mainstay of therapy in Europe. This compound has a crystal lattice structure, which binds thallium ions and interrupts enterohepatic recycling. The recommended dose is 250 mg/kg/d via a nasogastric tube in 2–4 divided doses, and administration is continued until urinary thallium excretion is less than 0.5 mg/24 h. Prussian blue appears to be nontoxic at these doses. Unfortunately, it is not available as a pharmaceutical-grade product in the United States, although it can be found as a common chemical laboratory reagent.
  2. **Activated charcoal** is readily available and has been shown to bind thallium in vitro. Multiple-dose charcoal is recommended because thallium apparently undergoes enterohepatic recirculation. In one study, charcoal was shown to be superior to Prussian blue in eliminating thallium.
  3. BAL (see p 341) and other chelators have been tried with varying success. Penicillamine and diethyldithiocarbamate should be avoided because of studies suggesting they contribute to redistribution of thallium to the brain.
- **C. Decontamination** (see p 43)
  1. **Prehospital.** Administer activated charcoal if available. Ipecac-induced vomiting may be useful for initial treatment at the scene (eg, children at home) if it can be given within a few minutes of exposure.
  2. **Hospital.** Administer activated charcoal. Consider gastric lavage for large recent ingestion.
- **D. Enhanced elimination.** Repeat-dose activated charcoal may enhance fecal elimination by binding thallium secreted into the gut lumen or via the biliary system, interrupting enterohepatic or enteroenteric recirculation. Forced diuresis, dialysis, and hemoperfusion are of no proven benefit.

► **THEOPHYLLINE**

Kent R. Olson, MD

Theophylline is a methylxanthine used for the treatment of asthma. Intravenous infusions of aminophylline, the ethylenediamine salt of theophylline, are used to treat bronchospasm, congestive heart failure, and neonatal apnea. Theophylline is most commonly used orally in sustained-release preparations (eg, Theo-Dur, Slo-Phyllin, Theobid, and many others).

I. **Mechanism of toxicity.** The exact mechanism of toxicity is not known. Theophylline is an antagonist of adenosine receptors, and it inhibits phosphodiesterase at high levels, increasing intracellular cyclic adenosine monophosphate (cAMP). It also is known to release endogenous catecholamines at therapeutic concentrations and may itself stimulate beta-adrenergic receptors.

  Pharmacokinetics. Absorption may be delayed with sustained-relese preparations. The volume of distribution (Vd) is approximately 0.5 L/kg. The normal elimination half-life is 4–6 hours; this may be doubled by illnesses or interacting drugs that slow hepatic metabolism, such as liver disease, congestive heart failure, influenza, erythromycin, or cimetidine, and may increase to as much as 20 hours after overdose. (See also Table II–55, p 331.)

II. **Toxic dose.** An acute single dose of 8–10 mg/kg will raise the serum level by up to 15–20 mg/L. Acute oral overdose of more than 50 mg/kg may potentially result in a level above 100 mg/L and severe toxicity.

III. **Clinical presentation.** Two distinct syndromes of intoxication may occur, depending on whether the exposure is **acute** or **chronic.**

  A. **Acute single overdose** is usually a result of a suicide attempt or accidental childhood ingestion but may also be caused by accidental or iatrogenic misuse (therapeutic overdose).

   1. Usual manifestations include vomiting (sometimes with hematemesis), tremor, anxiety, and tachycardia. Metabolic effects include pronounced hypokalemia, hypophosphatemia, hyperglycemia, and metabolic acidosis.

   2. With serum levels above 90–100 mg/L, hypotension, ventricular arrhythmias, and seizures are common; status epilepticus is frequently resistant to anticonvulsant drugs.

   3. Seizures and other manifestations of severe toxicity may be delayed 12–16 hours or more after ingestion, in part owing to delayed absorption of drug from sustained-release preparations.

  B. **Chronic intoxication** occurs when excessive doses are administered repeatedly over 24 hours or longer or when intercurrent illness or an interacting drug interferes with hepatic metabolism of theophylline. The usual victims are very young infants or elderly patients, especially those with chronic obstructive lung disease.

   1. Vomiting may occur but is not as common as in acute overdose. Tachycardia is common, but hypotension is rare. Metabolic effects such as hypokalemia and hyperglycemia do not occur.

   2. Seizures may occur with lower serum levels (eg, 40–60 mg/L) and have been reported with levels as low as 20 mg/L.

IV. **Diagnosis** is based on a history of ingestion or the presence of tremor, tachycardia, and other manifestations in a patient known to be on theophylline. Hypokalemia strongly suggests acute overdose rather than chronic intoxication.

  A. **Specific levels.** Serum theophylline levels are essential for diagnosis and determination of emergency treatment. After acute oral overdose, obtain repeated levels every 2–4 hours; single determinations are not sufficient, because continued absorption from sustained-release preparations may result in peak levels 12–16 hours or longer after ingestion.

   1. Levels less than 90–100 mg/L after acute overdose are not usually associated with severe symptoms such as seizures or ventricular arrhythmias.

   2. However, with chronic intoxication, severe toxicity may occur with levels of 40–60 mg/L. **Note:** Acute caffeine overdose (see p 118) will cause a similar clinical picture and will produce falsely elevated theophylline concentrations with most commercial immunoassays.

  B. **Other useful laboratory studies** include electrolytes, glucose, BUN, creatinine, hepatic function tests, and ECG monitoring.

V. **Treatment.**

  A. **Emergency and supportive measures**

   1. Maintain an open airway and assist ventilation if necessary (see pp 1–7).

    2. Treat seizures (p 21), arrhythmias (pp 10–14), and hypotension (p 15) if they occur. Tachyarrhythmias and hypotension are best treated with a beta–adrenergic agent (see **B**, below).

    3. Hypokalemia is caused by intracellular movement of potassium and does not reflect a significant total body deficit; it usually resolves spontaneously without aggressive treatment.

    4. Monitor vital signs, ECG, and serial theophylline levels for at least 16–18 hours after a significant oral overdose.

B. Specific drugs and antidotes. Hypotension, tachycardia, and ventricular arrhythmias are caused primarily by excessive beta-adrenergic stimulation. Treat with low-dose **propranolol** (see p 405), 0.01–0.03 mg/kg IV, or **esmolol** (see p 366), 25–50 µg/kg/min. Use beta blockers cautiously in patients with a prior history of asthma or wheezing.

C. Decontamination (see p 43)

    1. Prehospital. Administer activated charcoal if available. Ipecac-induced vomiting may be useful for initial treatment at the scene (eg, children at home) if it can be given within a few minutes of exposure.

    2. Hospital. Administer activated charcoal. Gastric emptying is not necessary for small ingestions if activated charcoal can be given promptly.

    3. Undissolved sustained-release tablets may not be removed with even the largest (40F) gastric tube. For significant ingestions, consider the following special techniques:

      a. Administer repeated doses of activated charcoal (p 54).

      b. Perform whole-bowel irrigation (p 50).

D. Enhanced elimination (see p 51). Theophylline has a small volume of distribution (0.5 L/kg) and is efficiently removed by dialysis, charcoal hemoperfusion, or repeat-dose activated charcoal.

    1. Hemoperfusion should be performed if the patient is in status epilepticus or if the serum theophylline concentration is greater than 100 mg/L. **Hemodialysis** is almost as effective and may be used if hemoperfusion is not readily available.

    2. Repeat-dose activated charcoal (see p 54) is not as effective as hemoperfusion but may be used for stable patients with levels below 100 mg/L.

▶ THYROID HORMONE

Paul D. Pearigen, MD

Thyroid hormone is available as synthetic triiodothyronine (T_3, or liothyronine), synthetic tetraiodothyronine (T_4, levothyroxine, or Synthroid), or natural dessicated animal thyroid (containing both T_3 and T_4; Table II–53). Despite concern over the potentially life-threatening manifestations of thyrotoxicosis, serious toxicity rarely occurs after acute thyroid hormone ingestion.

  I. Mechanism of toxicity. Excessive thyroid hormone potentiates adrenergic activity in the cardiovascular, gastrointestinal, and neurologic systems. The effects of T_3 overdose are manifested within the first 6 hours after ingestion. In contrast,

TABLE II–53. DOSAGE EQUIVALENTS OF THYROID HORMONE

Thyroid USP	65 mg (1 grain)
l-Thyroxine (T_4, levothyroxine, synthroid)	0.1 mg (100 µg)
l-Triiodothyronine (T_3)	0.025 mg (25 µg)

symptoms of T_4 overdose may be delayed 2–5 days after ingestion while metabolic conversion to T_3 occurs.

II. **Toxic dose.**
   A. An acute ingestion of more than 3 mg of **levothyroxine** (T_4) or 0.75 mg of **tri-
      iodothyronine** (T_3) is considered potentially toxic. An adult has survived an
      ingestion of 48 g of unspecified thyroid tablets; a 15-month-old child had mod-
      erate symptoms after ingesting 1.5 g of desiccated thyroid.
   B. Euthyroid persons and children appear to have a high tolerance to the effects
      of an acute overdose. Patients with pre-existing cardiac disease and those
      with chronic overmedication have a lower threshold of toxicity. Sudden deaths
      have been reported after chronic thyroid hormone abuse in healthy adults.

III. **Clinical presentation.** The effects of an acute T_4 overdose may not be evident
   for several days because of a delay for metabolism of T_4 to more active T_3.
   A. **Mild to moderate intoxication** may cause sinus tachycardia, elevated tem-
      perature, diarrhea, vomiting, headache, anxiety, agitation, psychosis, and
      confusion.
   B. **Severe toxicity** may include supraventricular tachycardia, hyperthermia, and
      hypotension. There is one case report of a seizure after acute overdose.

IV. **Diagnosis** is based on a history of ingestion and signs and symptoms of increased sympathetic activity.
   A. **Specific levels**
      1. **Levothyroxine (T_4).** Serious poisoning is very unlikely, and blood levels
         may not be required unless symptoms develop over 5–7 days after the in-
         gestion. In this case, obtain free T_3 and T_4 concentrations and total T_3 and
         T_4 levels with T_3 resin uptake.
      2. **Thyroid USP or triiodothyronine (T_3).** Serious poisoning is more likely.
         Obtain free and total T_3 levels approximately 2–6 hours after an acute in-
         gestion; repeat over the following 5–7 days. There is a reasonable qualita-
         tive relationship between the presence of elevated levels and the presence
         of symptoms.
   B. **Other useful laboratory studies** include electrolytes, glucose, BUN, creati-
      nine, and ECG monitoring.

V. **Treatment.**
   A. **Emergency and supportive measures**
      1. Maintain an open airway and assist ventilation if necessary (see pp 1–7).
      2. Treat seizures (p 21), hyperthermia (p 20), hypotension (p 15), and ar-
         rhythmias (pp 10–14) if they occur.
      3. Repeated evaluation over several days is recommended after T_4 or com-
         bined ingestions, because serious symptoms may be delayed.
      4. Most patients will suffer no serious toxicity or will recover with simple sup-
         portive care.
   B. **Specific drugs and antidotes**
      1. Treat serious tachyarrhythmias with **propranolol** (see p 405), 0.01–0.1
         mg/kg IV repeated every 2–5 minutes to desired effect, or **esmolol** (see
         p 366), 25–100 µg/kg/min IV. Simple sinus tachycardia may be treated
         with oral propranolol, 0.1–0.5 mg/kg every 4–6 hours.
      2. Peripheral metabolic conversion of T_4 to T_3 can be partially inhibited by
         propylthiouracil, 6–10 mg/kg/d (maximum 1 g) divided into three oral
         doses, for 5–7 days.
   C. **Decontamination** (see p 43)
      1. **Prehospital.** Administer activated charcoal if available. Ipecac-induced
         vomiting may be useful for initial treatment at the scene (eg, children at
         home) if it can be given within a few minutes of exposure.
      2. **Hospital.** Administer activated charcoal. Gastric emptying is not neces-
         sary after small ingestions if activated charcoal can be given promptly.
   D. **Enhanced elimination.** Diuresis and hemodialysis are not useful because
      thyroid hormones are extensively protein bound. Charcoal hemoperfusion
      may be effective, but limited data are available. Exchange transfusion has
      been performed in children and adults, but data on its efficacy are limited.

▶ TOLUENE AND XYLENE

Janet Weiss, MD

Toluene (methylbenzene) and xylene (dimethylbenzene and xylol) are very common aromatic solvents widely used in glues, inks, dyes, lacquers, varnishes, paints, paint removers, pesticides, cleaners, and degreasers. The largest source of exposure to toluene is in the production and use of gasoline. Toluene is also frequently abused intentionally by inhaling paints containing toluene to induce a "sniffer's high."

I. **Mechanism of toxicity.** Toluene and xylene cause generalized central nervous system depression. Like other aromatic hydrocarbons, they may sensitize the myocardium to the arrhythmogenic effects of catecholamines. They are mild mucous membrane irritants affecting the eyes and respiratory and gastrointestinal tracts. Pulmonary aspiration can cause a hydrocarbon pneumonitis (see p 183). Chronic abuse of toluene can cause diffuse CNS demyelination, renal tubular damage, and myopathy.

Kinetics. Toluene is metabolized by alcohol dehydrogenase, and the presence of ethanol can inhibit toluene metabolism and prolong systemic toxicity.

II. **Toxic dose.**
A. **Ingestion.** As little as 15–20 mL of toluene is reported to cause serious toxicity. A 60-mL dose was fatal in an adult male, with death occurring within 30 minutes.
B. **Inhalation.** The recommended workplace limits (ACGIH TLV-TWA) are 50 ppm (188 mg/m^3) for toluene and 100 ppm (434 mg/m^3) for xylene, as 8-hour time-weighted averages, with a "skin" notation indicating the potential for appreciable skin absorption. The air levels considered immediately dangerous to life or health (IDLH) are 500 ppm for toluene and 900 ppm for xylene.
C. Prolonged **dermal** exposure may cause chemical burns; both toluene and xylene are well-absorbed across the skin.

III. **Clinical presentation.** Toxicity may be a result of ingestion, pulmonary aspiration, or inhalation.
A. **Ingestion** of toluene or xylene may cause vomiting and diarrhea, and if pulmonary aspiration occurs, chemical pneumonitis may result. Systemic absorption may lead to CNS depression.
B. **Inhalation** produces euphoria, dizziness, headache, nausea, and weakness. Exposure to high concentrations may rapidly cause delirium, coma, pulmonary edema, respiratory arrest, and death. Arrhythmias may occasionally occur due to cardiac sensitization. Both tachydysrhythmias and bradydysrhythmias have been reported.
C. **Chronic exposure** to toluene may cause permanent CNS impairment, including tremors; ataxia; brainstem, cerebellar and cerebral atrophy; and cognitive and neurobehavioral abnormalities. Myopathy, hypokalemia, and renal tubular acidosis are also common. Animal studies suggest that toluene may cause adverse reproductive effects.

IV. Diagnosis is based on a history of exposure and typical manifestations of acute CNS effects such as euphoria or "drunkenness." After acute ingestion, pulmonary aspiration is suggested by coughing, choking, tachypnea, or wheezing and is confirmed by chest x-ray.
A. **Specific levels.** In acute symptomatic exposures, toluene or xylene may be detectable in blood drawn with a gas-tight syringe, but usually only for a few hours. The metabolites hippuric acid, ortho-cresol (toluene), and methylhippuric acid (xylene) are excreted in the urine and can be used to document exposure, but urine levels do not correlate with systemic effects.
B. **Other useful laboratory studies** include electrolytes, glucose, BUN, creatinine, liver transaminases, CPK, and urinalysis.

V. **Treatment.**
A. **Emergency and supportive measures**
1. Maintain an open airway and assist ventilation if necessary (see pp 1–7). Administer supplemental oxygen, and monitor arterial blood gases and chest x-rays.

    a. If the patient is coughing or dyspneic, aspiration pneumonia is likely. Treat as for hydrocarbon pneumonia (see p 183).

    b. If the patient remains asymptomatic after a 6-h observation period, chemical pneumonia is unlikely and further observation or chest x-ray is not needed.

  2. Treat coma (p 18), arrhythmias (pp 10–14), and bronchospasm (p 8) if they occur. *Caution:* Epinephrine and other sympathomimetic amines can provoke or aggravate cardiac arrhythmias. Tachyarrhythmias may be treated with **propranolol** (p 405), 1–2 mg IV, or **esmolol** (p 366), 25–100 μg/kg/min IV.

B. Specific drugs and antidotes. There is no specific antidote.

C. Decontamination. Rescuers should treat heavily contaminated victims in a well-ventilated area or should use self-contained breathing apparatus or other appropriate respiratory protection, as well as chemical-resistant clothing and gloves.

  1. Inhalation. Remove the victim from exposure and give supplemental oxygen if available.

  2. Skin and eyes. Remove contaminated clothes and wash exposed skin with soap and water. Irrigate exposed eyes with copious tepid water or saline.

  3. Ingestion (see p 45)

    a. Prehospital. Administer activated charcoal if available. Do *not* induce vomiting because of the risk of rapidly progressive CNS depression.

    b. Hospital. Administer activated charcoal. Consider gastric lavage for large ingestions (> 1–2 oz) if it can be performed within 30 minutes of ingestion.

D. Enhanced elimination. There is no role for enhanced elimination.

▶ TRICHLOROETHANE AND TRICHLOROETHYLENE

Diane Liu, MD, MPH

Trichloroethane and trichloroethylene are widely used solvents found as ingredients in many products including typewriter correction fluid ("white-out"), color film cleaners, insecticides, spot removers, fabric cleaning solutions, adhesives, and paint removers. They are used extensively in industry as degreasers. Trichloroethane is available in 2 isomeric forms, 1,1,2- and 1,1,1-, with the latter (also known as methyl chloroform) being the most common.

I. Mechanism of toxicity.

  A. Trichloroethane and trichloroethylene act as respiratory and central nervous system depressants and skin and mucous membrane irritants. They have rapid anesthetic action, and both were used for this purpose medically until the advent of safer agents.

  B. Trichloroethane, trichloroethylene, and their metabolite trichloroethanol may sensitize the myocardium to the arrhythmogenic effects of catecholamines.

  C. Trichloroethylene or a metabolite may act to inhibit acetaldehyde dehydrogenase, blocking the metabolism of ethanol and causing "degreaser's flush."

  D. NIOSH considers 1,1,2-trichloroethane and trichloroethylene possible carcinogens.

II. Toxic dose.

  A. Trichloroethane. The acute lethal oral dose to humans is reportedly between 0.5–5 mL/kg. The recommended workplace limits (ACGIH TLV-TWA) in air for the 1,1,1- and 1,1,2-isomers are 350 and 10 ppm, respectively, and the air levels considered immediately dangerous to life or health (IDLH) are 700 and 100 ppm, respectively. Anesthetic levels are in the range of 10,000–26,000 ppm. The odor is detectable by a majority of people at 500 ppm, but olfactory fatigue commonly occurs.

    B. **Trichloroethylene.** The acute lethal oral dose is reported to be approximately 3–5 mL/kg. The recommended workplace limit (ACGIH TLV-TWA) is 50 ppm (269 mg/m³), and the air level considered immediately dangerous to life or health (IDLH) is 1000 ppm.

III. **Clinical presentation.** Toxicity may be a result of inhalation, skin contact, or ingestion.

    A. **Inhalation or ingestion** may cause nausea, euphoria, ataxia, dizziness, agitation, and lethargy, and if intoxication is significant, respiratory arrest, seizures, and coma. Hypotension and cardiac arrhythmias may occur. With severe overdose, renal and hepatic injury may be apparent 1–2 days after exposure.

    B. **Local effects** of exposure to liquid or vapors include irritation of the eyes, nose, and throat. Prolonged skin contact can cause defatting and dermatitis.

    C. **Ingestion.** Aspiration into the tracheobronchial tree may result in hydrocarbon pneumonia (see p 183).

    D. **Degreaser's flush.** Workers exposed to these vapors may have acute flushing and orthostatic hypotension if they ingest alcohol, owing to a disulfiramlike effect (see Disulfiram, p 158).

IV. **Diagnosis** is based on a history of exposure and typical symptoms. Addictive inhalational abuse of typewriter correction fluid suggests trichloroethylene poisoning.

    A. **Specific levels**

        1. Although trichloroethane can be measured in expired air, blood, and urine, levels are not routinely rapidly available and are not needed for evaluation or treatment. Confirmation of exposure might be possible by detecting the metabolite trichloroethanol in the blood or urine. Hospital laboratory methods are not usually sensitive to these amounts.

        2. Breath analysis is becoming more widely used for workplace exposure control, and serial measurements may allow for estimation of the amount absorbed.

    B. **Other useful laboratory studies** include electrolytes, glucose, BUN, creatinine, liver transaminases, arterial blood gases, and ECG monitoring.

V. **Treatment.**

    A. **Emergency and supportive measures**

        1. Maintain an open airway and assist ventilation if necessary (see pp 1–7). Administer supplemental oxygen, and treat hydrocarbon aspiration pneumonitis (p 183) if it occurs.

        2. Treat seizures (p 21), coma (p 18), and arrhythmias (pp 10–14) if they occur. *Caution:* Avoid the use of epinephrine or other sympathomimetic amines because of the risk of inducing or aggravating cardiac arrhythmias. Tachyarrhythmias caused by myocardial sensitization may be treated with **propranolol** (p 405), 1–2 mg IV, or **esmolol** (p 366), 25–100 µg/kg/min IV.

        3. Monitor for a minimum of 4–6 hours after significant exposure.

    B. **Specific drugs and antidotes.** There is no specific antidote.

    C. **Decontamination** (see p 43)

        1. **Inhalation.** Remove the victim from exposure and administer supplemental oxygen, if available.

        2. **Skin and eyes.** Remove contaminated clothing and wash exposed skin with soap and water. Irrigate exposed eyes with copious tepid water or saline.

        3. **Ingestion** (see p 45)

            a. **Prehospital.** Administer activated charcoal if available. Do *not* induce vomiting because of the danger of rapid absorption and abrupt onset of seizures or coma.

            b. **Hospital.** Administer activated charcoal orally or by gastric tube. Consider gastric lavage; for small ingestions (< 30 mL), oral activated charcoal alone without gut emptying may be sufficient.

    D. **Enhanced elimination.** These procedures are not effective or necessary.

▶ TRICYCLIC ANTIDEPRESSANTS

Neal L. Benowitz, MD

Tricyclic antidepressants are commonly taken in overdose by suicidal patients and represent a major cause of poisoning hospitalizations and deaths. Currently available tricyclic antidepressants are described in Table II–54. Amitriptyline is also marketed in combination with chlordiazepoxide (Limbitrol) or perphenazine (Etrafon or Triavil).

Cyclobenzaprine (Flexeril), a centrally acting muscle relaxant (see p 291), is structurally related to the tricyclic antidepressants but exhibits minimal cardiotoxic and variable CNS effects. **Newer, noncyclic antidepressants** are discussed on p 79. **Monoamine oxidase inhibitors** are discussed on page 225.

I. **Mechanism of toxicity.** Tricyclic antidepressant toxicity affects primarily the cardiovascular and central nervous systems.

    A. **Cardiovascular effects.** Several mechanisms contribute to cardiovascular toxicity.

        1. Anticholinergic effects and inhibition of neuronal reuptake of catecholamines result in tachycardia and mild hypertension.

        2. Peripheral alpha-adrenergic blockade induces vasodilation.

        3. Membrane-depressant (quinidinelike) effects cause myocardial depression and cardiac conduction disturbances by inhibition of the fast sodium channel that initiates the cardiac cell action potential. Metabolic or respiratory acidosis may contribute to cardiotoxicity by further inhibiting the fast sodium channel.

    B. **Central nervous system effects.** These result in part from anticholinergic toxicity (eg, sedation and coma), but seizures are probably a result of inhibition of reuptake of norepinephrine or serotonin in the brain or other central effects.

    C. **Pharmacokinetics.** Anticholinergic effects of the drugs may retard gastric emptying, resulting in slow or erratic absorption. Most of these drugs are extensively bound to body tissues and plasma proteins, resulting in very large volumes of distribution and long elimination half-lives (Table II–54 and II–55). Tricyclic antidepressants are primarily metabolized by the liver, with only a small fraction excreted unchanged in the urine. Active metabolites may con-

TABLE II–54. TRICYCLIC ANTIDEPRESSANTS

Drug	Usual Adult Daily Dose (mg)	Usual Half-Life (h)	Toxicity[a]
Amitriptyline	75–200	9–25	A, C, S
Amoxapine	150–300	8–30	S
Clomipramine	100–250	20–40	A, C, S
Desipramine	75–200	12–24	A, C, S
Doxepin	75–300	8–15	A, C, S
Imipramine	75–200	11–25	A, C, S
Maprotiline	75–300	21–50	C, S
Nortriptyline	75–150	18–35	A, C, S
Protriptyline	20–40	54–92	A, C, S
Trimipramine	75–200	15–30	A, C, S

[a]A = anticholinergic; C = cardiovascular; S = seizures.

tribute to toxicity; several drugs are metabolized to other well-known tricyclic antidepressants (eg, amitriptyline to nortriptyline and imipramine to desipramine).

II. **Toxic dose.** Most of the tricyclic antidepressants have a narrow therapeutic index so that doses of less than 10 times the therapeutic daily dose may produce severe intoxication. In general, ingestion of 10–20 mg/kg is potentially life threatening.

III. **Clinical presentation.** Triyclic antidepressant poisoning may produce any of three major toxic syndromes: anticholinergic effects, cardiovascular effects, and seizures. Depending on the dose and the drug, patients may experience some or all of these toxic effects. Symptoms usually begin within 30–40 minutes of ingestion but may be delayed owing to erratic gut absorption. Patients who are initially awake may abruptly lose consciousness or develop seizures without warning.

  A. **Anticholinergic** effects include sedation, delirium, coma, dilated pupils, dry skin and mucous membranes, diminished sweating, tachycardia, diminished or absent bowel sounds, and urinary retention. Myoclonic or myokymic jerking is common with anticholinergic intoxication and may be mistaken for seizure activity.

  B. **Cardiovascular** toxicity manifests as abnormal cardiac conduction, arrhythmias, and hypotension.

    1. Typical electrocardiographic findings include sinus tachycardia with prolongation of the PR, QRS, and QT intervals. Various degrees of atrioventricular (AV) block may be seen. Prolongation of the QRS complex to 0.12 s or longer is a fairly reliable predictor of serious cardiovascular and neurologic toxicity (except in the case of amoxapine, which causes seizures and coma with no change in the QRS interval).

    2. Sinus tachycardia accompanied by QRS interval prolongation may resemble ventricular tachycardia (see Figure I–4, p 11). True ventricular tachycardia and fibrillation may also occur. Atypical or polymorphous ventricular tachycardia (torsades de pointes; see Figure I–5, p 12) associated with QT interval prolongation may occur with therapeutic dosing, but is actually uncommon in overdose. Development of bradyarrhythmias usually indicates a severely poisoned heart and carries a poor prognosis.

    3. Hypotension caused by venodilation is common and usually mild. In severe cases, hypotension results from myocardial depression and may be refractory to treatment; some patients die with progressive intractable cardiogenic shock. Pulmonary edema is also common in severe poisonings.

  C. **Seizures** are common with tricyclic antidepressant toxicity and may be recurrent or persistent. The muscular hyperactivity from seizures and myoclonic jerking, combined with diminished sweating, can lead to severe hyperthermia (see p 20), resulting in rhabdomyolysis, brain damage, multisystem failure, and death.

  D. **Death** from tricyclic antidepressant overdose usually occurs within a few hours of admission and may result from ventricular fibrillation, intractable cardiogenic shock, or status epilepticus with hyperthermia. Sudden death several days after apparent recovery has occasionally been reported, but in all such cases there was evidence of continuing cardiac toxicity within 24 hours of death.

IV. **Diagnosis.** Tricyclic antidepressant poisoning should be suspected in any patient with lethargy, coma, or seizures accompanied by QRS interval prolongation. QRS interval prolongation greater than 0.12 s in the limb leads suggests severe poisoning. However, with amoxapine, seizures and coma may occur with no widening of the QRS interval.

  A. **Specific levels**

    1. Plasma levels of some of the tricyclic antidepressants can be measured by clinical laboratories. Therapeutic concentrations are usually less than 0.3 μg/mL (300 ng/mL). Total concentrations of parent drug plus metabolite of 1 μg/mL (1000 ng/mL) or greater are usually associated with serious poisoning. Generally, plasma levels are not used in emergency management

because the QRS interval and clinical manifestations of overdose are reliable and more readily available indicators of toxicity.

2. Most tricyclics are detectable on comprehensive urine toxicology screening. Some rapid immunologic techniques are available and have sufficiently broad cross-reactivity to detect several tricyclics. However, use of these assays for rapid screening in the hospital laboratory is not recommended because they may miss some important drugs and give positive results for others present in therapeutic concentrations.

B. **Other useful laboratory studies** include electrolytes, glucose, BUN, creatinine, CPK, urinalysis for myoglobin, arterial blood gases or oximetry, 12-lead ECG and continuous ECG monitoring, and chest x-ray.

V. **Treatment.**

A. **Emergency and supportive measures**
1. Maintain an open airway and assist ventilation if necessary (see pp 1–7). *Caution:* Respiratory arrest can occur abruptly and without warning.
2. Treat coma (p 18), seizures (p 21), hyperthermia (p 20), hypotension (p 15), and arrhythmias (pp 10–14) if they occur. *Note:* Do not use procainamide or other Type Ia or Ic antiarrhythmic agents for ventricular tachycardia, because these drugs may aggravate cardiotoxicity.
3. Consider cardiac pacing for bradyarrhythmias and high-degree AV block, and overdrive pacing for Torsades de pointes.
4. Mechanical support of the circulation (eg, cardiopulmonary bypass) may be useful (based on anecdotal reports) to stabilize patients with refractory shock, allowing time for the body to eliminate some of the drug.
5. If seizures are not immediately controlled with usual anticonvulsants, paralyze the patient with a neuromuscular blocker such as pancuronium (p 386) to prevent hyperthermia, which may induce further seizures, and lactic acidosis, which aggravates cardiotoxicity. *Note:* Paralysis abolishes the muscular manifestations of seizures, but has no effect on brain seizure activity. After paralysis, ECG monitoring is necessary to determine the efficacy of anticonvulsant therapy.
6. Continuously monitor the temperature, other vital signs, and ECG in asymptomatic patients for a minimum of 6 hours, and admit patients to an intensive care setting for at least 24 hours if there are any signs of toxicity.

B. **Specific drugs and antidotes**
1. In patients with QRS interval prolongation or hypotension, administer **sodium bicarbonate** (see p 345), 1–2 mEq/kg IV, and repeat as needed to maintain the arterial pH between 7.45 and 7.55. Sodium bicarbonate may reverse membrane-depressant effects by increasing extracellular sodium concentrations and by a direct effect of pH on the fast sodium channel.
2. Hyperventilation, by inducing a respiratory alkalosis (or reversing respiratory acidosis), may also be of benefit but works only transiently and may provoke seizures.
3. Although **physostigmine** has been widely advocated in the past, it should *not* be routinely administered to patients with tricyclic antidepressant poisoning; it may aggravate conduction disturbances, causing asystole, further impair myocardial contractility, worsening hypotension, and contribute to seizures.

C. **Decontamination** (see p 43)
1. **Prehospital.** Administer activated charcoal if available. Do *not* induce vomiting because of the risk of abrupt onset of seizures.
2. **Hospital.** Administer activated charcoal. Perform gastric lavage for large ingestions (eg, > 20–30 mg/kg). Gastric emptying is probably not necessary for smaller ingestions if activated charcoal can be given promptly.

D. **Enhanced elimination.** Owing to extensive tissue and protein binding with a resulting large volume of distribution, dialysis and hemoperfusion are not effective. Although repeat-dose charcoal has been reported to accelerate tricyclic antidepressant elimination, the data are not convincing.

▶ VACOR (PNU)

Neal L. Benowitz, MD

Vacor rat killer (2% *N*-3-pyridylmethyl-*N'*-*p*-nitrophenylurea; PNU) is a unique rodenticide that causes irreversible insulin-dependent diabetes and autonomic nervous system injury. It was removed from general sale in the United States in 1979 but is still available in some homes and for use by licensed exterminators. The product was sold in 39-g packets of cornmeal-like material containing 2% PNU.

I. **Mechanism of toxicity.** PNU is believed to antagonize the actions of nicotinamide and, in a manner similar to that of alloxan and streptozocin, injure pancreatic beta cells. The mechanisms of autonomic neuropathy and central nervous system effects are unknown. Adrenergic neurons acting on blood vessels but not the heart are affected. As a result, orthostatic hypotension associated with an intact reflex tachycardia is the usual picture.

II. **Toxic dose.** Acute toxicity has usually occurred after ingestion of one 39-g packet of Vacor (approximately 8 g of PNU). The smallest dose reported to cause toxicity was 390 mg.

III. **Clinical presentation.** Initial symptoms include nausea and vomiting. Occasionally, confusion, stupor, and coma occur after several hours. After a delay of several hours to days, irreversible autonomic neuropathy, peripheral neuropathy, and diabetes may occur.

   A. **Autonomic dysfunction.** Dizziness or syncope or both caused by severe orthostatic hypotension occur with an onset from 6 hours to 2 days after ingestion. Orthostatic hypotension is usually accompanied by intact reflex tachycardia. Other manifestations of autonomic neuropathy include dysphagia, recurrent vomiting, and constipation.

   B. **Insulin-dependent diabetes mellitus**, with polyuria, polydipsia, hyperglycemia, and ketoacidosis, occurs after a few days. Hypoglycemia, resulting from insulin release, occasionally precedes hyperglycemia.

   C. **Peripheral neuropathy** may cause paresthesias and muscle weakness.

IV. **Diagnosis.** Sudden onset of orthostatic hypotension or diabetes mellitus should suggest the possibility of Vacor ingestion. A careful investigation should be performed to determine what rat-killing chemicals may be present in the home.

   A. **Specific levels.** PNU levels are not available.

   B. **Other useful laboratory studies** include electrolytes, glucose, BUN, and creatinine.

V. **Treatment.**

   A. **Emergency and supportive measures**

     1. Maintain an open airway and assist ventilation if necessary (see pp 1–7).

     2. Orthostatic hypotension usually responds to supine positioning and intravenous fluids. Chronic therapy includes a high-salt diet and fludrocortisone (0.1–1 mg/d).

     3. Treat diabetes in the usual manner with fluids and insulin.

   B. **Specific drugs and antidotes.** Immediately administer **nicotinamide** (see p 389). Although its efficacy in humans is not proved, nicotinamide can prevent PNU-induced diabetes in rats.

   C. **Decontamination** (see p 43)

     1. **Prehospital.** Administer activated charcoal if available. Ipecac-induced vomiting may be useful for initial treatment at the scene (eg, children at home) if it can be given within a few minutes of exposure.

     2. **Hospital.** Administer activated charcoal. For large ingestions (eg, more than 1 packet), consider gastric lavage and extra doses of charcoal (ie, to maintain 10:1 ratio of charcoal to PNU).

   D. **Enhanced elimination.** Forced diuresis, dialysis, and hemoperfusion are not effective. Repeat-dose charcoal treatment has not been studied.

▶ VALPROIC ACID

Thomas E. Kearney, PharmD

Valproic acid (Depakene or Depakote [divalproex sodium]) is a structurally unique anticonvulsant. It is used alone or in combination with other agents for the treatment of absence seizures, partial complex, and generalized seizure disorders and is a secondary agent for refractory status epilepticus. It is also commonly used for the propylaxis and treatment of acute manic episodes and other affective disorders.

I. Mechanism of toxicity.

   A. Valproic acid is a small-molecular-weight (144.21), branched-chain carboxylic acid (pK_a = 4.8) that increases levels of the inhibitory neurotransmitter γ-aminobutyric acid (GABA) and prolongs the recovery of inactivated sodium channels. These properties may be responsible for its action as a general central nervous system depressant. Valproic acid also alters amino acid and fatty acid metabolism and can cause hepatotoxicity and metabolic pertubations.

   B. Pharmacokinetics

   1. Valproic acid is rapidly and completely absorbed from the gastrointestinal tract. There is a delay in the absorption with the preparation Depakote (divalproex sodium), because of its delayed-release formulation as well as the intestinal conversion of divalproex to 2 molecules of valproic acid.

   2. At therapeutic levels, valproic acid is highly protein bound (80–95%) and primarily confined to the extracellular space with a small (0.13–0.22 L/kg) volume of distribution (Vd). In overdose and at levels exceeding 90 mg/mL, saturation of protein-binding sites occurs, resulting in a greater circulating free fraction of valproic acid and a larger Vd.

   3. Valproic acid is predominantly metabolized by the liver and may undergo some degree of enterohepatic recirculation. The elimination half-life is 5–20 hours (average 10.6 hours). In overdose, the half-life may be prolonged to as long as 30 hours. A level exceeding 1000 mg/mL may not drop into the therapeutic range for at least 3 days. In addition, active metabolites (eg, the neurotoxic 2-en-valproic acid) may contribute to prolonged or delayed toxicity.

II. Toxic dose. The usual daily dose for adults is 1.2–1.5 g, to achieve therapeutic serum levels of 50–100 mg/mL, and the suggested maximum daily dose is 60 mg/kg. Acute ingestions exceeding 200 mg/kg are associated with high risk for significant CNS depression. The lowest published fatal dose is 15 g (750 mg/kg) in a 20-month-old child, but adult patients have survived after ingestions of 75 g.

III. Clinical presentation.

   A. Acute overdose

   1. Acute ingestion commonly causes gastrointestinal upset, variable CNS depression (confusion, disorientation, obtundation, and coma with respiratory failure), and occasionally hypotension with tachycardia. The pupils may be miotic, and the presentation may mimic an opiate poisoning. Cardiorespiratory arrest has been associated with severe intoxication; and the morbidity and mortality from valproic acid poisoning seem to be related primarily to hypoxia.

   2. Paradoxic seizures may occur in patients with a pre-existing seizure disorder.

   3. Transient rises of transaminase levels have been observed, without evidence of liver toxicity. Hyperammonemia with encephalopathy has been observed with therapeutic levels and in overdose.

   4. At very high serum levels (> 1000 mg/mL) after large ingestions, other metabolic and electrolyte abnormalities may be observed, including an increased anion gap acidosis, hypocalcemia, and hypernatremia.

   5. Other complications or late sequelae (days after ingestion) associated with severe intoxication may include optic nerve atrophy, cerebral edema, noncardiogenic pulmonary edema, anuria, and pancreatitis (in one fatal case).

B. **Adverse effects of chronic valproic acid therapy** include hepatic failure (high-risk patients are less than 2 years of age, receiving multiple anticonvulsants, or have other long-term neurologic complications) and weight gain. Hepatitis is not dose-related and is not usually seen after an acute overdose. Pancreatitis is usually considered a non-dose-related effect. Alopecia, red cell aplasia, thrombocytopenia, and neutropenia have been associated with both acute and chronic valproic acid intoxication.

C. Valproic acid is a known human teratogen.

IV. **Diagnosis** is based on the history of exposure and typical findings of CNS depression and metabolic disturbances. The differential diagnosis is broad and includes most CNS depressants. Encephalopathy and hyperammonemia may mimic Reye's syndrome.

A. **Specific levels.** Obtain a stat serum valproic acid level. Serial valproic acid level determinations should be obtained, particularly after ingestion of divaloproex-containing preparations (Depakote), owing to the potential for delayed absorption.

1. In general, serum levels exceeding 500 mg/mL are associated with drowsiness or obtundation, and levels greater than 1000 mg/mL are associated with coma with metabolic pertubations. However, there appears to be poor correlation of serum levels with outcome.

2. Death from acute valproic acid poisoning has been associated with peak levels ranging from 106–2728 mg/mL, and survival was reported in a patient with a peak level of 2120 mg/mL.

B. **Other useful laboratory studies** include electrolytes, glucose, BUN, creatinine, calcium, ammonia, liver transaminases, bilirubin, prothrombin time (PT), amylase, serum osmolality and osmolar gap (see p 30; serum levels > 1500 mg/mL may increase the osmolar gap by 10 mOsm/L or more), arterial blood gases or oximetry, and ECG monitoring. Valproic acid may cause a false-positive urine ketone determination.

V. **Treatment.**

A. **Emergency and supportive measures**

1. Maintain an open airway and assist ventilation if needed (see pp 1–7). Administer supplemental oxygen.

2. Treat coma (p 18), hypotension (p 15), and seizures (p 21) if they occur. Corticosteroids, hyperventilation, barbiturates, and osmotic agents have been used anecdotally to treat cerebral edema.

3. Treat acidosis, hypocalcemia, or hypernatremia if they are severe and symptomatic.

4. Monitor patients for at least 6 hours after ingestion and for up to 12 hours after ingestion of Depakote (divalproex sodium) because of the potential for delayed absorption.

B. **Specific drugs and antidotes.** There is no specific antidote. Naloxone (see p 384) has been reported to increase arousal, but inconsistently, with greatest success in patients with serum valproic acid levels of 185–190 mg/L. L-Carnitine has been used to treat valproic acid-induced hyperammonemia.

C. **Decontamination** (see p 43)

1. **Prehospital.** Administer activated charcoal if available. Do **not** induce vomiting, because valproic acid may cause abrupt onset of CNS depression and, in some patients, paradoxic seizures.

2. **Hospital.** Administer activated charcoal. Consider gastric lavage for large ingestions. Moderately large ingestions (eg, > 5–10 g) theoretically require extra doses of activated charcoal to maintain the desired charcoal:drug ratio of 10:1. The charcoal is not given all at once, but in repeated 25- to 50-g quantities over the first 12–24 hours. The addition of **whole bowel irrigation** (p 50) may be helpful in large ingestions of sustained release products such as divalproex (Depakote).

D. Enhanced elimination (see p 51). Although valproic acid is highly protein bound at therapeutic serum levels, saturation of protein binding in overdose makes valproic acid favorably disposed to enhanced removal methods.

1. **Hemodialysis and hemoperfusion.** Hemodialysis may result in a four- to fivefold decrease in elimination half-life in overdose patients. Dialysis also corrects metabolic disturbances and removes valproic acid metabolites. Consider dialysis in patients with serum valproic acid levels exceeding 1000 mg/L, since these cases are associated with higher morbidity and mortality. Charcoal hemoperfusion has also been utilized with clearances similar to those observed with hemodialysis.

2. **Repeat-dose activated charcoal.** Theoretically, repeated doses of charcoal may enhance clearance by interruption of enterohepatic recirculation, but no data exist to confirm or quantify this benefit. Another benefit is enhanced gastrointestinal decontamination after large or massive ingestion, since single doses of charcoal are inadequate to adsorb all ingested drug.

▶ VASODILATORS

Brett Roth, MD

A variety of vasodilators and alpha-receptor blockers are used in clinical medicine. Nonselective alpha-adrenergic blocking agents (eg, phenoxybenzamine, phentolamine, and tolazoline) have been used in clinical practice since the 1940s. The first selective α_1 blocker, prazosin, was introduced in the early 1970s; doxazosin, indoramin, terazosin, trimazosin, and urapidil are newer α_1-selective agents. Serious acute overdoses of these agents seldom occur. Nitroprusside (see p 235) and nitrates (see p 233) are discussed elsewhere.

I. **Mechanism of toxicity.** All these drugs dilate peripheral arterioles to lower blood pressure. A reflex sympathetic response results in tachycardia and occasionally cardiac arrhythmias. Prazosin and other newer α_1-specific agents are associated with little or no reflex tachycardia; however, postural hypotension is common, especially in patients with hypovolemia.

II. **Toxic dose.** The minimum toxic or lethal doses of these drugs have not been established. No fatalities have been reported except with indoramin overdose and excessive intravenous doses of phentolamine.

A. **Indoramin.** A 43-year-old woman died 6 hours after ingesting 2.5 g; central nervous system stimulation and seizures were also reported.

B. **Prazosin.** A young man developed priapism 24 hours after an overdose of 150 mg. A 19-year-old man became hypotensive after taking 200 mg and recovered within 36 hours. Two elderly men ingesting 40–120 mg were found comatose with Cheyne-Stokes breathing and recovered after 15–18 hours.

C. **Pharmacokinetics.** See Table II–55, p 319.

III. **Clinical presentation.** Acute overdose may cause headache, nausea, dizziness, weakness, syncope, orthostatic hypotension, warm flushed skin, and palpitations. Lethargy and ataxia may occur in children. Severe hypotension may result in cerebral and myocardial ischemia and acute renal failure. First-time users of α_1 blockers may experience syncope after therapeutic dosing.

IV. **Diagnosis** is based on a history of exposure and the presence of orthostatic hypotension, which may or may not be accompanied by reflex tachycardia.

A. **Specific levels.** Blood levels of these drugs are not routinely available or clinically useful.

B. **Other useful laboratory studies** include electrolytes, glucose, BUN, creatinine, and ECG and ECG monitoring.

V. **Treatment.**

A. **Emergency and supportive measures**

1. Maintain an open airway and assist ventilation if necessary (see pp 1–7).

2. Hypotension usually responds to supine positioning and intravenous crystalloid fluids. Occasionally, pressor therapy is needed (p 15).
B. Specific drugs and antidotes. There is no specific antidote.
C. Decontamination (see p 43)
1. **Prehospital.** Administer activated charcoal if available. Do **not** induce vomiting, because of the risk of hypotension and syncope.
2. **Hospital.** Administer activated charcoal. Gastric emptying is not necessary if activated charcoal can be given promptly.
D. Enhanced elimination. There is no clinical experience with extracorporeal drug removal for these agents. Terazosin and doxazosin are long-acting and eliminated 60% in feces; thus, repeat-dose activated charcoal may enhance their elimination.

▶ VITAMINS

Gerald Joe, PharmD

Acute toxicity is unlikely after ingestion of vitamin products that do not contain iron (when iron is present, see p 192). Vitamins A and D may cause toxicity but usually only after chronic use. The essential amino acid L-tryptophan is not a vitamin, but has been considered a dietary supplement and was widely used for treatment of depression, premenstrual symptoms, and insomnia until it was linked to the eosinophilia myalgia syndrome and its sale was banned by the FDA.

I. **Mechanism of toxicity.**
A. **Vitamin A.** The mechanism by which excessive amounts of vitamin A produce increased intracranial pressure is not known.
B. **Vitamin C.** Chronic excessive use and large intravenous doses can produce increased levels of the metabolite oxalic acid. Urinary acidification promotes calcium oxalate crystal formation, which can result in nephropathy or acute renal failure.
C. **Vitamin D.** Chronic ingestion of excessive amounts of vitamin D enhances calcium absorption and produces hypercalcemia.
D. **Niacin.** Histamine release results in cutaneous flushing and pruritus.
E. **Pyridoxine.** Chronic overdose may alter neuronal conduction, resulting in paresthesias and muscular incoordination.
F. **Tryptophan.** L-Tryptophan can enhance brain serotonin levels, especially in patients taking monoamine oxidase (MAO) inhibitors (see p 225). The mechanism involved in causing an epidemic of eosinophilia-myalgia syndrome is unknown, but appears to have been related to a contaminant associated with mass production of the amino acid by one Japanese producer.

II. **Toxic dose.**
A. **Vitamin A.** Acute ingestion of more than 12,000 IU/kg is considered toxic. Chronic ingestion of more than 25,000 IU/d for 2–3 weeks may produce toxicity.
B. **Vitamin C.** Acute intravenous doses of more than 1.5 g and chronic ingestion of more than 4 g/d have produced nephropathy.
C. **Vitamin D.** Acute ingestion is highly unlikely to produce toxicity. Chronic ingestion in children of more than 5000 IU/d for several weeks (adults > 25,000 IU/d) may result in toxicity.
D. **Niacin.** Acute ingestion of more than 100 mg may cause dermal flushing reaction.
E. **Pyridoxine.** Chronic ingestion of 2–5 g/d for several months has resulted in neuropathy.

III. **Clinical presentation.** Most acute overdoses of multivitamins are associated with nausea, vomiting, and diarrhea.
A. Chronic **vitamin A** toxicity is characterized by dry, peeling skin and signs of increased intracranial pressure (headache, altered mental status, and blurred

vision). Bulging fontanelles have been described in infants. Liver injury may cause jaundice and ascites.

B. Vitamin C. Calcium oxalate crystals may cause acute renal failure or chronic nephropathy.

C. Chronic excessive use of **vitamin D** is associated with hypercalcemia, producing weakness, altered mental status, gastrointestinal upset, renal tubular injury, and occasionally cardiac arrhythmias.

D. Chronic excessive use of **vitamin E** can cause nausea, headaches, and weakness.

E. Vitamin K can cause hemolysis in newborns (particularly if they are G6PD deficient).

F. Acute ingestion of **niacin** but not niacinamide (nicotinamide) may produce unpleasant dramatic cutaneous flushing and pruritus, which may last for a few hours. Chronic excessive use (particularly the sustained-release form) has been associated with hepatitis.

G. Chronic excessive **pyridoxine** use may result in peripheral neuropathy.

H. Large doses of **B vitamins** may intensify the yellow color of urine, and **riboflavin** may produce yellow perspiration.

I. Tryptophan
  1. Use of L-tryptophan by persons taking monoamine oxidase (MAO) inhibitors may cause myoclonus and hyperthermia ("serotonin syndrome," see p 20).
  2. Chronic use of L-tryptophan has been associated with development of eosinophilia-myalgia syndrome, characterized by high eosinophil counts (> 1000/μL), severe generalized myalgias, and swelling and induration of the skin. Fever, polyneuropathy, and death have also been reported.

IV. Diagnosis of vitamin overdose is usually based on a history of ingestion. Cutaneous flushing and pruritus suggest a niacin reaction but may be caused by other histaminergic agents.

A. Specific levels. Serum vitamin A (retinol) or carotenoid assays may assist in the diagnosis of hypervitaminosis A. Other serum vitamin concentration measurements are not useful.

B. Other useful laboratory studies include CBC, electrolytes, glucose, BUN, calcium, creatinine, liver transaminases, and urinalysis.

V. Treatment.
  A. Emergency and supportive measures
    1. Treat fluid losses caused by gastroenteritis with intravenous crystalloid solutions (see p 15).
    2. Treat vitamin A-induced elevated intracranial pressure and vitamin D-induced hypercalcemia if they occur.
    3. Antihistamines may alleviate niacin-induced histamine release.
  B. Specific drugs and antidotes. There is no specific antidote.
  C. Decontamination (see p 43). Usually, gut decontamination is unnecessary unless a toxic dose of vitamin A or D has been ingested, or if the product contains a toxic amount of iron.
    1. Prehospital. Administer activated charcoal if available. Ipecac-induced vomiting may be useful for initial treatment at the scene (eg, children at home) if it can be given within 30 minutes of exposure.
    2. Hospital. Administer activated charcoal. Gastric emptying is not necessary if activated charcoal can be given promptly.
  D. Enhanced elimination. Forced diuresis, dialysis, and hemoperfusion are of no clinical benefit.

TABLE II-55. PHARMACOKINETIC DATA[a]

Drug	Half-Life (h)	Vd (L/kg)	Onset (h)	Peak (h)	Duration (h)	Protein Binding %	Comments[b]
Acebutolol	3–6	3		2–4		20	
Acetaminophen	1–3	0.8–1	<1	0.5–2	4–6	25	S
Acetazolamide	1.5–8		1	1–4	8–12		
Acetohexamide			2	4	12–24		
Acrivastine	1.5		Rapid	1–2	6–8		M
Albuterol	2–5	2	0.25–0.5	1–2	4–8		S
Alfentenyl	1–2	0.3–1	<0.25	0.5–1		92	
Alprazolam	6–15	0.8–1.3		1–2		65–80	
Alprenolol	2–3 1 (metabolite)	3–6	0.5	2–4		85	M
Amantadine	7–37	4–8	1–4	1–4		60–70	
Amikacin	2–4	0.3		0.5–1.5		4–11	
Amiloride	21–144	5	2	3–10	24	23	
Amiodarone	35–68 days 60–90d (metabolite)	22–100	3–21 days	3–8	25–100 days	96–99	M Half-life 3–80 h after single dose.
Amitriptyline	9–25	8	1–2	4		95	D, M Metabolized to nortriptyline
Amlodipine	30–50	21	0.5–1	6–12	24	95	
Amobarbital	15–40	0.9–1.4	<1	2	6–8	59	
Amoxapine	8–16 30 (metabolite)	0.9–1.2		1–2		90	M
Amphetamine	7–14	6		2	4–24	16	Route-dependent kinetics

[a]Data provided are based on therapeutic dosing, not overdose. In general, after overdose the peak effect is delayed and the half-life and duration of effect are prolonged. Changes may occur in the volume of distribution and the percent protein bound.
[b]Key to abbreviations: D = delayed absorption may result in prolonged effect; M = active metabolite; S = sustained release formulations are available, and may lead to delayed absorption and prolonged effect. Kinetics may vary depending on the formulation.
Table compiled by Ilene B. Anderson, PharmD.

(continued)

TABLE II–55. PHARMACOKINETIC DATA[a] (CONTINUED)

Drug	Half-Life (h)	Vd (L/kg)	Onset (h)	Peak (h)	Duration (h)	Protein Binding %	Comments[b]
Amphotericin	24–48	4		1	20	95	
Aprobarbital	14–34		<1		6–8	55	
Aspirin0.5–10	0.1–0.3	0.5	1–2		49		D, S, Dose-dependent kinetics
Astemizole	1–9 days	250	<24	1–4	30–60 days	97	M
Atenolol	4–10	1	2	2–4		10	M
Atropine	2–4	2	Rapid	1	4	18	
Azithromycin	10–40	23–31	2–3	2–3			M
Baclofen	2.5–4	1–2.5	0.5–1	2–3	8	30–36	
Benazepril	0.6 11 (metabolite)	8.7		0.5–1 1–4 (metabolite)	24		M
Bendroflumethiazide	3–4		2	4	6–12		
Benzphetamine	6–12			3–4	4		M Metabolized to methamphetamine
Benzthiazide			2	4–6	6–18		
Benztropine	24	8	1–2	12	24	14–22	
Bepridil	24		1	2–3		99	
Betaxolol	12–22	5–13	1	2	12	55	M
Biperiden	18			1.5			
Bisoprolol	8–12	3		2–4		30	
Bretylium	5–14	5.4	<0.1	1–2	6–24	8	
Bromfenac	1–2						
Brompheniramine	25	12		2–5	4–6		
Bumetanide	2	13–25	0.5–1		6	95	S

Drug							
Bupivacaine	2–5	0.4–1	5 min	0.5–1	2–8	82–96	
Buprenorphine	2–3		0.5	1–3	6	10	
Bupropion	16	20–47	1–3	1–3		75–85	M
Buspirone	2–4	6		1		95	
Butabarbital	66–140		<1	0.5–1.5	6–8	26	
Butorphanol	3–4		<0.2	0.5–1	3–4	83	
Caffeine	3–6	0.6	0.5–1	0.5–2			
Captopril	<2	0.7	0.5	0.5–1.5		25–30	
Carbamazepine	15–24 / 5–10 (metabolite)	1.4–3		6–24+		75	D, M, S
Carbinoxamine	1–2				3–4		
Carisoprodol	1.5–8 / 8–17 (metabolite)	0.25	0.5	1–4	4–8	0	M — Metabolized to meprobamate
Carteolol	6		1	2	12–24	25	M
Cetrizine	8		Rapid	1	24	93	
Chloral hydrate	0.1 / 8–10 (metabolite)	0.7	0.5	0.5–1	4–8	35	M — Rapidly converted to trichloroethanol
Chloramphenicol	1.5–4	0.6–1.5		1–3		50–60	
Chlordiazepoxide	5–30	0.3		0.5–4		96	
Chloroquine	3–14 days	200		0.5–2		55	
Chlorothiazide	1–2	0.2	2	4	6–12		
Chlorpheniramine	12–43	2.5–7.5	1	2–6	4–6	70	S
Chlorpromazine	6–30	8–160	1	2–4	4–12	99	M
Chlorpropamide			1	3–6	24–72		
Chlorprothixene	8–12	4–20		4		99	
Chlorthalidone	40–65	3.9	2–3	2–6	24–72	99	

(continued)

TABLE II–55. PHARMACOKINETIC DATA[a] (CONTINUED)

Drug	Half-Life (h)	Vd (L/kg)	Onset (h)	Peak (h)	Duration (h)	Protein Binding %	Comments[b]
Chlorzoxazone	1		1	1–2	3–4		
Clemastine	4–6	13	Rapid	3–5	10–12		
Clidinium	2–20		1		3		
Clomipramine	20–40	10–20		3–4	93		D, M
Clonazepam	20–60	1.5–4.4		1–4		80	M
Clonidine	5–13	3–5.5	0.5–1	2–3	6–10	30	
Clorazepate	1–3 50–100 (metabolite)	1.5	Fast	1–2			M
Clozapine	5–13	0.5–3		2		95	
Cocaine	1–2.5	2–2.7	0.5 (oral)		0.5–1	10	Route-dependent kinetics
Codeine	2–4	3.5	< 0.5	0.5–1	4–6	20	M
Colchicine	1	2		0.5–2		30–50	
Coumadin (warfarin)	36–72	0.15	24–72	3–7 days	2–7 days	99	
Cyclobenzaprine	24–72		1	3–8	12–24	93	D
Cyproheptadine	16			6–9	8		
Dapsone	10–50	1.5	2–7	2–6	3–14 days	70–90	M
Desipramine	12–24	22–60		3–6		80	D
Dexbrompheniramine	22				6–8		
Dexfenfluramine	17–20			1.5–8			M
Dextroamphetamine	10–12	6	1–1.5	3		16	S
Dextromethorphan	3	6	0.5	2	6		M, S
Dezocine	2	10	< 0.5	0.5–1.5	2–4		
Diazepam	20–70 50–100 (metabolite)	0.7–2.6	Very fast	0.5–2.5		96	M

Drug							
Diazoxide	24	0.9–0.25	1	3–6	8	90	
Dichlorphenamide				2–4	6–12		
Diclofenac	2	0.1–0.5	0.2	1–3		99	S
Dicyclomine	2–10	3.7	1–2	1.5	4		
Diethylproprion	2.5–6				4		S
Diflunisal	8–12	0.1	1	2–3		99	
Digitoxin	4–10 days	0.6	2–4	10		95	
Digoxin	30–60	7	1–2	2–6	3–4 days	25	
Dihydroergotamine	2–4	15	0.5	0.75	3–4*	90	*In overdose may see vasospasm for up to 2 weeks.
Diltiazem	4–6	2–5	0.5–3	2–3	6–10	85	S
Dimenhydrinate			<0.5		4–6		
Diphenhydramine	2–8	5	<0.5	1–4	4–6	85	S
Disopyramide	4–10	0.5–1.3	0.5–3.5	1–2	2–9	40	M
Disulfiram	7		3–12	10	1–2 weeks		M
Doxazosin	22	1–1.7	1 min	2–3	0.2		
Doxepin	8–15	9–20		2		80	D, M
Doxylamine	10			2–3	4–6		
Dronabinol	20–30*		<1	2–4	4–6		M *Longer in chronic users.
Enalapril	1, 11 (metabolite)		1	1, 4–8 (metabolite)	12–24	50–60	M
Encainide	2–11	2.7–4.3		1		70–85	M
Ephedrine	3–4		0.25–1		3–6		
Ergotamine	3–21	1.8		1–3	24*		*In overdose may see vasospasm for up to 2 weeks.

(continued)

TABLE II-55. PHARMACOKINETIC DATA[a] (CONTINUED)

Drug	Half-Life (h)	Vd (L/kg)	Onset (h)	Peak (h)	Duration (h)	Protein Binding %	Comments[b]
Esmolol	9 min	3	2–10 min	0.5	0.5	55	
Estazolam	10–24			2		93	M
Ethacrynic acid	2–4		0.5	2	12		
Ethchlorvynol	10–30	3–4	0.5–1	1–2	5	35–60	
Etidocaine	1.5	1.9	5 min	0.25–0.5	5–12	96	
Etodolac	7		0.5	1–2	6–8		
Felodipine	11–16	10	2–5	3–5	16–24	99	
Fenfluramine	10–30		1–2	3	2–6		
Fenoprofen	3		0.5	2		99	
Fentanyl	1–5	4	< 0.25	< 0.5	0.5–2	80	M
Fexofenadine	14		Rapid	2–3	24	60–70	
Flecainide	14–15	9		3		40–68	
Fluoride	2–9	0.5–0.7	0.5–1	1		0	
Fluoxetine	70	11–88	6–8	4–8		95	M
Fluphenazine	12–20		<1	1–2	6–8	99	S
Flurazepam	1–3 75 (metabolite)	3.4–5.5	< 0.5	0.5–1 10 (metabolite)	7–8	97	M
Fosinopril	3–4 12 (metabolite)			2–4			M
Fosphenytoin	0.25 22 (metabolite)	0.65		< 0.5		90	M Converted rapidly to phenytoin
Furosemide	1	0.11	0.5–1	1–2	6–8	99	
Gamma hydroxy-butyrate (GHB)	0.5*		0.25	0.5–1*	2–6*	0	*Dose-dependent kinetics

Drug								
Gentamicin	2–4	0.25–0.3				10		S
Glipizide	10–15		0.25–0.5	0.5–2	<24			
Glutethimide		2.7	0.5	1–6	4–8	35–55		M
Glyburide			0.25–1	4	24*			*Duration may be >24h after overdose
Guanabenz	7–14	7.4–14	1	2–5	12	90		
Guanfacine	12–24	6.3		1.5–4				
Haloperidol	14–35	18–30	1–3	1–6	3–4	>90		S
Heroin	1–2			0.2		40		M — Rapidly hydrolyzed to morphine
Hydralazine	2–8	1.6	<0.5	0.5–1	2–6	90		M
Hydrochlorothiazide	5–15	0.83	2	4	6–12	64		
Hydrocodone	3–4	3–5		1–2	4–8	6–8		M
Hydroflumethiazide	17		2	4	6–24			
Hydromorphone	1–4	1.2	0.5	1	4–5	35		
Hydroxyzine	20–25	19	<0.5	2–4	6–24			M
Hyoscyamine	3–12		0.5	0.5–1	4–6			
Ibuprofen	2–4	0.12–0.2	0.5	1–2	4–6	50		
Imipramine	11–25	15		1–2		90–99		D
Indapamide	14–16		1–2	2–3	36	70–90	75	
Indomethacin	3–11	0.3–0.9	0.5	1–2	4–6	99		S
Indoramin	1–2	7.4		1–2		72–92		
Insulin, isophane (NPH)			1–2	8–12	18–24			
Insulin, prolonged zinc			4–8	16–18	36			
Insulin, protamine zinc			4–8	14–20	36			
Insulin, rapid zinc			0.5	4–7	12–16			
Insulin, regular			0.5–1	2–3	5–7			

(continued)

TABLE II–55. PHARMACOKINETIC DATA[a] (CONTINUED)

Drug	Half-Life (h)	Vd (L/kg)	Onset (h)	Peak (h)	Duration (h)	Protein Binding %	Comments[b]
Insulin, zinc			1-2	8-12	18-24		
Isoniazid	1-5	0.6-0.7	<1	1-2		10-15	
Isradipine	8	3	1-2	1.5		95	
Kanamycin	1.5-3.2	0.2-0.3		0.5-1.5		3	
Ketoprofen	2-4	0.1		1-2		99	
Ketorolac	4-6	0.15-0.3		1		99	
Labetalol	6-8	3-16	0.5-2	1-4	8	50	
Levobunolol	5-6		1	2-6	24		
Levorphanol	12-16		0.5-1.5	0.5-1	6-8		
Lidocaine	1-2 h	1.2			0.5-2	40-80	
Lisinopril	12	1.6	1	7	12-24	60	
Lithium	14-30	0.7-0.9		2-5			S
Loperamide	9-14		0.5-1	3-5		97	M
Loratadine	8-18	120	1-3		>24	97	M
Lorazepam	9-20	0.9-1.3	0.5	1-6	6-8	93	
Loxapine	5-19		0.5	2	12		M
Lysergic acid (LSD)	3	0.27	0.5-2	1	8-12	80	
Magnesium	*		3	<6	*	33	*Depends on renal function
Maprotiline	21-50	18		8-16		90	
Mazindol	10		0.5-1		8-15		
Meclizine	6		1-2		12-24		
Meclofenamate	1-3	0.3		0.5-1	2-4	99	
Mefenamic acid	2			2-4		99	

Drug							Comments
Mefloquine	20 days					98	
Meperidine	2–5 15–30 (metabolite)	3.7–4.2	<1	1–2	2–4	55–75	M
Mephobarbital	11–67	2.6	0.5–2		10–16	40–60	
Meprobamate	8–17	0.7	<1	1–3	6–8	20	D
Mesoridazine	5–15	3–6		4	4–6	95	
Metaproterenol			0.25	1–2	4–6		
Metformin	4–9	0.8–8		3–6		Negligible	
Methadone	20–30	3.6	0.5–1	2–4	4–8*	80	*In overdose toxicity may last 2–3 days
Methamphetamine	4–5	3.5			>24		
Methaqualone	20–40	3–6	<1	2		80	
Methazolamide	14		2–4	6–8	10–18	55	
Methocarbamol	1–2		0.5	2			
Methohexital	1–2	1–2.6		<0.1	<0.5	83	
Methyclothiazide			1–2	6	24		
Methyldopa	4–14	0.24	1–2	3–4	12–24	10	
Methylphenidate	2–7	12–33	1–2	1–3	3–6		S
Methysergide	10		24–48		*		*In overdose may see vasospasm for up to 2 weeks.
Methyprylon	3–11	1	0.75	1–2	5–8	60	M
Metoprolol	3–7	6	1	2	10–20	10	S
Mexiletine	10–12	5–7		2–3		50–66	
Mibefradil	17–25	2		1–2	24	99	M
Midazolam	1–5	1–2.5	0.1	0.5–1	2	95	
Minoxidil	3–4	2.8–3.3	1	2–8	75	Negligible	

(continued)

TABLE II–55. PHARMACOKINETIC DATA[a] (CONTINUED)

Drug	Half-Life (h)	Vd (L/kg)	Onset (h)	Peak (h)	Duration (h)	Protein Binding %	Comments[b]
Moexipril	>1 2–9 (metabolite)			1.5			M
Morphine	2–4	3–4	<1	<1	3–6	95	S
Morizicine	1.5–3.5	>4	2	0.5–2	10–24	95	
Nabumetone	24			4–12	24	99	M
Nadolol	10–24	1–3		2–4	24	30	
Nalbuphine	5	3–14	<0.2	0.5–1	3–6		
Naloxone	1–1.5	3.6	1 min	0.25–0.5	1–4	54	
Naltrexone	4–10	3		1	24–72	20	M
Naproxen	10–20	0.16	1	2–4		99	
Niacin 1		<1	1–2	3–4			
Nicardipine	8	0.7	0.3	0.5–2		95	
Nifedipine	2–5	0.8–1.4	0.5–2	0.5–2		95	S
Nitrendipine	2–20	4–8		1.5		90	
Nitroprusside	2 min		1 min	1 min	2–10 min		
Nortriptyline	18–35	18		7		93	D
Orphenadrine	14–16			2–4	4–6	20	
Oxaprozin	42–50			2–4		99	
Oxazepam	5–20	0.7–1.3	Slow	2–4		86–99	
Oxybutynin	2		0.5–1	1–3	6–10		
Oxycodone	2–5		<0.5	1	4–6		
Oxymetazoline			0.25–1		6–12		

Oxyphenbutazone	27–64					90	
Oxyphencyclimine	13			4			
Oxprenolol	1–3	0.8		1–2	8–12	80	
Paraldehyde	6–7	0.9	<0.1	0.5–1			
Paroxetine	21	12–16		2–8		95	
Pemoline	9–14	0.2–0.6	2–4	1–5		50	M
Penbutolol	17–26	2		1–3		85	
Pentazocine	2–3		<0.5	1–2	2–3	65	
Pentobarbital	15–50	0.5–1	0.25	0.5–2	3–4	45–70	
Perphenazine	8–12	10–35		3–6			M
Phencyclidine	1 (30–100 in adipose)	6.2	<0.1	0.5	4–12	65	
Phendimetrazine	5–12			3		15	
Phenobarbital	80–120	0.88	<1	0.5–2	10–16	20–50	
Phenoxybenzamine	24					72–96	
Phentermine	7–24	3–4		4			
Phentolamine	2.5		1 min IV				
Phenylbutazone	50–100	0.14		2–3		98	
Phenylephrine	2–3	5					S
Phenylpropanolamine	4–7	2.5–5	1	2–3	6–8	90	
Phenytoin	22	0.65		1.5–3 (12*)		90	D, S*
Pindolol	3–4	2		1–2		50	
Piroxicam	45–50	0.13	1	0.5	48–72	99	
Prazepam	1–2 / 5–10 (metabolite)	9–19	Very slow	6		97	M
Prazosin	2–4	0.6–1.7	2–4	2–4	10–24	95	

(continued)

TABLE II–55. PHARMACOKINETIC DATA[a] (CONTINUED)

Drug	Half-Life (h)	Vd (L/kg)	Onset (h)	Peak (h)	Duration (h)	Protein Binding %	Comments[b]
Primaquine	4–10	3		1–2			
Procainamide 6–8 metabolite	3–5	1.5–2.5		1–2		15	M, S
Procainamide/ NAPA*	3.5 5–7 (metabolite)	1.5–2.4 1.4	0.5	1–2 1–8		15 10	M, S *Active metabolite: N-acetyl procainamide
Procaine	7–8 min	0.3–0.8	2–5 min		0.25–1	6	
Prochlorperazine	7–23		0.5	1–5	3–4		S
Promethazine	7–16	13	0.5	2–3	4–8	93	
Propafenone	2–10	1.9–3		2–3		77–97	
Propantheline	1–9		<1	6	6		M
Propoxyphene	6–12		0.5–1	2–3	4–6		S
Propranolol	2–6	3.6	1–2	1	6	93	D
Protriptyline	54–92	22		25		92	S
Pseudoephedrine	5–8	2.5–3	0.5	3	4–6	20	
Pyridoxine	15–20 days		<1	1–2	1–2 months		M
Quinapril	1–2 2 (metabolite)			1–2			
Quinidine	6–8	2–3	0.5	1–3	6–8	70–90	M, S
Quinine	8–14	1.2–1.7		1–3		80	
Ramipril	5 3–17 (metabolite)		2	1 2–4 (metabolite)	24		M
Rifampin	2–5	1.6	1–4	1–4		90	M
Ritodrine	1–2 15 (metabolite)	0.7		1		32	M

Scopolamine	3	1.5		1			
Secobarbital	19–34	1.5–1.9	0.25	1–6	3–4	45–70	
Sertraline	28	20	4–8	4–8		98	
Sotalol	5–15	2	1–2	3–4		0	
Spironolactone	2		24	2–4	24–48	95	
Strychnine	10	13	0.5				
Sufentanyl	1–3		<0.1		<0.2	90	
Sulindac	7–16			2		98	
Temazepam	10–12	0.7–1.4	Intermediate	0.5–2		97	M
Terazosin	9–12		1–2	1–2	18+	95	
Terbutaline	4–16	1.5	0.5–1	3	4–8	15	
Terfenadine	8–23		Rapid	1–2	12	97	M
Tetrahydrozoline			0.25–1		4–8		
Theophylline	2–16	0.5				40	S
Thiopental	3–11	1.4–6.7	<0.1	<0.1	0.5	72–86	
Thioridazine	10–36	18		1–2	96	96	M
Thiothixene	3–34			1–3			
Timolol	2–4	3.5	0.5	1–2	12–24	10–60	
Tizanidine	2.7–4.2	2.4		1–2			
Tobramycin	1.6–3	0.26		0.5–1.5	8	3	
Tocainide	11–15	2–4		1–2		10–20	
Tolazamide				4–6	14–20		
Tolbutamide			1	5–8	6–12		
Tolmetin	1	0.13	1	1		99	

(continued)

TABLE II-55. PHARMACOKINETIC DATA^a (CONTINUED)

Drug	Half-Life (h)	Vd (L/kg)	Onset (h)	Peak (h)	Duration (h)	Protein Binding %	Comments^b
Trandolapril	16–24 (metabolite)			1 4–10 (metabolite)			
Trazodone	3–9	1.3	1–2	1–2		95	
Triamterene	1.5–2	2.5	2–4	2–8	8–12	65	
Triazolam	1–6	0.8–1.8	0.5	1–2	6	90	M
Trichlormethiazide	2–7		2	4	12–24		
Trifluoperazine	5–18			2–5			
Trihexyphenidyl	5–10		1	2–3	6–12		
Trimethobenzamide	1	0.5	0.5	1	3–4		
Trimipramine	15–30	31		2		95	D
Tripelennamine			05.	2–3	4–6		S
Urapidil	5					80	
Valproic acid	5–20	0.13–22				80–95	D, S
Verapamil	2–8	4.7	1–2	2–5	6–8	92	M, S
Vitamin A	50–100 days		8–12	1–3 days	> 2 months		
Vitamin C	8–10 days		< 1	1–2	3–4 weeks		
Vitamin D	19 days		10–24	3–4 weeks	> 2 months		
Zolpidem	2–3	0.5	0.5	1–2	6–8	95	

^{a}Data provided are based on therapeutic dosing, not overdose. In general, after overdose the peak effect is delayed and the half-life and duration of effect are prolonged. Changes may occur in the volume of distribution and the percent protein bound.
^{b}Key to abbreviations: D = delayed absorption may result in prolonged effect; M = active metabolite; S = sustained release formulations are available, and may lead to delayed absorption and prolonged effect. Kinetics may vary depending on the formulation.
Table compiled by Ilene B. Anderson, PharmD.

SECTION III. Therapeutic Drugs and Antidotes

Thomas E. Kearney, PharmD

INTRODUCTION

This section provides detailed descriptions of antidotes and other therapeutic agents used in the management of a poisoned patient. For each agent, a summary is provided of its pharmacologic effects, clinical indications, adverse effects and contraindications, usage in pregnancy, dosage, available formulations, and recommended minimum stocking levels for the hospital pharmacy. This information was obtained from a variety of resources, as noted in the bibliography.

I. **Use of antidotes in pregnancy.** It is always prudent to avoid or minimize drug exposure during pregnancy, and physicians are often reluctant to use an antidote for fear of potential fetal harm. This reluctance, however, must be tempered with a case-by-case risk-benefit analysis of use of the particular therapeutic agent. An acute drug overdose or poisoning in pregnancy may threaten the life of the mother as well as the fetus, and the antidote or therapeutic agent, despite unknown or questionable effects on the fetus, may have lifesaving benefit. The inherent toxicity and large body burden of the drug or toxic chemical involved in the poisoning may far exceed that of the indicated therapeutic agent or antidote.

With most agents discussed in this section, there is little or no information regarding their use in pregnant patients. The **Food and Drug Administration (FDA)** has established five categories of required labeling to indicate the potential for teratogenicity (see Table III–1). The distinction between categories depends mainly on the amount and reliability of animal and human data and the risk-benefit assessment for use of the agent. Note that the categorization may be based on anticipated chronic or repeated use and may not be relevant to a single or brief antidotal treatment.

TABLE III–1. FDA PREGNANCY CATEGORIES FOR TERATOGENIC EFFECTS

FDA Pregnancy Category	Definition
A	Adequate and well-controlled studies in pregnant women have failed to demonstrate a risk to the fetus in the first trimester, and there is no evidence of a risk in later pregnancy. The possibility of fetal harm appears remote.
B	Either (1) animal reproduction studies have failed to demonstrate any adverse effect (other than a decrease in fertility), but there are no adequate and well-controlled studies in pregnant women or (2) animal studies have shown an adverse effect that was not confirmed by adequate and well-controlled studies in pregnant women. The possibility of fetal harm is probably remote.
C	Either (1) animal reproduction studies have shown an adverse effect on the fetus and there are no adequate and well-controlled human studies or (2) there are no animal or human studies. The drug should be given only if the potential benefit outweighs the potential risk to the fetus.
D	There is positive evidence of human fetal risk based on adverse reaction data from investigational or marketing experience or human studies, but the potential risks may be acceptable in light of potential benefits (eg, use in a life-threatening situation for which safer drugs are ineffective or unavailable).
X	Studies in animals or humans have demonstrated fetal abnormalities, or there is positive evidence of fetal risk based on human experience, or both, and the risk of using the drug in a pregnant patient outweighs any possible benefit. The drug in contraindicated in women who are or may become pregnant.

Reference: *Code of Federal Regulations,* title 21, section 201.57 (4/1/90).

II. **Hospital stocking.** The hospital pharmacy should maintain the medical staff-approved stock of antidotes and other emergency drugs. Many antidotes are used only infrequently, have a short shelf life, or are expensive. Optimal case management, however, requires having adequate supplies of antidotes readily available. Fortunately, only a minimal acquisition and maintenance cost is required to adequately stock many of these drugs.

    A. The basis for our **suggested minimum stocking level** is a combination of factors to anticipate the highest total dose of a drug generally given during a 24-hour period as quoted in the literature, the maximum manufacturer's recommended or tolerated daily dose, and estimation of these quantities for a 70-kg adult.

    B. Larger quantities of a drug might be needed in unusual situations, particularly if multiple patients are treated simultaneously or for extended periods of time. Hospitals in close proximity may wish to explore the practicality of sharing stocks, but should carefully consider the logistics of such arrangements (eg, transferring stocks after hours or on weekends).

▶ ACETYLCYSTEINE (N-ACETYLCYSTEINE [NAC])

Thomas E. Kearney, PharmD

I. **Pharmacology.** Acetylcysteine (*N*-acetylcysteine [NAC]) is a mucolytic agent that acts as a sulfhydryl group donor, substituting for the liver's usual sulfhydryl donor, glutathione. It rapidly binds (detoxifies) the highly reactive electrophilic intermediates of metabolism. It is most effective in preventing acetaminophen-induced liver injury when given early in the course of intoxication (within 8 to 10 hours), but may also be of benefit in reducing the severity of liver injury even when given after 24 hours. It may be used empirically when the severity of ingestion is unknown or serum concentrations of the ingested drug are not immediately available.

II. **Indications.**
    A. Acetaminophen overdose.
    B. Carbon tetrachloride and chloroform poisoning.
    C. Pennyroyal oil (one case report). The mechanism of hepatic injury by pennyroyal oil is similar to that of acetaminophen, and empiric use of NAC seems justified for any significant pennyroyal oil ingestion.

III. **Contraindications.** Known hypersensitivity (rare).

IV. **Adverse effects.**
    A. Acetylcysteine typically causes nausea and vomiting when given **orally.** If the dose is vomited, it should be repeated. Use of a gastric tube, slower rate of administration, and a strong antiemetic agent (eg, metoclopramide, p 382; ondansetron, p 395) may be necessary.
    B. Rapid **intravenous** administration can cause flushing, hypotension, and bronchospasm (anaphylactoid reaction). One death was reported in a small child rapidly receiving a large dose intravenously. Reactions can be minimized by giving each dose slowly over 45–60 minutes in a dilute (3%) solution.
    C. **Use in pregnancy.** There is no evidence for teratogenicity. Use of this drug to treat acetaminophen overdose is considered beneficial to both mother and developing fetus.

V. **Drug or laboratory interactions.**
    A. Activated charcoal adsorbs acetylcysteine and may interfere with its systemic absorption when both are given orally together; data suggest that peak acetylcysteine levels are decreased by about 30% and that the time to reach peak level may be delayed. However, these effects are not considered clinically important.
    B. NAC can produce a false-positive test for ketones in the urine.

VI. **Dosage and method of administration.**

A. Oral loading dose. Give 140 mg/kg of the 10% or 20% solution diluted to 5% in juice or soda.

B. Maintenance oral dose. Give 70 mg/kg every 4 hours. The commonly accepted protocol for treatment of acetaminophen poisoning in the United States calls for 17 doses of oral NAC given over approximately 72 hours. However, successful protocols in Canada, the United Kingdom, and Europe utilize intravenous NAC for only 20 hours. We give NAC orally until 36 hours have passed since the time of ingestion. Then, if the serum acetaminophen level is below the limits of detection and liver transaminase levels are normal, NAC can be stopped. If there is evidence of hepatic toxicity, NAC should be continued until resolution of toxic effects (ie, liver function tests are clearly improving).

C. Intravenous administration is *not* approved in the United States and is generally used only when recurrent vomiting prevents oral administration despite generous doses of antiemetics. Contact a medical toxicologist or regional poison center (see p 55) for advice. A 48-hour investigational protocol showed safety and efficacy with the same doses and intervals as for oral administration. In the United Kingdom, the dosing regimen is 150 mg/kg in 200 mL of 5% dextrose in water (D5W) over 15 minutes, followed by 50 mg/kg in 500 mL of D5W over 4 hours and then 100 mg/kg in 1000 mL of D5W over 16 hours.

D. Dosage during dialysis. Although acetylcysteine is removed during dialysis, no change in dosage is necessary.

VII. Formulations.

A. The usual formulation is as a 10% (100-mg/mL) or 20% (200-mg/mL) solution, supplied as an inhaled mucolytic agent (Mucomyst or Mucosil). This form is available through most hospital pharmacies or respiratory therapy departments. This preparation is *not* approved for parenteral use. In rare circumstances when intravenous administration of this preparation is required, a 3% solution and a micropore filter should be used, and the dose should be given over 45–60 minutes.

B. In the United States, an investigational intravenous formulation is available only at medical centers participating in an approved study.

C. Suggested minimum stocking level for treatment of a 70-kg adult for the first 24 hours: 20% solution, 7 vials (30 mL each).

▶ **AMRINONE**

Anthony S. Manoguerra, PharmD

I. Pharmacology. Amrinone is a positive inotropic agent with vasodilator activity. It is not a beta-adrenergic receptor agonist, and its exact mechanism of action is unknown. It appears to work by inhibition of myocardial cell phosphodiesterase activity, thereby increasing cellular concentrations of cyclic AMP. Cardiac afterload and preload are reduced owing to a direct vasodilator effect.

II. Indications. Amrinone may be useful as a third-line inotropic agent for patients with beta-blocker or calcium antagonist overdose, when intravenous fluids, atropine, beta-agonists, and glucagon have failed to restore cardiac output and blood pressure.

III. Contraindications. Known hypersensitivity to amrinone or sulfites (used as a preservative).

IV. Adverse effects.

A. Hypotension may result from direct vasodilator effects, especially in patients who are volume depleted. Give adequate intravenous fluids prior to and with amrinone administration.

B. The formulation contains sodium metabisulfite as a preservative, which can cause acute allergiclike reactions in patients (especially asthmatics) who are sensitive to sulfites.

C. Amrinone may aggravate outflow obstruction in patients with hypertrophic subaortic stenosis.

D. Amrinone affects platelet survival time resulting in a dose- and time-dependent thrombocytopenia.

E. Use in pregnancy. FDA category C. Animal studies are conflicting, and there are no good human data. Use only if benefit justifies the potential risk (eg, a severe beta-blocker or calcium antagonist overdose unresponsive to other measures).

V. Drug or laboratory interactions. The positive inotropic effects of amrinone are additive with other inotropic agents, including digitalis glycosides. These drugs can be used together but the patient should be monitored for cardiac dysrhythmias.

VI. Dosage and method of administration.

A. The initial dose is 0.75 mg/kg as a bolus over 2–3 minutes. This is followed by an infusion at 5–10 μg/kg/h.

B. The manufacturer recommends that the total daily dose not exceed 10 mg/kg. However, up to 18 mg/kg/d has been given in some patients.

VII. Formulations.

A. Amrinone lactate (Inocor): 5 mg/mL in 20-mL ampules containing 0.25 mg/mL sodium metabisulfite as a preservative.

B. Suggested minimum stocking level to treat a 70-kg adult for the first 24 hours is 10 ampules.

▶ ANTIVENIN, CROTALIDAE (RATTLESNAKE)

Richard F. Clark, MD

I. Pharmacology. To produce the antivenin for rattlesnake venom, horses are hyperimmunized with the pooled venom of *Crotalus adamanteus* (eastern diamondback rattlesnake), *Crotalus atrox* (western diamondback), *Crotalus durissus terrificus* (tropical rattlesnake, cascabel), and *Bothrops atrox* (fer-de-lance). The lyophilized protein product from these pooled equine sera is a combination of several antibodies against venom constituents and also contains residual serum components. After intravenous administration, the antivenin is distributed widely throughout the body, where it binds to venom.

II. Indications. Antivenin is used for treatment of significant envenomation by Crotalidae species (see Section II, p 293).

III. Contraindications. Known hypersensitivity to the antivenin or to horse serum is a relative contraindication; antivenin may still be indicated for severe envenomation despite a patient history of allergic reaction.

IV. Adverse effects.

A. Immediate hypersensitivity reactions (including life-threatening anaphylaxis) may occur, even in patients with no history of horse serum sensitivity and negative skin test results.

B. Mild flushing and wheezing often occur within the first 30 minutes of intravenous administration and often improve after slowing the rate of infusion.

C. Delayed hypersensitivity (serum sickness) occurs in over 75% of patients receiving more than four vials of antivenin and in virtually all patients who receive more than 12 vials. Onset occurs in 5–14 days.

D. Use in pregnancy. There are no data on teratogenicity. Anaphylactic reaction resulting in shock or hypoxemia in the mother could conceivably adversely affect the fetus.

V. Drug or laboratory interactions. There are no known interactions.

VI. Dosage and method of administration. The initial dose is based on severity of symptoms, not on body weight (Table III–2). Children may require doses as large as or larger than those for adults. The end point of antivenin therapy is the rever-

TABLE III–2. INITIAL DOSE OF CROTALIDAE ANTIVENIN

Severity of Envenomation	Initial Dose (vials)
None or minimal	None
Mild (local pain and swelling)	5
Moderate (proximal progression of swelling, ecchymosis, mild systemic symptoms)	10
Severe (hypotension, rapidly progressive swelling and ecchymosis, coagulopathy	15

sal of systemic manifestations (eg, shock, coagulopathy, and paresthesias) and the halting of progressive edema and pain. Antivenin may be effective up to 3 days or more after envenomation.

If you suspect envenomation by the Mojave rattlesnake (*Crotalus scutulatus*) and symptoms are present, especially an increased serum creatine phosphokinase (CPK) level, administer 10 vials of antivenin even when there is minimal swelling or local pain.

A. Treat all patients in an intensive care setting.

B. Before skin tests or antivenin administration, insert at least one and preferably two secure intravenous lines.

C. Perform the skin test for horse serum sensitivity, using a 1:10 dilution of antivenin (some experts prefer this method) or the sample of horse serum provided in the antivenin kit (follow package instructions). Do *not* perform the skin test unless signs of envenomation are present and imminent antivenin therapy is anticipated. If the skin test is positive, reconsider the need for antivenin as opposed to supportive care, but do not abandon antivenin therapy if it is needed. Even if the skin test is negative, anaphylaxis may still occur unpredictably.

D. If antivenin is used in a patient with a positive skin test, pretreat with intravenous diphenhydramine (see p 359) and cimetidine (or another H_2 blocker, see p 353), and have ready at the bedside a preloaded syringe containing epinephrine (1:10,000 for intravenous use) in case of anaphylaxis. Dilute the antivenin 1:10 to 1:1000 before administration, and give each vial very slowly at first (ie, over 30–45 minutes), increasing the rate of infusion as tolerated.

E. Reconstitute the lyophilized product with the 10 mL of diluent provided and gently swirl for 10–30 minutes to solubilize the material. Avoid shaking, which may destroy the immunoglobulins (indicated by foam formation). Further dilution with 50–200 mL of saline may facilitate solubilization.

F. Administer antivenin by the intravenous route only. Start slowly, increasing the rate as tolerated. In nonallergic individuals, 5–10 vials can be diluted in 250–500 mL saline and given over 60–90 minutes.

VII. Formulations.

A. Antivenin (Crotalidae) polyvalent. Supplies can be located by a regional poison center (see Table I–42, p 55).

B. The **suggested minimum stocking level** to treat a 70-kg adult for the first 24 hours is 20 vials.

▶ **ANTIVENIN, *LATRODECTUS MACTANS* (BLACK WIDOW SPIDER)**

Richard F. Clark, MD

I. Pharmacology. To produce the antivenin, horses are hyperimmunized with *Latrodectus mactans* (black widow spider) venom. The lyophilized protein product from pooled equine sera contains antibody specific to certain venom fractions, as well as residual serum proteins such as albumin and globulins. After intravenous administration, the antivenin distributes widely throughout the body, where it binds to venom.

II. **Indications.**
  A. Severe hypertension or muscle cramping not alleviated by muscle relaxants, analgesics, or sedation, particularly in patients at the extremes of age (ie, younger than 1 year or older than 65 years).
  B. Black widow envenomation in **pregnancy** may cause abdominal muscle spasms severe enough to threaten spontaneous abortion or early onset of labor.

III. **Contraindications.** Known hypersensitivity to horse serum.

IV. **Adverse effects.**
  A. Immediate hypersensitivity may occur rarely, including life-threatening anaphylaxis.
  B. Delayed-onset serum sickness may occur after 10–14 days, but is rare owing to the small volume of antivenin used in most cases.
  C. **Use in pregnancy.** There are no data on teratogenicity. An anaphylactic reaction resulting in shock or hypoxemia in the mother could conceivably adversely affect the fetus.

V. **Drug or laboratory interactions.** No known interactions.

VI. **Dosage and method of administration.** Generally, one vial of antivenin is sufficient to treat black widow envenomation in adults or children.
  A. Treat all patients in an emergency department or intensive care setting.
  B. Before a skin test or antivenin administration, insert at least one and preferably two secure intravenous lines.
  C. Perform a skin test for horse serum sensitivity, by using a 1:10 dilution of antivenin (some experts prefer this method) or the sample of horse serum provided in the antivenin kit (according to package instructions). Do **not** perform the skin test unless signs of envenomation are present and imminent antivenin therapy is anticipated. If the skin test is positive, reconsider the need for antivenin as opposed to supportive care, but do not abandon antivenin therapy if it is needed. Even if the skin test is negative, anaphylaxis may still occur unpredictably.
  D. If antivenin is used in a patient with horse serum sensitivity, pretreat with intravenous diphenhydramine (see p 359) and cimetidine (or another H_2 blocker; see p 353), and have ready at the bedside a preloaded syringe containing epinephrine (1:10,000 for intravenous use) in case of anaphylaxis. Dilute the antivenin (1:10 to 1:1000) and administer it very slowly.
  E. Reconstitute the lyophilized product to 2.5 mL with the supplied diluent, using gentle swirling for 15–30 minutes to avoid shaking and destroying the immunoglobulins (indicated by the formation of foam).
  F. Dilute this solution to a total volume of 10–50 mL with normal saline.
  G. Administer the diluted antivenin slowly over 15–30 minutes. One or two vials are sufficient in most cases.

VII. **Formulations.**
  A. Lyophilized antivenin (L mactans), 6000 units.
  B. The **suggested minimum stocking level** to treat a 70-kg adult for the first 24 hours is one vial.

▶ **ANTIVENIN, *MICRURUS FULVIUS* (CORAL SNAKE)**

Richard F. Clark, MD

I. **Pharmacology.** To produce the antivenin, horses are hyperimmunized with venom from *Micrurus fulvius,* the eastern coral snake. The lyophilized protein preparation from pooled equine sera contains antibody to venom fractions as well as residual serum proteins. Administered intravenously, the antibody distributes widely throughout the body where it binds the target venom.

II. **Indications.**
  A. Envenomation by the eastern coral snake (*M fulvius*) or the Texas coral snake (*M fulvius tenere*).
  B. ***Not*** effective for envenomation by the western, Arizona, or Sonora coral snake (*M euryxanthus.*)

III. **Contraindications.** Known hypersensitivity to the antivenin or to horse serum is a relative contraindication; if a patient with significant envenomation needs the antivenin, it should be given with caution.

IV. **Adverse effects.**
  A. Immediate hypersensitivity, including life-threatening anaphylaxis, may occur even after a negative skin test for horse serum sensitivity.
  B. Delayed hypersensitivity (serum sickness) may occur 1–3 weeks after antivenin administration, the severity depending on the total quantity of antivenin administered.
  C. **Use in pregnancy.** There are no data on teratogenicity. Anaphylactic reactions resulting in shock or hypoxemia in expectant mothers could conceivably adversely affect the fetus.

V. **Drug or laboratory interactions.** There are no known interactions.

VI. **Dosage and method of administration.** Generally, the recommended initial dose is three to five vials. The drug is most effective if given before the onset of signs or symptoms of envenomation. An additional three to five vials may be given, depending on the severity of neurological manifestations but not on body weight (children may require doses as large as or even larger than those for adults).
  A. Treat all patients in an intensive care unit setting.
  B. Before a skin test or antivenin administration, insert at least one and preferably two secure intravenous lines.
  C. Perform a skin test for horse serum sensitivity, using a 1:10 dilution of antivenin (some experts prefer this method) or the sample of horse serum provided in the antivenin kit (according to package instructions). If the skin test is positive, reconsider the need for antivenin as opposed to supportive care, but do not abandon antivenin therapy if it is needed. Even if the skin test is negative, anaphylaxis may still occur unpredictably.
  D. If antivenin is used in a patient with a positive skin test, pretreat with intravenous diphenhydramine (see p 359) and cimetidine (or another H_2 blocker, see p 353) and have ready at the bedside a preloaded syringe containing epinephrine (1:10,000 for intravenous use) in case of anaphylaxis. Dilute the antivenin (1:10 to 1:1000) and administer very slowly.
  E. Reconstitute the lyophilized material with 10 mL of the diluent supplied, gently swirling for 10–30 minutes. Avoid shaking the preparation because this may destroy the immunoglobulins (indicated by the formation of foam). Dilution with 50–200 mL of saline may aid solubilization.
  F. Administer the antivenin intravenously over 15–30 minutes per vial.

VII. **Formulations.**
  A. Antivenin (*M fulvius.*)
  B. **Suggested minimum stocking level** to treat a 70-kg adult for the first 24 hours is 5–10 vials.

▶ **APOMORPHINE**

Thomas E. Kearney, PharmD

I. **Pharmacology.** Apomorphine is an alkaloid salt derived from morphine that has minimal analgesic properties but marked emetic efficacy. Vomiting is produced by direct stimulation of the medullary chemoreceptor trigger zone. After subcutaneous administration, emesis occurs within an average of 5 minutes; oral admin- istration is *not* recommended because of erratic absorption.

II. **Indications.** Apomorphine was previously used for induction of emesis in the acute management of oral poisoning, but it has been abandoned because of its potential for respiratory depression and its inconvenient formulation (soluble tablets for parenteral injection). The drug is not discussed further in this book, but it remains popular in veterinary practice.

▶ ATROPINE

Brent R. Ekins, PharmD

I. **Pharmacology.** Atropine is a parasympatholytic agent that competitively blocks the action of acetylcholine at muscarinic receptors. Desired therapeutic effects for treating poisoning include decreased secretions from salivary and other glands, decreased bronchorrhea and wheezing, decreased intestinal peristalsis, increased heart rate, and enhanced atrioventricular conduction.

II. **Indications.**
   A. Correction of bronchorrhea and excessive salivation associated with organophosphate and carbamate insecticide intoxication.
   B. Acceleration of the rate of sinus node firing and atrioventricular nodal conduc- tion velocity in the presence of drug-induced atrioventricular conduction im- pairment (eg, caused by digitalis, beta blockers, calcium antagonists, organo- phosphate or carbamate insecticides, or physostigmine).
   C. Reversal of central and peripheral muscarinic symptoms in patients with in- toxication by *Clitocybe* or *Inocybe* mushroom species.

III. **Contraindications.**
   A. Angle-closure glaucoma in which pupillary dilation may increase intraocular pressure.
   B. Patients with hypertension, tachyarrhythmias, thyrotoxicosis, congestive heart failure, coronary artery disease, and other illnesses, who might not tol- erate a rapid heart rate.
   C. Partial or complete obstructive uropathy.
   D. Myasthenia gravis.

IV. **Adverse effects.**
   A. Some adverse effects include dry mouth, blurred vision, cycloplegia, mydria- sis, urinary retention, palpitations, tachycardia, aggravation of angina, and constipation. Duration of effects may be prolonged (several hours).
   B. Doses less than 0.5 mg (in adults) and those administered by very slow intra- venous push may result in paradoxic slowing of heart rate.
   C. **Use in pregnancy.** FDA category C (indeterminate). It readily crosses the placenta. However, this does not preclude its acute, short-term use for a seri- ously symptomatic patient (see p 333).

V. **Drug or laboratory interactions.**
   A. Atropinization may occur more rapidly if atropine and pralidoxime are given concurrently to patients with organophosphate or carbamate insecticide poi- soning.
   B. Atropine has an additive effect with other antimuscarinic and antihistaminic compounds.
   C. Slowing of gastrointestinal motility may delay absorption of orally ingested materials.

VI. **Dosage and method of administration.**
   A. **Organophosphate or carbamate insecticide poisoning.** For adults, begin with 1–5 mg IV; for children, give 0.02 mg/kg IV. (The drug may also be given via the intratracheal route: dilute the dose in normal saline to a total volume of 1–2 mL.) Repeat this dose every 5–10 minutes until satisfactory atropiniza- tion is achieved. The goal of therapy is drying of bronchial secretions (this

end point may be reached prematurely if the patient is dehydrated) and reversal of wheezing and significant bradycardia. Recrudescence of symptoms may occur, and in severe poisonings several grams of atropine may be required and may be administered by constant intravenous infusion.
- **B. Drug-induced bradycardia.** For adults, give 0.5–1 mg IV; for children, give 0.02 mg/kg IV up to a maximum of 0.5 mg in children and 1 mg in adolescents. Repeat as needed. Note that 3 mg is a fully vagolytic dose in adults. If response is not achieved by 3 mg, the patient is unlikely to benefit from further treatment unless bradycardia is caused by excessive cholinergic effects (eg, carbamate or organophosphate overdose).

VII. Formulations.
- **A. Parenteral.** Atropine sulfate injection, 0.05-, 0.1-, 0.3-, 0.4-, 0.5-, 0.6-, 0.8-, 1-, and 1.2-mg/mL solutions. Use preservative-free formulations when massive doses are required.
- **B.** The **suggested minimum stocking level** to treat a 70-kg adult for the first 24 hours is 1 g.

▶ BAL (DIMERCAPROL)

Saralyn R. Williams, MD

I. Pharmacology. BAL (British anti-Lewisite, Dimercaprol) is a dithiol-chelating agent used in the treatment of poisoning by the heavy metals arsenic, mercury, lead, and gold. It is of no value for the treatment of poisoning by selenium, iron, or cadmium; in fact, it is contraindicated in these poisonings because the BAL-metal (mercaptide) complex may be more toxic than the metal alone. Adequate doses of BAL must be given to ensure an excess of free BAL. An insufficient concentration of BAL may allow dissociation of the BAL-metal complex. This chelate dissociates more rapidly in an acidic urine; adequate renal function must exist to allow elimination of the mercaptide complex.

II. Indications.
- **A.** Arsenic poisoning (except arsine, for which BAL is ineffective).
- **B.** Mercury poisoning (except monoalkyl mercury). BAL is most effective in preventing renal damage if administered within 2 hours after ingestion; it is not effective in reversing neurologic damage caused by chronic mercury poisoning.
- **C.** Lead poisoning (except alkyl lead compounds). Calcium EDTA (p 363) and DMSA (p 360) are the preferred chelating agents, but BAL is commonly used as adjunctive therapy in patients with acute lead encephalopathy.
- **D. Other indications.** Possibly effective for poisoning caused by antimony, bismuth, chromium, copper, gold, nickel, tungsten, or zinc.

III. Contraindications.
- **A.** Heavy metal poisoning resulting from iron, cadmium, selenium, or uranium (BAL-metal complex is more toxic than the metal alone).
- **B.** Poisoning caused by thallium, tellurium, or vanadium (BAL is ineffective).
- **C. Glucose-6-phosphate dehydrogenase (G6PD) deficiency.** BAL may cause hemolysis; use only in life-threatening situations.
- **D. Hepatic impairment** (except arsenic-induced jaundice).
- **E. Renal impairment.** Avoid BAL or use only with extreme caution.

IV. Adverse effects.
- **A.** Local pain at injection site; sterile or pyogenic abscess formation.
- **B.** Dose-related hypertension, with or without tachycardia. Onset, 15–30 minutes; duration, 2 hours. Use with caution in hypertensive patients.
- **C.** BAL can induce hemolysis in patients with G6PD deficiency.
- **D.** Thrombocytopenia and increased prothrombin time, which may limit intramuscular administration.
- **E. Nephrotoxicity.** Urine should be kept alkaline to protect renal function and to prevent dissociation of metal-BAL complex.

F. Effects on the brain. Despite its capacity to increase survival in acutely intoxicated animals, use of BAL is associated with redistribution of mercury and arsenic into the brain.

G. Other adverse symptoms. Nausea, vomiting, headache, lacrimation, rhinorrhea, salivation, urticaria, myalgias, paresthesias, dysuria, fever (particularly in children), central nervous system depression, seizures.

H. Use in pregnancy. BAL is embryotoxic in mice. The safety of BAL in human pregnancy is not established, although it has been used in a pregnant patient with Wilson's disease without apparent harm. It should be used in pregnancy only for life-threatening acute intoxication.

V. Drug or laboratory interactions.

  A. BAL forms toxic complexes with iron, cadmium, selenium, and uranium. Avoid concurrent iron replacement therapy.

  B. BAL may abruptly terminate gold therapy-induced remission of rheumatoid arthritis.

  C. BAL interferes with iodine accumulation by the thyroid.

VI. Dosage and method of administration (adults and children).

  A. Arsenic, mercury, and gold poisoning. Give BAL, 3 mg/kg deep intramuscularly (IM) every 4–6 hours for 2 days, then every 12 hours for 7–10 days or until recovery. In patients with severe arsenic or mercury poisoning, an initial dose of up to 5 mg/kg may be used.

  B. Lead poisoning (in conjunction with calcium EDTA therapy [see p 363]). For symptomatic acute encephalopathy or blood lead greater than 100 μg/dL, give BAL, 4–5 mg/kg deep IM every 4 hours for 3–5 days.

VII. Formulations.

  A. Parenteral (for deep IM injection only; must *not* be given as IV). BAL in oil, 100 mg/mL, 3-mL ampules.

  B. The **suggested minimum stocking level** to treat a 70-kg adult for the first 24 hours is 1200 mg (4 ampules).

▶ BENZODIAZEPINES (DIAZEPAM, LORAZEPAM, AND MIDAZOLAM)

Thomas E. Kearney, PharmD

I. Pharmacology.

  A. Benzodiazepines potentiate inhibitory γ-aminobutyric acid (GABA) neuronal activity in the central nervous system. Pharmacologic effects include reduction of anxiety, suppression of seizure activity, central nervous system depression (possible respiratory arrest when given rapidly intravenously), and inhibition of spinal afferent pathways to produce skeletal muscle relaxation.

  B. In addition, diazepam has been reported to antagonize the cardiotoxic effect of chloroquine (the mechanism is unknown, but diazepam may compete with chloroquine for fixation sites on cardiac cells).

  C. Benzodiazepines generally have little effect on the autonomic nervous system or cardiovascular system.

  D. Pharmacokinetics. All agents are well absorbed orally, but diazepam is not well absorbed intramuscularly. The drugs are eliminated by hepatic metabolism, with serum elimination half-lives of 1–50 hours. The duration of central nervous system effects is determined by the rate of drug redistribution from the brain to peripheral tissues. Active metabolites further extend the duration of effect of diazepam.

    1. Diazepam. Onset of action is fast after intravenous (IV) injection, but slow to intermediate after oral or rectal administration. The half-life is greater than 24 hours, although anticonvulsant effects and sedation are often shorter as a result of redistribution from the central nervous system.

2. **Lorazepam.** Onset is intermediate after intramuscular (IM) dosing. The elimination half-life is 10–20 hours, and anticonvulsant effects are generally longer than for diazepam.

3. **Midazolam.** Onset is rapid after intramuscular or intravenous injection and intermediate after nasal application or ingestion. The half-life is 1.5–3 hours and the duration of effects is very short due to rapid redistribution from the brain. However, sedation may persist for 10 hours or longer after prolonged infusions due to saturation of peripheral sites and slowed redistribution.

II. **Indications.**

A. **Anxiety and agitation.** Benzodiazepines are often used for the treatment of anxiety or agitation (eg, caused by sympathomimetic or hallucinogenic drug intoxication).

B. **Convulsions.** All three drugs can be used for the treatment of acute seizure activity or status epilepticus resulting from idiopathic epilepsy or convulsant drug overdose. Midazolam and lorazepam have the advantage of rapid absorption after intramuscular injection. Lorazepam also has a longer duration of anticonvulsant action than the other two agents.

C. **Muscle relaxant.** These drugs can be used for relaxation of excessive muscle rigidity and contractions (eg, caused by strychnine poisoning or black widow spider envenomation).

D. **Chloroquine poisoning.** Diazepam may antagonize cardiotoxicity.

E. **Alcohol or sedative-hypnotic withdrawal.** Diazepam and lorazepam are used to abate symptoms and signs of alcohol and hypnosedative withdrawal (eg, anxiety, tremor, and seizures).

F. **Conscious sedation.** Midazolam is used to induce sedation and amnesia during brief procedures and in conjunction with neuromuscular paralysis for endotracheal intubation.

III. **Contraindications.** Do not use in patients with a known sensitivity to benzodiazepines.

IV. **Adverse effects.**

A. Central nervous system-depressant effects may interfere with evaluation of neurologic function.

B. Excessive or rapid intravenous administration may cause respiratory arrest.

C. The drug may precipitate or worsen hepatic encephalopathy.

D. Rapid or large volume IV administration may cause cardiotoxicity similar to that seen with phenytoin (see p 401) because of the diluent propylene glycol. Several products also contain up to 2% benzyl alcohol as a presentative.

E. **Use in pregnancy.** FDA category D. All of these drugs readily cross the placenta. However, this does not preclude their acute, short-term use for a seriously symptomatic patient (see p 333).

V. **Drug or laboratory interactions.**

A. Benzodiazepines will potentiate the central nervous system-depressant effects of opioids, ethanol, and other sedative-hypnotic and depressant drugs.

B. **Flumazenil** (see p 369) will reverse the effects of benzodiazepines and may trigger an acute abstinence syndrome in patients using the drugs chronically. Patients who have received flumazenil will have an unpredictable but reduced or absent response to benzodiazepines.

C. Diazepam may produce a false-positive glucose reaction with Clinistix and Diastix test strips.

VI. **Dosage and method of administration.**

A. **Anxiety or agitation; muscle spasm or hyperactivity**

1. **Diazepam.** Give 0.1–0.2 mg/kg IV initially (no faster than 5 mg/min in adults; administer over 3 minutes in children), depending on severity; may repeat every 1–4 hours as needed. The oral dose is 0.1–0.3 mg/kg. Do *not* give intramuscularly.

2. **Lorazepam.** Give 1–2 mg (children: 0.04 mg/kg IV) not to exceed 2 mg/min, or 0.05 mg/kg IM (maximum 4 mg). The usual adult oral dose is 2–6 mg daily.

3. **Midazolam.** Give 0.05 mg/kg IV over 20–30 seconds or 0.1 mg/kg IM. Repeat after 10–20 minutes if needed. *Caution:* There have been several reports of respiratory arrest and hypotension after rapid intravenous injection, especially when midazolam is given in combination with opioids. Prolonged continuous infusion is not recommended because midazolam accumulates in tissues, leading to persistent sedation after the drug is discontinued.

B. **Convulsions.** *Note:* If convulsions persist after initial doses of benzodiazepines, consider alternate anticonvulsant drugs such as phenobarbital (p 399), phenytoin (p 401), or pentobarbital (p 398).
   1. **Diazepam** Give 0.1–0.2 mg/kg IV, not to exceed 5 mg/min, every 5–10 minutes (usual initial doses: adult, 5–10 mg; children >5 years, 1–2 mg; children < 5 years, 0.2–0.5 mg), to a maximum total of 30 mg (adults) or 5 mg (young children) or 10 mg (older children).
   2. **Lorazepam** Give 1–2 mg (neonates, 0.05–0.1 mg/kg; older children, 0.04 mg/kg) IV, not to exceed 2 mg/min; repeat if needed after 5–10 minutes. Usual dose for status epilepticus is up to 4 mg slow IV push over 2 min (dilute with an equal volume of saline). The drug can also be given IM (0.05 mg/kg, maximum 4 mg), with onset of effects after 6–10 minutes.
   3. **Midazolam** Give 0.05 mg/kg IV over 20–30 seconds, or 0.1–0.2 mg/kg IM; this may be repeated if needed, after 5–10 minutes. The drug is rapidly absorbed after IM injection and can be used when IV access is not readily available.

C. **Chloroquine and hydroxychloroquine intoxication.** There is reported improvement of cardiotoxicity with high-dose administration of **diazepam** at 1 mg/kg IV. *Caution:* This will likely cause apnea; the patient must be intubated, and ventilation must be controlled.

E. **Alcohol withdrawal syndrome**
   1. **Diazepam.** Administer 5–10 mg IV initially, then 5 mg every 10 minutes until the patient is calm. Large doses may be required to sedate patients with severe withdrawal. The oral dose is 10–20 mg initially, repeated every 1–2 hours until calm.
   2. **Lorazepam.** Administer 1–2 mg IV initially, then 1 mg every 10 minutes until the patient is calm. Large doses may be required to sedate patients in severe withdrawal. The oral dose is 2–4 mg, repeated every 1–2 hours until calm.

VII. **Formulations**
A. **Parenteral**
   1. **Diazepam** (Valium, others): 5-mg/mL solution, 2-mL prefilled syringes.
   2. **Lorazepam** (Ativan, others): 2- and 4-mg/mL solutions; 1 mL in 2 mL syringe for dilution.
   3. **Midazolam** (Versed): 1- and 5-mg/mL solutions; 1-, 2-, 5-, and 10-mL vials.
B. **Oral**
   1. **Diazepam** (Valium, others): 2-, 5-, and 10-mg tablets.
   2. **Lorazepam** (Ativan, others): 0.5-, 1-, and 2-mg tablets; 2 mg/mL oral solution.
C. **Suggested minimum stocking levels** to treat a 70-kg adult for the first 24 hours:
   1. **Diazepam,** 200 mg.
   2. **Lorazepam,** 24 mg.
   3. **Midazolam,** 50 mg (two vials of 5 mg/mL, 5 mL each, or equivalent).

▶ **BENZTROPINE**

Thomas E. Kearney, PharmD

I. **Pharmacology.** Benztropine is an antimuscarinic agent with pharmacologic activity similar to that of atropine. The drug also exhibits antihistaminic properties. Benztropine is used for the treatment of parkinsonism and for the control of extrapyramidal side effects associated with neuroleptic use.

II. Indications. Benztropine is an alternative in adults to diphenhydramine (the drug of choice for children) for the treatment of acute dystonic reactions associated with neuroleptics or metoclopramide. **Note:** It is not effective for tardive dyskinesia or neuroleptic malignant syndrome (see p 20).

III. Contraindications.
 A. Angle-closure glaucoma.
 B. Obstructive uropathy (prostatic hypertrophy).
 C. Myasthenia gravis.
 D. Not recommended for children under 3 years (use diphenhydramine; see p 359).

IV. Adverse effects.
 A. Adverse effects include sedation, blurred vision, tachycardia, urinary hesitancy or retention, and dry mouth. Adverse effects are minimal after single doses.
 B. **Use in pregnancy.** FDA category C (indeterminate). However, this does not preclude its acute, short-term use for a seriously symptomatic patient (see p 333).

V. Drug or laboratory interactions.
 A. Benztropine has additive effects with other drugs exhibiting antimuscarinic properties (eg, antihistamines, phenothiazines, cyclic antidepressants, and disopyramide).
 B. Slowing of gastrointestinal motility may delay or inhibit absorption of certain drugs.

VI. Dosage and method of administration.
 A. **Parenteral.** Give 1–2 mg IV or IM (children >3 years old, 0.02 mg/kg and 1 mg maximum).
 B. **Oral.** Give 1–2 mg PO every 12 hours (children >3 years old, 0.02 mg/kg, and 1 mg maximum) for 2–3 days to prevent recurrence of symptoms.

VII. Formulations.
 A. **Parenteral.** Benztropine mesylate (Cogentin), 1 mg/mL, 2-mL ampules.
 B. **Oral.** Benztropine mesylate (Cogentin), 0.5-, 1-, and 2-mg tablets.
 C. The **suggested minimum stocking level** to treat a 70-kg adult for the first 24 hours is 6 mg (3 ampules, 2 mL each).

▶ BICARBONATE, SODIUM

Thomas E. Kearney, PharmD

I. Pharmacology.
 A. Sodium bicarbonate is a buffering agent that reacts with hydrogen ions to correct acidemia and produce alkalemia. Urinary alkalinization from renally excreted bicarbonate ions enhances the renal elimination of certain acidic drugs (eg, salicylate and phenobarbital) and helps prevent renal tubular myoglobin deposition in patients with rhabdomyolysis. In addition, maintenance of a normal or high serum pH may prevent intracellular distribution of salicylate.
 B. The sodium ion load and alkalemia produced by hypertonic sodium bicarbonate reverse the sodium channel-dependent membrane-depressant ("quinidinelike") effects of several drugs (eg, tricyclic antidepressants, type Ia and type Ic antiarrhythmic agents, and diphenhydramine).
 C. Alkalinization causes an intracellular shift of potassium and is used for the acute treatment of hyperkalemia.
 D. Sodium bicarbonate given orally or by gastric lavage forms an insoluble salt with iron and may theoretically help prevent absorption of ingested iron tablets (unproved).

II. Indications.
 A. Severe metabolic acidosis resulting from intoxication by methanol, ethylene glycol, or salicylates or from excessive lactic acid production (eg, resulting from status epilepticus or shock).

B. To produce urinary alkalinization, to enhance elimination of salicylate or phenobarbital, or to prevent renal deposition of myoglobin after severe rhabdomyolysis.

C. Cardiotoxicity with impaired ventricular depolarization (as evidenced by a prolonged QRS interval) caused by tricyclic antidepressants, type Ia or type Ic antiarrhythmics, and other membrane-depressant drugs (see Table I–5, p 11). *Note:* Not effective for dysrhythmias associated with abnormal repolarization (prolonged QT interval and Torsades de pointes).

D. Sodium bicarbonate has been used in lavage fluid to treat excessive iron ingestion (effectiveness unproved).

III. **Contraindications.** The following contraindications are relative.

A. Significant metabolic or respiratory alkalemia or hypernatremia.

B. Severe pulmonary edema.

IV. **Adverse effects.**

A. Excessive alkalemia: impaired oxygen release from hemoglobin, hypocalcemic tetany, and paradoxic intracellular acidosis (from elevated pCO_2 concentrations) and hypokalemia.

B. Hypernatremia and hyperosmolality.

C. Aggravation of congestive heart failure and pulmonary edema.

D. Extravasation leading to tissue inflammation and necrosis (product is hypertonic).

E. May exacerbate QT prolongation and associated dysrhythmias (eg, Torsades de pointes) as a result of electrolyte shifts (hypokalemia).

F. **Use in pregnancy.** FDA category C (indeterminate). However, this does not preclude its acute, short-term use for a seriously symptomatic patient (see p 333).

V. **Drug or laboratory interactions.** Do not mix with other parenteral drugs because of the possibility of drug inactivation or precipitation.

VI. **Dosage and method of administration (adults and children).**

A. **Metabolic acidemia.** Give 0.5–1 mEq/kg IV bolus; repeat as needed to correct serum pH to at least 7.2. For salicylates, methanol, or ethylene glycol, raise the pH to at least 7.4–7.5.

B. **Urinary alkalinization.** Give 50-100 mEq in 1 L of 5% dextrose in 0.25% normal saline at 2–3 mL/kg/h. Check urine pH frequently and adjust flow rate to maintain urine pH level at 7–8. *Note:* Hypokalemia and fluid depletion prevent effective urinary alkalinization: add 20 mEq of potassium to each liter, unless renal failure is present.

C. **Cardiotoxic drug intoxication.** Give 1–2 mEq/kg IV bolus; repeat as needed to improve cardiotoxic manifestations and to maintain serum pH at 7.45–7.5. There is no evidence that constant infusions are as effective as boluses given as needed.

D. **Gastric iron complexation.** Make a 1–2% solution by diluting sodium bicarbonate with normal saline, and use 4–5 mL/kg as a gastric lavage solution.

VII. **Formulations.**

A. Several products are available, ranging from 4.2% (0.5 mEq/mL) to 8.4% (1 mEq/mL) in volumes of 10–500 mL. The most commonly used formulation available in most emergency "crash carts" is 8.4% ("hypertonic") sodium bicarbonate, 1 mEq/mL, in 50-mL ampules or prefilled syringes.

B. The **suggested minimum stocking level** to treat a 70-kg adult for the first 24 hours is 10 ampules or syringes (approximately 500 mEq).

▶ **BOTULIN ANTITOXIN**

Thomas E. Kearney, PharmD

I. **Pharmacology.** Botulin antitoxin contains concentrated equine-derived antibodies directed against the toxins produced by the various strains of *Clostridium botulinum* (A, B, and E). The trivalent form (A, B, E) provides the greatest degree of coverage and is preferred over the older bivalent (A, B) type. The antibodies bind and inactivate freely circulating botulin toxins but do *not* remove toxin that is already bound to nerve terminals. Because antitoxin will not reverse established paralysis once it occurs, it must be administered before paralysis sets in. Treatment within 24 hours of the onset of symptoms may shorten the course of intoxication and prevent progression to total paralysis.

II. Indications. Botulin antitoxin is used to treat clinical botulism to prevent progression of neurologic manifestations. It is generally not recommended for treatment of infant botulism; however, open-label clinical trials have been under way in California with human-derived botulism immune globulin (BIG) and may be extended nationwide. For information, call the California Department of Health Services at (510) 540-2646.

III. Contraindications. No absolute contraindications. Known hypersensitivity to botulin antitoxin or horse serum requires extreme caution if this product is given.

IV. Adverse effects.
- **A.** Immediate hypersensitivity reactions (anaphylaxis) resulting from the equine source of antibodies.
- **B.** Delayed arthus reaction (serum sickness) 1–2 weeks after antitoxin administration.
- **C. Use in pregnancy.** There are no data on teratogenicity. Anaphylactic reaction resulting in shock or hypoxemia in the mother could conceivably adversely affect the fetus.

V. Drug or laboratory interactions. No known interactions.

VI. Dosage and method of administration.
- **A.** For established clinical botulism, give one to two vials IV every 4 hours for four to five doses (for suspected botulism, one to two vials are usually given empirically). Intramuscular administration is not recommended. Duration of therapy depends on clinical response, particularly any progression of muscular paralysis.
- **B.** Perform a skin test prior to administration according to the package instructions. Should the patient have known sensitivity to horse serum or demonstrate a positive skin test, provide desensitization as indicated in the package insert. Even if the skin test is negative, anaphylaxis may still occur unpredictably. Pretreat the patient with diphenhydramine (see p 359), 1–2 mg/kg IV, and cimetidine 300 mg IV (or other H_2 blocker, see p 353), also have epinephrine (see p 365) ready in case anaphylaxis occurs.

VII. Formulations.
- **A. Parenteral.** Trivalent botulin antitoxin (7500 IU type A, 5500 IU type B, 8500 IU type E); available through the Centers for Disease Control (CDC), telephone (404) 639-3356 (weekdays) or (404) 639-2888 (after hours). To obtain BIG for suspected infant botulism in the state of California, call (510) 540-2646 (24 hours).
- **B. Suggested minimum stocking level.** Not relevant—available only through federal (CDC) or state (California) government.

▶ **BRETYLIUM**

Thomas E. Kearney, PharmD

I. Pharmacology. Bretylium is a quaternary ammonium compound that is an effective type III antifibrillatory drug and also suppresses ventricular ectopic activity. It increases the threshold for ventricular fibrillation and reduces the disparity in action potential duration between normal and ischemic tissue, which is believed to abolish boundary currents responsible for reentrant arrhythmias. Its pharmacologic actions are complex. Initially, norepinephrine is released from sympathetic neurons; this is followed by a block of further norepinephrine release. In addition, norepinephrine uptake is inhibited at adrenergic neurons. The result is a transient increase in heart rate, blood pressure, and cardiac output that may last from a few minutes to 1 hour. Subsequent adrenergic blockade produces vasodilation, which may result in hypotension.

II. **Indications.**
   A. **Prophylaxis and treatment of ventricular fibrillation.** Bretylium may be particularly effective in hypothermic patients.
   B. **Ventricular tachycardia resistant to other antiarrhythmic agents.** However, it has not been proved beneficial for drug- or chemical-induced ventricular dysrhythmias.

III. **Contraindications.**
   A. Use with extreme caution in patients with intoxication by digitalis, chloral hydrate, or halogenated hydrocarbons, because the initial release of catecholamines may aggravate arrhythmias.
   B. Use with extreme caution in patients with arrhythmias caused by intoxication with cyclic antidepressants or type Ia or type Ic antiarrhythmic agents because of additive cardiac depression.
   C. Use with extreme caution in patients with severe pulmonary hypertension or aortic stenosis.
   D. Not recommended for children under 12 years old.

IV. **Adverse effects.**
   A. Hypotension (both supine and orthostatic).
   B. Nausea and vomiting from rapid intravenous administration.
   C. Transient hypertension and worsening of arrhythmias may be caused by initial catecholamine release .
   D. **Use in pregnancy.** FDA category C (indeterminate). However, this does not preclude its acute, short-term use for a seriously symptomatic patient (see p 333).

V. **Drug or laboratory interactions.**
   A. The pressor effect of sympathomimetic amines may be enhanced with initial catecholamine release.
   B. Cardiac-depressant effects may be additive with other antiarrhythmic drugs, particularly type Ia and type Ic drugs.

VI. **Dosage and method of administration.**
   A. **For ventricular fibrillation,** give 5 mg/kg IV over 1 minute (in addition to cardiopulmonary resuscitation and defibrillation). If not effective, administration may be repeated with 10 mg/kg.
   B. **For ventricular tachycardia,** give adults and children older than 12 years 5–10 mg/kg IV over 8–10 minutes or IM, repeated as necessary at 15-minute intervals to a maximum dose of 30 mg/kg; repeat every 6 hours as needed.
   C. **The continuous infusion rate** after the loading dose is 1–2 mg/min (children >12 years old, 20–30 μg/kg/min).

VII. **Formulations.**
   A. **Parenteral.** Bretylium tosylate (Bretylol, others), 50 mg/mL: 10-mL ampules, vials, and syringes and 20-mL single-use vials; 500 and 1000 mg premixed in 250-mL 5% dextrose solutions.
   B. The **suggested minimum stocking level** to treat a 70-kg adult for the first 24 hours is six 10-mL vials.

▶ BROMOCRIPTINE

Thomas E. Kearney, PharmD

I. **Pharmacology.** Bromocriptine mesylate is a semisynthetic derivative of the ergopeptide group of ergot alkaloids with dopaminergic agonist effects. It also has minor α-adrenergic antagonist properties. The dopaminergic effects account for its inhibition of prolactin secretion and its beneficial effects in the treatment of parkinsonism, neuroleptic malignant syndrome (NMS; see p 20), and cocaine craving, as well as its adverse effect profile and drug interactions. A key limitation is the inability to administer bromocriptine by the parenteral route coupled with poor bioavailability (only about 6% of an oral dose is absorbed). In addition, the onset of therapeutic effects (eg, alleviation of muscle rigidity, hypertension, and hyperthermia) in the treatment of NMS may take several hours to days.

II. **Indications.**
   A. Treatment of NMS caused by neuroleptic drugs (eg, haloperidol and other antipsychotics) or levodopa withdrawal.

   Note: If the patient has significant hyperthermia (eg, rectal or core temperature >40 (C), bromocriptine should be considered secondary and adjunctive therapy to immediate measures such as neuromuscular paralysis and aggressive external cooling.

   B. Bromocriptine has been used experimentally to alleviate craving for cocaine. *Caution:* There is one case report of a severe adverse reaction (hypertension, seizures, and blindness) when bromocriptine was used in a cocaine abuser during the postpartum period.

   C. *Note:* Bromocriptine is *not* considered appropriate first-line therapy for acute drug-induced extrapyramidal or parkinsonian symptoms (see p 24).

III. **Contraindications.**
   A. Uncontrolled hypertension or toxemia of pregnancy.
   B. Known hypersensitivity to the drug.
   C. A relative contraindication is a history of angina, myocardial infarction, stroke, vasospastic disorders (eg, Raynaud's disease), or bipolar affective disorder. In addition, there is no published experience in children.

IV. **Adverse effects.** Most adverse effects are dose-related and of minor clinical consequence; some are unpredictable.
   A. The most common side effect is nausea. Epigastric pain, dyspepsia, and diarrhea also have been reported.
   B. Hypotension (usually transient) and syncope may occur at the initiation of treatment, and hypertension may occur later. Other cardiovascular effects include dysrhythmias (with high doses), exacerbation of angina and vasospastic disorders such as Raynaud's disease, and intravascular thrombosis resulting in acute myocardial infarction (one case report).
   C. Nervous system side effects vary considerably and include headache, drowsiness, fatigue, hallucinations, mania, psychosis, agitation, seizures, and cerebrovascular accident. Multiple interrelated risk factors include dose, concurrent drug therapy, and preexisting medical and psychiatric disorders.
   D. Rare effects include pulmonary toxicity (infiltrates, pleural effusion and thickening) and myopia with long-term, high-dose treatment (months). There has been one case of retroperitoneal fibrosis.
   E. Sulfite preservatives in some preparations may cause hypersensitivity reactions. SnapTabs tablets do not contain sulfites.
   F. **Use in pregnancy.** No FDA category. This drug has been used therapeutically during the last trimester of pregnancy for treatment of a pituitary tumor. It has been shown to inhibit fetal prolactin secretion, and it may precipitate premature labor and inhibit lactation in the mother.

V. **Drug or laboratory interactions.**
   A. Bromocriptine may accentuate hypotension in patients receiving antihypertensive drugs.
   B. Theoretically, this drug may have additive effects with other ergot alkaloids, and its potential to cause peripheral vasospasm may be exacerbated by propranolol.
   C. Bromocriptine may reduce ethanol tolerance.
   D. There has been one case report of apparent serotonin syndrome (see p 20) in a patient with Parkinson's disease receiving levodopa and carbidopa.

VI. **Dosage and method of administration for NMS.** In adults, administer 2.5–10 mg orally or by gastric tube 2–6 times daily. The pediatric dose is unknown. Use small, frequent dosing to minimize nausea.

A. A therapeutic response is usually achieved with total daily doses of 5–30 mg.

B. Continue treatment until rigidity and fever have completely resolved, then slowly taper the dose. Several days of therapy may be required for complete reversal of NMS.

VII. Formulations.

  A. Oral. Bromocriptine mesylate (Parlodel), 2.5- and 5-mg capsules and scored (SnapTabs) tablets.

  B. The **suggested minimum stocking level** to treat a 70-kg adult for the first 24 hours is 30 mg, or one 30-tablet (SnapTabs) package. SnapTabs tablets do not contain sulfite preservatives.

▶ CALCIUM

Thomas E. Kearney, PharmD

I. Pharmacology.

  A. Calcium is a cation necessary for the normal functioning of a variety of enzymes and organ systems, including muscle and nerve tissue. Hypocalcemia, or a blockade of calcium's effects, may cause muscle cramps, tetany, and ventricular fibrillation. Antagonism of calcium-dependent channels results in hypotension, bradycardia, and atrioventricular block.

  B. Calcium ions rapidly bind to fluoride ions, abolishing their toxic effects.

  C. The neuromuscular effects of black widow spider venom can be antagonized to some degree by the administration of calcium, through a mechanism not fully understood.

  D. Calcium can reverse the negative inotropic effects of calcium antagonists; however, depressed automaticity and atrioventricular nodal conduction velocity and vasodilation may not respond to calcium administration.

  E. Calcium is directly antagonistic to the cardiotoxic effects of hyperkalemia.

II. Indications.

  A. Symptomatic hypocalcemia resulting from intoxication by fluoride, oxalate, or the intravenous anticoagulant citrate.

  B. Topical hydrofluoric acid exposure.

  C. Black widow spider envenomation with muscle cramping or rigidity.

  D. Calcium antagonist (eg, verapamil) overdose with hypotension.

  E. Severe hyperkalemia with cardiotoxic manifestations (except in patients with digitalis toxicity, see part III.B, below).

III. Contraindications.

  A. Hypercalcemia.

  B. Digitalis intoxication (may aggravate digitalis-induced ventricular tachyarrhythmias).

  C. *Note:* Calcium *chloride* salt should *not* be used for intradermal or subcutaneous injection because it is too concentrated and may result in further tissue damage.

IV. Adverse effects.

  A. Tissue irritation, particularly with calcium chloride salt; extravasation may cause local cellulitis or necrosis.

  B. Hypercalcemia, especially in patients with diminished renal function.

  C. Hypotension, bradycardia, syncope, and cardiac arrhythmias caused by rapid intravenous administration.

  D. Constipation caused by orally administered calcium salts.

  E. Use in pregnancy. FDA category C (indeterminate). This does not preclude its acute, short-term use for a seriously symptomatic patient (see p 333).

V. Drug or laboratory interactions.

  A. Inotropic and arrhythmogenic effects of digitalis are potentiated by calcium.

B. A precipitate will form with solutions containing soluble salts of carbonates, phosphates, or sulfates and with various antibiotics.

VI. Dosage and method of administration. *Note:* Calcium chloride contains nearly threefold the milliequivalents of Ca^{2+} per milliliter of 10% solution compared with calcium gluconate.

   A. Oral fluoride ingestion. Administer calcium-containing antacid (calcium carbonate) orally to complex fluoride ions.

   B. Symptomatic hypocalcemia, hyperkalemia, or black widow spider envenomation. Give 10% calcium gluconate, 10–20 mL (children, 0.2–0.3 mL/kg), or 10% calcium chloride, 5–10 mL (children, 0.1–0.2 mL/kg), slowly IV. Repeat as needed.

   C. Calcium antagonist poisoning. Start with doses as described above. *High-dose calcium* therapy has been reported effective in some cases of severe calcium channel blocker overdose. As much as 12 g of calcium chloride has been given over 2 hours. Administer calcium as multiple boluses (eg, 1 g every 10–20 minutes) or as a continuous infusion (eg, 20–50 mg/kg/h).

   C. Dermal hydrofluoric acid exposure. For any exposure involving the hand or fingers, obtain immediate consultation from an experienced hand surgeon.

     1. Topical Calcium concentrations for topical therapy have ranged from 2.5 to 33%; the optimal concentration has not been determined. Most commonly, a 2.5% gel is prepared by combining 1 g of calcium gluconate per 40 g (approximately 40 mL) of water-soluble base material (Surgilube, K-Y Jelly). A 32.5% gel can be made by compounding a slurry of ten 650-mg calcium carbonate tablets in 20 mL of water-soluble lubricant. For exposures involving the hand or fingers, place the gel into a large surgical latex glove to serve as an occlusive dressing to maximize skin contact.

     2. For **subcutaneous** injection (when topical treatment fails to relieve pain), inject 5–10% calcium gluconate (*not* chloride) SC, 0.5 mL/cm^2 of affected skin, using a 27-gauge or smaller needle. This can be repeated two to three times at 1- to 2-hour intervals if pain is not relieved.

     3. For **intra-arterial** administration, infuse 20 mL of 10% calcium gluconate (*not* chloride) diluted in 250 mL D5W via the radial or brachial artery proximal to the injury over 3–4 hours. Alternately, dilute 10 mL of 10% calcium gluconate with 40–50 mL of D5W.

     4. Nebulized inhalation and **ocular** administration of 2.5% calcium gluconate solutions are of unproved efficacy.

VII. Formulations.

   A. Oral. Calcium carbonate; suspension, tablets, or chewable tablets; 300–800 mg.

   B. Parenteral. Calcium gluconate (10%), 10 mL (1 g contains 4.5 mEq calcium); calcium chloride (10%), 10 mL (1 g contains 13.6 mEq).

   C. Topical. No commercial formulation is approved currently in the United States.

   D. The **suggested minimum stocking level** to treat a 70-kg adult for the first 24 hours is 5–10 vials (1 g each) of 10% calcium gluconate.

▶ CHARCOAL, ACTIVATED

Thomas E. Kearney, PharmD

I. Pharmacology. Activated charcoal, by virtue of its large surface area, adsorbs many drugs and toxins. Highly ionic salts (eg, iron, lithium, and cyanide) or small polar molecules (eg, alcohols) are poorly adsorbed. Repeated oral doses of activated charcoal can increase the rate of elimination of some drugs that have a small volume of distribution (Vd) and that undergo enterogastric or enterohepatic recirculation (eg, digitoxin) or diffuse into the gastrointestinal lumen from the intestinal circulation (eg, phenobarbital and theophylline). See also discussion in Section I, p 54.

II. **Indications.**
    A. Activated charcoal is used orally after an ingestion to limit drug or toxin absorption. Although traditionally given after the stomach has been emptied by ipecac-induced emesis or gastric lavage, recent studies suggest that it may be used alone for most ingestions. Use in the home after a childhood exposure is controversial.
    B. Repeated doses of activated charcoal may be indicated to enhance elimination of some drugs if (1) more rapid elimination will benefit the patient (and the benefits outweigh the risks of repeated doses; see parts IV.C and V.C, below), and (2) more aggressive means of removal (eg, hemodialysis or hemoperfusion) are not immediately indicated or available (see p 51). However, it has not been proven to improve patient outcome in clinical studies.
    C. Repeated doses of activated charcoal may be useful when the quantity of drug or toxin ingested is greater than one-tenth of the usual charcoal dose (eg, an aspirin ingestion of more than 6–10 g) or when surface contact with the drug is hindered (eg, pharmacobezoars and wrapped or packaged drugs).

III. **Contraindications.**
    A. Gastrointestinal ileus or obstruction may prevent the administration of more than one or two doses.
    B. Acid or alkali ingestions, unless other drugs have also been ingested (charcoal makes endoscopic evaluation more difficult).

IV. **Adverse effects.**
    A. Constipation (may be prevented by coadministration of a cathartic).
    B. Distention of the stomach, with potential risk of aspiration.
    C. Diarrhea, dehydration, hypermagnesemia, and hypernatremia resulting from coadministered cathartics, especially with repeated doses of charcoal and cathartics, or even after a single large dose of a premixed, sorbitol-containing charcoal product.
    D. Intestinal bezoar with obstruction.
    E. **Use in pregnancy.** Activated charcoal is not systemically absorbed. Diarrhea resulting in shock or hypernatremia in the mother could conceivably adversely affect the fetus.

V. **Drug or laboratory interactions.**
    A. Activated charcoal may reduce, prevent, or delay the absorption of orally administered antidotes or other drugs (eg, nifedipine and acetylcysteine).
    B. The adsorptive capacity of activated charcoal may be diminished by the concurrent ingestion of ice cream, milk, or sugar syrup; the clinical significance is unknown but is probably minor.
    C. Repeated doses of charcoal may enhance the elimination of some necessary therapeutic drugs (eg, anticonvulsants).

VI. **Dosage and method of administration.**
    A. **Initial dose.** Activated charcoal, 1 g/kg orally or via gastric tube, is administered, or if the quantity of toxin ingested is known, 10 times the amount of ingested toxin by weight is given. For massive overdoses (eg, 60–100 g aspirin), this may need to be given in divided doses over 1–2 days.
    B. **Repeat-dose charcoal.** Activated charcoal, 15–30 g (0.25–0.5 g/kg) every 2–4 hours is given orally or by gastric tube. (The optimal regimen and dose are unknown.) Administer a small dose of cathartic with every second or third charcoal dose. Do *not* use cathartic with every activated charcoal dose.
        End points for repeat-dose charcoal therapy include clinical improvement and declining serum drug level; the usual empiric duration is 24–48 hours.
    C. For patients with nausea or vomiting, administer antiemetics (metoclopramide, p 382; or ondansetron, p 395) and consider giving the charcoal by gastric tube.

VII. **Formulations.**
    A. There are a variety of formulations and a large number of brands of activated charcoal. It is available as a powder, a liquid aqueous suspension, and a liquid suspension in sorbitol or propylene glycol.

B. The **suggested minimum stocking level** to treat a 70-kg adult for the first 24 hours is three bottles containing 50 g of activated charcoal each. Preferred stock is the plain aqueous suspension.

▶ CIMETIDINE AND OTHER H₂ BLOCKERS

Thomas E. Kearney, PharmD

I. Pharmacology. Cimetidine, ranitidine, and famotidine are selective competitive inhibitors of histamine on H_2 receptors. These receptors modulate smooth muscle, vascular tone, and gastric secretions and may be involved in clinical effects associated with anaphylactic and anaphylactoid reactions, as well as ingestion of histamine or histamine-like substances (eg, Scombroid fish poisoning).

II. Indications.

A. Adjunctive with H_1 blockers such as diphenhydramine (see p 359) in the management and prophylactic treatment of anaphylactic and anaphylactoid reactions (see Antivenins, pp 336–339).

B. Adjunctive with H_1 blockers such as diphenhydramine (see p 359) in the management of Scombroid fish poisoning (see p 175).

C. Ranitidine has been used to reduce vomiting associated with theophylline poisoning. Because cimetidine may interfere with hepatic elimination of theophylline it should not be used.

III. Contraindications. Known hypersensitivity to H_2 blockers.

IV. Adverse effects.

A. Headache, drowsiness, fatigue, and dizziness have been reported, but are usually mild.

B. Confusion, agitation, hallucinations, and even seizures have been reported with cimetidine use in the elderly, severely ill, and patients with renal failure.

C. A reversible, dose-dependent rise in serum alanine aminotransferase (ALT) activity has been reported with nizatidine, a related agent. Hepatitis has also occurred with ranitidine.

D. Cardiac dysrhythmias (bradycardia, tachycardia) and hypotension have been associated with rapid IV bolus of cimetidine and ranitidine (rare).

E. Preparations containing the preservative benzyl alcohol have been associated with "gasping syndrome" in premature infants.

V. Drug or laboratory interactions.

A. Cimetidine, and to a lesser extent ranitidine, reduces hepatic clearance and prolongs the elimination half-life of several drugs as a result of inhibition of cytochrome P-450 activity and reduction of hepatic blood flow. Examples of drugs affected include phenytoin, theophylline, phenobarbital, cyclosporin, morphine, lidocaine, calcium channel blockers, tricyclic antidepressants, and warfarin.

B. Cimetidine, ranitidine, and nizatidine inhibit gastric mucosal alcohol dehydrogenase and therefore increase the systemic absorption of ethyl alcohol.

C. Increased gastric pH may inhibit the absorption of some pH-dependent drugs such as ketoconazole, ferrous salts, and tetracyclines.

VI. Dosage and method of administration. In general, there are no clinically proven advantages of any one of the H_2 blockers, although cimetidine is more likely to be associated with drug-drug interactions. See Table III–3 for oral and parenteral doses.

VII. Formulations.

A. Cimetidine (Tagamet, others)

1. Oral. 100-, 200-, 300-, 400-, and 800-mg tablets; 300 mg/5 mL oral solution.

2. Parenteral. 150 mg/mL in 2- and 8-mL vials; premixed 300 mg in 50 mL saline.

B. Famotidine (Pepcid)

1. Oral. 10-, 20-, and 40-mg tablets; 40 mg/5mL oral suspension.

TABLE III–3. CIMETIDINE, FAMOTIDINE, AND RANITIDINE

Drug	Route	Dose[a]
Cimetidine	PO	300 mg every 6–8 h or 400 mg every 12 h (maximum 2400 mg/d). Children: 10 mg/kg single dose; 20–40 mg/kg/d.
	IV, IM	300 mg IV or IM every 6–8 h. For IV administration, dilute in normal saline to a total volume of 20 mL and give over 2 min or longer. Children: 10 mg/kg.
Famotidine	PO	20–40 mg once or twice daily (as much as 160 mg every 6 h has been used).
	IV	20 mg IV every 12 h (dilute in normal saline to a total volume of 5–10 mL).
Ranitidine	PO	150 mg twice daily (up to 6 g/d has been used).
	IV, IM	50 mg IV or IM every 6–8 h. For IV use, dilute in normal saline to a total volume of 20 mL, and inject over 5 min or longer.

[a]Note: May need to reduce dose in patients with renal dysfunction.

    2. **Parenteral.** 10 mg/mL in 2- and 4-mL vials; premixed 20 mg in 50 mL saline.
  C. Ranitidine (Zantac, others)
    1. **Oral** 75-, 150-, and 300-mg tablets and capsules; 15 mg/mL in 10 mL syrup; and 150 mg effervescent granules.
    2. **Parenteral.** 0.5 mg/mL in 100-mL container; 25 mg/mL in 2-, 10-, and 40-mL vials and 2-mL syringe.
  D. The **suggested minimum stocking levels** to treat a 70-kg adult for the first 24 hours (all are parenteral dose form) are the following:
    1. **Cimetidine.** 1200 mg (8-mL vial).
    2. **Famotidine.** 40 mg (4-mL multidose vial).
    3. **Ranitidine.** 250 mg (10-mL vial).

▶ CYANIDE ANTIDOTE PACKAGE

See Nitrite (p 390) and Thiosulfate (p 408).

▶ DANTROLENE

Thomas E. Kearney, PharmD

  I. Pharmacology. Dantrolene relaxes skeletal muscle by inhibiting the release of calcium from the sarcoplasmic reticulum, thereby reducing actin-myosin contractile activity. Dantrolene can help control hyperthermia that results from excessive muscle hyperactivity, particularly when hyperthermia is caused by a defect within the muscle cell (eg, malignant hyperthermia). Dantrolene is not a substitute for other temperature-controlling measures (eg, sponging and fanning).
  II. Indications.
    A. The primary indication for dantrolene is malignant hyperthermia (see p 20).
    B. Dantrolene may be useful in treating hyperthermia and rhabdomyolysis caused by drug-induced muscular hyperactivity not controlled by usual cooling measures or neuromuscular paralysis.
    C. Dantrolene is not likely to be effective for hyperthermia caused by conditions other than muscular hyperactivity, such as increased metabolic rate (eg, sali-

cylate or dinitrophenol poisoning), impaired heat dissipation (eg, anticholinergic syndrome), or environmental exposure (heat stroke).

III. Contraindications. No absolute contraindications exist. Patients with muscular weakness or respiratory impairment must be observed closely for possible respiratory arrest.

IV. Adverse effects.
  A. Muscle weakness, which may aggravate respiratory depression.
  B. Drowsiness or diarrhea.
  C. Hypersensitivity hepatitis, occasionally fatal, reported after chronic therapy. Transaminases are elevated in about 10% of patients treated with dantrolene.
  D. Use in pregnancy. FDA category C (indeterminate). This does not preclude its acute, short-term use for a seriously symptomatic patient (see p 333).

V. Drug or laboratory interactions.
  A. Dantrolene may have additive central nervous system-depressant effects with sedative and hypnotic drugs.
  B. Each 20-mg vial of Dantrium contains 3 g of mannitol; this should be taken into consideration as it may have additive effects with any mannitol given to treat rhabdomyolysis.

VI. Dosage and method of administration (adults and children).
  A. Parenteral. Give 1–2 mg/kg rapidly IV; this may be repeated as needed every 5–10 minutes, to a total dose of 10 mg/kg. Satisfactory response is usually achieved with 2–5 mg/kg.
  B. Oral. To prevent recurrence of hyperthermia, administer 1–2 mg/kg intravenously or orally (up to 100 mg maximum) 4 times a day for 2–3 days.

VII. Formulations.
  A. Parenteral. Dantrolene sodium (Dantrium), 20 mg of lyophilized powder for reconstitution (after reconstitution, protect from light and use within 6 hours to ensure maximal activity). Each 20-mg vial contains 3 g of mannitol.
  B. Oral. Dantrolene sodium (Dantrium) in 25-, 50-, and 100-mg capsules.
  C. The **suggested minimum stocking level** to treat a 70-kg adult for the first 24 hours is thirty-five 20-mg vials.

▶ DEFEROXAMINE

Anthony S. Manoguerra, PharmD

I. Pharmacology. Deferoxamine is a specific chelating agent for iron. It binds free iron and, to some extent, loosely bound iron (eg, from ferritin or hemosiderin). Iron bound to hemoglobin, transferrin, cytochrome enzymes, and all other sites is unaffected. The red iron-deferoxamine (ferrioxamine) complex is water-soluble and is excreted renally, where it imparts an orange-pink, or "vin rosé" color to the urine. One hundred milligrams of deferoxamine is capable of binding 8.5 mg of elemental iron.

II. Indications.
  A. Deferoxamine is used to treat iron intoxication when the serum iron is greater than 450–500 µg/dL or when clinical signs of significant iron intoxication exist (eg, shock, acidosis, severe gastroenteritis, or numerous radiopaque tablets visible in the gastrointestinal tract by x-ray).
  B. Deferoxamine is sometimes used as a "test dose" to determine the presence of free iron by observing for the characteristic "vin rosé" color in the urine; however, a change in urine color change is not a reliable indicator.

III. Contraindications. No absolute contraindications to deferoxamine use in patients with serious iron poisoning. The drug should be used with caution in patients with known sensitivity to deferoxamine.

IV. Adverse effects.
  A. Hypotension or an anaphylactoid-type reaction may occur from very rapid intravenous bolus administration; this may be avoided by limiting the rate of administration to 15 mg/kg/h.

B. Local pain, induration, and sterile abscess formation may occur at intramuscular injection sites. Large intramuscular injections may also cause hypotension.

C. The ferrioxamine complex may itself cause hypotension and may accumulate in patients with renal impairment; hemodialysis may be necessary to remove the ferrioxamine complex.

D. Deferoxamine, as a siderophore, promotes the growth of certain bacteria such as *Yersinia enterocolitica* and may predispose patients to *Yersinia* sepsis.

E. Infusions exceeding 24 hours have been associated with pulmonary complications (acute respiratory distress syndrome [ARDS]).

F. Use in pregnancy. FDA category C (indeterminate). Although deferoxamine is a teratogen in animals, it has relatively poor placental transfer, and there is no evidence that short-term treatment is harmful in human pregnancy (see p 333). More importantly, failure to treat a serious acute iron intoxication may result in maternal and fetal morbidity or death.

V. Drug or laboratory interactions. Deferoxamine may interfere with determinations of serum iron (falsely low) and total iron-binding capacity (falsely high) It may chelate and remove aluminum from the body.

VI. Dosage and method of administration.

A. The intravenous route is preferred in all cases. In children or adults, give deferoxamine at an infusion rate generally not to exceed 15 mg/kg/h (although rates up to 40–50 mg/kg/h have been given in patients with massive iron intoxication). The maximum cumulative daily dose should generally not exceed 6 g (doses up to 16 g have been tolerated). The end points of therapy include loss of "vin rosé"-colored urine, a serum iron level less than 350 μg/dL, and resolution of clinical signs of intoxication.

B. Oral complexation is *not* recommended.

C. "Test dose" intramuscular injection is *not* recommended. If the patient is symptomatic, use the intravenous route. If the patient is not symptomatic but serious toxicity is expected to occur, intravenous access is essential (eg, for fluid boluses), and intravenous dosing provides more reliable administration.

VII. Formulations.

A. Parenteral. Deferoxamine mesylate (Desferal), vials containing 500 mg of lyophilized powder.

B. The **suggested minimum stocking level** to treat a 70-kg adult for the first 24 hours is 12 vials.

▶ DIAZOXIDE

Thomas E. Kearney, PharmD

I. Pharmacology.

A. Diazoxide, a nondiuretic thiazide, is a direct arterial vasodilator formerly used to treat severe hypertension. Heart rate and cardiac output increase owing to a reflex response to decreased peripheral vascular resistance. The duration of the hypotensive effect ranges from 3 to 12 hours, although the elimination half-life is 20–40 hours.

B. Diazoxide is currently used in the treatment of oral hypoglycemic overdose because it increases serum glucose by inhibiting insulin secretion, diminishing peripheral glucose utilization, and enhancing hepatic glucose release (see also Octreotide, p 394).

II. Indications.

A. Management of an acute hypertensive crisis, although other newer antihypertensive agents generally are preferred (see Nifedipine [p 389], Phentolamine [p 400], Nitroprusside [p 392], and Labetalol [p 377]).

B. Oral hypoglycemic overdose, when serum glucose concentrations cannot be adequately maintained by intravenous 5% dextrose infusions.

III. **Contraindications.**
   A. Hypertension associated with aortic stenosis, aortic coarctation, hypertrophic cardiomyopathy, or arteriovenous shunt.
   B. Known hypersensitivity to thiazides.

IV. **Adverse effects.**
   A. Hypotension or excessive blood pressure reduction must be avoided in patients with compromised cerebral or cardiac circulation.
   B. Fluid retention from prolonged therapy may compromise patients with congestive heart failure.
   C. Hyperglycemia may occur, particularly in patients with diabetes or hepatic dysfunction.
   D. **Use in pregnancy.** FDA category C (indeterminate). This drug has caused skeletal, cardiac, and pancreatic abnormalities in animals, but no adequate human data exist. Use of this drug near term may cause hyperbilirubinemia and altered carbohydrate metabolism in the fetus or neonate, and intravenous administration during labor may cause cessation of uterine contractions. These cautions, however, do not necessarily preclude acute, short-term use of the drug for a seriously symptomatic patient (see p 333).

V. **Drug or laboratory interactions.**
   A. The hypotensive effect is potentiated by concomitant therapy with diuretics or β-adrenergic blockers.
   B. Diazoxide displaces warfarin from protein-binding sites and may transiently potentiate its anticoagulant effects.
   C. Diazoxide can increase phenytoin metabolism.

VI. **Dosage and method of administration (adults and children).**
   A. **For oral hypoglycemic-induced hypoglycemia.**
      1. Give a 0.1–2 mg/kg/h infusion; initiate at a lower infusion rate and titrate up as needed. Hypotension is minimized by keeping the patient supine and increasing the infusion rate slowly. Duration of therapy has ranged from 22 to 60 hours.
      2. An oral dosing regimen of 200 mg every 4 hours has also been used.
   B. **For hypertensive crisis,** give 1–3 mg/kg IV (150 mg maximum) every 5–15 minutes as needed. *Note:* The use of a 300-mg rapid bolus is no longer recommended.

VII. **Formulations.**
   A. **Parenteral.** Diazoxide (Hyperstat), 15 mg/mL in 20-mL ampules.
   B. **Oral.** Diazoxide (Proglycem), 50-mg capsules, or 50-mg/mL oral suspension.
   C. The **suggested minimum stocking levels** to treat a 70-kg adult for the first 24 hours: parenteral, 2 vials (20 mL each); oral, 1 bottle (100 tablets) or 30 mL of suspension.

▶ DIGOXIN-SPECIFIC ANTIBODIES

Thomas E. Kearney, PharmD

I. **Pharmacology.** Digoxin-specific antibodies are produced in immunized sheep and have a high binding affinity for digoxin and (to a lesser extent) digitoxin and other cardiac glycosides. The Fab fragments used to treat poisoning are derived by cleaving the whole antibodies. Once the digoxin-Fab complex is formed, the digoxin molecule is no longer pharmacologically active. The complex enters the circulation, is renally eliminated, and has a half-life of 16–20 hours. Reversal of signs of digitalis intoxication occurs within 30–60 minutes of administration, with complete reversal by 4 hours.

II. Indications. Digoxin-specific antibodies are used for life-threatening arrhythmias or hyperkalemia (>5 mEq/L) caused by cardiac glycoside intoxication (see p 128).

III. Contraindications. No contraindications are known. Caution is warranted in patients with known sensitivity to ovine (sheep) products; a skin test for hypersensitivity may be performed in such patients, using diluted reconstituted drug. There are no reports of hypersensitivity reactions in patients who have received the drug more than once.

IV. Adverse effects.
   A. Monitor the patient for potential hypersensitivity reactions and serum sickness.
   B. In patients with renal insufficiency and impaired clearance of the digitalis-Fab complex, the complex may theoretically degrade, slowly releasing active glycoside (this has not been reported).
   C. Removal of the inotropic effect of digitalis may exacerbate preexisting heart failure.
   D. With removal of digitalis effect, patients with preexisting atrial fibrillation may develop accelerated ventricular response.
   E. Removal of the digitalis effect may reactivate sodium-potassium ATPase and shift potassium into cells, causing a drop in the serum potassium level.
   F. Use in pregnancy. FDA category C (indeterminate). This does not preclude its acute, short-term use for a seriously symptomatic patient (see p 333).

V. Drug or laboratory interactions.
   A. Digoxin-specific Fab fragments will bind other cardiac glycosides including digitoxin, ouabain, oleander glucosides, and possibly glycosides in lily of the Nile, strophanthus, and toad venom (*Bufo* species cardenolides).
   B. The digoxin-Fab complex cross-reacts with the antibody commonly utilized in quantitative immunoassay techniques. This results in falsely high serum concentrations of digoxin owing to measurement of the inactive Fab complex.

VI. Dosage and method of administration. Each vial (38 mg) of digoxin-immune Fab binds 0.5 mg of digoxin.
   A. Estimation of the dose of Fab is based on the body burden of digitalis. This may be calculated if the approximate amount ingested is known (Table III–4) or if the steady-state (postdistributional) serum drug concentration is known (Table III–5). (The steady-state serum drug concentration should be determined at least 12–16 hours after the last dose.) *Note:* The calculation of digoxin body burden is based on an estimated volume of distribution for digoxin of approximately 5–6 L/kg; however, other estimates for the Vd range as high as 8 L/kg. If the patient fails to respond to the initial treatment, the dose may need to increase by an additional 50%.
   B. If the amount ingested or the postdistributional level is not known and the patient has life-threatening dysrhythmias, dosing may have to be empiric. Average dose requirements are 10 and 5 vials for acute and chronic digoxin intoxication, respectively.

TABLE III–4. APPROXIMATE DIGOXIN-FAB DOSE IF AMOUNT INGESTED IS KNOWN

Tablets ingested (0.125-mg size)	Tablets ingested (0.25-mg size)	Approximate dose absorbed (mg)	Recommended dose (no. of vials)
5	2.5	0.5	1
10	5	1	2
20	10	2	4
50	25	5	10
100	50	10	20

TABLE III–5. APPROXIMATE DIGOXIN-FAB DOSE BASED ON SERUM CONCENTRATION AT STEADY STATE (AFTER EQUILIBRATION)

Digoxin: [a] number of digoxin-Fab vials $\cong \dfrac{\text{Serum digoxin (ng/mL)} \times \text{Body weight (kg)}}{100}$

Digitoxin: number of digoxin-Fab vials $\cong \dfrac{\text{Serum digoxin (ng/mL)} \times \text{Body weight (kg)}}{100}$

[a]This calculation provides a quick estimate of the number of vials needed, but could underestimate the actual need, because of variations in the volume of distribution (5–7 L/kg). Be prepared to increase dose by 50% if clinical response to initial dose is not satisfactory.

    C. Theoretically, Fab may be used to neutralize a *portion* of the digoxin body burden to reverse toxicity but maintain therapeutic benefits. The Fab dose can be estimated by subtracting the desired digoxin level from the measured postdistributional level before completing the calculation. Alternately, if the patient is hemodynamically stable, the drug can be given empirically, a vial at a time, titrating to clinical effect. However, partial dosing has been associated with recurrences of symptoms in some digoxin-poisoned patients.

    D. Reconstitute the drug according to package instructions, and administer intravenously over 30 minutes using a 0.22-μm membrane filter. It may be given as a rapid bolus for immediately life-threatening arrhythmias.

VII. Formulations.

    A. **Parenteral.** Digibind, 38 mg of lyophilized digoxin-specific Fab fragments per vial.

    B. The **suggested minimum stocking level** to treat a 70-kg adult for the first 24 hours is 20 vials.

▶ DIPHENHYDRAMINE

Thomas E. Kearney, PharmD

I. Pharmacology. Diphenhydramine is an antihistamine with anticholinergic, antitussive, antiemetic, and local anesthetic properties. The antihistaminic property affords relief from itching and minor irritation caused by plant-induced dermatitis and insect bites and, when used as pretreatment, provides partial protection against anaphylaxis caused by animal serum-derived antivenins or antitoxins. Drug-induced extrapyramidal symptoms respond to the anticholinergic effect of diphenhydramine. The effects of diphenhydramine are maximal at 1 hour after intravenous injection, and they last up to 7 hours. The drug is eliminated by hepatic metabolism, with a serum half-life of 3–7 hours.

II. Indications.

    A. Relief of symptoms caused by excessive histamine effect (eg, ingestion of scombroid-contaminated fish or niacin and rapid intravenous administration of acetylcysteine). Diphenhydramine may be combined with cimetidine or another H_2 histamine receptor blocker (see p 353).

    B. Pretreatment before administration of animal serum-derived antivenins or antitoxins, especially in patients with a history of hypersensitivity or with a positive skin test. Diphenhydramine can be combined with cimetidine or another H_2 histamine receptor blocker.

    C. Neuroleptic drug-induced extrapyramidal symptoms and priapism (one case report).

    D. Pruritus caused by poison oak, poison ivy, or minor insect bites.

III. Contraindications.

   A. Angle-closure glaucoma.
   B. Prostatic hypertrophy with obstructive uropathy.
   C. Concurrent therapy with monoamine oxidase inhibitors.
IV. Adverse effects.
   A. Sedation, drowsiness, and ataxia may occur. Paradoxic excitation is possible in small children.
   B. Excessive doses may cause flushing, tachycardia, blurred vision, delirium, toxic psychosis, urinary retention, and respiratory depression.
   C. Some preparations may contain sulfite preservatives, which can cause allergic-type reactions in susceptible persons.
   D. Use in pregnancy. FDA category B (see p 333). Fetal harm is extremely unlikely.
V. Drug or laboratory interactions.
   A. Additive sedative effect with opioids, ethanol, and other sedatives.
   B. Additive anticholinergic effect with other antimuscarinic drugs.
VI. Dosage and method of administration.
   A. Pruritus. Give 25–50 mg PO every 6–8 hours (children, 5 mg/kg/d in divided doses); maximum adult daily dose, 300 mg. The drug may also be applied topically, although systemic absorption and toxicity have been reported, especially when used on large areas with blistered or broken skin.
   B. Pretreatment before antivenin administration. Give 50 mg (children, 0.5–1 mg/kg) IV; if possible, it should be given at least 15–20 minutes before antivenin use.
   C. Drug-induced extrapyramidal symptoms. Give 50 mg (children, 0.5–1 mg/kg) IV or IM; if there is no response within 30–60 minutes, repeat dose to a maximum 100 mg (adults). Provide oral maintenance therapy, 25–50 mg (children, 0.5–1 mg/kg) every 4–6 hours for 2–3 days to prevent recurrence.
VII. Formulations.
   A. Oral. Diphenhydramine hydrochloride (Benadryl, others), 25- and 50-mg tablets and capsules; elixir, 12.5 mg/5 mL.
   B. Parenteral. Diphenhydramine hydrochloride (Benadryl, others), 10- and 50-mg/mL solutions.
   C. The **suggested minimum stocking level** to treat a 70-kg adult for the first 24 hours is five vials (10 mg/mL, 10 mL each).

▶ DMSA (SUCCIMER)

Saralyn R. Williams, MD

I. Pharmacology. DMSA (meso-2,3-dimercaptosuccinic acid [succimer]) is a chelating agent used in the treatment of intoxication from several heavy metals. A water-soluble analog of dimercaprol (BAL; see p 341), DMSA enhances the urinary excretion of lead and mercury. Its effect on elimination of the endogenous minerals calcium, iron, and magnesium is insignificant. Minor increases in zinc and copper excretion may occur. In an animal model, oral DMSA was not associated with a significant increas in gastrointestinal absorption of lead; the effect of oral DMSA on gastrointestinal absorption of mercury and arsenic is not known.
   DMSA is rapidly but variably absorbed after oral administration, with peak levels occurring between 1 and 2 hours. The drug is eliminated primarily by the kidneys, with peak urinary excretion of the parent drug and its metabolites after 2–4 hours.
II. Indications.
   A. DMSA is approved for treatment of intoxication by lead and mercury, where it is associated with increased urinary excretion of the metals and concurrent reversal of metal-induced enzyme inhibition. Oral DMSA is comparable to

parenteral calcium EDTA (see p 363) in decreasing blood lead concentrations. Although DMSA treatment has been associated with subjective clinical improvement, controlled clinical trials demonstrating therapeutic efficacy have yet to be reported.
  B. DMSA is protective against acute lethal effects of arsenic in animal models and may have potential utility in human arsenic poisoning.
III. Contraindications. History of allergy to the drug.
IV. Adverse effects.
  B. Gastrointestinal disturbances including anorexia, nausea, vomiting, and diarrhea are the most common side effects and occur in less than 10% of patients. There may be a mercaptanlike odor to the urine, which has no clinical significance.
  B. Mild, reversible increases in liver transaminases have been observed in 6–10% of patients.
  C. Rashes, some requiring discontinuation of treatment, have been reported in less than 5% of patients.
  D. Mild to moderate neutropenia has been noted occasionally.
  E. Minimal increases (less than twofold) in urinary excretion of zinc and copper have been observed and have minor or no clinical significance.
  F. Hyperglycemia and pancreatic injury were reported in early animal studies.
  G. Use in pregnancy. FDA category C (indeterminate). DMSA has produced adverse fetal effects when administered to pregnant animals in amounts 1–2 orders of magnitude greater than recommended human doses; its effect on human pregnancy has not been determined (see p 333).
V. Drug or laboratory interactions. No known interactions. Concurrent administration with other chelating agents has not been adequately studied.
VI. Dosage and method of administration (adults and children).
  A. Lead poisoning. Availability in the United States is limited to an oral formulation (100-mg capsules) officially approved by the FDA for use in children with blood lead levels > 45 μg/dL. However, DMSA can also lower lead concentrations in adults. **Note:** Administration of DMSA should never be a substitute for removal from lead exposure. In adults, the federal OSHA Lead Standard requires removal from occupational lead exposure of any worker with a single blood lead concentration in excess of 60 μg/dL or an average of three successive values in excess of 50 μg/dL. **Prophylactic chelation,** defined as the routine use of chelation to prevent elevated blood lead concentrations or to lower blood lead levels below the standard in asymptomatic workers, **is not permitted.** Consult the local or state health department or OSHA (see Table IV–3, p 426) for more detailed information.
    1. Give 10 mg/kg (or 350 mg/m²) PO every 8 hours for 5 days, and then give the same dose every 12 hours for 2 weeks.
    2. An additional course of treatment may be considered based on post-treatment blood lead levels and on the persistence or recurrence of symptoms. Although blood lead levels may decline by more than 50% during treatment, patients with high body lead burdens may experience rebound to within 20% of pretreatment levels as bone stores equilibrate with tissue levels. An interval of 2 or more weeks may be needed to assess the extent of post-treatment rebound.
    3. Experience with oral DMSA for severe lead intoxications (ie, lead encephalopathy) is very limited. In such cases, consideration should be given to parenteral therapy with calcium EDTA (see p 363).
  B. Mercury and arsenic poisoning
    1. Intoxication by inorganic mercury compounds and arsenic compounds may result in severe gastroenteritis and shock. In such circumstances, the capacity of the gut to absorb orally administered DMSA may be severely impaired, and use of an available parenteral agent such as BAL (see p 341) may be preferable.

2. Give 10 mg/kg (or 350 mg/m^2) orally every 8 hours for 5 days, and then give the same dose every 12 hours for 2 weeks. The value of extending the duration of treatment in the presence of continuing symptoms or high levels of urinary metal excretion is undetermined.

VII. Formulations.
- **A. Oral.** DMSA, *meso*-2,3-dimercaptosuccinic acid, Succimer (Chemet), 100-mg capsules in bottles of 100.
- **B. Parenteral.** A parenteral form of DMSA (sodium 2,3-dimercaptosuccinate), infused at a dose of 1–2 g per day, has been in use in the People's Republic of China, but is not available in the United States.
- **C.** The **suggested minimum stocking level** to treat a 70-kg adult for the first 24 hours is 20 capsules.

▶ DOPAMINE

Neal L. Benowitz, MD

I. Pharmacology. Dopamine is an endogenous catecholamine and the immediate metabolic precursor of norepinephrine. It stimulates α- and β-adrenergic receptors directly and indirectly. In addition, it acts on specific dopaminergic receptors. Its relative activity at these various receptors is dose-related. At low infusion rates (1–5 µg/kg/min), dopamine stimulates β$_1$ activity (increased heart rate and contractility) and increases renal and mesenteric blood flow through dopaminergic agonist activity. At high infusion rates (>10–20 µg/kg/min), α-adrenergic stimulation predominates, resulting in increased peripheral vascular resistance. Dopamine is not effective orally. After IV administration, its onset of action occurs within 5 minutes, and the duration of effect is less than 10 minutes. The plasma half-life is about 2 minutes.

II. Indications.
- **A.** Dopamine is used to increase blood pressure, cardiac output, and urine flow in patients with shock who have not responded to intravenous fluid challenge, correction of hypothermia, or reversal of acidosis.
- **B.** Low-dose infusion is most effective for hypotension caused by venodilation or reduced cardiac contractility; high-dose dopamine is indicated for shock resulting from decreased peripheral arterial resistance.

III. Contraindications.
- **A.** Uncorrected tachyarrhythmias or ventricular fibrillation and uncorrected hypovolemia.
- **B.** High-dose infusion is relatively contraindicated in the presence of peripheral arterial occlusive disease with thrombosis or in patients with ergot poisoning (see p 160).

IV. Adverse effects.
- **A.** Severe hypertension, which may result in intracranial hemorrhage, pulmonary edema, or myocardial necrosis.
- **B.** Aggravation of tissue ischemia, resulting in gangrene (with high-dose infusion).
- **C.** Ventricular arrhythmias, especially in patients intoxicated by halogenated or aromatic hydrocarbon solvents or anesthetics.
- **D.** Tissue necrosis after extravasation (see part VI.A, below, for treatment of extravasation).
- **E.** Anaphylactoid reaction induced by sulfite preservatives in sensitive patients.
- **F. Use in pregnancy.** FDA category C (indeterminate). There may be a dose-related effect on uterine blood flow. This does not preclude its acute, short-term use for a seriously symptomatic patient (see p 333).

V. Drug or laboratory interactions.
- **A.** Enhanced pressor response may occur in the presence of cocaine and cyclic antidepressants owing to inhibition of neuronal reuptake.

B. Enhanced pressor response may occur in patients taking monoamine oxidase inhibitors, owing to inhibition of neuronal metabolic degradation.

C. Chloral hydrate and halogenated hydrocarbon anesthetics may enhance the arrhythmogenic effect of dopamine, owing to sensitization of the myocardium to effects of catecholamines.

D. Alpha- and beta-blocking agents antagonize the adrenergic effects of dopamine; haloperidol and other dopamine antagonists may antagonize the dopaminergic effects.

E. There may be a reduced pressor response in patients with depleted neuronal stores of catecholamines (eg, chronic disulfiram or reserpine use).

VI. Dosage and method of administration (adults and children).

A. Avoid extravasation. *Caution:* The intravenous infusion must be free flowing, and the infused vein should be observed frequently for signs of subcutaneous infiltration (pallor, coldness, or induration). If extravasation occurs, immediately infiltrate the affected area with phentolamine (see p 400), 5–10 mg in 10–15 mL of normal saline (children, 0.1–0.2 mg/kg; maximum 10 mg total) via a fine (25- to 27-gauge) hypodermic needle; improvement is evidenced by hyperemia and return to normal temperature. Topical nitrates and infiltration of terbutaline have also been reported successful for treatment of extravasation involving other catecholamines.

B. For **predominantly inotropic effects,** begin with 1 μg/kg/min and increase infusion rate as needed to 5–10 μg/kg/min.

C. For **predominantly vasopressor effects,** infuse 10–20 μg/kg/min and increase as needed. Doses above 50 μg/kg/min may result in severe peripheral vasoconstriction and gangrene.

VII. Formulations.

A. Dopamine hydrochloride (Intropin and others): as a concentrate for admixture to intravenous solutions (40-, 80-, and 160-mg/mL in 5-mL vials) or premixed parenteral product for injection (0.8-, 1.6-, and 3.2-mg/mL in 5% dextrose). All contain sodium bisulfite as a preservative.

B. The **suggested minimum stocking level** to treat a 70-kg adult for the first 24 hours is approximately 1800–2000 mg (2–3 vials, 160 mg/mL, 5 mL each).

▶ **EDTA, CALCIUM (CALCIUM DISODIUM EDTA, CALCIUM DISODIUM EDETATE, CALCIUM DISODIUM VERSENATE)**

Michael J. Kosnett, MD, MPH

I. Pharmacology. Calcium EDTA has been used as a chelating agent to enhance elimination of certain toxic metals, principally lead. The elimination of endogenous metals, including zinc, manganese, iron, and copper, may also occur to a lesser extent. The plasma half-life of the drug is 20–60 minutes, and 50% of the injected dose is excreted in the urine within 1 hour. Increased urinary excretion of lead begins within 1 hour of EDTA administration and is followed by a decrease in whole blood lead concentration over the course of treatment. Calcium EDTA mobilizes lead from soft tissues and from a fraction of the larger lead stores present in bone. In persons with high body lead burdens, cessation of EDTA chelation is often followed by an upward rebound in blood lead levels as bone stores equilibrate with lower soft tissue levels. *Note:* Calcium EDTA should *not* be confused with sodium EDTA (edetate disodium), which is occasionally used to treat life-threatening severe hypercalcemia.

II. Indications.

A. Calcium EDTA has been used to decrease blood lead concentrations and increase urinary lead excretion in individuals with symptomatic lead intoxication (see p 199) and in asymptomatic persons with high blood lead levels. Although clinical experience associates calcium EDTA chelation with relief of symptoms (particularly lead colic) and decreased mortality, controlled clinical trials demonstrating therapeutic efficacy are lacking, and treatment recommendations have been largely empiric.

   B. Calcium EDTA may have possible utility in poisoning by zinc, manganese, and certain heavy radioisotopes.

III. Contraindications. Since calcium EDTA increases renal excretion of lead, anuria is a contraindication. Use reduced doses, with extreme caution, in patients with renal dysfunction, because accumulation of EDTA increases the risk of nephropathy, especially in volume-depleted patients.

IV. Adverse effects.

   A. Nephrotoxicity (eg, acute tubular necrosis, proteinuria, and hematuria) may be minimized by adequate hydration, establishment of adequate urine flow, avoidance of excessive doses, and limitation of continuous administration to 5 or fewer days. Laboratory assessment of renal function should be performed daily during treatment for severe intoxication and after the second and fifth days in other cases.

   B. In individuals with lead encephalopathy, rapid or high-volume infusions may exacerbate increased intracranial pressure. In such cases, the use of intramuscular injections or lower-volume, more concentrated intravenous infusions may be preferable.

   C. Local pain may occur at intramuscular injection sites. Lidocaine (1 mL of 1% lidocaine per mL of EDTA concentrate) may be added to intramuscular injections to decrease discomfort.

   D. Inadvertent use of sodium EDTA (edetate disodium) may cause serious hypocalcemia.

   E. Calcium EDTA may result in short-term zinc depletion, which has uncertain clinical significance.

   F. Use in pregnancy. The safety of calcium EDTA in human pregnancy has not been established. Fetal malformations with high doses have been noted in animal studies.

V. Drug or laboratory interactions. Intravenous infusions may be incompatible with 10% dextrose solutions, amphotericin, or hydralazine.

VI. Dosage and method of administration for lead poisoning (adults and children). *Note:* Administration of EDTA should never be a substitute for removal from lead exposure. In adults, the federal OSHA Lead Standard requires removal from occupational lead exposure of any worker with a single blood lead concentration in excess of 60 μg/dL or an average of three successive values in excess of 50 μg/dL. *Prophylactic chelation,* defined as the routine use of chelation to prevent elevated blood lead concentrations or to lower blood lead levels below the standard in asymptomatic workers, *is not* **permitted.** Consult the local or state health department or OSHA (see Table IV–3, p 426) for more detailed information.

   A. Lead poisoning with encephalopathy, or blood lead levels greater than 100 mg/dL. Administer calcium EDTA at a dose of 1500 mg/m^2/d (approximately 30 mg/kg) in two to three divided doses (every 8–12 hours) deep IM or as a continuous slow IV infusion (diluted to 2–4 mg/mL in 5% dextrose or normal saline). Treatment is usually continued for 5 days. Some clinicians advocate that treatment of patients with lead encephalopathy be initiated with a single dose of BAL (dimercaprol; see p 341), followed 4 hours later by the concomitant administration of BAL and calcium EDTA.

   B. Symptomatic lead poisoning without encephalopathy, and blood lead levels 50–100 mg/dL. Administer calcium EDTA at a dose of 1000–1500 mg/m^2/d (approximately 20–30 mg/kg) in two to three divided doses via deep IM or as a continuous IV infusion (diluted to 2–4 mg/mL) for 3–5 days.

   C. An additional course of treatment may be considered based on post-treatment blood lead concentrations and the persistence or recurrence of symptoms. Treatment courses should be separated by a minimum of 2 days, and

an interval of 2 or more weeks may be indicated to assess the extent of post-treatment rebound in blood lead levels.
  D. Single-dose EDTA chelation lead mobilization tests have been advocated by some clinicians to evaluate body lead burden or to assess the need for a full course of treatment in patients with moderately elevated blood lead levels, but the value and necessity of these tests are controversial.
  E. Oral EDTA therapy is *not* recommended for prevention or treatment of lead poisoning, because it may increase the absorption of lead from the gastrointestinal tract.
VII. **Formulations.**
  A. **Parenteral.** Calcium disodium edetate (Versenate), 200 mg/mL, 5-mL ampules. For intravenous infusion, dilute to 2–4 mg/mL in normal saline or 5% dextrose solution.
  B. The **suggested minimum stocking level** to treat a 70-kg adult for the first 24 hours is three boxes (six ampules per box, 18 g).

▶ EPINEPHRINE

Neal L. Benowitz, MD

  I. **Pharmacology.** Epinephrine is an endogenous catecholamine with α- and β-adrenergic agonist properties, used primarily in emergency situations to treat anaphylaxis or cardiac arrest. Beneficial effects include inhibition of histamine release from mast cells and basophils, bronchodilation, positive inotropic effects, and peripheral vasoconstriction.
     Epinephrine is not active after oral administration. Subcutaneous injection produces effects within 5–10 minutes, with peak effects at 20 minutes. Intravenous or inhalational administration produces much more rapid onset. Epinephrine is rapidly inactivated in the body, with an elimination half-life of 2 minutes.
  II. **Indications.**
  A. Anaphylaxis and anaphylactoid reactions.
  B. Epinephrine is occasionally used for hypotension resulting from overdose by beta blockers, calcium antagonists, and other cardiac-depressant drugs.
  III. **Contraindications.**
  A. Uncorrected tachyarrhythmias or ventricular fibrillation and uncorrected hypovolemia.
  B. Epinephrine is relatively contraindicated in patients with organic heart disease, peripheral arterial occlusive vascular disease with thrombosis, or ergot poisoning (see p 160).
  C. Narrow-angle glaucoma.
  IV. **Adverse effects.**
  A. Anxiety, restlessness, tremor, headache.
  B. Severe hypertension, which may result in intracranial hemorrhage, pulmonary edema, or myocardial necrosis or infarction.
  C. Use with caution in patients intoxicated by halogenated or aromatic hydrocarbon solvents and anesthetics, because these may sensitize the myocardium to the arrhythmogenic effects of epinephrine.
  D. Tissue necrosis after extravasation or intra-arterial injection.
  E. Aggravation of tissue ischemia, resulting in gangrene.
  F. Anaphylactoid reaction, which may occur owing to the bisulfite preservative in patients with sulfite hypersensitivity.
  G. Hypokalemia, hypophosphatemia, hyperglycemia, and leukocytosis may occur owing to β-adrenergic effects of epinephrine.
  H. **Use in pregnancy.** FDA category C (indeterminate). It is teratogenic in animals, crosses the placenta, can cause placental ischemia, and may suppress

uterine contractions, but these effects do not preclude its acute, short-term use for a seriously symptomatic patient (see p 333).

V. Drug or laboratory interactions.

   A. An enhanced arrhythmogenic effect may occur when epinephrine is given to patients with chloral hydrate overdose or anesthetized with cyclopropane or halogenated general anesthetics.

   B. Use in patients taking propranolol and other nonselective beta blockers may produce severe hypertension owing to blockade of β_2-mediated vasodilation, resulting in unopposed α-mediated vasoconstriction.

   C. Cocaine and cyclic antidepressants may enhance stimulant effects owing to inhibition of neuronal epinephrine reuptake.

   D. Monoamine oxidase inhibitors may enhance pressor effects because of decreased neuronal epinephrine metabolism.

   E. Digitalis intoxication may enhance arrhythmogenicity of epinephrine.

VI. Dosage and method of administration.

   A. *Caution:* **Avoid extravasation.** The intravenous infusion must be free flowing, and the infused vein should be observed frequently for signs of subcutaneous infiltration (pallor, coldness, or induration).

      1. If extravasation occurs, immediately infiltrate the affected area with phentolamine (see p 400), 5–10 mg in 10–15 mL of normal saline (children, 0.1–0.2 mg/kg; maximum 10 mg total) via a fine (25- to 27-gauge) hypodermic needle; improvement is evidenced by hyperemia and return to normal temperature.

      2. Alternately, topical application of nitroglycerin paste and infiltration of terbutaline have been reported successful.

   B. **Mild to moderate allergic reaction.** Give 0.3–0.5 mg subcutaneously (SC) or IM (children, 0.01 mg/kg of 1:1000 solution or 1:200 suspension; maximum 0.5 mg). May be repeated after 10–15 minutes if needed.

   C. **Severe anaphylaxis.** Give 0.05–0.1 mg IV (0.5–1 mL of a 1:10,000 solution) every 5–10 minutes (children, 0.01 mg/kg; maximum 0.1 mg), or an IV infusion at 1–4 µg/min. If intravenous access is not available, the endotracheal route may be used; give 0.5 mg (5 mL of a 1:10,000 solution) down the endotracheal tube.

   D. **Hypotension.** Infuse at 1 µg/min; titrate upward every 5 minutes as necessary. If the patient has refractory hypotension and is on a beta-adrenergic blocking drug, consider glucagon (see p 371).

VII. Formulations.

   A. Parenteral. Epinephrine hydrochloride (Adrenalin, others), 0.01 mg/mL (1:100,000), 0.1 mg/mL (1:10,000), 0.5 mg/mL (1:2000), and 1 mg/mL (1:1000), in 1-, 2-, and 30-mL ampules, vials, and prefilled syringes. Most preparations contain sodium bisulfite or sodium metabisulfite as a preservative.

   B. The **suggested minimum stocking level** to treat a 70-kg adult for the first 24 hours is 10 mg (10 ampules, 1:1000, 1 mL, or equivalent).

▶ ESMOLOL

Thomas E. Kearney, PharmD

   I. Pharmacology. Esmolol is a short-acting, IV, cardioselective β-adrenergic blocker with no intrinsic sympathomimetic or membrane-depressant activity. In usual therapeutic doses, it causes little or no bronchospasm in patients with asthma. Esmolol produces peak effects within 6–10 minutes of administration of an intravenous bolus. It is rapidly hydrolyzed by red blood cell esterases, with an elimination half-life of 9 minutes; therapeutic and adverse effects disappear within 30 minutes after the infusion is discontinued.

   I. Indications

    A. Rapid control of supraventricular and ventricular tachyarrhythmias and hypertension, especially if caused by excessive sympathomimetic activity (eg, stimulant drugs, hyperthyroid state).

    B. Reversal of hypotension and tachycardia caused by excessive β-adrenergic activity resulting from theophylline or caffeine overdose.

    C. Control of ventricular tachyarrhythmias caused by excessive myocardial catecholamine sensitivity (eg, chloral hydrate and chlorinated hydrocarbon solvents).

III. Contraindications.

    A. Contraindications include hypotension, bradycardia, or congestive heart failure secondary to intrinsic cardiac disease or cardiac-depressant effects of drugs and toxins (eg, cyclic antidepressants and barbiturates).

    B. Hypertension caused by α-adrenergic or generalized stimulant drugs, unless coadministered with a vasodilator (eg, nitroprusside or phentolamine).

IV. Adverse effects.

    A. Hypotension and bradycardia may occur, especially in patients with intrinsic cardiac disease or cardiac-depressant drug overdose.

    B. Bronchospasm may occur in patients with asthma or chronic bronchospasm, but it is less likely than with propranolol or other nonselective beta blockers and it is rapidly reversible after the infusion is discontinued.

    C. Esmolol may mask physiologic responses to hypoglycemia (tremor, tachycardia, and glycogenolysis) and therefore should be used with caution in patients with diabetes.

    D. Use in pregnancy. FDA category C (indeterminate). This does not preclude its short-term use for a seriously symptomatic patient (see p 333). High-dose infusion may contribute to placental ischemia.

V. Drug or laboratory interactions.

    A. Esmolol may transiently increase the serum digoxin level by 10–20%, but the clinical significance of this is unknown.

    B. Recovery from succinylcholine-induced neuromuscular blockade may be slightly delayed (5–10 minutes). Similarly, esmolol metabolism may be inhibited by anticholinesterase agents (eg, organophosphates).

    C. Esmolol is not compatible with sodium bicarbonate solutions.

VI. Dosage and method of administration.

    A. Dilute before intravenous injection to a final concentration of 10 mg/mL, with 5% dextrose, lactated Ringer's injection, or saline solutions.

    B. Give as an intravenous infusion, starting at 50 μg/kg/min and increasing as needed up to 100 μg/kg/min. Steady-state concentrations are reached approximately 30 minutes after each infusion adjustment. A loading dose of 500 μg/kg should be given if more rapid onset of clinical effects (5–10 minutes) is desired.

    C. Infusion rates greater than 200 μg/kg/min are likely to produce excessive hypotension.

VII. Formulations.

    A. Parenteral. Esmolol hydrochloride (Brevibloc), 2.5 g in 10-mL ampules (250 mg/mL) and 100 mg in 10-mL vials (10 mg/mL).

    B. The **suggested minimum stocking level** to treat a 70-kg adult for the first 24 hours is 2 ampules (250 mg/mL, 10 mL) or 25 vials (10 mg/mL, 10 mL).

▶ ETHANOL

Thomas E. Kearney, PharmD

I. Pharmacology. Ethanol (ethyl alcohol) acts as a competitive substrate for the enzyme alcohol dehydrogenase, preventing the metabolic formation of toxic metabolites from methanol or ethylene glycol. Blood ethanol concentrations of 100 mg/dL effectively saturate alcohol dehydrogenase and prevent further methanol and ethylene glycol metabolism (see also fomepizole, p 370). Ethanol is well absorbed from the gastrointestinal tract when given orally, but the onset is more rapid and predictable when it is given intravenously. The elimination of ethanol is zero order; the average rate of decline is 15 mg/dL/h; however, this is highly variable and will be influenced by prior chronic use of alcohol, recruitment of alternate metabolic pathways, and concomitant hemodialysis (eg, to remove methanol or ethylene glycol).

II. **Indications.** Suspected **methanol** (methyl alcohol, see p 218) or **ethylene glycol** (see p 166) poisoning with:
  A. A suggestive history of ingestion but no available blood concentration measurements;
  B. Metabolic acidosis and an unexplained elevated osmolar gap (see p 30); or
  C. A serum methanol or ethylene glycol concentration > 20 mg/dL.
     Note: Since the introduction of fomepizole (4-methylpyrazole, see p 370), a potent inhibitor of alcohol dehydrogenase, confirmed cases of ethylene glycol or methanol poisoning will probably be treated with this drug instead of ethanol.

III. **Contraindications.** Use of interacting drugs, which may cause disulfiram-type reaction (see part V.B, below).

IV. **Adverse effects.**
  A. Nausea, vomiting, and gastritis may occur with oral administration. Ethanol may also exacerbate pancreatitis.
  B. Inebriation, sedation, and hypoglycemia (particularly in children and malnourished adults) may occur.
  C. Intravenous use is sometimes associated with local phlebitis (especially with ethanol solutions > 10%). Hyponatremia may result from large doses of sodium-free intravenous solutions.
  D. Acute flushing, palpitations, and postural hypotension may occur in patients with atypical aldehyde dehydrogenase enzyme (up to 50–80% of Japanese, Chinese, and Korean individuals).
  E. **Use in pregnancy.** FDA category C (indeterminate). Ethanol crosses the placenta. Chronic overuse in pregnancy is associated with birth defects (fetal alcohol syndrome). The drug reduces uterine contractions and may slow or stop labor. However, these effects do not preclude its acute, short-term use for a seriously symptomatic patient (see p 333).

V. **Drug or laboratory interactions.**
  A. Ethanol potentiates the effect of central nervous system-depressant drugs and hypoglycemic agents.
  B. **Disulfiram reaction** (see p 158), including flushing, palpitations, and postural hypotension, may occur in patients taking disulfiram as well as a variety of other medications (eg, metronidazole, furazolidone, procarbazine, chlorpropamide, some cephalosporins, and *Coprinus* mushrooms). In such cases, hemodialysis is the recommended alternative to ethanol treatment.

VI. **Dosage and method of administration.** Obtain serum ethanol levels after the loading dose and frequently during maintenance therapy to ensure a concentration of 100 mg/dL.
  A. Ethanol may be given orally or intravenously. The desired serum concentration is 100 mg/dL (20 mmol/L); this can be achieved by giving approximately 750 mg/kg (Table III–6) as a loading dose, followed by a maintenance infusion of approximately 100–150 mg/kg/h (give a larger dose to chronic alcoholics).
  B. Increase the infusion rate to 175–250 mg/kg/h (larger dose for chronic alcoholics) during hemodialysis to offset the increased rate of ethanol elimination. Alternately, ethanol may be added to the dialysate.

VII. **Formulations.**
  A. **Oral.** Pharmaceutical-grade ethanol (96% USP). *Note:* Commercial liquor may be used orally if pharmaceutical-grade ethanol is not available: administer 200 mL/kg divided by the "proof" of the liquor, eg, if using 80 proof liquor give 2.5 mL/kg.
  B. **Parenteral.** Ethanol, 5% in 5% dextrose solution; 10% in 5% dextrose solution.
  C. The **suggested minimum stocking level** to treat a 70-kg adult for the first 24 hours is 3 bottles (10% ethanol, 1 L each).

TABLE III–6. ETHANOL DOSING (ADULTS AND CHILDREN)

Dose	Intravenous[c]		Oral
	5%	10%	50%
Loading[a]	15 mL/kg	7.5 mL/kg	2 mL/kg
Maintenance[b]	2–4 mL/kg/h	1–2 mL/kg/h	0.2–0.4 mL/kg/h
Maintenance during hemodialysis[b]	4–7 mL/kg/h	2–3.5 mL/kg/h	0.4–0.7 mL/kg/h

[a]If the patients serum ethanol level is greater than 0, reduce the loading dose in a proportional manner. Multiply the calculated loading dose by the following factor:

$$\frac{100 - [\text{patient's serum ethanol in mg/dL}]}{100}$$

[b]Doses may vary depending on the idividual. Chronic alcoholics have a higher rate of ethanol elimination, and maintenance doses should be adjusted to maintain an ethanol level of approximately 100 mg/dL.
[c]Infuse intravenous loading dose over 20–30 minutes or longer

▶ FLUMAZENIL

Walter H. Mullen, PharmD

I. **Pharmacology.** Flumazenil (Romazicon) is a highly selective competitive inhibitor of central nervous system benzodiazepine receptors. It has no demonstrable benzodiazepine agonist activity and no significant toxicity even in high doses. It has no effect on alcohol or opioid receptors, and it does not reverse alcohol intoxication. Flumazenil is most effective parenterally (high first-pass effect with oral administration). After intravenous administration, the onset of benzodiazepine reversal occurs within 1–2 minutes, peaks at 6–10 minutes, and lasts for 1–5 hours, depending on the dose of flumazenil and the degree of preexisting benzodiazepine effect. It is eliminated by hepatic metabolism with a serum half-life of approximately 1 hour.

II. **Indications.**
   A. Rapid reversal of benzodiazepine overdose-induced coma and respiratory depression, both as a diagnostic aid and potential substitute for endotracheal intubation.
   B. Postoperative or postprocedure reversal of benzodiazepine sedation.

III. **Contraindications.**
   A. Known hypersensitivity to flumazenil or benzodiazepines.
   B. Suspected serious cyclic antidepressant overdose.
   C. Benzodiazepine use for control of a potentially life-threatening condition (eg, status epilepticus or increased intracranial pressure).

IV. **Adverse effects.**
   A. Anxiety, agitation, headache, dizziness, nausea, vomiting, tremor, and transient facial flushing.
   B. Rapid reversal of benzodiazepine effect in patients with benzodiazepine addiction or high tolerance may result in an acute withdrawal state, including hyperexcitability, tachycardia, and seizures (rarely reported).
   C. Seizures or arrhythmias may be precipitated in patients with a serious cyclic antidepressant overdose.
   D. Flumazenil has precipitated arrhythmias in a patient with a mixed benzodiazepine and chloral hydrate overdose.
   E. **Use in pregnancy.** FDA category C (indeterminate). This does not preclude its acute, short-term use for a seriously symptomatic patient (see p 333).

V. **Drug or laboratory interactions.** No known interactions. Flumazenil does not appear to alter kinetics of benzodiazepines or other drugs.

VI. Dosage and method of administration.
   A. Benzodiazepine overdose. Titrate the dosage until desired response is achieved.
   1. Administer 0.2 mg IV over 30 seconds (pediatric dose not established; start with 0.01 mg/kg). If there is no response, give 0.3 mg. If there still is no response, give 0.5 mg, and repeat every 30 seconds if needed to a total maximum dose of 3 mg (1 mg in children).
   2. Because effects last only 1–5 hours, continue to monitor the patient closely for resedation. If multiple repeated doses are needed, consider a continuous infusion (0.2–1 mg/h).
   B. Reversal of conscious sedation or anesthetic doses of benzodiazepine. A dose of 0.2 mg given intravenously is usually sufficient and may be repeated, titrating up to 1 mg.
VII. Formulations.
   A. Parenteral. Flumazenil (Romazicon), 0.1 mg/mL, 5- and 10-mL vials.
   B. The **suggested minimum stocking level** to treat a 70-kg adult for the first 24 hours is 10 vials (0.1 mg/mL, 10 mL).

► FOLIC ACID

Kathryn H. Keller, PharmD

I. Pharmacology. Folic acid is a B-complex vitamin that is essential for protein synthesis and erythropoiesis. In addition, the administration of folate to patients with methanol (and possibly ethylene glycol) poisoning may enhance the elimination of the toxic metabolite formic acid, based on studies in folate-deficient primates. *Note:* Folic acid requires metabolic activation and is not effective for treatment of poisoning by dihydrofolate reductase inhibitors (eg, methotrexate and trimethoprim). Leucovorin (see p 378) is the proper agent in these situations.
II. Indications.
   A. Adjunctive treatment for methanol poisoning.
   B. May be administered in ethylene glycol poisoning.
III. Contraindications. No known contraindications.
IV. Adverse effects.
   A. Rare allergic reactions have been reported after intravenous administration.
   B. Use in pregnancy. Folic acid is a recommended supplement.
V. Drug or laboratory interactions. This agent may increase metabolism of phenytoin.
VI. Dosage and method of administration. The dose required for methanol or ethylene glycol poisoning is not established, although 50 mg IV (children, 1 mg/kg) every 4 hours for 6 doses has been recommended.
VII. Formulations.
   A. Parenteral. Sodium folate (Folvite), 5 and 10 mg/mL, 10-mL vials.
   B. The **suggested minimum stocking level** to treat a 70-kg adult for the first 24 hours is 6 vials (5 mg/mL, 1 mL each).

► FOMEPIZOLE (4-MP)

Thomas E. Kearney, PharmD

I. Pharmacology.
   A. Fomepizole (4-methylpyrazole) is a potent competitive inhibitor of alcohol dehydrogenase, the first enzyme in the metabolism of ethanol and other alcohols. Fomepizole can prevent the formation of toxic metabolites after methanol or ethylene glycol ingestion.

   B. Fomepizole is eliminated mainly via zero-order kinetics, but P-450 metabolism can undergo autoinduction within 2–3 days. The drug is dialyzable.

II. Indications are similar to those for ethanol (see p 367): suspected or confirmed **methanol** (methyl alcohol; see p 218) or **ethylene glycol** (see p 166) poisoning with one or more of the following:

   A. A reliable history of ingestion of a toxic dose but no available blood concentration measurements;

   B. Metabolic acidosis and an unexplained elevated osmolar gap (see p 30); or

   C. Serum methanol or ethylene glycol concentration > 20 mg/dL.

     Note: Owing to the high cost of fomepizole, the drug's role in the routine management of suspected methanol or ethylene glycol poisoning is uncertain. Ethanol (p 367) remains a less expensive treatment.

III. Contraindications. History of allergy to the drug or to other pyrazoles.

IV. Adverse effects.

   A. Venous irritation and phlebosclerosis after intravenous injection of the undiluted product.

   B. Headache, nausea and dizziness are the most commonly reported side effects.

   C. Transient non–dose-dependent elevation of hepatic transaminases has been reported after multiple doses.

   D. Safety and effectiveness in children has not been established.

   E. Use in pregnancy. FDA category C (indeterminant).

V. Drug or laboratory interactions.

   A. Drugs or chemicals metabolized by alcohol dehydrogenase (eg, chloral hydrate, ethanol, isopropyl alcohol) will also have impaired elimination.

   B. Drugs or chemicals metabolized by cytochrome P-450 enzymes may compete with fomepizole for elimination. Also, induction of P-450 activity by these drugs or by fomepizole may alter metabolism.

VI. Dosage and method of administration. *Note:* The interval between the initial dose and subsequent maintenance doses, 12 hours, provides the opportunity to confirm the diagnosis with laboratory testing.

   A. Initial dose. Give a loading dose of 15 mg/kg (up to 1 g). Dilute in at least 100 mL of normal saline or 5% dextrose and infuse slowly over 30 minutes. *Note:* The drug may solidify at room temperature and should be visually inspected prior to administration. If there is any evidence of solidification, hold the vial under a stream of warm water or roll between the hands.

   B. Maintenance therapy. Give 10 mg/kg every 12 hours for 4 doses, then increase to 15 mg/kg (to offset increased metabolism resulting from autoinduction) until methanol or ethylene glycol serum levels are below 20 mg/dL.

   C. Adjustment for hemodialysis. To offset loss of fomepizole during dialysis, increase the frequency of dosing to every 4 hours.

VII. Formulations.

   A. Parenteral. Fomepizole (Antizol, Orphan Drug Corp.): 1 g/mL in 1.5-mL vials, prepackaged in tray packs containing four vials.

   B. The **suggested minimum stocking level** to treat a 70-kg adult for the first 24 hours is four vials. *Note:* Orphan Drug Corp. has announced that it will replace free of charge any expired vials of fomepizole.

▶ **GLUCAGON**

Thomas E. Kearney, PharmD

I. Pharmacology. Glucagon is a polypeptide hormone that stimulates the formation of adenyl cyclase, which in turn increases the intracellular concentration of cyclic adenosine monophosphate (cAMP). This results in enhanced glycogenolysis and an elevated serum glucose concentration; vascular smooth muscle relaxation; and positive inotropic, chronotropic, and dromotropic effects. These effects occur independently of β-adrenergic stimulation. Glucagon is destroyed in the gastrointestinal tract and must be given parenterally. After intravenous administration, effects are seen within 1–2 minutes and persist for 10–20 minutes. The serum half-life is about 3–10 minutes.

II. Indications.
   A. Hypotension, bradycardia, or conduction impairment caused by beta-adrenergic blocker intoxication (see p 107). Also consider in patients with hypotension associated with anaphylactic or anaphylactoid reactions who may be on β-adrenergic blocking agents.
   B. Possibly effective for severe cardiac depression caused by intoxication with calcium antagonists, quinidine, or other types Ia and Ic antiarrhythmic drugs.
   C. Because of the benign side effect profile of glucagon, consider its early empiric use in any patient with myocardial depression (bradycardia, hypotension, or low cardiac output) who does not respond rapidly to usual measures.

III. Contraindications. Known hypersensitivity to the drug (rare), or pheochromocytoma.

IV. Adverse effects.
   A. Hyperglycemia.
   B. Nausea and vomiting.
   C. Use in pregnancy. FDA category B. Fetal harm is extremely unlikely (see p 333).

V. Drug or laboratory interactions. Concurrent administration of epinephrine potentiates and prolongs the hyperglycemic and cardiovascular effects of glucagon.

VI. Dosage and method of administration. Give 5–10 mg IV, followed by 1–5 mg/h infusion (children, 0.15 mg/kg IV, followed by 0.05–0.1 mg/kg/h). For very large doses, consider using sterile water or saline to reconstitute, rather than the phenol-containing diluent provided with the drug.

VII. Formulations.
   A. Parenteral. Glucagon for injection, 1 unit (approximately 1 mg, with 1 mL diluent) and 10 units (approximately 10 mg, with 10 mL diluent). Diluent contains phenol 0.2%.
   B. The **suggested minimum stocking level** to treat a 70-kg adult for the first 24 hours is 100 mg (10 vials, 10 units each).

▶ GLUCOSE

Thomas E. Kearney, PharmD

I. Pharmacology. Glucose is an essential carbohydrate used as a substrate for energy production within the body. Although many organs use fatty acids as an alternative energy source, the brain is totally dependent on glucose as its major energy source; thus, hypoglycemia may rapidly cause serious brain injury.

II. Indications.
   A. Hypoglycemia.
   B. Empiric therapy for patients with stupor, coma, or seizures who may have unsuspected hypoglycemia.

III. Contraindications. No absolute contraindications for empiric treatment of comatose patients with possible hypoglycemia. However, hyperglycemia and (possibly) recent ischemic brain injury may be aggravated by excessive glucose administration.

IV. Adverse effects.
   A. Hyperglycemia and serum hyperosmolality.
   B. Local phlebitis and cellulitis after extravasation (occurs with concentrations > 10%) from the intravenous injection site.

C. Administration of a large glucose load may precipitate acute Wernicke-Korsakoff syndrome in thiamine-depleted patients. For this reason, thiamine (see p 408) is routinely given along with glucose to alcoholic or malnourished patients.

D. Administration of large volumes of sodium-free dextrose solutions may contribute to hyponatremia.

E. **Use in pregnancy.** FDA category C (indeterminate). This does not preclude its acute, short-term use for a seriously symptomatic patient (see p 333).

V. **Drug or laboratory interactions.** No known interactions.

VI. **Dosage and method of administration.**

A. As empiric therapy for coma, give 50–100 mL of 50% dextrose via a secure intravenous line (children, 2–4 mL/kg of 25% dextrose; do *not* use 50% dextrose in children).

B. Persistent hypoglycemia (eg, resulting from poisoning by hypoglycemic agent) may require repeated boluses of 25% (for children) or 50% dextrose and infusion of 5–10% dextrose, titrated as needed. Consider use of diazoxide (see p 356) or octreotide (see p 394) in such situations.

VII. **Formulations.**

A. **Parenteral.** Dextrose injection, 50%, 50-mL prefilled injector; 25% dextrose, 10 mL; various solutions of 5–10% dextrose, some in combination with saline or other crystalloids.

B. The **suggested minimum stocking level** to treat a 70-kg adult for the first 24 hours is four prefilled injectors (50% and 25%) and four bottles or bags (5% and 10%, 1 L each).

▶ HALOPERIDOL

Thomas E. Kearney, PharmD

I. **Pharmacology.** Haloperidol is a butyrophenone neuroleptic drug useful for the management of acutely agitated psychotic patients. It has strong central antidopaminergic activity and weak anticholinergic effects. Haloperidol is well absorbed from the gastrointestinal tract and by the intramuscular route. Peak pharmacologic effects occur within 30–40 minutes of an intramuscular injection. The drug is metabolized and excreted slowly in the urine and feces. The serum half-life is 12–24 hours.

II. **Indications.** Haloperidol is used for the management of acute agitated functional psychosis or extreme agitation induced by stimulants or hallucinogenic drugs, especially when drug-induced agitation has not responded to a benzodiazepine.

III. **Contraindications.**

A. Severe central nervous system depression in the absence of airway and ventilatory control.

B. Severe parkinsonism.

C. Known hypersensitivity to haloperidol.

IV. **Adverse effects.**

A. Haloperidol produces less sedation and less hypotension than chlorpromazine but is associated with a higher incidence of extrapyramidal side effects.

B. Rigidity, diaphoresis, and hyperpyrexia may be a manifestation of **neuroleptic malignant syndrome** (see p 20) induced by haloperidol and other neuroleptic agents.

C. Haloperidol lowers the seizure threshold and should be used with caution in patients with known seizure disorder or who have ingested a convulsant drug.

D. Large doses can prolong the QT interval and cause Torsades de pointes.

    E. Some oral haloperidol tablets contain tartrazine dye, which may precipitate allergic reactions in susceptible patients.

    F. Use in pregnancy. This drug is teratogenic and fetotoxic in animals, and it crosses the placenta. Its safety in human pregnancy has not been established.

V. Drug or laboratory interactions.

    A. Haloperidol potentiates central nervous system-depressant effects of opioids, antidepressants, phenothiazines, ethanol, barbiturates, and other sedatives.

    B. Combined therapy with lithium may increase the risk of neuroleptic malignant syndrome (see p 20).

VI. Dosage and method of administration.

    A. Oral. Give 2–5 mg of haloperidol PO; repeat once if necessary; usual daily dose is 3–5 mg two to three times daily (children > 3 years old, 0.05–0.15 mg/kg/d or 0.5 mg in 2–3 divided doses).

    B. Parenteral. Give 2–5 mg of haloperidol IM; may repeat once after 20–30 minutes and hourly if necessary (children > 3 years old, same as orally). Haloperidol is not approved for intravenous use in the United States, but that route has been widely used and is reportedly safe (except the decanoate salt formulation).

VII. Formulations.

    A. Oral. Haloperidol (Haldol), 0.5-, 1-, 2-, 5-, 10-, and 20-mg tablets.

    B. Parenteral. Haloperidol (Haldol), 2 and 5 mg/mL, 10-mL vials.

    C. The **suggested minimum stocking level** to treat a 70-kg adult for the first 24 hours is two vials (5 mg/mL, 10 mL each).

▶ HYDROXOCOBALAMIN

Kathryn H. Keller, PharmD

I. Pharmacology. Hydroxocobalamin and cyanocobalamin are synthetic forms of vitamin B_{12} used for the treatment of pernicious anemia. When administered to patients with cyanide poisoning, hydroxocobalamin exchanges its hydroxyl group with free cyanide in the plasma to produce the nontoxic cyanocobalamin.

II. Indications.

    A. Acute cyanide poisoning (concentrated formulation for this use has orphan drug status in the United States [orphan drug status means the drug is not commercially available for stocking]). This drug may be synergistic with sodium thiosulfate (see p 408).

    B. Prophylaxis against cyanide poisoning during nitroprusside infusion.

III. Contraindications. Do not use in patients with a known hypersensitivity to the drug.

IV. Adverse effects.

    A. Urine, sweat, tears, and other secretions become brownish-red after hydroxocobalamin administration.

    B. Nausea, vomiting, hypertension, and mild muscle twitching or spasms.

    C. Allergic reactions have been reported.

    D. Use in pregnancy. No assigned FDA category; no reported experience with use during pregnancy is available. This does not preclude its acute, short-term use for a seriously symptomatic patient (see p 333), and it may be preferable to nitrite administration for cyanide poisoning.

V. Drug or laboratory interactions. Coloration of the serum sample may interfere with some general laboratory tests (AST, bilirubin, creatinine, magnesium).

VI. Dosage and method of administration. *Note:* In the United States, the only readily available formulation of hydroxocobalamin contains 1 mg/mL, which is

impractical for acute cyanide poisoning because of the preparation time and the large volume (up to 4 g or 4,000 mL) that would need to be administered.
   A. **Acute cyanide poisoning.** Administer hydroxocobalamin intravenously in a dose equivalent to 50 times the amount of the cyanide exposure. If the amount of cyanide exposure is unknown, the recommended empiric dose is 4 g (or 50 mg/kg).
   B. **Prophylaxis during nitroprusside infusion.** Administer 25 mg/h IV. Sodium thiosulfate (p 408) may also be given.
VII. **Formulations.**
   A. **Parenteral (United States).** Hydroxocobalamin, 1 mg/mL IM; 10- and 30-mL vials.
   B. A preparation of 2 g of hydroxocobalamin is manufactured by Groupe Lipha and is available in France, Sweden, and a few other European countries, but is not sold in the US.
   C. The **suggested minimum stocking level** to treat a 70-kg adult for nitroprusside prophylaxis for the first 24 hours is 4 g; however, for acute cyanide poisoning, a concentrated form of the drug is not commercially available in the US.

▶ **IPECAC SYRUP**

Anthony S. Manoguerra, PharmD

   I. **Pharmacology.** Ipecac syrup is a mixture of plant-derived alkaloids, principally emetine and cephaeline, that produce emesis by direct irritation of the stomach and by stimulation of the central chemoreceptor trigger zone. Vomiting occurs in 90% of patients, usually within 20–30 minutes. Depending on the time after ingestion of the toxin, ipecac-induced emesis removes 30–50% of the stomach contents.
  II. **Indications.** For a more complete discussion of gastric decontamination, see p 45.
   A. Early on-scene management of oral poisonings, immediately after ingestion, in the home or at industrial on-site health care facilities without access to activated charcoal or the capacity to perform gastric lavage.
   B. In health care facilities, ipecac is rarely indicated but may find occasional use in patients with recent ingestions involving substances poorly adsorbed by activated charcoal (eg, iron, lithium, potassium, and sodium) or sustained-release or enteric-coated tablets.
 III. **Contraindications.**
   A. Comatose or obtunded mental state.
   B. Ingestion of a caustic or corrosive substance or sharp object.
   C. Ingestion of most petroleum distillates or hydrocarbons (see p 183).
   D. Ingestion of a drug or toxin likely to result in abrupt onset of seizures or coma (eg, tricyclic antidepressants, strychnine, camphor, nicotine, cocaine, amphetamines, or isoniazid).
   E. Severe hypertension.
   F. Patient at high risk for hemorrhagic diathesis (eg, coagulopathy or esophageal varices).
 IV. **Adverse effects.**
   A. Persistent gastrointestinal upset after emesis may significantly delay administration of activated charcoal or other oral antidotes, or food or fluids, for up to several hours.
   B. Severe and repeated vomiting may cause Mallory-Weiss tear, pneumomediastinum, hemorrhagic gastritis, or intracranial hemorrhage.
   C. Vomiting may stimulate vagal reflex, resulting in bradycardia or atrioventricular block.

D. Drowsiness occurs in about 20% and diarrhea in 25% of children.

E. Single ingestions of therapeutic doses of ipecac syrup are not toxic (the former fluid extract was more potent), and failure to induce vomiting does not require removal of the ipecac. However, **chronic repeated ingestion** of ipecac (eg, in bulemics) may result in accumulation of cardiotoxic alkaloids and may lead to fatal cardiomyopathy and arrhythmias.

F. Use in pregnancy. FDA category C (indeterminate). There is minimal systemic absorption, but it may induce uterine contractions in late pregnancy.

V. Drug or laboratory interactions.

A. Ipecac syrup potentiates nausea and vomiting associated with the ingestion of other gastric irritants.

B. Ipecac syrup is adsorbed in vitro by activated charcoal; however, ipecac still produces vomiting when given concurrently with charcoal.

C. Ipecac syrup contains 1.5–2% ethanol, which may cause an adverse reaction in patients taking disulfiram (see p 158) or other agents that have disulfiram-like effects (eg, metronidazole or *Coprinus* mushrooms).

VI. Dosage and method of administration.

A. Children 6–12 months old. Give 5–10 mL. *Note:* Not recommended for non-health-care facility use in this age group.

B. Children 1–12 years old. Give 15 mL.

C. Adults and children over 12 years old. Give 30 mL.

D. Follow ipecac administration with 4–8 oz of water or clear liquid (not essential for emetic effect). If emesis does not occur within 30 minutes, repeat the dose of ipecac and fluid.

VII. Formulations.

A. Ipecac syrup, 30 mL.

B. The **suggested minimum stocking level** to treat a 70-kg adult for the first 24 hours is two 30-mL bottles.

▶ ISOPROTERENOL

Thomas E. Kearney, PharmD

I. Pharmacology. Isoproterenol is a catecholaminelike drug that stimulates β-adrenergic receptors (β_1 and β_2). Pharmacologic properties include positive inotropic and chronotropic cardiac effects, peripheral vasodilation, and bronchodilation. Isoproterenol is not absorbed orally and shows variable and erratic absorption from sublingual and rectal sites. The effects of the drug are rapidly terminated by tissue uptake and metabolism; effects persist only a few minutes after intravenous injection.

II. Indications.

A. Severe bradycardia or conduction block resulting in hemodynamically significant hypotension. *Note:* After beta-blocker overdose, even exceedingly high doses of isoproterenol may not overcome the pharmacologic blockade of β-receptors, and glucagon (see p 371) is the preferred agent.

B. Use isoproterenol to increase heart rate and normalize conduction to abolish polymorphous ventricular tachycardia (Torsades de pointes) associated with QT interval prolongation (see p 14).

III. Contraindications.

A. Do not use isoproterenol for ventricular fibrillation or ventricular tachycardia (other than Torsades de pointes).

B. Use with extreme caution in the presence of halogenated or aromatic hydrocarbon solvents or anesthetics, or chloral hydrate.

IV. Adverse effects.

A. Increased myocardial oxygen demand may result in angina pectoris or acute myocardial infarction.

B. Peripheral β_2-mediated vasodilation may worsen hypotension.

C. The drug may precipitate ventricular arrhythmias.

D. Sulfite preservative in some parenteral preparations may cause hypersensitivity reactions.

E. Hypokalemia may occur secondary to β-adrenergic-mediated intracellular potassium shift.

F. Use in pregnancy. FDA category C (indeterminate). This does not preclude its acute, short-term use for a seriously symptomatic patient (see p 333). However, it may cause fetal ischemia and also can reduce or stop uterine contractions.

V. Drug or laboratory interactions.

A. Additive β-adrenergic stimulation occurs in the presence of other sympathomimetic drugs, theophylline, or glucagon.

B. Administration in the presence of cyclopropane, halogenated anesthetics, or other halogenated or aromatic hydrocarbons may enhance risk of ventricular arrhythmias because of sensitization of the myocardium to the arrhythmogenic effects of catecholamines.

C. Digitalis-intoxicated patients are more prone to develop ventricular arrhythmias when isoproterenol is administered.

D. Beta blockers may interfere with the action of isoproterenol by competitive blockade at β-adrenergic receptors.

VI. Dosage and method of administration.

A. For intravenous infusion, use a solution containing 2–4 μg/mL, and begin with 0.5- to 1-μg/min infusion (children, 0.1 μg/kg/min) and increase as needed for desired effect or as tolerated (by monitoring for arrhythmias). The usual upper dosage is 20 μg/min (1.5 μg/kg/min in children), but as high as 200 μg/min has been given in adults with propranolol overdose.

B. If a dilute solution is not available, make a solution of 1:50,000 (20 μg/mL) by diluting 1 mL of the 1:5000 solution to a volume of 10 mL with normal saline.

VII. Formulations.

A. Parenteral. Isoproterenol hydrochloride (Isuprel), 0.02 mg/mL (1:50,000) or 0.2 mg/mL (1:5000), which contains sodium bisulfite or sodium metabisulfite as a preservative.

B. The **suggested minimum stocking level** to treat a 70-kg adult for the first 24 hours is 10 ampules.

▶ LABETALOL

Thomas E. Kearney, PharmD

I. Pharmacology. Labetalol is a mixed α- and β-adrenergic antagonist; after intravenous administration, the nonselective β-antagonist properties are approximately sevenfold greater than the α_1-antagonist activity. Hemodynamic effects generally include decreases in heart rate, blood pressure, and systemic vascular resistance. Atrioventricular conduction velocity may be decreased. After intravenous injection, hypotensive effects are maximal within 10–15 minutes and persist about 2–4 hours. The drug is eliminated by hepatic metabolism and has a half-life of 5–6 hours.

II. Indications. Labetalol may be used to treat hypertension and tachycardia associated with stimulant drug overdose (eg, cocaine or amphetamines). *Note:* Hypertension with bradycardia suggests excessive α-mediated vasoconstriction (see pp 17, 259); in this case, a pure alpha blocker such as phentolamine (see p 400) is preferable, because the reversal of β_2-mediated vasodilation may worsen hypertension.

III. Contraindications.

A. Asthma.

B. Congestive heart failure.
C. Atrioventricular block.
IV. Adverse effects.
  A. Paradoxic hypertension may result when labetalol is used in the presence of stimulant intoxicants possessing strong mixed α- and β-adrenergic agonist properties (eg, cocaine, amphetamines) owing to the relatively weak α-antagonist properties of labetalol compared with its beta-blocking ability. (This has been reported with propranolol but not with labetalol.)
  B. Orthostatic hypotension and negative inotropic effects may occur.
  C. Dyspnea and bronchospasm may result, particularly in asthmatics.
  D. Nausea, abdominal pain, diarrhea, and lethargy have been reported.
  E. Use in pregnancy. FDA category C (indeterminate). This does not preclude its acute, short-term use for a seriously symptomatic patient (see p 333).
V. Drug or laboratory interactions.
  A. Additive blood pressure lowering with other antihypertensive agents, halothane, or nitroglycerin.
  B. Cimetidine increases oral bioavailability of labetalol.
  C. Labetalol is incompatible with 5% sodium bicarbonate injection (forms a precipitate).
  D. Labetalol may cause false-positive elevation of urinary catecholamine levels, and it can produce a false-positive test for amphetamines on urine drug screening.
VI. Dosage and method of administration.
  A. Adult. Give 20 mg slow IV bolus initially; repeat with 40- to 80-mg doses at 10-minute intervals until blood pressure is controlled or a cumulative dose of 300 mg is achieved (most patients will respond to total doses of 50–200 mg). Alternatively, administer a constant infusion of 2 mg/min until blood pressure is controlled or a 300-mg cumulative dose is reached. After this, give oral labetalol starting at 100 mg twice daily.
  B. Children older than 12 years. Initial 0.25 mg/kg dose is given intravenously over 2 minutes.
VII. Formulations.
  A. Parenteral. Labetalol hydrochloride (Normodyne, Trandate), 5 mg/mL, 40-mL vials.
  B. Oral. Labetalol hydrochloride (Normodyne, Trandate), 100-, 200-, 300-mg tablets.
  C. The **suggested minimum stocking level** to treat a 70-kg adult for the first 24 hours is two vials (5 mg/mL, 40 mL each).

▶ LEUCOVORIN CALCIUM

Kathryn H. Keller, PharmD

I. Pharmacology. Leucovorin (folinic acid or citrovorum factor) is a metabolically functional form of folic acid. Unlike folic acid, leucovorin does not require reduction by dihydrofolate reductase, and therefore it can participate directly in the one-carbon transfer reactions necessary for purine biosynthesis and cellular DNA and RNA production. In animal models of methanol intoxication, replacement of a deficiency of leucovorin and folic acid can reduce morbidity and mortality by catalyzing the oxidation of the highly toxic metabolite formic acid to nontoxic products. However, there is no evidence that administration of these agents in the absence of a deficiency is effective.
II. Indications.
  A. Folic acid antagonists (eg, methotrexate, trimethoprim, and pyrimethamine). *Note:* Leucovorin treatment is essential because cells are incapable of utilizing folic acid owing to inhibition of dihydrofolate reductase.

    B. Methanol poisoning. Leucovorin is an alternative to folic acid.
III. Contraindications. No known contraindications.
IV. Adverse effects.
    A. Allergic reactions as a result of prior sensitization have been reported.
    B. Hypercalcemia from the calcium salt may occur (limit infusion rate to 16 mL/min).
    C. Use in pregnancy. FDA category C (indeterminate). This does not preclude its acute, short-term use for a seriously symptomatic patient (see p 333).
V. Drug or laboratory interactions. Leucovorin bypasses the antifolate effect of methotrexate.
VI. Dosage and method of administration.
    A. Methotrexate poisoning. *Note:* Efficacy depends on early administration; **the drug should be given within 1 hour of poisoning** if possible. Administer intravenously a dose equal to or greater than the dose of methotrexate. If the dose is large but unknown, administer 75 mg (children, 10 mg/m^2/dose) and then 12 mg every 6 hours for 4 doses. Serum methotrexate levels can be used to guide subsequent leucovorin therapy (Table III–7). Do not use oral therapy.
    B. Other folic acid antagonists. Administer 5–15 mg/d IM, IV, or PO for 5–7 days.
    C. Methanol poisoning. For adults and children, give 1 mg/kg (up to 50–70 mg) IV every 4 hours for 1–2 doses. Oral folic acid is given thereafter at the same dosage every 4–6 hours until resolution of symptoms and adequate elimination of methanol from the body (usually 2 days). Although leucovorin could be used safely for the entire course of treatment, it is no more effective than folic acid and its cost does not justify such prolonged use in place of folic acid.
VII. Formulations.
    A. Parenteral. Leucovorin calcium (Wellcovorin, others), 3- and 10-mg/mL vials; and 50, 100, and 350 mg for reconstitution (use sterile water rather than diluent provided, which contains benzyl alcohol).
    B. Oral. Leucovorin calcium (Wellcovorin, others), 5-, 10-, 15-, and 25-mg tablets.
    C. The **suggested minimum stocking level** to treat a 70-kg adult for the first 24 hours is two 100-mg vials or one 350-mg vial.

▶ LIDOCAINE

Thomas E. Kearney, PharmD

I. Pharmacology.
    A. Lidocaine is a local anesthetic and a type Ib antiarrhythmic agent. It inhibits fast sodium channels, depresses automaticity within the His-Purkinje system and the ventricles, and prolongs the effective refractory period and action po-

TABLE III–7. LEUCOVORIN DOSE DETERMINATION (AFTER THE FIRST 24 HOURS)

Methotrexate Concentration (10^{-6} μmol/L)	Hours After Methotrexate Exposure	Leucovorin Dose[a] (Adults and Children)
0.1–1	24	10–15 mg/m^2 q6h for 12 doses
1–5	24	50 mg/m^2 q6h until serum level is $< 1 \times 10^{-7}$ mol/L
5–10	24	100 mg/m^2 q6h until serum level is $< 1 \times 10^{-7}$ mol/L

Reference: Methotrexate Management, in Rumack, B H et al (eds); Poisindex. Denver, 1989.
[a]If serum creatinine increases by 50% in the first 24 hours after methotrexate, increase the dose frequency to every 3 hours until the methotrexate level is less than 5×10^{-6} mol/L

tential duration. Conduction within ischemic myocardial areas is depressed, abolishing reentrant circuits. Unlike quinidine and related drugs, lidocaine exerts minimal effect on the automaticity of the sino-atrial node and on conduction through the atrioventricular node and does not decrease myocardial contractility or blood pressure in usual doses.

    B. The oral bioavailability of lidocaine is poor owing to extensive first-pass hepatic metabolism. After intravenous administration of a single dose, the onset of action is within 60–90 seconds and the duration of effect is 10–20 minutes. The elimination half-life of lidocaine is approximately 1.5–2 hours; active metabolites have elimination half-lives of 2–10 hours. Drug accumulation may occur in patients with congestive heart failure or liver or renal disease.

II. Indications. Lidocaine is used for the control of ventricular arrhythmias arising from poisoning by a variety of cardioactive drugs and toxins (eg, digoxin, cyclic antidepressants, stimulants, and theophylline). Patients with atrial arrhythmias do not usually respond to this drug.

III. Contraindications.

    A. The presence of nodal or ventricular rhythms in the setting of third-degree atrioventricular or intraventricular block. These are usually reflex escape rhythms that may provide lifesaving cardiac output, and abolishing them may result in asystole.

    B. Hypersensitivity to lidocaine or other amide-type local anesthetics (rare).

IV. Adverse effects.

    A. Excessive doses produce dizziness, confusion, agitation, and seizures.

    B. Conduction defects, bradycardia, and hypotension may occur with extremely high serum concentrations or in patients with underlying conduction disease.

    C. Use in pregnancy. FDA category B. Fetal harm is extremely unlikely (see p 333).

V. Drug or laboratory interactions.

    A. Cimetidine and propranolol may decrease the hepatic clearance of lidocaine.

    B. Lidocaine may produce additive effects with other local anesthetics. In severe cocaine intoxication, lidocaine theoretically may cause additive neuronal depression.

VI. Dosage and method of administration (adults and children). Administer 1 mg/kg IV bolus over 1 minute, followed by infusion of 1–4 mg/min (20–50 µg/kg/min) to maintain serum concentrations of 1.5–5 mg/L. If significant ectopy persists after the initial bolus, repeat doses of 0.5 mg/kg IV can be given if needed at 10-minute intervals (to a maximum 300 mg or 3 mg/kg total dose). In patients with congestive heart failure or liver disease, use half the recommended dose.

VII. Formulations.

    A. Parenteral. Lidocaine hydrochloride (Xylocaine, others), 50-mg (5-mL) and 100-mg (5-mL) prefilled syringes without preservatives; 1- and 2-g single-use vials or additive syringes for preparing intravenous infusions.

    B. The **suggested minimum stocking level** to treat a 70-kg adult for the first 24 hours is 10 prefilled 100-mg syringes and six 1-g vials for infusions.

▶ METHOCARBAMOL

Thomas E. Kearney, PharmD

  I. Pharmacology. Methocarbamol is a centrally acting muscle relaxant. It does not directly relax skeletal muscle, and it does not depress neuromuscular transmission or muscle excitability; muscle relaxation is probably related to its sedative effects. After intravenous administration, the onset of action is nearly immediate. Elimination occurs by hepatic metabolism, with a serum half-life of 0.9–2.2 hours.

II. Indications.

A. Control of painful muscle spasm caused by black widow spider envenomation (see p 296). Methocarbamol should be used as an adjunct to other medications (eg, calcium or diazepam) that are considered more effective.

B. Management of muscle spasm caused by mild tetanus (see p 301) or strychnine (see p 298) poisoning.

III. Contraindications.

A. Known hypersensitivity to the drug.

B. History of epilepsy (intravenous methocarbamol may precipitate seizures).

IV. Adverse effects.

A. Dizziness, drowsiness, nausea, flushing, and metallic taste may occur.

B. Extravasation from an intravenous site may cause phlebitis and sloughing. Do not administer subcutaneously.

C. Hypotension, bradycardia, and syncope have occurred after intramuscular or intravenous administration. Keep patient in a recumbent position for 10–15 minutes after injection.

D. Urticaria and anaphylactic reactions have been reported.

E. **Use in pregnancy.** There is no reported experience, and no FDA category has been assigned.

V. Drug or laboratory interactions.

A. Methobarbamol produces additive sedation with alcohol and other central nervous system depressants.

B. Methocarbamol may cause false-positive urine 5-HIAA and VMA results.

C. The urine may turn brown, black, or blue after it stands.

VI. Dosage and method of administration.

A. Parenteral

1. Administer 1 g (children, 15 mg/kg) IV over 5 minutes, followed by 0.5 g in 250 mL of 5% dextrose (children, 10 mg/kg in 5 mL of 5% dextrose) over 4 hours. Repeat every 6 hours to a maximum of 3 g daily.

2. For tetanus, higher doses are usually recommended. Give 1–2 g IV initially, no faster than 300 mg/min; if needed, use a continuous infusion up to a total of 3 g.

3. The usual intramuscular dose is 500 mg every 8 hours for adults and 10 mg/kg every 8 hours for children. Do not give subcutaneously.

B. **Oral.** Switch to oral administration as soon as tolerated. Give 0.5–1 g (children, 10–15 mg/kg) PO or by gastric tube every 6 hours. The maximum dose is 1.5 g every 6 hours; for tetanus, the maximum adult dose is 24 g/d.

VII. Formulations.

A. **Parenteral.** Methocarbamol (Robaxin), 100 mg/mL.

B. **Oral.** Methocarbamol (Robaxin, others), 500- and 750-mg tablets.

C. The **suggested minimum stocking level** to treat a 70-kg adult for the first 24 hours is 24 vials (100 mg/mL, 10 mL each).

▶ METHYLENE BLUE

Kathryn H. Keller, PharmD

I. Pharmacology. Methylene blue is a redox dye that reverses drug-induced methemoglobinemia by increasing the conversion of methemoglobin to hemoglobin. This requires the presence of adequate amounts of the enzymes methemoglobin reductase and glucose-6-phosphate dehydrogenase (G6PD). The onset is rapid, with a maximum effect within 30 minutes. Methylene blue is excreted in the urine and bile, which turn blue or green.

II. Indications. Methylene blue is used to treat methemoglobinemia (see p 220), in which the patient has symptoms or signs of hypoxemia (eg, dyspnea, confusion, or chest pain) or has a methemoglobin level greater than 30%. **Note:** Methylene blue is not effective for sulfhemoglobinemia.

III. **Contraindications.**
  A. G6PD deficiency. Treatment with methylene blue is ineffective and may cause hemolysis.
  B. Severe renal failure.
  C. Known hypersensitivity to methylene blue.
  D. Methemoglobin reductase deficiency.
  E. Reversal of nitrite-induced methemoglobinemia for treatment of cyanide poisoning.

IV. **Adverse effects.**
  A. Gastrointestinal upset, headache, and dizziness may occur.
  B. Excessive doses of methylene blue (> 7 mg/kg) can actually cause methemoglobinemia by directly oxidizing hemoglobin. Doses greater than 15 mg/kg are associated with hemolysis, particularly in neonates.
  C. Long-term administration may result in marked anemia.
  D. Extravasation may result in local tissue necrosis.
  E. **Use in pregnancy.** There is no reported experience, and no FDA category has been assigned. This does not preclude its acute, short-term use for a seriously symptomatic patient (see p 333).

V. **Drug or laboratory interactions.**
  A. No known drug interactions, but the intravenous preparation should not be mixed with other drugs.
  B. Transient false-positive methemoglobin levels of about 15% are produced by dosages of 2 mg/kg of methylene blue.

VI. **Dosage and method of administration (adults and children).**
  A. Administer 1–2 mg/kg (0.1–0.2 mL/kg of 1% solution) IV slowly over 5 minutes. May be repeated in 30–60 minutes.
  B. If no response after 2 doses, do not repeat dosing; consider G6PD deficiency or methemoglobin reductase deficiency.
  C. Patients with continued production of methemoglobin from a long-acting oxidant stress (eg, dapsone) may require repeated dosing every 6–8 hours for 2–3 days.

VII. **Formulations.**
  A. **Parenteral.** Methylene blue injection 1% (10 mg/mL).
  B. The **suggested minimum stocking level** to treat a 70-kg adult for the first 24 hours is 5 ampules (10 mg/mL, 10 mL each).

▶ **METOCLOPRAMIDE**

Judith A. Alsop, PharmD

I. **Pharmacology.** Metoclopramide is a dopamine antagonist with antiemetic activity at the chemoreceptor trigger zone. It also accelerates gastrointestinal motility and facilitates gastric emptying. The onset of effect is 1–3 minutes after intravenous administration, and therapeutic effects persist for 1–2 hours after a single dose. The drug is excreted primarily by the kidney. The elimination half-life is about 5–6 hours but may be as long as 14 hours in patients with renal insufficiency.

II. **Indications.**
  A. Metoclopramide is used to prevent and control persistent nausea and vomiting, particularly when the ability to administer activated charcoal (eg, treatment of theophylline poisoning) or other oral antidotal therapy (eg, acetylcysteine for acetaminophen poisoning) is compromised.
  B. Theoretical (unproved) use to stimulate bowel activity in patients with ileus who require repeat-dose activated charcoal or whole-bowel irrigation.

III. Contraindications.
A. Known hypersensitivity to the drug; possible cross-sensitivity with procainamide.
B. Mechanical bowel obstruction or intestinal perforation.
C. Pheochromocytoma (metoclopramide may cause hypertensive crisis).

IV. Adverse effects.
A. Sedation, restlessness, fatigue, and diarrhea may occur.
B. Extrapyramidal reactions may result, particularly with high-dose treatment. Pediatric patients appear to be more susceptible. These reactions may be prevented by pretreatment with diphenhydramine (see p 359).
C. May increase the frequency and severity of seizures in patients with seizure disorders.
D. Parenteral formulations that contain sulfite preservatives may precipitate bronchospasm in susceptible individuals.
E. Use in pregnancy. FDA category B. Not likely to cause harm when used as short-term therapy.

V. Drug or laboratory interactions.
A. Additive sedation in the presence of other central nervous system depressants.
B. Risk of extrapyramidal reactions may be increased in the presence of other dopamine antagonist agents (eg, haloperidol or phenothiazines).
C. In one study involving hypertensive patients, metoclopramide enhanced the release of catecholamines. As a result, the manufacturer advises cautious use in hypertensive patients and suggests that the drug should not be used in patients taking monoamine oxidase (MAO) inhibitors.
D. The drug may enhance the absorption of ingested drugs by promoting gastric emptying.
E. Anticholinergic agents may inhibit bowel motility effects.

VI. Dosage and method of administration.
A. Low-dose therapy. Effective for mild nausea and vomiting. Give 10–20 mg IM or slowly IV (children, 0.1 mg/kg).
B. High-dose therapy. For control of severe or persistent vomiting. For adults and children, give 1–2 mg/kg IV infusion over 15 minutes in 50 mL dextrose or saline. May be repeated twice at 2- to 3-hour intervals.
   1. Metoclopramide is most effective if given before emesis or 30 minutes before administration of a nausea-inducing drug (eg, acetylcysteine).
   2. If no response to initial dose, may give additional 2 mg/kg, and repeat every 2–3 hours up to maximum 12 mg/kg total dose.
   3. Pretreatment with 50 mg (children, 1 mg/kg) of diphenhydramine (see p 359) helps to prevent extrapyramidal reactions.
   4. Reduce dose by one-half in patients with renal insufficiency.

VII. Formulations.
A. Parenteral. Metoclopramide hydrochloride (Reglan), 5 mg/mL; 2-, 10-, 30-, 50-, and 100-mL vials. Also available in preservative-free 2-, 10-, and 30-mL vials and 2- and 10-mL ampules.
B. The **suggested minimum stocking level** to treat a 70-kg adult for the first 24 hours is 1,000 mg (4 vials, 50 mL each, or equivalent).

▶ MORPHINE
Thomas E. Kearney, PharmD

I. Pharmacology. Morphine is the principal alkaloid of opium and is a potent analgesic and sedative agent. In addition, it decreases venous tone and systemic vascular resistance, resulting in reduced preload and afterload. Morphine is variably absorbed from the gastrointestinal tract and is usually used parenterally. After intravenous injection, peak analgesia is attained within 20 minutes and usually lasts 3–5 hours. Morphine is eliminated by hepatic metabolism, with a serum half-life of about 3 hours; however, the clearance of morphine is slowed and duration of effect is prolonged in patients with renal failure.

II. **Indications.**
   A. Severe pain associated with black widow spider envenomation, rattlesnake envenomation, or other bites or stings.
   B. Pain caused by corrosive injury to the eyes, skin, or gastrointestinal tract.
   C. Pulmonary edema resulting from congestive heart failure. Chemical-induced noncardiogenic pulmonary edema is *not* an indication for morphine therapy.

III. **Contraindications.**
   A. Known hypersensitivity to morphine.
   B. Respiratory or central nervous system depression with impending respiratory failure, unless the patient is intubated or equipment and trained personnel are standing by for intervention if necessary.
   C. Suspected head injury. Morphine may obscure or cause exaggerated central nervous system depression.

IV. **Adverse effects.**
   A. Respiratory and central nervous system depression may result in respiratory arrest. Depressant effects may be prolonged in patients with liver disease and chronic renal failure.
   B. Hypotension may occur owing to decreased systemic vascular resistance and venous tone.
   C. Nausea, vomiting, and constipation may occur.
   D. Bradycardia, wheezing, flushing, pruritus, urticaria, and other histaminelike effects may occur.
   E. **Use in pregnancy.** FDA category C (indeterminate). This does not preclude its acute, short-term use for a seriously symptomatic patient (see p 333).

V. **Drug or laboratory interactions.**
   A. Additive depressant effects with other opioid agonists, ethanol and other sedative-hypnotic agents, tranquilizers, and antidepressants.
   B. Morphine is physically incompatible with solutions containing a variety of drugs, including aminophylline, phenytoin, phenobarbital, and sodium bicarbonate.

VI. **Dosage and method of administration.**
   A. Morphine may be injected subcutaneously, intramuscularly, or intravenously. The oral and rectal routes produce erratic absorption and are not recommended for use in acutely ill patients.
   B. The usual initial dose is 5–10 mg IV or 10–15 mg SC or IM, with maintenance analgesic doses of 5–20 mg every 4 hours. The pediatric dose is 0.1–0.2 mg/kg every 4 hours.

VII. **Formulations.**
   A. **Parenteral.** Morphine sulfate for injection; variety of available concentrations from 0.5 to 15 mg/mL.
   B. The **suggested minimum stocking level** to treat a 70-kg adult for the first 24 hours is 150 mg.

▶ **NALOXONE AND NALMEFENE**

Brett Roth, MD

I. **Pharmacology.** Naloxone and nalmefene are pure opioid antagonists that competitively block μ, κ, and σ opiate receptors within the central nervous system. They have no opioid agonist properties and can be given safely in large doses without producing respiratory or central nervous system depression. *Naltrexone* is another potent competitive opioid antagonist that is active orally and is used to prevent recidivism in patients detoxified from opioid abuse. It has also been used to reduce craving for alcohol. It is *not* used for the acute reversal of opioid intoxication, and will not be discussed further in this handbook.

    A. **Naloxone** is not effective orally but may be given subcutaneously, intramuscularly, intravenously, or even endotracheally. After intravenous administration, opioid antagonism occurs within 1–2 minutes and persists for approximately 1–4 hours. The plasma half-life is about 60 minutes.

    B. **Nalmefene** was approved in 1995. It is 4 times more potent than naloxone at mu receptors and slightly more potent at kappa receptors. It has a longer elimination half-life, and has a duration of action of 1–4 hours (see Table III–8).

II. Indications.

    A. Reversal of acute opioid intoxication manifested by coma, respiratory depression, or hypotension.

    B. Empiric therapy for stupor or coma suspected to be caused by opioid overdose.

    C. Anecdotal reports suggest that high-dose naloxone may partially reverse the central nervous system and respiratory depression associated with clonidine (see p 141), ethanol (see p 162), benzodiazepine (see p 106), or valproic acid (see p 314) overdoses, although these effects are inconsistent.

III. Contraindications. Do not use in patients with a known hypersensitivity to either agent (may have cross-sensitivity).

IV. Adverse effects. Human studies have documented an excellent safety record for both drugs. Volunteers have received up to 24 mg nalmefene intravenously and 50 mg orally.

    A. Use in opiate-dependent patients may precipitate acute withdrawal syndrome. This may be more protracted with nalmefene. Neonates of addicted mothers may suffer more severe withdrawal symptoms, including seizures.

    B. Pulmonary edema or ventricular fibrillation has occasionally occurred shortly after naloxone administration in opioid-intoxicated patients. Pulmonary edema has also been associated with post-anesthetic use of naloxone, especially when catecholamines and large fluid volumes have been administered.

    C. Reversing the sedative effects of an opioid may amplify the toxic effects of other drugs. For example, agitation, hypertension, and ventricular irritability have occurred after naloxone administration to persons high on "speedball" (heroin plus cocaine or methamphetamine).

    D. Seizures have been associated with nalmefene use in animals but have not been reported in humans.

    E. There has been one case report of hypertension following naloxone administration in a patient with clonidine overdose.

    F. **Use in pregnancy.** FDA category B (see p 333). Naloxone or nalmefene-induced drug withdrawal syndrome may precipitate labor in an opioid-dependent mother.

TABLE III–8. CHARACTERISTICS OF NALOXONE AND NALMEFENE

	Naloxone	Nalmefene
Elimination half-life	60–90 min	10–13 h
Duration of action	1 h	1–4 h*
Metabolism	Liver (glucuronidation)	Liver (glucuronidation)
Cost (equivalent doses)	$0.91/0.4 mg	$4.38/0.25 mg
Advantages	Lower cost; shorter action; more human experience	Longer duration lowers risk of recurrent respiratory depression for most (but not all) opioids
Disadvantages	More frequent dosing or constant infusion	Cost; may cause prolonged opioid withdrawal

*High doses (eg, > 6 mg) may increase the duration of action but are not recommended at this time. (Clinical studies suggest that a single 50-mg oral dose of nalmefene may block opioid effects for 48 h.)

V. **Drug or laboratory interactions.** Naloxone and nalmefene antagonize the analgesic effect of opioids.

VI. **Dosage and method of administration for suspected opioid-induced coma.**

A. **Naloxone.** Administer 0.4–2 mg IV; repeat at 2- to 3-minute intervals until desired response is achieved. Titrate carefully in opioid-dependent patients. The dose for children is the same as for adults.

1. The total dose required to reverse the effects of the opioid is highly variable and is dependent on the concentration and receptor affinity of the opioid. Some drugs (eg, propoxyphene) do not respond to usual doses of naloxone. However, if no response is achieved by a total dose of 10–15 mg, the diagnosis of opioid overdose should be questioned.

2. *Caution:* Resedation can occur when the naloxone wears off in 1–2 hours. Repeated doses of naloxone may be required to maintain reversal of the effects of opioids with prolonged elimination half-lives (eg, methadone) or sustained-release formulations or when packets or vials have been ingested.

3. **Infusion** Give 0.4–0.8 mg/h in normal saline or 5% dextrose, titrated to clinical effect (in infants, start with 0.04–0.16 mg/kg/h). Another method is to estimate two-thirds of the initial dose needed to awaken the patient and give this amount each hour.

B. **Nalmefene.** Give 0.25 mg incrementally every 2–5 minutes to a total dose of 1.5 mg. To treat opioid-induced respiratory arrest, start with 0.5 mg and repeat in 0.5-mg increments until spontaneous respiration is reestablished.

1. Dosage, safety, and efficacy in children have not been established.

2. As with naloxone, the total dose required to reverse the effects of the opioid is highly variable.

3. *Caution:* The duration of action of nalmefene will vary depending on the half-life and concentration of the opioid being reversed, the presence of other sedating drugs, and the dose of nalmefene. Smaller doses of nalmefene may have a shorter duration because of rapid redistribution of the drug out of the brain. Fully reversing doses (1–1.5 mg in a 70-kg person) have been shown to last several hours. However, this may not be long enough for patients who have overdosed on a long-acting opioid such as methadone or propoxyphene or who have ingested a drug-containing condom or packet with unpredictable breakage and absorption.

C. *Note:* While both drugs can be given by the intramuscular or subcutaneous route, absorption is erratic and incomplete. Naloxone is not effective orally. Huge doses of nalmefene have been used orally in experimental studies, but this route is not recommended at this time.

VII. **Formulations.**

A. **Naloxone** hydrochloride (Narcan): 0.02, 0.4, or 1 mg/mL; 1-, 2-, or 10-mL syringes, ampules, or vials. The **suggested minimum stocking level** to treat a 70-kg adult for the first 24 hours is 30 mg (3 vials, 1 mg/mL, 10 mL each, or equivalent).

B. **Nalmefene** hydrochloride (Revex): 100 μg in 1-mL ampules; 1 mg/mL in 2-mL vials; syringes containing 2 mL of 1 mg/mL nalmefene. The **suggested minimum stocking level** to treat a 70-kg adult for the first 24 hours is 16 mg (8 vials, 1 mg/mL, 2 mL each, or equivalent).

▶ NEUROMUSCULAR BLOCKERS

Thomas E. Kearney, PharmD

I. **Pharmacology**

A. Neuromuscular-blocking agents produce skeletal muscle paralysis by inhibiting the action of acetylcholine at the neuromuscular junction. **Depolarizing agents** (eg, succinylcholine; Table III–9) depolarize the motor end plate and

TABLE III–9. SELECTED NEUROMUSCULAR BLOCKERS

Drug	Onset	Duration[a]	Dose (all are intravenous)
Depolarizing			
Succinylcholine	0.5–1 min	2–3 min	0.6 mg/kg[b] (children: 1 mg/kg[c]) over 10–20 seconds; repeat as needed.
Nondepolarizing			
Atracurium	3–5 min	20–45 min	0.4–0.5 mg/kg (children < 2 years: 0.3–0.4 mg/kg)
Cisatracurium	1.5–2 min	55–61 min	0.15–0.2 mg/kg (children 2–12 years: 0.1 mg/kg), then 1–3 µg/kg/min to maintain blockade.
Pancuronium	2–3 min	35–45 min	0.06–0.1 mg/kg; then 0.01–0.02 mg/kg every 20–40 min as needed to maintain blockade.
Rocuronium	0.5–3 min	22–94 min	0.6–1 mg/kg; then 10–12 µg/kg/min to maintain blockade.
Vecuronium	1–2 min	25–40 min	For children > 1 year and adults: 0.08–0.1 mg/kg bolus, then 0.01–0.02 mg/kg every 10–20 min to maintain blockade.

[a]For most agents, duration is dose- and age-dependent. With succinylcholine or mivacurium, effects may be prolonged in patients who have genetic plasma cholinesterase deficiency or organophosphate intoxication.
[b]To prevent fasciculations, administer a small dose of a nondepolarizing agent (eg, pancuronium, 0.01 mg/kg) 2–3 min before the succinylcholine.
[c]Pretreat children with atropine at 0.005–0.01 mg/kg to prevent bradycardia or atrioventricular block.

block recovery; transient muscle fasciculations occur with the initial depolarization. **Nondepolarizing agents** (eg, atracurium, pancuronium, and others; Table III-9) competitively block the action of acetylcholine at the motor end plate; therefore, no initial muscle fasciculations occur. They also block acetylcholine at sympathetic ganglia, which may result in hypotension.

B. The neuromuscular blockers produce complete muscle paralysis with no depression of central nervous system function. Thus, patients who are conscious will remain awake but unable to move and patients with status epilepticus may continue to have central nervous system seizure activity despite flaccid paralysis.

C. Succinylcholine produces the most rapid onset of effects, with total paralysis within 30–60 seconds after intravenous administration. It is rapidly hydrolyzed by plasma cholinesterases, and its effects dissipate in 10–20 minutes. Onset and duration of several other neuromuscular blockers is described in Table III-9.

II. **Indications.**

A. Neuromuscular blockers are used to abolish excessive muscular activity, rigidity, or peripheral seizure activity when continued hyperactivity may produce or aggravate rhabdomyolysis and hyperthermia. Examples of such situations include the following. **Note:** The preferred agent for these conditions is a nondepolarizing agent.

1. Drug overdoses involving stimulants (eg, amphetamines, cocaine, phencyclidine, monoamine oxidase inhibitors) or strychnine.

2. Tetanus.

3. Hyperthermia associated with muscle rigidity or hyperactivity (eg, status epilepticus, neuroleptic malignant syndrome, or serotonin syndrome [see p 20]). **Note:** Neuromuscular blockers are not effective for malignant hyperthermia (see p 20); in fact, inability to induce paralysis with these agents should suggest the diagnosis of malignant hyperthermia.

   B. Neuromuscular blockers provide prompt flaccid paralysis to facilitate orotracheal intubation. The preferred agents for this purpose are rapid onset agents such as succinylcholine, rocuronium, and vecuronium.
III. Contraindications.
   A. Lack of preparedness or inability to intubate the trachea and ventilate the patient after total paralysis ensues. Proper equipment and trained personnel must be assembled before the drug is given.
   B. Known history of malignant hyperthermia. Succinylcholine use is associated with malignant hyperthermia in susceptible patients (incidence, approximately 1 in 50,000).
IV. Adverse effects.
   A. Complete paralysis results in respiratory depression and apnea.
   B. Succinylcholine can stimulate vagal nerves, resulting in sinus bradycardia and atrioventricular block. Children are particularly sensitive to vagotonic effects.
   C. Muscle fasciculations may cause increased intraocular and intragastric pressure (the latter of which may result in emesis and aspiration of gastric contents). Rhabdomyolysis and myoglobinuria may be observed, especially in children.
   D. Succinylcholine may produce hyperkalemia in patients with myopathy, recent severe burns, or spinal cord injury (this risk is maximal a few months after the injury).
   E. Clinically significant histamine release with bronchospasm may occur, especially with succinylcholine.
   F. Neuromuscular blockade is potentiated by hypokalemia and hypocalcemia (nondepolarizing agents) and by hypermagnesemia (depolarizing and nondepolarizing agents).
   G. Prolonged effects may occur after succinylcholine use in patients with genetic deficiency of plasma cholinesterase.
   H. Prolonged effects may occur in patients with neuromuscular disease (eg, myasthenia gravis, Eaton-Lambert syndrome).
   I. Use in pregnancy. FDA category C (indeterminate). This does not preclude their acute, short-term use for a seriously ill patient (see p 333).
V. Drug or laboratory interactions.
   A. Actions of the nondepolarizing agents are potentiated by ether, methoxyflurane, and enflurane and are inhibited or reversed by anticholinesterase agents (eg, neostigmine, physostigmine, and carbamate and organophosphate insecticides).
   B. Organophosphate or carbamate (see p 244) insecticide intoxication may potentiate or prolong the effect of succinylcholine.
   C. Numerous drugs may potentiate neuromuscular blockade. These include calcium antagonists, aminoglycoside antibiotics, propranolol, membrane-stabilizing drugs (eg, quinidine), magnesium, lithium, and thiazide diuretics.
   D. Anticonvulsants (carbamazepine and phenytoin) and theophylline may delay the onset and shorten the duration of action of some nondepolarizing agents. Carbamazepine has additive effects, and reduction of the neuromuscular blocker dose may be required.
VI. Dosage and method of administration (see Table III–9).
VII. Formulations.
   A. Succinylcholine chloride (Anectine and others), 20, 50, and 100 mg/mL; 5- and 10-mL vials and ampules. The **suggested minimum stocking level** to treat a 70-kg adult for the first 24 hours is two vials of each concentration.
   B. Atracurium besylate (Tracrium), 10 mg/mL in 5-mL single-dose and 10-mL multidose vials. The **suggested minimum stocking level** to treat a 70-kg adult for the first 24 hours is four 10-mL vials .
   C. Cisatracurium besylate (Nimbex), 2 mg/mL in 5- and 10-mL vials; 10 mg/mL in 20-mL vials. The **suggested minimum stocking level** to treat a 70-kg adult for the first 24 hours is one 20-mL vial or equivalent.

D. Pancuronium bromide (Pavulon), 1 and 2 mg/mL in 2-, 5-, and 10-mL vials and ampules. The **suggested minimum stocking level** to treat a 70-kg adult for the first 24 hours is eight vials (2 mg/mL, 5 mL each).

E. Rocuronium bromide (Zemuron), 10 mg/mL in 5-mL vials. The **suggested minimum stocking level** to treat a 70-kg adult for the first 24 hours is seven vials.

F. Vecuronium bromide (Norcuron), 10-mg vials of lyophilized powder for reconstitution. The **suggested minimum stocking level** to treat a 70-kg adult for the first 24 hours is three vials.

▶ NICOTINAMIDE (NIACINAMIDE)

Thomas E. Kearney, PharmD

I. **Pharmacology.** Nicotinamide (niacinamide, vitamin B_3), one of the B vitamins, is required for the functioning of the coenzymes nicotinamide adenine dinucleotide (NAD) and nicotinamide adenine dinucleotide phosphate (NADP). NAD and NADP are responsible for energy transfer reactions. Niacin deficiency, which results in pellagra, can be corrected with nicotinamide.

II. **Indications.** Nicotinamide is used to prevent the neurologic and endocrinologic toxicity associated with the ingestion of Vacor (PNU), a rodenticide that is believed to act by antagonizing nicotinamide (see p 313). Best results are achieved when nicotinamide therapy is instituted within 3 hours of ingestion. It may also be effective for treatment of Vacor analogs such as alloxan and streptozocin.

III. **Contraindications.** No known contraindications.

IV. **Adverse effects.**

    A. Headache and dizziness.

    B. Hyperglycemia.

    C. Hepatotoxicity (reported after chronic use with daily dose > 3 g).

    D. Use in pregnancy. No assigned FDA category. This does not preclude its acute, short-term use for a seriously symptomatic patient (see p 333).

V. **Drug or laboratory interactions.** No known interactions.

VI. **Dosage and method of administration (adults and children).** *Note:* The parenteral preparation is no longer available in the United States. The oral form may be substituted, but is of unknown efficacy.

    1. Give 500 mg IV initially, followed by 100–200 mg IV every 4 hours for 48 hours. Then give 100 mg orally 3–5 times daily for 2 weeks. If clinical deterioration from the Vacor progresses during initial therapy with nicotinamide, change dosing interval to every 2 hours. The maximum suggested daily dose is 3 g.

    2. *Note:* Nicotinic acid (niacin) is *not* a substitute for nicotinamide in the treatment of Vacor ingestions.

VII. **Formulations.**

    A. Parenteral. Niacinamide, 100 mg/mL (not available in the United States).

    B. Oral. Niacinamide, 50-, 100-, 125-, 250-, and 500-mg tablets. The **suggested minimum stocking level** to treat a 70-kg adult for the first 24 hours is 3 g.

▶ NIFEDIPINE

Thomas E. Kearney, PharmD

I. **Pharmacology.** Nifedipine is a calcium antagonist that inhibits the influx of calcium ions through calcium channels. It acts primarily by dilating systemic and coronary arteries. Unlike some calcium antagonists (eg, verapamil and diltiazem), nifedipine has minimal effects on cardiac conduction and contractility. Nifedipine is administered orally. The rapid onset of effect (15–30 minutes) after sublingual administration of the capsule contents appears to be caused by swallowing of the liquid rather than actual buccal absorption. The drug is metabolized by the liver and has a serum half-life of 2–5 hours.

II. **Indications.**
  A. Hypertension after overdose with vasoconstrictive substances such as phenylpropanolamine, cocaine, amphetamines, phencyclidine, or other stimulants. However, for rapid and titratable effect in patients with severe hypertension, a parenteral vasodilator such as phentolamine (see p 400) or nitroprusside (see p 392) is preferred.
  B. Adjunctive use as a vasodilator for treatment of arterial spasm (ie, ergot poisoning).

III. **Contraindications.**
  A. Known hypersensitivity to the drug.
  B. Volume depletion (relative contraindication).

IV. **Adverse effects.** The main disadvantage of nifedipine is that it is administered orally, with less titratability than other agents and the potential to "overshoot" the desired drop in blood pressure.
  A. Hypotension may result, especially in volume-depleted patients.
  B. Tachycardia, headache, and flushing may occur.
  C. Cerebral perfusion may be compromised if blood pressure is lowered too rapidly in a patient with intracranial hypertension resulting from stroke or hypertensive encephalopathy.
  D. Use with extreme caution in patients with obstructive cardiomyopathy or aortic stenosis; increased gradient across the aortic valve may cause pulmonary edema and hypotension.
  E. **Use in pregnancy.** FDA category C (indeterminate). However, this does not preclude its acute, short-term use for a seriously symptomatic patient (see p 333).

V. **Drug or laboratory interactions.** Nifedipine has an additive blood pressure-lowering effect when given with other antihypertensives or beta blockers.

VI. **Dosage and method of administration.** The usual dose is a 10-mg capsule, punctured, chewed, and contents swallowed (do not use extended-release formulations). It may be repeated as needed. Most hypertensive patients respond to 10–20 mg. For childhood hypertensive emergencies, give 0.25–0.5 mg/kg/dose.

VII. **Formulations.**
  A. **Oral.** Nifedipine (Procardia, Adalat, and others), 10- and 20-mg fluid-filled capsules.
  B. The **suggested minimum stocking level** to treat a 70-kg adult for the first 24 hours is 1 bottle (10 mg, 100 capsules).

▶ NITRITE, SODIUM AND AMYL

Kathryn H. Keller, PharmD

I. **Pharmacology.** Sodium nitrite injectable solution and amyl nitrite crushable ampules for inhalation are components of the cyanide antidote package. The value of nitrites as an antidote to cyanide poisoning is twofold: they oxidize hemoglobin to methemoglobin, which binds free cyanide, and they may enhance endothelial cyanide detoxification by producing vasodilation. Inhalation of an ampule of amyl nitrite produces a methemoglobin level of about 5%. Intravenous administration of a single dose of sodium nitrite is anticipated to produce a methemoglobin level of about 20–30%.

II. **Indications.**

A. Symptomatic cyanide poisoning (see p 150). Nitrites are not usually used for empiric treatment unless cyanide is very strongly suspected, and they are not recommended for smoke inhalation victims.

B. Nitrites are possibly effective for hydrogen sulfide poisoning, if given within 30 minutes of exposure (see p 188).

III. Contraindications.

A. Significant pre-existing methemoglobinemia (>40%).

B. Severe hypotension is a relative contraindication, as it may be worsened by nitrites.

C. Administration to patients with concurrent carbon monoxide poisoning is a relative contraindication; generation of methemoglobin may further compromise oxygen transport to the tissues.

IV. Adverse effects.

A. Headache, facial flushing, dizziness, nausea, vomiting, tachycardia, and sweating may occur. These side effects may be masked by the symptoms of cyanide poisoning.

B. Rapid intravenous administration may result in hypotension.

C. Excessive and potentially fatal methemoglobinemia may result.

D. Use in pregnancy. No assigned FDA category. These agents may compromise blood flow and oxygen delivery to the fetus, and they may induce fetal methemoglobinemia. Fetal hemoglobin is more sensitive to the oxidant effects of nitrites. However, this does not preclude their acute, short-term use for a seriously symptomatic patient (see p 333).

V. Drug or laboratory interactions.

A. Hypotension may be exacerbated by the concurrent presence of alcohol or other vasodilators, or any antihypertensive agent.

B. Methylene blue should not be administered to a cyanide-poisoned patient, because it may reverse nitrite-induced methemoglobinemia and theoretically result in release of free cyanide ions. However, it may be considered when severe and life-threatening excessive methemoglobinemia (eg, > 70%) is present.

C. Binding of methemoglobin to cyanide (cyanomethemoglobin) may lower the measured free methemoglobin level.

VI. Dosage and method of administration.

A. Amyl nitrite crushable ampules. Crush one to two ampules in gauze, cloth, or a sponge and place under the nose of the victim, who should inhale deeply for 30 seconds. Rest for 30 seconds, then repeat. Each ampule lasts about 2–3 minutes. If the victim is receiving respiratory support, place the ampules in the face mask or port access to the endotracheal tube. Stop ampule use when administering intravenous sodium nitrite.

B. Sodium nitrite parenteral.

1. Adults. Administer 300 mg of sodium nitrite (10 mL of 3% solution) IV over 3–5 minutes.

2. Children. Give 0.15–0.33 mL/kg to a maximum of 10 mL. Pediatric dosing should be based on the hemoglobin concentration, if known (see Table III–10). If anemia is suspected or hypotension is present, start with the lower dose, dilute in 50–100 mL of saline, and give over at least 5 minutes.

3. Oxidation of hemoglobin to methemoglobin occurs within 30 minutes. If no response to treatment occurs within 30 minutes, an additional half-sized dose of intravenous sodium nitrite may be given.

VII. Formulations.

A. Amyl nitrite. A component of the Cyanide Antidote Package, 0.3 mL in crushable ampules, 12 per kit. The drug may also be acquired separately in aspirols. *Note:* The ampules have a shelf life of only 1 year and may disappear because of the potential for abuse (as "poppers").

B. Sodium nitrite parenteral. A component of the Cyanide Antidote Package, 300 mg in 10 mL of sterile water (3%), 2 ampules per kit.

TABLE III–10. PEDIATRIC DOSING OF SODIUM NITRITE BASED ON HEMOGLOBIN CONCENTRATION

Hemoglobin (g//dL)	Initial Dose (mg/kg)	Initial Dose of 3% Sodium Nitrite (mL/kg)
7	5.8	0.19
8	6.6	0.22
9	7.5	0.25
10	8.3	0.27
11	9.1	0.3
12	10	0.33
13	10.8	0.36
14	11.6	0.39

C. The **suggested minimum stocking level** to treat a 70-kg adult for the first 24 hours is two Cyanide Antidote Packages, or equivalent (one package should be kept in the Emergency Department). Available from Taylor Pharmaceuticals.

► **NITROPRUSSIDE**

Thomas E. Kearney, PharmD

I. **Pharmacology.** Nitroprusside is an ultrashort-acting and titratable parenteral hypotensive agent that acts by directly relaxing vascular smooth muscle. Both arterial and venous dilation occurs; the effect is more marked in patients with hypertension. A small increase in heart rate may be observed in hypertensive patients. Intravenous administration produces nearly immediate onset of action, with a duration of effect of 1–10 minutes. Nitroprusside is rapidly metabolized, with a serum half-life of about 1–2 minutes. Cyanide is produced during metabolism and is converted to the less toxic thiocyanate. Thiocyanate has a half-life of 2–3 days and accumulates in patients with renal insufficiency.

II. **Indications.**
   A. Rapid control of severe hypertension (eg, in patients with stimulant intoxication or monoamine oxidase inhibitor toxicity).
   B. Arterial vasodilation in patients with ergot-induced peripheral arterial spasm.

III. **Contraindications.**
   A. Compensatory hypertension, for example, in patients with increased intracranial pressure (eg, hemorrhage or mass lesion) or in patients with coarctation of the aorta. If nitroprusside is required in such patients, use with extreme caution.
   B. Use with caution in patients with hepatic insufficiency, because cyanide metabolism may be impaired.

IV. **Adverse effects.**
   A. Nausea, vomiting, headache, and sweating may be caused by excessively rapid lowering of the blood pressure.
   B. **Cyanide toxicity,** manifested by altered mental status and metabolic acidosis, may occur with rapid high-dose infusion (> 10–15 µg/kg/min) for periods of 1 hour or longer. Continuous intravenous infusion of hydroxocobalamin, 25 mg/h (see p 374), or thiosulfate (see p 376) has been used to limit cyanide toxicity. If severe cyanide toxicity occurs, discontinue the nitroprusside infusion and give antidotal doses of thiosulfate and sodium nitrite (see p 390).

C. **Thiocyanate intoxication,** manifested by disorientation, delirium, muscle twitching, and psychosis, may occur with prolonged high-dose infusions (usually > 3 µg/kg/min for 48 hours or longer), particularly in patients with renal insufficiency (may occur at rates as low as 1 µg/kg/min). Thiocyanate production is also enhanced by coadministration of sodium thiosulfate. Monitor thiocyanate levels if the nitroprusside infusion lasts more than 1–2 days; toxicity is associated with thiocyanate levels of 50 mg/L or greater.

D. Rebound hypertension may be observed after sudden discontinuance.

E. **Use in pregnancy.** FDA category C (indeterminate; see p 333). It may cross the placenta, and it may affect uterine blood flow; however, it has been used successfully in pregnant women.

V. **Drug or laboratory interactions.** A hypotensive effect is potentiated by other antihypertensive agents and inhalational anesthetics.

VI. **Dosage and method of administration.**

A. Use only in an emergency or intensive care setting with the capability of frequent or continuous blood pressure monitoring.

B. Dissolve 50 mg of sodium nitroprusside in 3 mL of 5% dextrose; then dilute this solution in 250, 500, or 1000 mL of 5% dextrose to achieve a concentration of 200, 100, or 50 µg/mL, respectively. Protect the solution from light to avoid photodegradation (as evidenced by a color change) by covering the bottle and tubing with paper or aluminum foil.

C. Start with an intravenous infusion rate of 0.3 µg/kg/min with a controlled infusion device, and titrate to desired effect. The average dose is 3 µg/kg/min in children and adults (range, 0.5–10 µg/kg/min).

1. The maximum rate should not exceed 10 µg/kg/min to avoid risk of acute cyanide toxicity. If there is no response after 10 minutes at the maximum rate, discontinue the infusion and use an alternate vasodilator (eg, phentolamine; see p 400).

2. Sodium thiosulfate (see p 408) has been added in a ratio of 10 mg thiosulfate to 1 mg nitroprusside to reduce or prevent cyanide toxicity.

VII. **Formulations.**

A. **Parenteral.** Nitroprusside sodium (Nipride and others), 50 mg of lyophilized powder for reconstitution.

B. The **suggested minimum stocking level** to treat a 70-kg adult for the first 24 hours is 24 vials.

▶ NOREPINEPHRINE

Neal L. Benowitz, MD

I. **Pharmacology.** Norepinephrine is an endogenous catecholamine that stimulates mainly alpha-adrenergic receptors. It is used primarily as a vasopressor to increase systemic vascular resistance and venous return to the heart. Norepinephrine is also a weak beta-1-adrenergic receptor agonist, and it may increase heart rate and cardiac contractility in patients with shock.

Norepinephrine is not effective orally and is erratically absorbed after subcutaneous injection. After intravenous administration, the onset of action is nearly immediate, and the duration of effect is 1–2 minutes after the infusion is discontinued.

II. **Indications.** Norepinephrine is used to increase blood pressure and cardiac output in patients with shock caused by venodilation or low systemic vascular resistance, or both. Hypovolemia, depressed myocardial contractility, hypothermia, and electrolyte imbalance should be corrected first or concurrently.

III. **Contraindications.**

A. Uncorrected hypovolemia.

B. Norepinephrine is relatively contraindicated in patients with organic heart disease, peripheral arterial occlusive vascular disease with thrombosis, or ergot poisoning (see p 160).

IV. Adverse effects.
  A. Severe hypertension, which may result in intracranial hemorrhage, pulmonary edema, or myocardial necrosis.
  B. Aggravation of tissue ischemia, resulting in gangrene.
  C. Tissue necrosis after extravasation.
  D. Anxiety, restlessness, tremor, and headache.
  E. Anaphylaxis induced by sulfite preservatives in sensitive patients. Use with extreme caution in patients with known hypersensitivity to sulfite preservatives.
  F. Use with caution in patients intoxicated by chloral hydrate or halogenated or aromatic hydrocarbon solvents or anesthetics.
  G. **Use in pregnancy.** This drug crosses the placenta, and it can cause placental ischemia and reduce uterine contractions.

V. Drug or laboratory interactions.
  A. Enhanced pressor response may occur in the presence of cocaine and cyclic antidepressants, owing to inhibition of neuronal reuptake.
  B. Enhanced pressor response may occur in patients taking monoamine oxidase inhibitors, owing to inhibition of neuronal metabolic degradation.
  C. Alpha- and beta-blocking agents may antagonize the adrenergic effects of norepinephrine.
  D. Anticholinergic drugs may block reflex bradycardia, which normally occurs in response to norepinephrine-induced hypertension, enhancing the hypertensive response.
  E. Chloral hydrate overdose and cyclopropane and halogenated or aromatic hydrocarbon solvents and anesthetics may enhance myocardial sensitivity to arrhythmogenic effects of norepinephrine.

VI. Dosage and method of administration.
  A. *Caution:* **Avoid extravasation.** The intravenous infusion must be free flowing, and the infused vein should be observed frequently for signs of infiltration (pallor, coldness, or induration).
    1. If extravasation occurs, immediately infiltrate the affected area with phentolamine (see p 400), 5–10 mg in 10–15 mL of normal saline (children, 0.1–0.2 mg/kg; maximum 10 mg) via a fine (25- to 27-gauge) hypodermic needle; improvement is evidenced by hyperemia and return to normal temperature.
    2. Alternately, topical application of nitroglycerin paste and infiltration of terbutaline have been reported successful.
  B. **Intravenous infusion.** Begin at 4–8 μg/min (children, 1-2 μg/min or 0.1 μg/kg/min) and increase as needed every 5–10 minutes.

VII. Formulations.
Norepinephrine bitartrate is rapidly oxidized on exposure to air; it must be kept in its airtight ampule until immediately before use. If the solution appears brown or contains a precipitate, do not use it. The stock solution must be diluted in 5% dextrose or 5% dextrose-saline for infusion; usually, a 4-mg ampule is added to 1 L of fluid to provide 4 μg/mL of solution.
  A. **Parenteral.** Norepinephrine bitartrate (Levophed), 1 mg/mL, 4-mL ampule. Contains sodium bisulfite as a preservative.
  B. The **suggested minimum stocking level** to treat a 70-kg adult for the first 24 hours is 5 ampules.

▶ OCTREOTIDE

Thomas E. Kearney, PharmD

I. Pharmacology.
  A. Octreotide is a synthetic polypeptide and a long-acting analogue of somatostatin. It significantly antagonizes pancreatic insulin release and is useful for the management of oral sulfonylurea hypoglycemic poisoning.
  B. Octreotide also suppresses pancreatic function, gastric acid secretion, and biliary- and gastrointestinal-tract motility.

C. As a polypeptide, it is bioavailable only by parenteral administration (intravenously or subcutaneously). Approximately 30% of octreotide is excreted unchanged in the urine, and it has an elimination half-life of 1.7 hours. Its half-life may be increased in patients with renal dysfunction and in the elderly.
II. **Indications.** Oral sulfonylurea hypoglycemic overdose when serum glucose concentrations cannot be maintained by an intravenous 5% dextrose infusion. This agent is preferred over diazoxide (see p 356).
III. **Contraindications.** Hypersensitivity to the drug (anaphylactic shock has occurred).
IV. **Adverse effects.** In general, the drug is well tolerated. Patients may experience pain or burning at the injection site. For the most part, the adverse-effect profile is based on long-term therapy for other disease states.
   A. The suppressive effects on the biliary tract may lead to significant gallbladder disease (cholelithiasis) and pancreatitis.
   B. Gastrointestinal effects (diarrhea, nausea, discomfort) may occur in 5–10% of users. Headache, dizziness, and fatigue have also been observed.
   C. Cardiac effects may include bradycardia, conduction abnormalities (QT prolongation), hypertension, and exacerbation of congestive heart failure.
   D. **Use in pregnancy.** FDA category B. Not likely to cause harm with short-term therapy.
V. **Drug or laboratory interactions.**
   A. Octreotide may inhibit the absorption of dietary fats.
   B. The drug depresses vitamin B_{12} levels and can lead to abnormal Schilling's Test results.
VI. **Dosage and method of administration.**
   A. **Oral sulfonylurea overdose.** Give 50 μg (children: 1–10 μg) by subcutaneous or intravenous injection every 12 hours.
   B. Subcutaneous injection sites should be rotated.
   C. For IV administration, dilute in 50 mL normal saline or 5% dextrose and infuse over 15–30 min. Alternately, the dose may be given IV push over 3 min.
   D. *Note:* Optimal dosage regimen is not known. For other indications, daily dosages up to 1500 μg are utilized (120 mg has been infused over 8 hours without severe adverse effects).
VII. **Formulations.**
   A. **Parenteral.** Octreotide acetate (Sandostatin): 0.05, 0.1, and 0.5 mg/mL in 1-mL ampules; 0.2 and 1 mg/mL in 5-mL multidose vials.
   B. The **suggested minimum stocking level** to treat a 70-kg adult for the first 24 hours is two (1-mL) ampules (0.1 mg/m) or one (5-mL) multidose vial (0.2 mg/mL).

▶ ONDANSETRON

Judith A. Alsop, PharmD

I. **Pharmacology.** Ondansetron is a selective serotonin 5-HT$_3$ receptor antagonist with powerful antiemetic activity, both centrally at the chemoreceptor trigger zone and peripherally at vagal nerve terminals. The onset is about 30 minutes after an intravenous dose and 60–90 minutes after an oral dose. The drug is extensively metabolized in the liver. The elimination half-life is 3–5.5 hours, increasing to as long as 20 hours in patients with severe liver disease.
II. **Indications.** Ondansetron is used to treat intractable nausea and vomiting, particularly when the ability to administer activated charcoal or antidotal therapy (eg, N-acetylcysteine) is compromised.
III. **Contraindications.** Known hypersensitivity to the drug.
IV. **Adverse effects.**
   A. Anxiety, headache, drowsiness, fatigue, fever, and dizziness.
   B. Extrapyramidal reactions may occur.
   C. Diarrhea and constipation are both reported.
   D. Seizures, hypoxia (rare).

    E. Use in pregnancy. FDA category B. Not likely to cause harm when used as short-term therapy.

V. Drug or laboratory interactions.

    A. Extrapyramidal reactions are more likely in patients who are also taking haloperidol or other central dopamine-blocking drugs.

    B. Anticholinergic agents may inhibit bowel motility.

    C. Increased liver transaminases have been reported.

VI. Dosage and method of administration. Give 8 mg (adults) or 0.15 mg/kg IV in 50 mL normal saline or 5% dextrose. This may be repeated twice at 4-hour intervals. *Alternate high-dose therapy:* 32 mg (adults) in 50 mL saline or dextrose administered over 15 minutes. (Do not repeat this dose.)

    A. Ondansetron is most effective when given at least 30 minutes before its antiemetic properties are needed.

    B. Do not exceed a total daily dose of 8 mg in patients with severe liver disease.

    C. Ondansetron does not require dilution and can be given by direct intravenous injection over a period of at least 30 seconds, preferably 2–3 minutes.

    D. Intramuscular use is not recommended.

VII. Formulations.

    A. Parenteral. Ondansetron hydrochloride (Zofran): 2 mg/mL in 2-mL single-dose vials and 20-mL multidose vials. Also available as 32 mg in a 50-mL premixed container.

    B. The **suggested minimum stocking level** to treat a 70-kg adult for the first 24 hours is 32 mg.

▶ OXYGEN

Thomas E. Kearney, PharmD

I. Pharmacology. Oxygen is a necessary oxidant to drive biochemical reactions. Room air contains 21% oxygen.

II. Indications.

    A. Supplemental oxygen is indicated when normal oxygenation is impaired because of pulmonary injury, which may result from aspiration (chemical pneumonitis) or inhalation of toxic gases. The PO_2 should be maintained at 70–80 mm Hg if possible.

    B. Supplemental oxygen is usually given empirically to patients with altered mental status or suspected hypoxemia.

    C. Oxygen (100%) is indicated for carbon monoxide poisoning to increase the conversion of carboxyhemoglobin and carboxymyoglobin to hemoglobin and myoglobin and to increase oxygen saturation of the plasma and subsequent delivery to tissues. It may also be of benefit in patients poisoned by inhibitors of cellular respiration such as cyanide or hydrogen sulfide.

    D. Hyperbaric oxygen (100% oxygen delivered to the patient in a pressurized chamber at 2–3 atm) is advocated by some clinicians in patients with carbon monoxide poisoning (see p 125) for rapid reversal of carbon monoxide binding to hemoglobin, intracellular myoglobin, and possibly cytochrome oxidase, and for its potentially beneficial effects on cerebral edema and postischemic cellular damage. It has also been advocated for treatment of poisoning by carbon tetrachloride, cyanide, and hydrogen sulfide, and for severe methemoglobinemia, but the experimental and clinical evidence is scanty.

III. Contraindications.

    A. In **paraquat** poisoning, oxygen may contribute to lung injury. In fact, slightly *hypoxic* environments (10–12% oxygen) have been advocated to reduce the risk of pulmonary fibrosis from paraquat.

    B. Relative contraindications to hyperbaric oxygen therapy include a history of recent middle ear or thoracic surgery, untreated pneumothorax, seizure disorder, or severe sinusitis.

IV. Adverse effects. *Caution:* Oxygen is extremely flammable.

A. Prolonged, high concentrations of oxygen are associated with pulmonary alveolar tissue damage. In general, the fraction of inspired oxygen (FIO_2) should not be maintained at greater than 80% for more than 24 hours.

B. Oxygen therapy may increase the risk of retrolental fibroplasia in neonates.

C. Administration of high oxygen concentrations to patients with severe chronic obstructive pulmonary disease and chronic carbon dioxide retention who are dependent on hypoxemia to provide a drive to breathe may result in respiratory arrest.

D. **Use in pregnancy.** No known adverse effects.

V. **Drug or laboratory interactions.**

A. May potentiate pulmonary toxicity associated with paraquat poisoning.

B. May potentiate toxicity via enhanced generation of free radicals with some chemotherapeutic agents (eg, bleomycin, adriamycin, and daunorubicin).

VI. **Dosage and method of administration.**

A. **Supplemental oxygen.** Provide supplemental oxygen to maintain a PO_2 of approximately 70–80 mm Hg. If a PO_2 greater than 50 mm Hg cannot be maintained with an FIO_2 of at least 60%, consider positive end-expiratory pressure or continuous positive airway pressure.

B. **Carbon monoxide poisoning.** Provide 100% oxygen via a tight-fitting face mask with a good seal or via an endotracheal tube and an oxygen reservoir. Consider hyperbaric oxygen if the patient does not respond rapidly or is pregnant (see p 125) and is stable enough for transport to a hyperbaric facility.

VII. **Formulations.**

A. **Nasal cannula.** See Table III–11.

B. **Ventimask.** Provides variable inspired oxygen concentrations from 24 to 40%.

C. **Non-rebreathing reservoir mask.** Provides 60–90% inspired oxygen concentrations.

D. **Hyperbaric oxygen.** One hundred percent oxygen can be delivered at a pressure of 2–3 atm.

▶ PENICILLAMINE

Thomas E. Kearney, PharmD

I. **Pharmacology.** Penicillamine is a derivative of penicillin that has no antimicrobial activity but effectively chelates some heavy metals such as lead, mercury, arsenic, and copper. It has been used as adjunctive therapy after initial treatment with calcium EDTA (see p 363) or BAL (dimercaprol; see p 341), although in recent years its use has largely been replaced by the oral chelator DMSA (succimer, see p 360). Penicillamine is well absorbed orally, and the penicillamine-metal complex is eliminated in the urine. No parenteral form is available.

II. **Indications.**

A. Penicillamine may be used to treat heavy metal poisoning caused by lead (penicillamine may be used alone for minor intoxication or as adjunctive therapy after calcium EDTA or BAL in moderate to severe intoxication), mercury (after initial BAL therapy), copper, and possibly gold.

TABLE III–11. AMOUNT OF OXYGEN PROVIDED BY NASAL CANNULA

Flow Rate (L/min)	Approximate Inspired Oxygen Concentration (%)
1	24
2	28
5	40

B. For lead or mercury poisoning, oral DMSA (see p 360) is preferable, as it may result in greater metal excretion with fewer adverse effects.

III. **Contraindications.**
   A. Penicillin allergy is a contraindication.
   B. Renal insufficiency is a relative contraindication because the complex is eliminated only through the urine.
   C. Concomitant administration with other hematopoietic-depressant drugs (eg, gold salts, immunosuppressants, antimalarial agents, and phenylbutazone) is not recommended.

IV. **Adverse effects.**
   A. Hypersensitivity reactions: rash, pruritus, drug fever, hematuria, anti-nuclear antibodies, and proteinuria.
   B. Leukopenia, thrombocytopenia, hemolytic anemia, and agranulocytosis.
   C. Hepatitis and pancreatitis.
   D. Anorexia, nausea, vomiting, epigastric pain, and impairment of taste.
   E. The requirement for pyridoxine is increased, and the patient may require daily supplementation.
   F. **Use in pregnancy.** Birth defects have been associated with its use during pregnancy. No assigned FDA category (see p 333).

V. **Drug or laboratory interactions.**
   A. Penicillamine may potentiate the hematopoietic-depressant effects of drugs such as gold salts, immunosuppressants, antimalarial agents, and phenylbutazone.
   B. Several drugs (eg, antacids and ferrous sulfate) and food can substantially reduce gastrointestinal absorption of penicillamine.
   C. Penicillamine may produce a false-positive test for ketones in the urine.

VI. **Dosage and method of administration.**
   A. Penicillamine should be taken on an empty stomach, at least 1 hour before or 3 hours after meals and at bedtime.
   B. The usual dose is 20–30 mg/kg/d, administered in 3–4 divided doses. The usual starting dose in adults is 250 mg four times daily. Initiating treatment at 25% of this dose and gradually increasing to the full dose over 2–3 weeks may minimize adverse reactions. Maximum adult daily dose is 2 g.
   C. Weekly measurement of urinary and blood concentrations of the intoxicating metal is indicated to assess the need for continued therapy. Treatment for as long as 3 months has been tolerated.

VII. **Formulations.** *Note:* Although the chemical derivative *N*-acetylpenicillamine may demonstrate better central nervous system and peripheral nerve penetration, it is not currently available in the USA.
   A. **Oral.** Penicillamine (Cuprimine, Depen), 125- and 250-mg capsules, 250-mg tablets.
   B. The **suggested minimum stocking level** to treat a 70-kg adult for the first 24 hours is 1500 mg.

▶ PENTOBARBITAL

Thomas E. Kearney, PharmD

I. **Pharmacology.** Pentobarbital is a short-acting barbiturate with anticonvulsant as well as sedative-hypnotic properties. It is used as a third-line drug in the treatment of status epilepticus. It may also reduce intracranial pressure in patients with cerebral edema. After intravenous administration of a single dose, the onset of effect occurs within about 1 minute and lasts about 15 minutes. Pentobarbital demonstrates a biphasic elimination pattern; the half-life of the initial phase is 4 hours, and the terminal phase half-life is 35–50 hours. Effects are prolonged after termination of a continuous infusion.

II. **Indications.**
   A. Pentobarbital is used for the management of status epilepticus that is unresponsive to conventional anticonvulsant therapy (eg, diazepam, phenytoin, or

phenobarbital). If the use of pentobarbital for seizure control is considered, consultation with a neurologist is recommended.
- **B.** It is used to manage elevated intracranial pressure, in conjunction with other agents.
- **C.** It may be used therapeutically or diagnostically for patients with suspected alcohol or sedative-hypnotic drug withdrawal syndrome.

III. Contraindications.
- **A.** Known sensitivity to the drug.
- **B.** Manifest or latent porphyria.

IV. Adverse effects.
- **A.** Central nervous system depression, coma, and respiratory arrest may occur, especially with rapid bolus or excessive doses.
- **B.** Hypotension may result, especially with rapid intravenous infusion.
- **C.** Laryngospasm and bronchospasm have been reported after rapid intravenous injection, although the mechanism is unknown.
- **D. Use in pregnancy.** FDA category D (possible fetal risk). Pentobarbital readily crosses the placenta, and chronic use may cause hemorrhagic disease of the newborn (owing to vitamin K deficiency) or neonatal dependency and withdrawal syndrome. However, these potential effects do not preclude its acute, short-term use for a seriously symptomatic patient (see p 333).

V. Drug or laboratory interactions.
- **A.** Pentobarbital has additive central nervous system and respiratory depression effects with other barbiturates, as well as sedative and opioid drugs.
- **B.** Hepatic enzyme induction is generally not encountered with acute pentobarbital overdose, although it may occur within 24–48 hours.
- **C.** Clearance may be enhanced by hemoperfusion, requiring supplemental doses during the procedure.

VI. Dosage and method of administration.
- **A. Intermittent intravenous bolus.** Give 100 mg IV slowly over at least 2 minutes; repeat as needed at 2-minute intervals, to a maximum dose of 300–500 mg (children, 1 mg/kg IV, repeated as needed to a maximum of 5–6 mg/kg).
- **B. Continuous intravenous infusion.** Administer a loading dose of 5–6 mg/kg IV over 1 hour (not to exceed 50 mg/min; children, 1 mg/kg/min), followed by maintenance infusion of 0.5–3 mg/kg/h titrated to the desired effect. Electroencephalographic achievement of burst suppression usually occurs with a serum pentobarbital concentration of 25–40 μg/mL.
- **C. Oral.** The oral regimen for treatment of barbiturate or other sedative-drug withdrawal syndrome is administration of 200 mg orally, repeated every hour until signs of mild intoxication appear (eg, slurred speech, drowsiness, or nystagmus). Most patients respond to 600 mg or less. Repeat the total initial dose every 6 hours as needed. Phenobarbital is an alternative (see below).

VII. Formulations.
- **A. Parenteral.** Pentobarbital sodium (Nembutal and others), 50 mg/mL in 1- and 2-mL tubes and vials, and 20- and 50-mL vials.
- **B. Oral.** Capsules and suppositories (50 and 100 mg). Also available as an elixir.
- **C.** The **suggested minimum stocking level** to treat a 70-kg adult for the first 24 hours is two vials, 50 mL each, or equivalent.

▶ PHENOBARBITAL

Thomas E. Kearney, PharmD

- **I. Pharmacology.** Phenobarbital is a barbiturate commonly used as an anticonvulsant. Because of the delay in onset of the therapeutic effect of phenobarbital, diazepam (see p 342) is usually the initial agent for parenteral anticonvulsant therapy. After an oral dose of phenobarbital, peak brain concentrations are achieved within 10–15 hours. Onset of effect after intravenous administration is usually within 5 minutes, although peak effects may take up to 30 minutes. Therapeutic plasma levels are 15–35 mg/mL. The drug is eliminated by metabolism and renal excretion, and the elimination half-life is 48–100 hours.

II. **Indications.**
   A. Control of tonic-clonic seizures and status epilepticus, generally as a second- or third-line agent after diazepam or phenytoin have been tried. *Note:* For treatment of drug-induced seizures, especially seizures caused by theophylline, phenobarbital is often tried before phenytoin.
   B. Management of withdrawal from ethanol and other sedative-hypnotic drugs.

III. **Contraindications.**
   A. Known sensitivity to barbiturates.
   B. Manifest or latent porphyria.

IV. **Adverse effects.**
   A. Central nervous system depression, coma, and respiratory arrest may result, especially with rapid bolus or excessive doses.
   B. Hypotension may result from rapid intravenous administration. This can be prevented by limiting the rate of administration to less than 50 mg/min (children, 1 mg/kg/min).
   C. **Use in pregnancy.** FDA category D (possible fetal risk). Phenobarbital readily crosses the placenta, and chronic use may cause hemorrhagic disease of the newborn (owing to vitamin K deficiency) or neonatal dependency and withdrawal syndrome. However, these potential effects do not preclude its acute, short-term use for a seriously symptomatic patient (see p 333).

V. **Drug or laboratory interactions.**
   A. Phenobarbital has additive central nervous system and respiratory depression effects with other sedative drugs.
   B. Hepatic enzyme induction with chronic use, although this is *not* encountered with acute phenobarbital dosing.
   C. Extracorporeal removal techniques (eg, hemodialysis, hemoperfusion, and repeat-dose activated charcoal; see p 51) may enhance the clearance of phenobarbital, possibly requiring supplemental dosing to maintain therapeutic levels.

VI. **Dosage and method of administration.**
   A. **Parenteral.** Administer slowly intravenously (rate < 50 mg/min; children, < 1 mg/kg/min) until seizures are controlled or the loading dose of 10–15 mg/kg is achieved (children have required as much as 30 mg/kg in the first 24 hours to treat status epilepticus). Slow the infusion rate if hypotension develops. Intermittent infusions of 2 mg/kg every 5–15 minutes may diminish the risk of respiratory depression or hypotension.
      1. If intravenous access is not immediately available, phenobarbital may be given intramuscularly; the initial dose in adults and children is 3–5 mg/kg IM.
      2. It may also be given by the intraosseous route.
   B. **Oral.** For treatment of barbiturate or sedative drug withdrawal, give 60–120 mg orally and repeat every hour until signs of mild intoxication appear (eg, slurred speech, drowsiness, or nystagmus).

VII. **Formulations.**
   A. **Parenteral.** Phenobarbital sodium (Luminal and others), 30, 60, 65, and 130 mg/mL in tubex syringes, vials, and ampules.
   B. **Oral.** 8-, 15-, 30-, 60-, 65-, and 100-mg tablets; also elixir.
   C. The **suggested minimum stocking level** to treat a 70-kg adult for the first 24 hours is 16 ampules (130 mg each) or equivalent.

▶ **PHENTOLAMINE**

Thomas E. Kearney, PharmD

I. **Pharmacology.** Phentolamine is a competitive presynaptic and postsynaptic alpha-adrenergic receptor blocker that produces peripheral vasodilation. By acting on both venous and arterial vessels, it decreases total peripheral resistance and venous return. It may also stimulate beta-adrenergic receptors, causing cardiac stimulation. Phentolamine has a rapid onset of action (usually 2 minutes) and short duration of effect (approximately 15–20 minutes).

II. Indications.

A. Hypertensive crisis associated with phenylpropanolamine or stimulant drug overdose (eg, amphetamines, cocaine, or ephedrine).

B. Hypertensive crisis resulting from interaction between monoamine oxidase inhibitors and tyramine or other sympathomimetic amines.

C. Hypertensive crisis associated with sudden withdrawal of sympatholytic antihypertensive drugs (eg, clonidine).

D. Extravasation of vasoconstrictive agents (eg, epinephrine, norepinephrine, or dopamine).

III. Contraindications. Use with extreme caution in patients with intracranial hemorrhage or ischemic stroke; excessive lowering of blood pressure may aggravate brain injury.

IV. Adverse effects.

A. Hypotension and tachycardia may occur from excessive doses.

B. Anginal chest pain and cardiac arrhythmias may occur.

C. Slow intravenous infusion (< 0.3 mg/min) may result in transient increased blood pressure caused by stimulation of beta-adrenergic receptors.

D. Use in pregnancy. No assigned FDA category. However, this does not preclude its acute, short-term use for a seriously symptomatic patient (see p 333).

V. Drug or laboratory interactions. Additive or synergistic effects may occur with other antihypertensive agents, especially other alpha-adrenergic antagonists (eg, prazosin, terazosin, or yohimbine).

VI. Dosage and method of administration.

A. Parenteral. Give 1–5 mg IV (children, 0.02–0.1 mg/kg) as a bolus; repeat at 5- to 10-minute intervals as needed to lower blood pressure to a desired level (usually < 100 mm Hg diastolic in adults and 80 mm Hg diastolic in children, but may vary depending on the clinical situation).

B. Catecholamine extravasation. Infiltrate 5–10 mg in 10–15 mL of normal saline (children, 0.1–0.2 mg/kg; maximum 10 mg) into an affected area with a fine (25- to 27-gauge) hypodermic needle; improvement is evidenced by hyperemia and return to normal temperature.

VII. Formulations.

A. Parenteral. Phentolamine mesylate (Regitine), 5 mg in 1-mL vials.

B. The **suggested minimum stocking level** to treat a 70-kg adult for the first 24 hours is 20 vials.

▶ PHENYTOIN AND FOSPHENYTOIN

Kathryn H. Keller, PharmD

I. Pharmacology. The neuronal membrane-stabilizing actions of phenytoin make this a popular drug for sustained control of acute and chronic seizure disorders and a useful drug for certain cardiac arrhythmias. Because of the relatively slow onset of anticonvulsant action, phenytoin is usually administered after diazepam. At serum concentrations considered therapeutic for seizure control, phenytoin acts similarly to lidocaine to reduce ventricular premature depolarization and suppress ventricular tachycardia. After intravenous administration, peak therapeutic effects are attained within 1 hour. The therapeutic serum concentration for seizure control is 10–20 mg/L. Elimination is nonlinear, with an apparent half-life averaging 22 hours. **Fosphenytoin,** a newly available prodrug of phenytoin for intravenous use, is converted to phenytoin after injection, with a conversion half-life of 8–32 minutes.

II. Indications.

A. Control of generalized tonic-clonic seizures or status epilepticus. However, benzodiazepines (p 342) and phenobarbital (p 399) are generally more effective for treating drug-induced seizures.

B. Control of cardiac arrhythmias, particularly those associated with digitalis intoxication.

III. Contraindications. Known hypersensitivity to phenytoin or other hydantoins.

IV. Adverse effects.

A. Rapid intravenous phenytoin administration (> 50 mg/min in adults or 1 mg/kg/min in children) may produce hypotension, atrioventricular block, and cardiovascular collapse, probably owing to the propylene glycol diluent. Fosphenytoin is readily soluble and does not contain propylene glycol. It can be given intravenously or intramuscularly.

B. Extravasation of phenytoin may result in local tissue necrosis and sloughing.

C. Drowsiness, ataxia, nystagmus, and nausea may occur.

D. Use in pregnancy. No assigned FDA category. Congenital malformations (fetal hydantoin syndrome) and hemorrhagic disease of the newborn have occurred with chronic use. However, this does not preclude its acute, short-term use for a seriously symptomatic patient (see p 333).

V. Drug or laboratory interactions.

A. The various drug interactions associated with chronic phenytoin dosing (ie, accelerated metabolism of other drugs) are not applicable to its acute emergency use.

B. Extracorporeal removal methods (eg, hemoperfusion and repeat-dose activated charcoal) will enhance phenytoin clearance. Supplemental dosing may be required during such procedures to maintain therapeutic levels.

VI. Dosage and method of administration.

A. Parenteral.

1. Phenytoin. Administer a loading dose of 15–20 mg/kg IV slowly at a rate not to exceed 50 mg/min (or 1 mg/kg/min in children). It may be diluted in 50–150 mL of normal saline with use of an in-line filter. Phenytoin has been administered via the intraosseous route in children. Do *not* administer by the intramuscular route.

2. Fosphenytoin. Dosage is based on the phenytoin equivalent: 750 mg of fosphenytoin is equivalent to 500 mg of phenytoin. (For example, a loading dose of 1 g phenytoin would require a dose of 1.5 g fosphenytoin.) Dilute twofold to tenfold in 5% dextrose or normal saline and administer no faster than 225 mg/min.

B. Maintenance oral phenytoin dose. Give 5 mg/kg/d as a single oral dose of capsules or twice daily for other dosage forms and in children. Monitor serum phenytoin levels.

VII. Formulations.

A. Parenteral. Phenytoin sodium, 50 mg/mL, 2- and 5-mL ampules and vials. Fosphenytoin sodium (Cerebyx), 150 mg (equivalent to 100 mg phenytoin) in 2-mL vials or 750 mg (equivalent to 500 mg phenytoin) in 10-mL vials.

B. Oral. Phenytoin sodium (Dilantin and others), 30- and 100-mg capsules.

C. The **suggested minimum stocking level** to treat a 70-kg adult for the first 24 hours is six vials (50 mg/mL, 5 mL each) or equivalent.

▶ PHYSOSTIGMINE

Thomas E. Kearney, PharmD

I. Pharmacology. Physostigmine is a reversible inhibitor of acetylcholinesterase, the enzyme that degrades acetylcholine. Physostigmine increases concentrations of acetylcholine, causing stimulation of both muscarinic and nicotinic receptors. The tertiary amine structure of physostigmine allows it to penetrate the blood-brain barrier and exert central cholinergic effects as well. Owing to cholinergic stimulation of the brain stem's reticular activating system, physostigmine has nonspecific analeptic (arousal) effects. After parenteral administration, the onset of action is within 3–8 minutes and the duration of effect is usually 30–60 minutes. The elimination half-life is 15–40 minutes.

II. **Indications.**

A. Physostigmine is used for the management of severe anticholinergic syndrome (agitated delirium, urinary retention, severe sinus tachycardia, or hyperthermia with absent sweating). Its overall utility is limited, because most patients with anticholinergic poisoning (see p 78) can be managed supportively.

B. Physostigmine is sometimes used diagnostically to differentiate functional psychosis from anticholinergic delirium.

III. **Contraindications.**

A. Physostigmine should *not* be used as an antidote for cyclic antidepressant overdose because it may worsen cardiac conduction disturbances, cause bradyarrhythmias or asystole, and aggravate or precipitate seizures.

B. Do not use physostigmine with concurrent use of depolarizing neuromuscular blockers (eg, succinylcholine or decamethonium).

IV. **Adverse effects.**

A. Bradycardia, heart block, and asystole.

B. Seizures (particularly with rapid administration or excessive dose).

C. Nausea, vomiting, and diarrhea.

D. Bronchorrhea and bronchospasm.

E. Fasciculations and muscle weakness.

F. **Use in pregnancy.** No assigned FDA category (see p 333). Transient weakness has been noted in neonates whose mothers were treated with physostigmine for myasthenia gravis.

V. **Drug or laboratory interactions.**

A. Physostigmine may potentiate depolarizing neuromuscular-blocking agents (eg, succinylcholine and decamethonium) and cholinesterase inhibitors (eg, organophosphate and carbamate insecticides).

B. It may inhibit or reverse the actions of nondepolarizing neuromuscular-blocking agents (eg, pancuronium, vecuronium, etc).

C. It may have additive depressant effects on cardiac conduction in patients with cyclic antidepressant overdose.

D. Through its nonspecific analeptic effects, it may induce arousal in patients with benzodiazepine or sedative-hypnotic intoxication.

VI. **Dosage and method of administration.** Parenteral: 0.5–2 mg slow IV push (children, 0.02 mg/kg) while a cardiac monitor is used to monitor the patient; repeat as needed every 20–30 minutes. Atropine (see p 340) should be kept nearby to reverse excessive muscarinic stimulation. Do *not* administer intramuscularly or as a continuous intravenous infusion.

VII. **Formulations.**

A. **Parenteral.** Physostigmine salicylate (Antilirium), 1 mg/mL in 1-mL syringes and 2-mL vials.

B. The **suggested minimum stocking level** to treat a 70-kg adult for the first 24 hours is 10 ampules (2 mL each).

▶ PRALIDOXIME (2-PAM)

Brent R. Ekins, PharmD

I. **Pharmacology.** Pralidoxime (2-PAM) reverses cholinesterase inhibition by reactivating the phosphorylated cholinesterase enzyme and protecting the enzyme from further inhibition. While this effect is most pronounced with organophosphate pesticides, positive clinical results have been seen with carbamate insecticides that have nicotinic toxicity. The clinical effect of pralidoxime is most apparent at nicotinic receptors, with reversal of skeletal muscle weakness and muscle fasciculations. Its impact on muscarinic symptoms (salivation, sweating, brady-

cardia, and bronchorrhea) is less pronounced than that of the antimuscarinic
agent atropine (see p 340).

    A. 2-PAM is most effective when given before the enzyme has been irreversibly
bound ("aged") by the organophosphate (the rate of aging varies with each
organophosphate: for most compounds, it occurs within 24 hours, but for
some chemical-warfare agents, it may occur in several minutes). However,
late therapy with 2-PAM is appropriate, especially in patients poisoned by fat-
soluble compounds (eg, fenthion, demeton, or sulfoton) that can be released
from tissue stores over days, causing continuous or recurrent intoxication.

    B. Inadequate dosing of 2-PAM may be linked to the "intermediate syndrome,"
which is characterized by prolonged muscle weakness.

    C. Peak plasma concentrations are reached within 5–15 minutes after intra-
venous administration. Pralidoxime is eliminated by renal excretion and hepatic metabolism, with a half-life of 0.8–2.7 hours.

II. Indications.

    A. Pralidoxime is used to treat poisoning caused by organophosphate
cholinesterase inhibitor insecticides, mixtures of organophosphate and carbamate insecticides, or pure carbamate insecticide intoxication with nicotinic-
associated symptoms. Because of its low toxicity, its possible ineffectiveness
if treatment is delayed until after the cholinesterase enzyme has aged, its
ability to reverse nicotinic as well as muscarinic effects, and its ability to reduce atropine requirements, it should be used early and empirically for suspected cholinesterase inhibitor poisoning.

    B. With carbamate poisoning, cholinesterase inhibition spontaneously resolves
without "aging" of the enzyme. As a result, many references state that pralidoxime is not needed for carbamate poisoning. However, spontaneous reversal of enzyme inhibition may take up to 30 hours, and case reports suggest
that pralidoxime is effective in human carbamate poisoning. Data suggesting
increased toxicity of pralidoxime in carbaryl (Sevin) poisoning are based on
limited animal studies and the results are not generalizable to humans.

III. Contraindications.

    A. Use in patients with myasthenia gravis may precipitate a myasthenic crisis.

    B. Use with caution and in reduced doses in patients with renal impairment.

IV. Adverse effects.

    A. Nausea, headache, dizziness, drowsiness, diplopia, and hyperventilation
may occur.

    B. Rapid intravenous administration may result in tachycardia, laryngospasm,
muscle rigidity, and transient neuromuscular blockade.

    C. Use in pregnancy. FDA category C (indeterminate). This does not preclude
its acute, short-term use for a seriously symptomatic patient (see p 333).

V. Drug or laboratory interactions.

    A. Symptoms of atropinization may occur more quickly when atropine and prali-
doxime are administered concurrently.

    B. RBC cholinesterase (ChE) activity is more readily reactivated by pralidoxime
compared with plasma ChE.

VI. Dosage and method of administration. The intravenous route is preferred. Intramuscular or subcutaneous injection is possible when the intravenous route is
not immediately available.

    A. Initial dose. Give 1–2 g (children, 25–50 mg/kg up to 1 g) IV over 5–10 minutes
(rate not to exceed 200 mg/min in adults or 4 mg/kg/min in children), or give as
a continuous intravenous infusion in 100 mL of saline (1–2 mL/kg) over 15–30
minutes. Repeat the initial dose after 1 hour if muscle weakness or fasciculations are not relieved. Several grams may be required in some cases.

    B. Maintenance infusion. Because of the short half-life of 2-PAM and the
longer duration of many organophosphate compounds, toxicity frequently re-
curs, requiring repeated doses.

        1. Discrete intermittent boluses may result in wide fluctuation in serum levels
and erratic clinical effects. Therefore, after the initial dose it is preferable
to give 2-PAM as a continuous intravenous infusion in a 1% solution (1 g

in 100 mL saline) at a rate of 200–500 mg/h (children, 5–10 mg/kg/h) and titrate to the desired clinical response.
2. Despite earlier recommendations that 2-PAM should be given for only 24 hours, therapy may need to be continued for several days, particularly when long-acting, lipid-soluble organophosphates are involved. Gradually reduce the dose and carefully observe the patient for signs of recurrent muscle weakness or other signs of toxicity.
3. *Note:* 2-PAM may accumulate in patients with renal insufficiency.
VII. Formulations.
  A. Parenteral. Pralidoxime chloride (Protopam), 1 g with 20 mL sterile water.
  B. The **suggested minimum stocking level** to treat a 70-kg adult for the first 24 hours is 12 vials.
    Note: In agricultural areas or in urbanized regions preparing for possible accidental or terrorist release of a large amount of cholinesterase inhibitor agent, much larger stockpiling may be appropriate.

▶ PROPRANOLOL

Thomas E. Kearney, PharmD

I. Pharmacology. Propranolol is a nonselective beta-adrenergic blocker that acts on β_1-receptors in the myocardium and β_2-receptors in the lung, vascular smooth muscle, and kidney. Within the myocardium, propranolol depresses heart rate, conduction velocity, myocardial contractility, and automaticity. Although propranolol is effective orally, for toxicological emergencies it is usually administered by the intravenous route. After intravenous injection, the onset of action is nearly immediate and the duration of effect is 10 minutes to 2 hours, depending on the cumulative dose. The drug is eliminated by hepatic metabolism, with a half-life of about 2–3 hours.
II. Indications.
  A. To control excessive sinus tachycardia or ventricular arrhythmias caused by catecholamine excess (eg, theophylline or caffeine), sympathomimetic drug intoxication (eg, amphetamines, pseudoephedrine, or cocaine), or excessive myocardial sensitivity (eg, chloral hydrate, freons, or chlorinated and other hydrocarbons).
  B. To control hypertension in patients with excessive β_1-mediated increases in heart rate and contractility; use in conjunction with a vasodilator (eg, phentolamine) in patients with mixed alpha- and beta-adrenergic hyperstimulation.
  C. To raise the diastolic blood pressure in patients with hypotension caused by excessive β_2–mediated vasodilation (eg, theophylline or metaproterenol).
  D. May ameliorate or reduce beta-adrenergic–mediated electrolyte and other metabolic abnormalities (eg, hypokalemia, hyperglycemia, or lactic acidosis).
III. Contraindications.
  A. Use with extreme caution in patients with asthma, congestive heart failure, sinus node dysfunction, or other cardiac conduction disease and in those receiving calcium antagonists and other cardiac-depressant drugs.
  B. Do not use as single therapy for hypertension resulting from sympathomimetic overdose. Propranolol produces peripheral vascular beta-blockade, which may abolish β_2–mediated vasodilation and allow unopposed alpha-mediated vasoconstriction, resulting in paradoxic worsening of hypertension.
IV. Adverse effects.
  A. Bradycardia and sinus and atrioventricular block.
  B. Hypotension and congestive heart failure.
  C. Bronchospasm in patients with asthma or bronchospastic chronic obstructive pulmonary disease. *Note:* Propranolol (in small intravenous doses) has been used successfully in asthmatic patients overdosed on theophylline or β_2 agonists, without precipitating bronchospasm.

D. Use in pregnancy. FDA category C (indeterminate). Propranolol may cross the placenta, and neonates delivered within 3 days of administration of this drug may have persistent beta-adrenergic blockade. However, this does not preclude its acute, short-term use for a seriously symptomatic patient (see p 333).

V. Drug or laboratory interactions.

  A. Propranolol may allow unopposed alpha-adrenergic stimulation in patients with mixed adrenergic stimulation (eg, epinephrine surge in patients with acute hypoglycemia, pheochromocytoma, or cocaine or amphetamine intoxication), resulting in severe hypertension or end-organ ischemia.

  B. Propranolol has an additive hypotensive effect with other antihypertensive agents.

  C. This drug may potentiate competitive neuromuscular blockers (see p 386).

  D. The drug has additive depressant effects on cardiac conduction and contractility when given with calcium antagonists.

  E. Cimetidine reduces hepatic clearance of propranolol.

  F. Propranolol may worsen vasoconstriction caused by ergot alkaloids.

VI. Dosage and method of administration.

  A. Parenteral. Give 0.5–3 mg IV (children, 0.01–0.02 mg/kg IV; maximum 1 mg/dose) while monitoring heart rate and blood pressure; dose may be repeated as needed after 5–10 minutes. The dose required for complete β-receptor blockade is about 0.2 mg/kg.

  B. Oral. Oral dosing may be initiated after the patient is stabilized; the dosage range is about 1–5 mg/kg/d in 3–4 divided doses for both children and adults.

VII. Formulations.

  A. Parenteral. Propranolol hydrochloride (Inderal), 1 mg/mL in 1-mL ampules and prefilled syringes.

  B. Oral. Propranolol hydrochloride (Inderal and others), 60-, 80-, 120-, and 160-mg capsules; 10-, 20-, 40-, 60-, 80-, and 90-mg tablets.

  C. The **suggested minimum stocking level** to treat a 70-kg adult for the first 24 hours is 10 ampules or syringes.

▶ PROTAMINE

Thomas E. Kearney, PharmD

I. Pharmacology. Protamine is a cationic protein that rapidly binds to and inactivates heparin. The onset of action after intravenous administration is nearly immediate (30–60 s).

II. Indications.

  A. Protamine is used for the reversal of the anticoagulant effect of heparin when an excessively large dose has been inadvertently administered. Protamine is generally not needed for treatment of bleeding during standard heparin therapy because discontinuance of the heparin infusion is generally sufficient.

  B. Protamine may be used for reversal of regional anticoagulation in the hemodialysis circuit in cases in which anticoagulation of the patient would be contraindicated (ie, active gastrointestinal or central nervous system bleeding).

III. Contraindications.

  A. Do not give protamine to patients with known sensitivity to the drug. Diabetic patients who have used protamine insulin may be at the greatest risk for hypersensitivity reactions.

  B. Protamine reconstituted with benzyl alcohol should not be used in neonates because of suspected toxicity from the alcohol.

IV. Adverse effects.

  A. Rapid intravenous administration is associated with hypotension, bradycardia, and anaphylactoid reactions. Have epinephrine (see p 365), diphenhydramine (see p 359), and cimetidine or another H_2 blocker (see p 353) ready.

     B. A rebound effect caused by heparin may occur within 8 hours of protamine administration.

     C. Use in pregnancy. FDA category C (indeterminate). Maternal hypersensitivity reaction or hypotension could result in placental ischemia. However, this does not preclude its acute, short-term use for a seriously symptomatic patient (see p 333).

V. Drug or laboratory interactions. No known drug interactions, other than the reversal of the effect of heparin.

VI. Dosage and method of administration.

     A. Administer protamine by slow intravenous injection, over at least 1–3 minutes, not to exceed 50 mg in a 10-minute period.

     B. The dose of protamine depends on the total dose and time since administration of heparin.

          1. Immediately after heparin administration, give 1–1.5 mg of protamine for each 100 units of heparin.

          2. At 30–60 minutes after heparin administration, give only 0.5–0.75 mg of protamine for each 100 units of heparin.

          3. Two hours or more after heparin administration, give only 0.25–0.375 mg of protamine for each 100 units of heparin.

          4. If heparin was administered by constant infusion, give 25–50 mg of protamine.

VII. Formulations.

     A. Parenteral. Protamine sulfate, 50 mg in 5-mL ampules and vials or 250 mg in 25-mL ampules and vials.

     B. The **suggested minimum stocking level** to treat a 70-kg adult for the first 24 hours is four ampules or one vial.

▶ PYRIDOXINE (VITAMIN B$_6$)

Thomas E. Kearney, PharmD

I. Pharmacology. Pyridoxine (vitamin B$_6$) is a water-soluble B-complex vitamin that acts as a cofactor in many enzymatic reactions. Overdose involving isoniazid or other monomethylhydrazines (eg, gyromitrin mushrooms) may cause seizures by interfering with pyridoxine utilization in the brain, and pyridoxine given in high doses can rapidly control these seizures. It can also correct the lactic acidosis secondary to isoniazid-induced impaired lactate metabolism. In ethylene glycol intoxication, pyridoxine theoretically may enhance metabolic conversion of the toxic metabolite glyoxylic acid to the nontoxic product, glycine. Pyridoxine is well absorbed orally but is usually given intravenously for urgent uses. The biologic half-life is about 15–20 days.

II. Indications.

     A. Acute management of seizures caused by intoxication with isoniazid (see p 195), *Gyromitra* mushrooms (see p 227), or possibly cycloserine. Pyridoxine may act synergistically with diazepam (see p 342).

     B. Adjunct to therapy for ethylene glycol intoxication.

III. Contraindications. No known contraindications.

IV. Adverse effects.

     A. Usually no adverse effects are noted from acute dosing of pyridoxine.

     B. Chronic excessive doses may result in peripheral neuropathy.

     C. Use in pregnancy. FDA category A (see p 333). However, chronic excessive use in pregnancy has resulted in pyridoxine withdrawal seizures in neonates.

V. Drug or laboratory interactions. No adverse interactions are associated with acute dosing.

VI. Dosage and method of administration.

     A. Isoniazid poisoning. Give 1 g of pyridoxine intravenously for each gram of isoniazid known to have been ingested (as much as 52 g have been administered and tolerated). Dilute in 50 mL dextrose or saline and give over 5 minutes. If the ingested amount is unknown, administer 4–5 g IV empirically and repeat as needed.

B. Monomethylhydrazine poisoning. Give 25 mg/kg IV; repeat as necessary.

C. Ethylene glycol poisoning. Give 50 mg IV or IM every 6 hours until intoxication is resolved.

D. Cycloserine poisoning. A dosage of 300 mg/d has been recommended.

VII. Formulations.

A. Parenteral. Pyridoxine hydrochloride (Beesix, others), 100 mg/mL (10% solution) in 10- and 30-mL vials.

B. The **suggested minimum stocking level** to treat a 70-kg adult for the first 24 hours is 20 g (20 vials, 10 mL each, or equivalent).

▶ THIAMINE (VITAMIN B₁)

Thomas E. Kearney, PharmD

I. Pharmacology. Thiamine (vitamin B_1) is a water-soluble vitamin that acts as an essential cofactor for various pathways of carbohydrate metabolism. Thiamine also acts as a cofactor in the metabolism of glyoxylic acid (produced in ethylene glycol intoxication). Thiamine deficiency may result in beriberi and Wernicke-Korsakoff syndrome. Thiamine is rapidly absorbed after oral, intramuscular, or intravenous administration.

II. Indications.

A. Empiric therapy to prevent and treat Wernicke-Korsakoff syndrome in alcoholic or malnourished patients. Thiamine should be given concurrently with glucose in such patients.

B. Adjunctive treatment in patients poisoned with ethylene glycol to possibly enhance the detoxification of glyoxylic acid.

III. Contraindications. Use caution in patients with known sensitivity to thiamine.

IV. Adverse effects.

A. Anaphylactoid reactions, vasodilation, hypotension, weakness, and angioedema after rapid intravenous injection.

B. Acute pulmonary edema in patients with beriberi, owing to sudden increase in vascular resistance.

C. Use in pregnancy. FDA category A (see p 333).

V. Drug or laboratory interactions. Theoretically, thiamine may enhance the effect of neuromuscular blockers, although the clinical significance is unclear.

VI. Dosage and method of administration. Parenteral, 100 mg (children, 50 mg) slow IV (over 5 minutes) or IM; repeat every 6 hours. Doses as high as 1 g over the first 12 hours have been given to patients with acute Wernicke-Korsakoff syndrome.

VII. Formulations.

A. Parenteral. Thiamine hydrochloride, 100 mg/mL, in 1-, 2-, 10-, and 30-mL ampules, vials, and prefilled syringes.

B. The **suggested minimum stocking level** to treat a 70-kg adult for the first 24 hours is 1 g (one 10-mL vial or equivalent).

▶ THIOSULFATE, SODIUM

Susan Kim, PharmD

I. Pharmacology. Sodium thiosulfate is a sulfur donor that promotes the conversion of cyanide to less toxic thiocyanate by the sulfur transferase enzyme rhodanese. Unlike nitrites, thiosulfate is essentially nontoxic and may be given empirically in suspected cyanide poisoning.

II. Indications.

A. May be given alone or in combination with nitrites (see p 390) in patients with acute cyanide poisoning.

B. Empiric treatment of possible cyanide poisoning associated with smoke inhalation.

C. Prophylaxis during nitroprusside infusions (see p 392).

D. Extravasation of mechlorethamine (infiltrate locally; see p 88).

E. Bromate salt ingestion (unproved).

III. Contraindications. No known contraindications.

IV. Adverse effects.

A. Intravenous infusion may produce burning sensation, muscle cramping and twitching, and nausea and vomiting.

B. Use in pregnancy. FDA category C (indeterminate). This does not preclude its acute, short-term use for a seriously symptomatic patient (see p 333).

V. Drug or laboratory interactions. Thiosulfate will falsely lower measured cyanide concentrations in several methods.

VI. Dosage and method of administration.

A. For cyanide poisoning. Administer 12.5 g (50 mL of 25% solution) IV at 2.5–5 mL/min. The pediatric dose is 400 mg/kg (1.6 mL/kg of 25% solution) up to 50 mL. Half the initial dose may be given after 30–60 minutes if needed.

B. For prophylaxis during nitroprusside infusions. Addition of 10 mg thiosulfate for each mg of nitroprusside in the intravenous solution has been reported to be effective, although physical compatibility data are not available.

VII. Formulations.

A. Parenteral. As a component of the Cyanide Antidote Package, thiosulfate sodium, 25% solution, 50 mL. Also available separately in vials and ampules containing 2.5 g/10 mL or 1 g/10 mL.

B. The **suggested minimum stocking level** to treat a 70-kg adult for the first 24 hours is two Cyanide Antidote Packages (one should be kept in the Emergency Department).

▶ VITAMIN K₁ (PHYTONADIONE)

Thomas E. Kearney, PharmD

I. Pharmacology. Vitamin K_1 is an essential cofactor in the hepatic synthesis of coagulation factors II, VII, IX, and X. In adequate doses, vitamin K_1 reverses the inhibitory effects of coumarin and indanedione derivatives on the synthesis of these factors. *Note:* Vitamin K_3**(menadione) is *not* effective** in reversing excessive anticoagulation caused by these agents. After parenteral vitamin K_1 administration, there is a 6- to 8-hour delay before vitamin K-dependent coagulation factors begin to achieve significant levels, and peak effects are not seen until 1–2 days after initiation of therapy. The duration of effect is 5–10 days. The response to vitamin K_1 is variable; it is influenced by the potency of the ingested anticoagulant and the patient's hepatic biosynthetic capability. Fresh frozen plasma or whole blood is indicated for immediate control of serious hemorrhage.

II. Indications.

A. Excessive anticoagulation caused by coumarin and indanedione derivatives, as evidenced by elevated prothrombin time. Vitamin K_1 is *not* indicated for empiric treatment of anticoagulant ingestion, as most cases do not require treatment.

B. Vitamin K deficiency (eg, malnutrition, malabsorption, or hemorrhagic disease of the newborn) with coagulopathy.

C. Hypoprothrombinemia resulting from salicylate intoxication.

III. Contraindications. Do not use in patients with known hypersensitivity.

IV. Adverse effects.

A. Anaphylactoid reactions have been reported after intravenous administration. Intravenous use should be restricted to true emergencies; the patient must be closely monitored in an intensive care setting.

B. Intramuscular administration in anticoagulated patients may cause large, painful hematomas. This can be avoided by using oral or subcutaneous routes.

C. Patients receiving anticoagulants for medical reasons (eg, deep vein thrombosis or prosthetic heart valves) may experience untoward effects from complete reversal of their anticoagulation status. Preferably, such patients should receive small quantities of fresh-frozen plasma or extremely small titrated doses (0.5–1 mg) until the prothrombin time is in the desired therapeutic range (eg, 1.5–2 times normal). Anticoagulation with heparin may be indicated until the desired prothrombin time is achieved.

D. Use in pregnancy. FDA category C (indeterminate). K_1 crosses the placenta readily. However, this does not preclude its acute, short-term use for a seriously symptomatic patient (see p 333).

V. Drug or laboratory interactions. Empiric use after an acute anticoagulant overdose will delay (for up to several days) the onset of elevation of prothrombin time, which may give a false impression of insignificant ingestion in a case of serious "superwarfarin" overdose (see p 148).

VI. Dosage and method of administration.

A. Oral administration may be considered for maintenance therapy after initial parenteral treatment of symptomatic "superwarfarin" poisonings. The usual oral dose of vitamin K_1 (*not* menadione or vitamin K_3) is 10–25 mg/d in adults and 5–10 mg/d in children. Recheck the prothrombin time after 48 hours, and increase the dose as needed. Daily doses of 50–200 mg have been required in some cases. Therapy may be required for several weeks or even months.

B. Subcutaneous administration is the preferred route. The adult dose is 5–10 mg, and that for children is 1–5 mg; this may be repeated in 6–8 hours. Switch to oral therapy as soon as possible.

C. Intravenous administration is rarely used, and only when hemorrhage is present or imminent (in such cases, consider fresh-frozen plasma for rapid replacement of coagulation factors). The usual dose is 10–50 mg (0.6 mg/kg in children under 12 years), depending on the severity of anticoagulation, diluted in preservative-free dextrose or sodium chloride solution. Give slowly at a rate not to exceed 1 mg/min or 5% of the total dose per minute, whichever is slower.

VII. Formulations.

A. Parenteral. Phytonadione (AquaMEPHYTON and others) 2 and 10 mg/mL, in 0.5-, 1-, 2.5-, and 5-mL ampules, vials, and prefilled syringes.

B. Oral. Phytonadione (Mephyton), 5-mg tablets.

C. The **suggested minimum stocking level** to treat a 70-kg adult for the first 24 hours is 100 mg (two 5-mL ampules, 10 mg/mL each, or equivalent).

REFERENCES

Hardman JG et al (editors): *Goodman & Gilman's The Pharmacological Basis of Therapeutics*, 9th ed. McGraw-Hill, 1996.

Kastrup EK et al (editors): *Drug Facts & Comparisons*. Facts and Comparisons, 1998.

Reynolds JEF (editor): *Martindale: The Extra Pharmacopoeia*, 31st ed. Royal Pharmaceutical Society of Great Britain, 1996.

McEvoy GK (editor): *American Hospital Formulary Service Drug Information 98*. American Society of Health-System Pharmacists, 1998.

SECTION IV. ENVIRONMENTAL AND OCCUPATIONAL TOXICOLOGY

▶ EMERGENCY MEDICAL RESPONSE TO HAZARDOUS MATERIALS INCIDENTS

Kent R. Olson, MD, and R. Steven Tharratt, MD

With the constant threat of accidental releases of hazardous materials and the potential use of chemical weapons by terrorists, local emergency response providers must be prepared to handle victims who may be contaminated with chemical substances. Many local jurisdictions have developed hazardous-materials (HazMat) teams, usually composed of fire and paramedical personnel who are trained to identify hazardous situations quickly and to take the lead in organizing a response. Health care providers, such as ambulance personnel, nurses, physicians, and local hospital officials, should participate in emergency response planning and drills with their local HazMat team before a chemical disaster occurs.

I. **General considerations.** The most important elements of successful medical management of a hazardous-materials incident are as follows:
   A. Use extreme caution when dealing with unknown or unstable conditions.
   B. Rapidly assess the potential hazard severity of the substances involved.
   C. Determine the potential for secondary contamination of downstream personnel and facilities.
   D. Perform any needed decontamination at the scene *before* victim transport, if possible.

II. **Organization.** Chemical accidents are managed under the **Incident Command System.** The Incident Commander or Scene Manager is usually the senior representative of the agency having primary traffic investigative authority, but authority may be delegated to a senior fire or health official. The first priorities of the Incident Commander are to secure the area, establish a command post, create hazard zones, and provide for the decontamination and immediate prehospital care of any victims. However, hospitals must be prepared to manage victims who leave the scene before teams arrive and who may arrive at the emergency department unannounced, possibly contaminated, and needing medical attention.
   A. **Hazard Zones** (Figure IV–1) are determined by the nature of the spilled substance and wind and geographic conditions. In general, the command post and support area are located upwind and uphill from the spill, with sufficient distance to allow rapid escape if conditions change.
      1. The **Exclusion Zone** (also known as the "hot" or "red" zone) is the area immediately adjacent to the chemical incident. This area may be extremely hazardous to persons without appropriate protective equipment. Only properly trained and equipped personnel should enter this zone, and they may require vigorous decontamination when leaving the area.
      2. The **Contamination Reduction Zone** (also known as the "warm" or "yellow" zone) is where victims and rescuers are decontaminated before undergoing further medical assessment and prehospital care. Patients in the Exclusion and Contamination Reduction Zones will generally receive only rudimentary first aid such as cervical spine stabilization and placement on a backboard.
      3. The **Support Zone** (also known as the "cold" or "green" zone) is where the Incident Commander, support teams, press, medical treatment areas, and ambulances are located. It is usually upwind, uphill, and a safe distance from the incident.

B. Medical officer. A member of the HazMat team should already have been designated to be in charge of health and safety. This person is responsible for determining the nature of the chemicals; the likely severity of their health effects; the need for specialized personal protective gear; the type and degree of decontamination required; and the need for triage and prehospital care. In addition, the medical officer supervises the safety of response workers at the emergency site and monitors entry to and exit from the spill site.

III. Assessment of hazard potential. Be prepared to recognize dangerous situations and to respond appropriately. The potential for toxic or other types of injury depends on the chemicals involved, their toxicity, their chemical and physical properties, the conditions of exposure, and the circumstances surrounding their release. Be aware that a substance's reactivity, flammability, explosiveness, or corrosiveness may be a source of greater hazard than its systemic toxicity. Do not depend on your senses for safety, even though sensory input (eg, smell) may give clues about the nature of the hazard.

   A. Identify the substances involved. Make inquiries and look for labels, warning placards, or shipping papers.

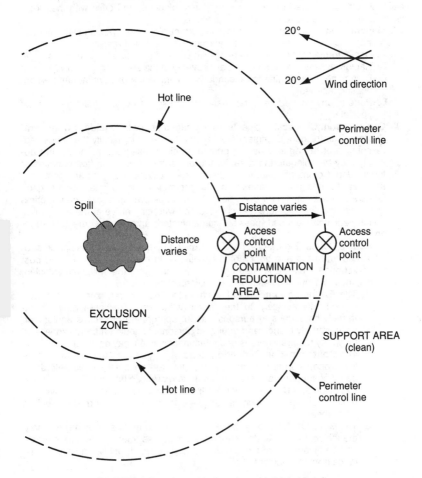

FIGURE IV–1. Control zones at a hazardous materials incident site.

NATIONAL FIRE PROTECTION ASSOCIATION
IDENTIFICATION OF THE FIRE HAZARDS OF MATERIALS

NFPA 704
Hazard Signal System

Flammability (Red)

4 – Highly flammable and volatile
3 – Highly flammable
2 – Flammable
1 – Low flammability
0 – Does not burn

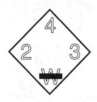

Health hazard (Blue)

4 – Extremely hazardous
3 – Moderately hazardous
2 – Hazardous
1 – Slightly hazardous
0 – No health hazard

Reactivity (Yellow)

4 – Highly explosive, detonates easily
3 – Explosive, less readily detonated
2 – Violently reactive but does not
    detonate
1 – Not violently reactive
0 – Normally stable

Other hazards

⚛ – Radioactive

OX – Oxidizer

🌊 – Water-reactive

FIGURE IV–2. National Fire Protection Association (NFPA) identification of the hazards of materials. (Modified and reproduced, with permission, from *Fire Protection Guide on Hazardous Materials,* 9th ed. National Fire Protection Association, 1986.) (*continued on p 414*)

1. The **National Fire Protection Association (NFPA)** has developed a labeling system for describing chemical hazards which is widely used (Figure IV–2).
2. The **US Department of Transportation (DOT)** has developed a system of warning placards for vehicles carrying hazardous materials. The DOT placards usually bear a 4-digit substance identification code and also a single-digit hazard classification code (Figure IV–3). Identification of the substance from the 4-digit code can be provided by the regional poison control center, CHEMTREC, or the DOT manual (see **B,** below).
3. **Shipping papers,** which may include Material Safety Data Sheets (MSDSs), are usually carried by a driver or pilot or may be found in the truck cab or pilot's compartment.

B. **Obtain toxicity information.** Determine the acute health effects and obtain advice on general hazards, decontamination procedures, and medical management of victims. Resources include the following:

1. **Regional poison control centers** (see Table I–42, p 55). The regional poison control center can provide information on immediate health effects, the need for decontamination or specialized protective gear, and specific treatment including the use of antidotes. The regional center can also provide consultation with a medical toxicologist.
2. **CHEMTREC** ([800] 424-9300). Operated by the Chemical Manufacturers' Association, this 24-hour hotline can provide information on the identity and hazardous properties of chemicals and, when appropriate, can put the caller in touch with industry representatives and medical toxicologists.

Signal	Identification of Health Hazard — Color Code: BLUE — Type of Possible Injury	Signal	Identification of Flammability — Color Code: RED — Susceptibility of Materials to Burning	Signal	Identification of Reactivity (Stability) — Color Code: YELLOW — Susceptibility to Release of Energy
4	Materials which on very short exposure could cause death or major residual injury even though prompt medical treatment were given.	4	Materials which will rapidly or completely vaporize at atmospheric pressure and normal ambient temperature, or which are readily dispersed in air and which will burn readily.	4	Materials which in themselves are readily capable of detonation or of explosive decomposition or reaction at normal temperatures and pressures.
3	Materials which on short exposure could cause serious temporary or residual injury even though prompt medical treatment were given.	3	Liquids and solids that can be ignited under almost all ambient temperature conditions.	3	Materials which in themselves are capable of detonation or explosive reaction but require a strong initiating source or which must be heated under confinement before initiation or which react explosively with water.
2	Materials which on intense or continued exposure could cause temporary incapacitation or possible residual injury unless prompt medical treatment is given.	2	Materials must be moderately heated or exposed to relatively high ambient temperatures before ignition can occur.	2	Materials that readily undergo violent chemical change at elevated temperatures and pressures; includes materials that react violently with water.
1	Materials which on exposure would cause irritation but only minor residual injury even if no treatment is given.	1	Materials that must be preheated before ignition can occur.	1	Materials which in themselves are normally stable, but which can become unstable at elevated temperatures and pressures.
0	Materials which on exposure under fire conditions would offer no hazard beyond that of ordinary combustible material.	0	Materials that will not burn.	0	Materials which in themselves are normally stable, even under fire exposure conditions, and which are not reactive with water.

FIGURE IV–2. (Continued). National Fire Protection Association (NFPA) identification of the hazards of materials.

EXAMPLE OF PLACARD AND PANEL WITH ID NUMBER

The Identification Number (ID No.) may be displayed on placards or on orange panels on tanks. Check the sides of the transport vehicle if the ID number is not displayed on the ends of the vehicle.

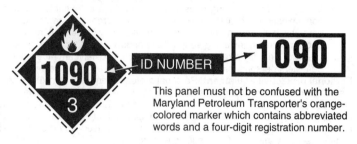

This panel must not be confused with the Maryland Petroleum Transporter's orange-colored marker which contains abbreviated words and a four-digit registration number.

FIGURE IV–3. Example of US Department of Transportation (DOT) vehicle warning placard and panel with DOT identification number.

3. **Table IV–4** (p 434) and specific chemicals covered in Section II of this manual.

4. A variety of texts, journals, and computerized information systems are available but are of uneven scope or depth. See the reference list at the end of this section (p 418).

C. **Recognize dangerous environments.** In general, environments likely to expose the rescuer to the same conditions that caused grave injury to the victim are not safe for unprotected entry. **These situations require trained and properly equipped rescue personnel.** Examples include the following:

1. Any indoor environment where the victim was rendered unconscious or otherwise disabled.

2. Environments causing acute onset of symptoms in rescuers, such as chest tightness, shortness of breath, eye or throat irritation, coughing, dizziness, headache, nausea, or loss of coordination.

3. Confined spaces such as large tanks or crawlspaces. (Their poor ventilation and small size can result in extremely high levels of airborne contaminants. In addition, such spaces permit only a slow or strenuous exit, which may become physically impossible for an intoxicated individual.)

4. Spills involving substances with poor warning properties or high vapor pressures (see p 431), especially when they occur in an indoor or enclosed environment. Substances with poor warning properties can cause serious injury without any warning signs of exposure such as smell or eye irritation. High vapor pressures increase the likelihood that dangerous air concentrations may be present. Also note that gases or vapors with a density greater than air may become concentrated in low-lying areas.

D. **Determine the potential for secondary contamination.** Although the threat of secondary contamination of emergency response personnel, equipment, and downstream facilities *may* be significant, it varies widely depending on the chemical, its concentration, and whether basic decontamination has already been performed. Not all toxic substances carry a risk of downstream contamination even though they may be extremely hazardous to rescuers in the hot zone. Exposures involving inhalation only and no external contamination do not pose a risk of secondary contamination.

1. Examples of substances with **no significant risk** for secondary contamination of personnel outside the hot zone are **gases,** such as carbon

monoxide, arsine, and chlorine, and **vapors,** such as those from xylene, toluene, or perchloroethylene.

2. Examples of substances with **significant potential** for secondary contamination and requiring aggressive decontamination and protection of downstream personnel include potent organophosphate insecticides, oily nitro compounds, and highly radioactive compounds such as plutonium.

3. In many cases involving substances with a high potential for secondary contamination, this risk can be minimized by removal of grossly contaminated clothing and thoroughly cleansing the body in the contamination reduction corridor, including soap or shampoo wash. After these measures are followed, only rarely will the downstream medical team face significant persistent personal threat to their health from an exposed victim.

IV. **Personal protective equipment.** Personal protective equipment includes chemical-resistant clothing and gloves and protective respiratory gear. The use of such equipment should be supervised by experts in industrial hygiene or others with appropriate training and experience. Equipment that is incorrectly selected, improperly fitted, poorly maintained, or inappropriately used may provide a false sense of security and may fail, resulting in serious injury.

A. **Protective clothing** may be as simple as a disposable apron or as sophisticated as a fully encapsulated chemical-resistant suit. However, no chemical-resistant clothing is completely impervious to all chemicals over the full range of exposure conditions. Each suit is rated for its resistance to specific chemicals, and many are also rated for chemical breakthrough time.

B. **Protective respiratory gear** may be a simple paper mask, a cartridge filter respirator, or a positive-pressure air-supplied respirator. Respirators must be properly fitted for each user.

1. **A paper mask** provides partial protection against gross quantities of airborne dust particles but does not prevent exposure to gases, vapors, or fumes.

2. **Cartridge filter respirators** filter certain chemical gases and vapors out of the ambient air. They are used only when the toxic substance is known to be adsorbed by the filter, the airborne concentration is low, and there is adequate oxygen in the ambient air.

3. **Air-supplied respirators** provide an independent source of clean air. They may be fully self-contained units or masks supplied with air by a long hose. **Self-contained breathing apparatus** (SCBA) has a limited duration of air supply, from 5 to 30 minutes. Users must be fitted for their specific gear.

V. **Victim management.** Victim management includes rapid stabilization and removal from the Exclusion Zone, initial decontamination, delivery to emergency medical services personnel at the Support Zone perimeter, and medical assessment and treatment in the support area. Usually only the HazMat team or other fire department personnel with appropriate training and protective gear will be responsible for rescue from the hot zone, where skin and respiratory protection may be critical. Emergency medical personnel without specific training and appropriate equipment must not enter the hot zone unless it is determined to be safe by the Incident Commander and the medical officer.

A. **Stabilization in the Exclusion Zone.** If there is suspicion of trauma, the patient should be placed on a backboard and a cervical collar applied if appropriate. Position the patient so that the airway remains open. Gross contamination may be brushed off the patient. No further medical intervention can be expected from rescuers who are wearing bulky suits, masks, and heavy gloves. Therefore, every effort should be made to get the seriously ill patient out of this area as quickly as possible. Victims who are ambulatory should be directed to walk to the contamination reduction area.

B. **Initial decontamination.** Gross decontamination may take place in the Exclusion Zone (eg, brushing off chemical powder and removing soaked clothing), but most decontamination occurs in the contamination reduction corridor before the victim is transferred to waiting emergency medical personnel in the support area. Do not delay critical treatment while decontaminating the victim unless the nature of the contaminant makes such treatment too dangerous. Consult a regional poison control center (see Table I–42, p 55) for specific advice on decontamination. See also Section I, p 43.

1. Pull or cut off contaminated clothing and flush exposed skin, hair, or eyes with copious plain water from a high-volume, low-pressure fire hose. For oily substances, additional washing with soap or shampoo may be required. Ambulatory, cooperative victims may be able to perform their own decontamination.
2. For eye exposures, remove contact lenses if present, and irrigate eyes with plain water or, if available, normal saline dribbled from an intravenous bag. Continue irrigation until symptoms resolve or, if the contaminant is an acid or base, until the pH of the conjunctival sac is nearly normal (pH 6–8).
3. Double bag and save all removed clothing and jewelry.
4. Collect run-off water if possible, but generally rapid flushing of exposed skin or eyes should not be delayed because of environmental concerns. Remember that protection of health takes precedence over environmental concerns at a hazardous-materials incident.
5. For ingestions, if the material ingested is a suspected corrosive substance or the patient is experiencing painful swallowing or has oral burns, give the patient a glass of water to drink. If available, administer activated charcoal (see p 351); even though this may obscure the view during later endoscopy, it can prevent absorption of systemic toxins.
6. In the majority of incidents, basic victim decontamination as outlined above will substantially reduce or eliminate the potential for secondary contamination of downstream personnel or equipment. Procedures for cleaning equipment are contaminant specific and depend on the risk of chemical persistence as well as toxicity.

C. **Treatment in the support area.** Once the patient is decontaminated (if required) and released into the support area, triage, basic medical assessment, and treatment by emergency medical providers may begin. In the majority of incidents, once the victim has been removed from the hot zone and is stripped and flushed, there is little or no risk of secondary contamination of these providers, and sophisticated protective gear is not necessary. Simple surgical latex gloves and a plain apron or disposable outer clothing is generally sufficient.

1. Maintain a patent airway and assist breathing if necessary (see pp 1–7). Administer supplemental oxygen.
2. Provide supportive care for shock (p 15), arrhythmias (pp 10–14), coma (p 18), or seizures (p 21).
3. Treat with specific antidotes if appropriate and available.
4. Further skin, hair, or eye washing may be necessary. If the victim ingested a toxic substance, consider oral administration of activated charcoal (p 351).
5. Take notes on the probable or suspected level of exposure for each victim, the initial symptoms and signs, and treatment provided. For chemicals with delayed toxic effects, this could be lifesaving.

VI. **Ambulance transport and hospital treatment.** For skin or inhalation exposures, no special precautions should be required if adequate decontamination has been carried out in the field prior to transport.

A. **Patients who have ingested toxic substances** may vomit en route; carry a large plastic bag-lined basin and extra towels to soak up and immediately isolate spillage. Vomitus may contain the original toxic material or even toxic gases created by action of stomach acid on the substance (eg, hydrogen cyanide from ingested cyanide salts). When performing gastric lavage in the emergency department, isolate gastric washings (eg, with a closed wall suction container system).

B. For those unpredictable situations in which **a contaminated victim arrives at the hospital before decontamination,** it is important to have a strategy ready that will minimize exposure of hospital personnel:

1. Ask the local HazMat team to set up a contamination reduction area outside the hospital emergency department entrance. However, keep in mind that all teams may already be committed and not available to assist.
2. Prepare in advance a hose with 85 °F water, soap, and an old gurney for rapid decontamination *outside* the emergency department entrance. Have a child's inflatable pool or another container ready to collect water runoff, if possible. However, do not delay patient decontamination if water runoff cannot be contained easily.
3. Do not bring patients soaked with liquids into the emergency department until they have been stripped and flushed outside, as the liquids may emit gas vapors and cause illness among hospital staff.
4. For incidents involving radioactive materials or other highly contaminating substances that are not volatile, utilize the hospital's radiation accident protocol, which will generally include the following:
   a. Restricted access zones.
   b. Isolation of ventilation ducts leading out of the treatment room to prevent spreading of the contamination throughout the hospital.
   c. Paper covering for floors, and use of absorbent materials if liquids are involved.
   d. Protective clothing for hospital staff (gloves, paper masks, shoe covers, caps, and gowns).
   e. Double bagging and saving all contaminated clothing and equipment.
   f. Monitoring to detect the extent and persistence of contamination (ie, using a Geiger counter for radiation incidents).
   g. Notifying appropriate local, state, and federal offices of the incident and obtaining advice on laboratory testing and decontamination of equipment.

VII. **Summary.** The emergency medical response to a hazardous-materials incident requires prior training and planning to protect the health of response personnel and victims.

A. Response plans and training should be flexible. The level of hazard and the required actions vary greatly with the circumstances at the scene and the chemicals involved.

B. First responders should be able to do the following:

1. Recognize potentially hazardous situations.
2. Take steps to protect themselves from injury.
3. Obtain accurate information about the identity and toxicity of each chemical substance involved.
4. Use appropriate protective gear.
5. Perform victim decontamination before transport to a hospital.
6. Provide appropriate first aid and advanced supportive measures as needed.
7. Coordinate their actions with other responding agencies such as the HazMat team, police and fire departments, and regional poison control centers.

REFERENCES

Agency for Toxic Substances and Disease Registry: *Medical Management Guidelines for Acute Chemical Exposures.* US Department of Health & Human Services, 1992.

Borak J, Callan M, Abbott W: *Hazardous Materials Exposure: Emergency Response and Patient Care.* Brady, 1991.

Bronstein AC, Currance PL: *Emergency Care for Hazardous Materials Exposure.* Mosby, 1988.

California Emergency Medical Services Authority: *Hazardous Materials Medical Management Protocols,* 2nd ed. California State Emergency Medical Services Authority, 1989.

Emergency Response Guidebook. US Department of Transportation, 1992.

Fire Protection Guide on Hazardous Materials, 9th ed. National Fire Protection Association, 1986.

NIOSH: *NIOSH Pocket Guide to Chemical Hazards.* US Department of Health and Human Services, 1990.

OSHA: Hazardous waste operations and emergency response: Interim final rule. 29 CFR Part 1910. *Fed Reg* 1986;**51**:45654.

Stutz DR, Ulin S: *Hazardous Materials Injuries: A Handbook for Prehospital Care,* 3rd ed. Bradford Communications, 1992.

Sullivan JB, Krieger GR: *Hazardous Materials Toxicology: Clinical Principles of Environmental Health.* Williams & Wilkins, 1992.

▶ EVALUATION OF THE PATIENT WITH OCCUPATIONAL CHEMICAL EXPOSURE

Paul D. Blanc, MD MSPH

This chapter highlights common toxicological problems in the workplace. Occupationally related disease is commonly seen in the outpatient setting. Estimates of the proportion of occupationally related medical problems in primary care practices range up to 15–20%, although this includes many patients with musculoskeletal complaints. However, approximately 5% of all symptomatic poison control center consultations are occupational in nature, suggesting a large number of chemical exposures. The largest single referring group for these calls is emergency medicine specialists.

I. **General considerations.**

A. **Occupational illness is rarely pathognomonic.** The connection between illness and workplace factors is typically obscure unless a specific effort is made to link exposure to disease.

1. Massive or catastrophic events leading to acute onset of symptoms, such as an irritant gas release, are relatively uncommon.

2. For most workplace exposures, symptom onset is more often insidious, following a subacute or chronic pattern, as in heavy metal poisoning.

3. Long latency, often years, between exposure and disease makes linking cause and effect even more difficult, for example in chronic lung disease or in occupationally related cancer.

B. **Occupational evaluation frequently includes legal and administrative components.**

1. Occupational illness, even if suspected but not established, may be a reportable illness in certain states (eg, in California through the Doctor's First Report system).

2. Establishing quantifiable documentation of adverse effects at the time of exposure may be critical to future attribution of impairment (for example, spirometric evaluation soon after an irritant inhalant exposure).

3. Although workers' compensation is in theory a straightforward "no-fault" insurance system, in practice it is often arcane and adversarial. It is important to remember that the person being treated is the patient, not the employer or a referring attorney.

II. **Components of the occupational-exposure history.**

A. **Job and job process.**

1. Ask specifics about the job. Do not rely on descriptions limited to a general occupation or trade such as "machinist," "painter," "electronics worker," or "farmer."

2. Describe the industrial process and equipment used on the job. If power equipment is used, ascertain how is it powered to assess carbon monoxide exposure risk.

3. Determine whether the work process utilizes a closed (eg, a sealed reaction vat) system or an open system and what other processes or work stations are nearby. Work under a lab hood may be an effectively "closed" system, but not if the window is raised too far or if the airflow is not calibrated.
4. Find out who does maintenance and how often it is done.

B. Level of exposure.
   1. Ask whether dust or mist can be seen in the air at the work site. If so, question whether coworkers or nearby objects can be seen clearly (very high levels will actually obscure sight). A history of dust-laden sputum or nasal discharge at the end of the work shift is also a marker of heavy exposure.
   2. Ask whether work surfaces are dusty or damp and whether the paint at the work site is peeling or discolored (eg, from a corrosive atmosphere).
   3. Determine whether strong smells or tastes are present and, if so, whether they diminish over time, suggesting olfactory fatigue.
   4. Find out whether there is any special ventilation system and where the fresh air intake is located (toxins can actually be recirculated by a poorly placed air intake system).
   5. Establish whether the person has direct skin contact with the materials worked with, especially solvents or other liquid chemicals.
   6. Confined-space work can be especially hazardous. Examples of such spaces include ship holds, storage tanks, and underground vaults.

C. Personal protective gear (see also p 416). Respiratory system and skin protection may be essential for certain workplace exposures. Just as important as availability of equipment are its proper selection and use.
   1. **Respiratory protection.** A disposable paper-type mask is inadequate for most exposures. A screw-in cartridge-type mask for which the cartridges are rarely changed is also unlikely to be effective. For an air-supplied respirator with an air supply hose, ascertain the location of the air intake.
   2. **Skin protection.** Gloves and other skin protection should be impervious to the chemical(s) used.

D. Temporal aspects of exposure.
   1. The most important question is whether there have been any changes in work process, products used, or job duties which could be temporally associated with the onset of symptoms.
   2. Patterns of recurring symptoms linked to the work schedule can be important, for example if symptoms are different on the first day of the work week, at the end of the first shift of the week, at the end of the work week, or on days off or vacation days.

E. Other aspects of exposure.
   1. It is critical to assess whether anyone else from the workplace is also symptomatic and, if so, to identify their precise job duties.
   2. Eating in work areas can result in exposure through ingestion; smoking on the job can lead to inhalation of native materials or of toxic pyrolysis products.
   3. Determine whether a uniform is provided and who launders it. For example, family lead poisoning can occur through work clothes brought home for laundering. After certain types of contamination (eg, with pesticides), a uniform should be destroyed, not laundered and reused.
   4. Find out how large the work site is, since small operations are often the most poorly maintained. An active work safety and health committee suggests that better general protection is in place.

F. Common toxic materials of frequent concern that are commonly addressed in the occupational exposure history.
   1. **Two-part glues, paints, or coatings** that must be mixed up just prior to use, such as urethanes and epoxides. These reactive polymers are often irritants or sensitizers.

    2. **Solvents or degreasers,** especially if exposure is high enough to cause dizziness, nausea, headache, or a sense of intoxication.

    3. **Respirable dusts,** including friable insulation or heat-resistant materials, and sand or quartz dust, especially from grinding or blasting.

    4. **Combustion products or fumes** from fires, flame cutting, welding, or other high-temperature processes.

  G. Identifying the specific chemical exposures involved may be difficult because the worker may not know or may not have been told their precise identification. Even the manufacturer may be uncertain because components of the chemical mixture were obtained elsewhere or because exposure is due to undetermined process byproducts. Finally, the exposure may have occurred long before. Aids to exposure identification include the following:

    1. **Product labels.** Obtain product labels as a first step. However, the label alone is unlikely to provide detailed information.

    2. **Material safety data sheets.** Contact the manufacturer directly for a material safety data sheet (MSDS). These must be provided upon a physician's request in cases of suspected illness. Do not take "no" for an answer. You may need to supplement the MSDS information through direct discussion with a technical person working for the supplier.

    3. **Computerized databases.** Consult computerized databases (eg, Poisindex, TOMES, NIOSHTIC, others) for further information. Regional Poison Control Centers (see p 54) can be extremely useful.

    4. **DOT identification placards.** In cases of transportation release, Department of Transportation (DOT) identification placards may be available (see p 413).

    5. **Industrial exposure data.** Rarely, detailed industrial hygiene data may be available to delineate specific exposures and exposure levels in cases of ongoing, chronic exposure.

    6. **Existing process exposure data.** Often, exposure is assumed on the basis of known specific exposures linked to certain work processes. Selected types of exposure are listed in Table IV–1.

III. **Organ-specific occupational toxidromes.** A list of *Ten Leading Causes of Occupational Injuries and Illnesses* has been published by the National Institute for Occupational Safety and Health (NIOSH). This list, organized generally by organ system, is included in Table IV–2, along with additional disorders not on the original NIOSH list.

  A. **Occupational lung diseases.**

    1. In acute pulmonary injury from **inhaled irritants,** exposure is typically brief and intense; initial symptom onset is within minutes to 24–48 hours after exposure. The responses to irritant exposure, in increasing severity, are mucous membrane irritation, burning eyes and runny nose, tracheobronchitis, hoarseness, cough, laryngospasm, bronchospasm, and pulmonary edema progressing to adult respiratory distress syndrome (ARDS). Lower water solubility gases (nitrogen dioxide, ozone, and phosgene) may produce little upper airway mucous membrane irritation. Any irritant (high or low solubility) can cause pulmonary edema after sufficient exposure.

    2. **Heavy metal** pneumonitis is clinically similar to irritant inhalation injury. As with low-solubility gases, upper-airway mucous membrane irritation is minimal, thus the exposure may have poor warning properties. Offending agents include cadmium, mercury, and, in limited industrial settings, nickel carbonyl.

    3. **Febrile inhalational syndromes** are acute, self-limited flulike syndromes including **metal fume fever** (caused by galvanized-metal fumes), **polymer fume fever** (after thermal breakdown of certain fluoropolymers), and **"organic dust toxic syndrome"** (ODTS) (after heavy exposure to high levels of organic dust such as occurs in shoveling wood chip mulch). In none of these syndromes is lung injury marked. The presence of hypoxemia or lung infiltrates suggests an alternative diagnosis.

TABLE IV-1. SELECTED JOB PROCESSES AT HIGH RISK OF SPECIFIC TOXIC EXPOSURES

Job Process	Exposure
Aerospace and other specialty metal work	Beryllium
Artificial nail application	Methacrylate
Artificial nail removal	Acetonitrile, nitroethane
Artificial leather making, fabric coating	Dimethylformamide
Auto body painting	Isocyanates
Battery recycling	Lead fumes and dust
Carburetor cleaning (car repair)	Methylene chloride
Cement manufacture	Sulfur dioxide
Commercial refrigeration	Ammonia, sulfur dioxide
Concrete application	Chromic acid
Custodial work	Chlorine (hypochlorite + acid mix)
Dry cleaning	Chlorinated hydrocarbon solvents
Explosives work	Nitrate oxidants
Epoxy glue and coatings use	Trimellytic anhydride
Fire fighting	Carbon monoxide, cyanide, acrolein
Fumigation	Methyl bromide, Vikane (sulfuryl fluoride), phosphine
Furniture refinishing	Methylene chloride
Gas-shielded welding	Nitrogen dioxide
Gold refining	Mercury vapor
Hospital sterilizer work	Ethylene oxide, glutaraldehyde
Indoor fork lift or compressor operation	Carbon monoxide
Manure pit operation	Hydrogen sulfide
Metal degreasing	Chlorinated hydrocarbon solvents
Metal plating	Cyanide, acid mists
Microelectronics chip etching	Hydrofluoric acid
Microelectronic chip doping	Arsine gas, diborane gas
Paper pulp work	Chlorine, chlorine dioxide
Pool and hot tub disinfection	Chlorine, bromine
Pottery glazing and glassmaking	Lead dust
Radiator repair	Lead fumes
Rayon manufacturing	Carbon disulfide
Rubber cement glue use	n-Hexane, other solvents
Rocket and jet fuel work	Hydrazine, monomethylhydrazine
Sandblasting	Silica dust
Sewage work	Hydrogen sulfide
Silo work with fresh silage	Nitrogen dioxide
Sheet-metal flame cutting or brazing	Cadmium fumes
Structural paint refurbishing	Lead dust
Water treatment or purification	Chlorine, ozone
Welding galvanized steel	Zinc oxide fumes
Welding solvent-contaminated metal	Phosgene

TABLE IV–2. LEADING WORK-RELATED DISEASES AND INJURIES AND THEIR RELEVANCE TO
CLINICAL TOXICOLOGY

Work-Related Conditions	NIOSH*	Relevance	Examples of Relevant Conditions
Occupational lung disease	Yes	High	Irritant inhalation
Musculoskeletal	Yes	Low	Chemical-related Raynaud's
Cancer	Yes	Low	Acute leukemia
Trauma	Yes	Low	High-pressure injury
Cardiovascular disease	Yes	Moderate	Carbon monoxide ischemia
Disorders of reproduction	Yes	Low	Spontaneous abortion
Neurotoxic disorders	Yes	High	Acetylcholinesterase inhibition
Noise-induced hearing loss	Yes	Low	Potential drug interactions
Dermatologic conditions	Yes	Moderate	Hydrofluoric acid burn
Psychologic disorders	Yes	Moderate	Postexposure stress disorder
Hepatic injury	No	High	Chemical hepatitis
Renal disease	No	Moderate	Acute tubular necrosis
Hematologic conditions	No	High	Methemoglobinemia
Physical exposures	No	Low	Radiation sickness
Systemic illness	No	High	Cyanide toxicity

*NIOSH = National Institute for Occupational Safety and Health list of 10 leading conditions.

4. **Work-related asthma** is a frequent occupational problem. Classic occupational asthma typically occurs after sensitization to either large-molecular-weight chemicals (eg, inhaled foreign proteins) or to small chemicals that appear to act as haptens (the most common of which are the urethane isocyanates such as **toluene diisocyanate** [TDI]). After acute, high-level irritant inhalations, for example of **chlorine,** a chronic irritant-induced asthma may persist (sometimes called Reactive Airways Dysfunction Syndrome or RADS).

5. **Chronic fibrotic occupational lung diseases** include **asbestosis** (see p 98), **silicosis, coal workers' pneumoconiosis,** and a few other less-common fibrotic lung diseases associated with occupational exposures to such substances as **beryllium** and hard metal (**cobalt-tungsten carbide**). These conditions occur after years of exposure and with long latency, although patients may present for evaluation after an acute exposure. Referral for follow-up surveillance is appropriate if exposure is anticipated to be long term.

6. **Hypersensitivity pneumonitis** (also called **allergic alveolitis**) includes a group of diseases caused by chronic exposure to organic materials, especially thermophylic bacteria. The most common of these is **"farmer's lung."** Although the process is chronic, acute illness can occur in a sensitized host after heavy exposure to the offending agent. In such cases the illness may need to be differentiated from exposure to an irritant inhalant leading to acute lung injury.

B. **Musculoskeletal** conditions, including acute mechanical trauma, are the most common occupational-medicine problem but rarely have direct toxicological implications.

1. **Raynaud's syndrome** may rarely be associated with chemical exposure (eg, vinyl chloride monomer).

2. **High-pressure injection injuries** (eg, from paint spray guns) are important not because of systemic toxicity due to absorption of an injected sub-

stance (eg, paint thinner) but because of extensive irritant-related tissue necrosis. Emergency surgical evaluation of such cases is mandatory.

C. **Occupational cancer** is a major public concern and often leads to referral for toxicological evaluation. A variety of different cancers have been associated with workplace exposure, some more strongly than others. Identifying the chemical causes of cancer has proved a great challenge for occupational toxicologists and epidemiologists. Often, the practitioner is faced with an individual patient who seeks an assessment of the relative attribution of disease due to chemical exposures in that particular case, for purposes of gaining compensation or establishing liability. This process, however, tends to be far removed from the acute care setting, and clinical oncology management is not impacted directly by such etiologic considerations.

D. **Cardiovascular disease.**
   1. **Atherosclerotic** cardiovascular disease is associated with **carbon disulfide.** This chemical solvent is used in rayon manufacturing and in specialty applications and research laboratories. It is also a principal metabolite of **disulfiram.**
   2. **Carbon monoxide** at high levels can cause myocardial infarction in otherwise healthy individuals and, at lower levels, can aggravate ischemia in the face of established atherosclerotic heart disease (ASHD). Chronic exposure to carbon monoxide may also be associated with ASHD. Many jurisdictions automatically grant workers' compensation to firemen or policemen with ASHD, regarding it as a "stress-related" occupational disease. This is related to social policy rather than established epidemiologic risk.
   3. **Nitrate-withdrawal-induced** coronary artery spasm has been reported among workers heavily exposed to nitrates during munitions manufacturing.
   4. **Hydrocarbon solvents,** especially chlorinated hydrocarbons, and chlorofluorocarbon propellants all enhance the sensitivity of the myocardium to catecholamine-induced dysrhythmias.

E. **Adverse reproductive outcomes** have been associated with or implicated in occupational exposures to **heavy metals** (lead and organic mercury), hospital chemical exposures (including **anesthetic and sterilizing gases**), and **dibromochloropropane** (a soil fumigant now banned in the United States).

F. **Occupational neurotoxins.**
   1. **Acute** central nervous system (CNS) toxicity can occur with many pesticides (including both cholinesterase-inhibiting and chlorinated hydrocarbons). The CNS is also the target of **methyl bromide** (a common structural fumigant; see p 222). Cytotoxic and anoxic asphyxiant gases (eg, carbon monoxide, cyanide, and hydrogen sulfide) all cause acute CNS injury. **Hydrocarbon solvents** (see p 183) are typically CNS depressants at high exposure levels.
   2. **Chronic** CNS toxicity is the hallmark of heavy metals. This includes inorganic forms (**arsenic, lead,** and **mercury**) and organic forms (tetraethyl lead and methyl mercury). Chronic **manganese** (see p 211) exposure can cause psychosis and parkinsonism. Postanoxic injury, especially from **carbon monoxide** (see p 125), can also lead to parkinsonism.
   3. Established causes of **peripheral neuropathy** include lead, arsenic, mercury, carbon disulfide (mentioned earlier in connection with ASHD), n-hexane, and certain organophosphates.

G. **Occupational ototoxicity** is common but is usually noise induced rather than chemical related. Preexisting noise-induced hearing loss may magnify the impact of common ototoxic drugs.

H. **Occupational skin disorders.**
   1. Allergic and irritant contact dermatitis and acute caustic-chemical or acid injuries are the most common toxin-related skin problems. Systemic toxicity may occur (see p 129) but is not a common complicating factor.
   2. **Hydrofluoric acid** burns present a specific set of management problems (see p 186). Relevant occupations include not only the microelectronics in-

dustry but maintenance or repair jobs in which hydrofluoric acid-containing rust removers are used.

I. **Work-related psychological disorders** include a heterogeneous mix of diagnoses. Of these, "post-traumatic stress disorder" and "mass psychogenic illness" can be extremely relevant to medical toxicology because the patients in these cases may believe that their symptoms have a chemical etiology. After reasonable toxicological causes have been excluded, psychological diagnoses should be considered when nonspecific symptoms or multiple somatic complaints cannot be linked to abnormal signs or physiologic effects.

J. **Occupational chemical hepatotoxins** (see also p 38).
   1. Causes of acute chemical hepatitis include exposure to industrial solvents such as **halogenated hydrocarbons** (methylene chloride, trichloroethylene, and trichloroethane; carbon tetrachloride (only rarely encountered in modern industry)); and **dimethylformamide, dinitropropane,** and **dimethylacetamide.** The jet and rocket fuel components **hydrazine** and **monomethylhydrazine** are also potent hepatotoxins.
   2. Other hepatic responses that can be occupationally related include steatosis, cholestatic injury, hepatoportal sclerosis, and hepatic porphyria. The acute care provider should always consider a toxic-chemical etiology in the differential diagnosis of liver disease.

K. **Renal diseases.**
   1. **Acute tubular necrosis** can follow high-level exposure to a number of toxins, although the more frequent exposure scenario is a suicide attempt rather than workplace inhalation.
   2. **Interstitial nephritis** is associated with chronic exposure to heavy metals, while hydrocarbon exposure has been associated epidemiologically with **glomerular nephritis,** in particular Goodpasture's disease.

L. **Hematologic toxicity.**
   1. Industrial oxidants are an important potential cause of chemically induced **methemoglobinemia** (see p 220), especially in the dyestuff and munitions industries.
   2. **Bone marrow** is an important target organ for certain chemicals, such as **benzene** and **methyl cellosolve.** Both can cause pancytopenia. Benzene exposure also causes leukemia in humans. **Lead** causes anemia through interference with hemoglobin synthesis.
   3. **Arsine gas** is a potent cause of massive hemolysis. It is of industrial importance in microelectronics manufacturing.

M. **Nonchemical physical exposures** in the workplace are important because they can cause systemic effects that mimic chemical toxidromes. The most important example is **heat stress,** which is a major occupational health issue. Other relevant nonchemical, work-related physical exposure types include **ionizing radiation, nonionizing radiation** (such as ultraviolet, infrared, and microwave exposure), and **increased barometric pressure** (eg, among caisson workers). Except for extremes of exposure, the adverse effects of these physical factors are generally associated with chronic conditions.

N. **Systemic poisons** fit poorly into organ system categories, but are clearly of major importance in occupational toxicology. Prime examples are the cytotoxic asphyxiants **hydrogen cyanide** (especially in metal plating and metal refining) (see p 150), **hydrogen sulfide** (important as a natural byproduct of organic-material breakdown) (see p 188), and **carbon monoxide** (principally encountered as a combustion byproduct, but also a metabolite of the solvent methylene chloride) (see p 224). **Arsenic** (see p 95) is a multiorgan toxin with a myriad of effects. It has been widely used in agriculture and is an important metal smelting byproduct. A systemic **disulfiram reaction** (see p 158) can occur as a drug interaction with coexposure to certain industrial chemicals. Toxicity from **dinitrophenol,** an industrial chemical that uncouples oxidative phosphorylation, is also best categorized as a systemic effect.

IV. Laboratory testing.
  A. Testing for specific occupational toxins has a limited, but important role. Selected tests are listed in the descriptions of specific substances in Section II of this book.
  B. For significant irritant inhalation exposures, in addition to assessing oxygenation and chest radiographic status, early spirometric assessment is often important.
  C. General laboratory testing for chronic exposure assessment should be driven by the potential organ toxicity delineated previously. Standard recommendations (eg, in NIOSH criteria documents) often include a complete blood count, electrolytes, tests of renal and liver function, and periodic chest radiographic and pulmonary-function studies.

V. Treatment.
  A. Elimination or reduction of further exposure is a key treatment intervention in occupational toxicology. This includes prevention of exposure of coworkers. The **Occupational Safety and Health Administration (OSHA)** may be of assistance and should be notified immediately about an ongoing, potentially life-threatening workplace exposure situation. Contact information for regional OSHA offices is listed in Table IV–3. Workplace modification and control, especially the substitution of less hazardous materials, should always be the first line of defense. Worker-required personal protective equipment is, in general, less preferred.
  B. The medical treatment of occupational toxic illness should follow the general principles outlined earlier in this section and in Sections I and II of this book. In particular, the use of specific antidotes should be undertaken in consultation with a regional poison control center (see p 54) or other specialists. This is particularly true before chelation therapy is initiated for heavy metal poisoning.

TABLE IV–3. REGIONAL OFFICES OF THE OCCUPATIONAL SAFETY AND HEALTH ADMINISTRATION (OSHA)

Region	Regional Office	Phone Number	States Served
I	Boston	(617) 565–7164	Connecticut, Maine, Massachusetts, New Hampshire, Rhode Island, Vermont
II	New York City	(212) 337–2378	New York, New Jersey, Puerto Rico, Virgin Islands
III	Philadelphia	(215) 596–1201	Delaware, District of Columbia, Maryland, Pennsylvania, Virginia, West Virginia
IV	Atlanta	(404) 347–3573	Alabama, Florida, Georgia, Kentucky, Mississippi, North Carolina, South Carolina, Tennessee
V	Chicago	(312) 353–2220	Illinois, Indiana, Michigan, Minnesota, Ohio, Wisconsin
VI	Dallas	(214) 767–4731	Arkansas, Louisiana, New Mexico, Oklahoma, Texas
VII	Kansas City	(816) 426–5861	Iowa, Kansas, Missouri, Nebraska
VIII	Denver	(303) 391–5858	Colorado, Montana, North Dakota, South Dakota, Utah, Wyoming
IX	San Francisco	(415) 975–4310	Arizona, California, Hawaii, Nevada, American Samoa, Guam
X	Seattle	(206) 553–5930	Alaska, Idaho, Oregon, Washington

REFERENCES

Blanc PD, Balmes JR. History and physical examination. In: Harber P, Schenker M, Balmes JR, eds: *Occupational and Environmental Respiratory Diseases*. Mosby Publishers, 1995 pp 28–38.

Blanc PD, Rempel D, Maizlish N, Hiatt O, Olson KR. Occupational illness: case detection by poison control surveillance. *Ann Intern Med* 1989;**111**:238–244.

Centers for Disease Control. Leading work-related diseases and injuries in the United States. *MMWR* 1983;**32**:25–26,32.

▶ THE TOXIC HAZARDS OF INDUSTRIAL AND OCCUPATIONAL CHEMICALS

Frank J. Mycroft, PhD, and Patricia Hess Hiatt, BS

Basic information on the toxicity of many of the most commonly encountered and toxicologically significant industrial chemicals is provided in Table IV–4. The table is intended to expedite the recognition of potentially hazardous exposure situations and therefore provides information such as vapor pressures, warning properties, physical appearance, occupational exposure standards and guidelines, and hazard classification codes, which may also be useful in the assessment of an exposure situation. Table IV–4 is divided into 3 sections: **health hazards, exposure guidelines,** and **comments.** To use the table correctly, it is important to understand the scope and limitations of the information it provides.

The chemicals included in Table IV–4 were selected based on the following criteria: (1) toxic potential; (2) prevalence of use; (3) public health concern; and (4) availability of adequate toxicologic, regulatory, and physical- and chemical-property information. Several governmental and industrial lists of "hazardous chemicals" were used. A number of chemicals were omitted because no toxicologic information could be found, there are no regulatory standards, or they have very limited use. Chemicals that were of specific interest, those with existing exposure recommendations, and those of high use (even if of low toxicity) were included.

I. **Health hazard information.** The health hazards section of Table IV–4 focuses primarily on the basic hazards associated with possible inhalation of or skin exposure to chemicals in a workplace. It is based almost entirely on the occupational health literature. Most of our understanding of the potential effects of chemicals on human health is derived from occupational exposures, the levels of which are typically many times greater than those of environmental exposures. Moreover, the information in Table IV–4 unavoidably emphasizes *acute* health effects. Much more is known about the acute effects of chemicals on human health than about their chronic effects. The rapid onset of symptoms after exposure makes the causal association more readily apparent for acute health effects.

    A. The table is *not* a comprehensive source of the toxicology and medical information needed to manage a severely symptomatic or poisoned patient. Medical management information and advice for specific poisonings are found in Section I (see pulmonary problems, pp 1–8, and pulmonary and skin decontamination, pp 43–45) and Section II (see caustics and corrosives, p 129; gases, p 181; and hydrocarbons, p 183).

    B. **Hydrocarbons,** broadly defined as chemicals containing carbon and hydrogen, make up the majority of substances in Table IV–4. Hydrocarbons have a wide range of chemical structures and, not surprisingly, a variety of toxic effects. There are a few common features of hydrocarbon exposure, and the reader is directed to Section II, p 183, for information on general diagnosis and treatment. Some common features include the following:

        1. **Skin.** Dermatitis caused by defatting or removal of oils in the skin is common, especially with prolonged contact. Some agents can cause frank burns.

2. **Arrhythmias.** Many hydrocarbons, most notably fluorinated, chlorinated, and aromatic compounds, can sensitize the heart to arrhythmogenic effects of epinephrine, resulting in premature ventricular contractions (PVCs), ventricular tachycardia, or fibrillation. Even simple aliphatic compounds such as butane occasionally can cause this effect.
   a. Because arrhythmias may not occur immediately, cardiac monitoring for 24 hours is recommended for all victims who have had significant hydrocarbon exposure (eg, syncope, coma, and arrhythmias).
   b. Ventricular arrhythmias are preferably treated with a beta-adrenergic blocker (eg, esmolol [p 366] or propranolol [p 405]) rather than lidocaine.
3. **Pulmonary aspiration** of most hydrocarbons, especially those with relatively high volatility and low viscosity (eg, gasoline, kerosene, and naphtha) can cause severe chemical pneumonitis.
C. **Carcinogens.** To broaden the scope of the table, findings from human and animal studies relating to the carcinogenic or reproductive toxicity of a chemical are included when available. The **International Agency for Research on Cancer (IARC)** is the foremost authority in evaluating the carcinogenic potential of chemical agents for humans. The overall IARC evaluations are provided, when available, in the health hazards section of the table. The following IARC ratings are based primarily upon human and animal data.
   1. **IARC 1** substances are considered human carcinogens; generally there is sufficient epidemiologic information to support a causal association between exposure and human cancer.
   2. **IARC 2** compounds are suspected of being carcinogenic to humans based on a combination of data from animal and human studies. Group IARC 2 is subdivided into two parts.
      a. An **IARC 2A** rating indicates that a chemical is *probably* carcinogenic to humans. Most often there is limited evidence of carcinogenicity in humans combined with sufficient evidence of carcinogenicity in animals.
      b. **IARC 2B** indicates that a chemical is *possibly* carcinogenic to humans. This category may be used when there is limited evidence from epidemiologic studies and less than sufficient evidence for carcinogenicity in animals. It also may be used when there is inadequate evidence of carcinogenicity in humans and sufficient evidence in animals.
   3. **IARC 3** substances cannot be classified in regard to their carcinogenic potential for humans because of inadequate data.
   4. If a chemical is described in the table as carcinogenic but an IARC category is not given, IARC has not classified the chemical, but other sources (eg, US Environmental Protection Agency and California Department of Health Services Hazard Evaluation Service and Information System) consider it carcinogenic.
D. **Problems in assessing health hazards.** The nature and magnitude of the health hazards associated with occupational or environmental exposures to any chemical depend on its intrinsic toxicity and the conditions of exposure.
   1. Characterization of these hazards is often difficult. Important considerations include the potency of the agent, the route of exposure, the level and temporal pattern of exposure, genetic susceptibility, overall health status, and life-style factors that may alter individual sensitivities (eg, alcohol consumption may cause "degreaser's flush" in workers exposed to trichloroethylene). Despite their value in estimating the likelihood and potential severity of an effect, quantitative measurements of the level of exposure are not often available.
   2. Hazard characterizations cannot address undiscovered or unappreciated health effects. The limited information available on the health effects of most chemicals makes this a major concern. For example, of the more than 5 million compounds known to science, only about 100,000 are listed in the *Registry of the Toxic Effects of Chemical Substances* (RTECS) pub-

lished by the National Institute for Occupational Safety and Health (NIOSH). Of these 100,000 substances, fewer than 5000 have any toxicity studies relating to their potential tumorigenic or reproductive effects in animals or humans. Because of these gaps, the absence of information does not imply the absence of hazard.

3. The predictive value of animal findings for humans is sometimes uncertain. For many effects, however, there is considerable concordance between test animals and humans.

4. The developmental toxicity information presented here is not a sufficient basis on which to make clinical judgments as to whether a given exposure might adversely affect a pregnancy. For most chemicals known to have adverse effects on fetal development in test animals, there are insufficient epidemiologic data in humans. The predictive value of these animal findings for humans, who are typically exposed to levels much lower than those used in animal tests, is thought to be poor. In general, so little is known about the effects of substances on fetal development that it is prudent to conservatively manage all chemical exposures. The information here is presented solely to identify those compounds for which available data further indicate the need to control exposures.

II. Exposure guidelines and National Fire Protection Association rankings.

A. **Threshold limit values (TLVs)** are workplace exposure guidelines established by the American Conference of Governmental Industrial Hygienists (ACGIH), a professional society. Although the ACGIH has no regulatory authority, its recommendations are highly regarded and widely followed by the occupational health community.

The toxicologic basis for each TLV varies. A TLV may be based on such diverse effects as respiratory sensitization, sensory irritation, narcosis, or asphyxia. Therefore, the TLV is not a relative index of toxicity. Because the degree of health hazard is a continuous function of exposure, TLVs are not fine lines separating safe from dangerous levels of exposure. The *Documentation of the Threshold Limit Values,* which is published by the ACGIH and describes in detail the rationale for each value, should be consulted for specific information on the toxicologic significance of a particular TLV. Common units for a TLV are parts of chemical per million parts of air (**ppm**) and milligrams of chemical per cubic meter of air (**mg/m^3**). **At standard temperature and pressure, TLV values in ppm can be converted to their equivalent concentrations in mg/m^3** by multiplying the TLV in ppm by the molecular weight (MW) in milligrams of the chemical and dividing the result by 22.4 (one mole of gas displaces 22.4 L of air at standard temperature and pressure):

$$mg/m^3 = \frac{ppm \times MW}{22.4}$$

1. The **threshold limit value time-weighted average (TLV-TWA)** refers to airborne contaminants and is the time-weighted average concentration to which nearly all workers may be repeatedly exposed during a normal 8-hour workday and 40-hour workweek, without adverse effect. Unless otherwise indicated, the values listed under the ACGIH TLV heading are the TLV-TWA values. Because TLV-TWA values are often set to protect against worker discomfort, nonspecific minor health complaints such as eye or throat irritation, cough, headache, or nausea may indicate overexposure.

2. The **threshold limit value ceiling (TLV-C)** is the airborne concentration that should not be exceeded during any part of a working exposure. Ceiling guidelines are often set for rapidly acting agents for which an 8-hour time-weighted average exposure limit would be inappropriate. TLV-Cs are listed under the ACGIH TLV heading and are noted by a "**(C).**"

3. Compounds for which **skin contact** is a significant route of exposure are designated with an "**S**." This could refer to potential corrosive effects or systemic toxicity owing to skin absorption.
4. The ACGIH classifies some substances as being *confirmed* (A1) or *suspected* (A2) **human carcinogens, or animal carcinogens (A3).** These designations are also provided in the table. The ACGIH does not consider A3 carcinogens likely to cause human cancer.
5. The TLVs are heavily based on workplace exposures and conditions occurring within the United States. Their application, which requires training in industrial hygiene, is therefore limited to similar exposures and conditions.
B. **OSHA regulations** are standards for exposure to airborne contaminants, set and enforced by OSHA, an agency of the federal government.
1. The **permissible exposure limit (PEL)** set by OSHA is closely analogous to the ACGIH TLV-TWA. In fact, when OSHA was established in 1971, it formally adopted the 1969 ACGIH TLVs for nearly all of its PELs. In 1988, OSHA updated the majority of its PELs by adopting the 1986 TLVs. These revised PELs were printed in the 1990 edition of this manual. However, in early 1993, the 1988 PEL revisions were voided as a result of legal challenges, and the earlier values were restored. Because these restored values cannot be reliably assumed to protect worker health, and because the values may change again as a result of further administrative or legislative action, the PELs are not printed in this edition.
2. Substances that are specifically **regulated as carcinogens** by OSHA are indicated by "**OSHA CA**" under the ACGIH TLV heading. For these carcinogens, additional regulations apply. The notation "**NIOSH CA**" in the TLV column identifies those chemicals that NIOSH recommends be treated as potential human carcinogens.
3. Some states operate their own occupational health and safety programs in cooperation with OSHA. In these states, stricter standards may apply.
C. **Immediately dangerous to life or health (IDLH)** represents "a maximum concentration from which one could escape within 30 minutes without any escape-impairing symptoms or any irreversible health effects." The IDLH values were originally jointly set by OSHA and NIOSH for the purpose of respirator selection. They have recently been updated by NIOSH.
D. **Emergency Response Planning Guidelines (ERPGs)** have been developed by the American Industrial Hygiene Association (AIHA) for 70 specific substances. The values are generally based upon limited human experience as well as available animal data and should be considered estimates. Although these values are printed in the IDLH column, they have different meanings:
1. **ERPG-1** is "the maximum air concentration below which it is believed nearly all individuals could be exposed for up to 1 hour without experiencing other than mild transient adverse health effects or perceiving a clearly defined objectionable odor."
2. **ERPG-2** is "the maximum air concentration below which it is believed that nearly all individuals could be exposed for up to 1 hour without experiencing or developing irreversible or other serious health effects or symptoms which could impair their abilities to take protective action."
3. **ERPG-3** is "the maximum air concentration below which it is believed that nearly all individuals could be exposed for up to 1 hour without experiencing or developing life-threatening health effects."
4. The ERPGs were developed for purposes of emergency planning and response. They are not exposure guidelines and do not incorporate the safety factors normally used in establishing acceptable exposure limits. Reliance on the ERPGs for exposures lasting longer than 1 hour is not safe.
E. **National Fire Protection Association (NFPA) codes** are part of the system created by the NFPA for identifying and ranking the potential fire hazards of materials. The system has 3 principal categories of hazard: **health (H), flam-**

mability **(F),** and reactivity **(R).** Within each category, hazards are ranked from four (4), indicating a severe hazard, to zero (0), indicating no special hazard. The NFPA rankings for each substance are listed under their appropriate headings. The criteria for rankings within each category are found in Figure IV–2, p 414.

1. The NFPA health hazard rating is based on both the intrinsic toxicity of a chemical and the toxicities of its combustion or breakdown products. The overall ranking is determined by the greater source of health hazard under fire or other emergency conditions. Common hazards from the ordinary combustion of materials are not considered in these rankings.

2. This system is intended to provide basic information to fire-fighting and emergency-response personnel. Its application to specific situations requires skill. Conditions at the scene, such as the amount of material involved and its rate of release, wind conditions, and the proximity to various populations and their health status, are as important as the intrinsic properties of a chemical in determining the magnitude of a hazard.

III. **Comments section.** The comment column of Table IV–4 provides supplementary information on the physical and chemical properties of substances, which would be helpful in assessing their health hazards. Information such as physical state and appearance, vapor pressures, warning properties, and potential breakdown products is included.

A. Information on **physical state and appearance** of a compound may help in its identification and indicate whether dusts, mists, vapors, or gases are likely means of airborne exposure. *Note:* For many products, especially pesticides, appearance and some hazardous properties may vary with the formulation.

B. The **vapor pressure** of a substance determines its potential maximum air concentration and influences the degree of inhalation exposure or airborne contamination. Vapor pressures fluctuate greatly with temperature.

1. Substances with high vapor pressures tend to volatilize more quickly and can reach higher maximum air concentrations than substances with low vapor pressures. Some substances have such low vapor pressures that airborne contamination is a threat only if they are finely dispersed in a dust or mist.

2. Substances with a **saturated-air concentration** below their TLVs do not pose a significant vapor inhalation hazard. Vapor pressures can be roughly converted to saturated-air concentrations expressed in parts per million by multiplying by a factor of 1300. This is equivalent to dividing by 760 mm Hg and then multiplying the result by 1 million to adjust for the original units of parts per million (a pressure of 1 equals 760 mm Hg):

$$ppm = \frac{\text{Vapor pressure (mm Hg)}}{760} \times 10^6$$

C. **Warning properties,** such as odor and sensory irritation, can be valuable indicators of exposure. However, because of olfactory fatigue and individual differences in odor thresholds, the sense of smell is often unreliable for detecting many compounds. There is no correlation between the quality of an odor and its toxicity. Pleasant-smelling compounds are not necessarily less toxic than foul-smelling ones.

1. The warning property assessments found in the table are based on OSHA evaluations. For the purpose of this manual, chemicals described as having *good* warning properties can be detected by smell or irritation at levels below the TLV by most individuals. Chemicals described as having *adequate* warning properties can be detected at air levels near the TLV. Chemicals described as having *poor* warning properties can be detected only at levels significantly above the TLV or not at all.

    2. Reported values for odor threshold in the literature vary greatly for many chemicals and are therefore uncertain. These differences make assessments of warning qualities difficult.

  D. Thermal-breakdown products. Under fire conditions, many organic substances will break down to other toxic substances. The amounts, kinds, and distribution of breakdown products vary with the fire conditions and are not easily modeled. Information on the likely thermal-decomposition products is included because of their importance in the assessment of health hazards under fire conditions.

    1. In general, incomplete combustion of *any* organic material will produce some carbon monoxide (see p 125).

    2. The partial combustion of compounds containing sulfur, nitrogen, or phosphorus atoms will also release their oxides (see pp 300, 234, and 181).

    3. Compounds with chlorine atoms will release some hydrogen chloride or chlorine (see p 134) when exposed to high heat or fire; some chlorinated compounds may also generate phosgene (see p 262).

    4. Compounds containing the fluorine atom are similarly likely to break down to yield some hydrogen fluoride (see p 186) and fluorine.

    5. Some compounds (eg, polyurethane) that contain an unsaturated carbon-nitrogen bond will release cyanide (see p 150) during their decomposition.

    6. Polychlorinated aromatic compounds may yield polychlorinated dibenzodioxins and polychlorinated dibenzofurans (see p 156) when heated.

    7. In addition, smoke from a chemical fire is likely to contain large amounts of the volatilized original chemical and still other poorly characterized partial-breakdown products.

    8. The thermal-breakdown product information found in Table IV–4 is derived primarily from data found in the literature and the general considerations described immediately above. Aside from the NFPA codes, Table IV–4 does not cover the chemical reactivity or compatibility of substances.

IV. Summary. Table IV–4 provides basic information that describes the potential health hazards associated with exposure to several hundred chemicals. The table is not a comprehensive listing of all the possible health hazards for each chemical. The information compiled here comes from a wide variety of respected sources (see references below) and focuses on the more likely or commonly reported health effects. Publications from NIOSH, OSHA, ACGIH, the Hazard Evaluation System and Information Service of the State of California, and NFPA; major textbooks in the fields of toxicology and occupational health; and major review articles were the primary sources of the information found here. Refer to the original sources for more complete information.

    Table IV–4 is intended primarily to guide users in the quick qualitative assessment of common toxic hazards. Its application to specific situations requires skill. Because of the many data gaps in the toxicology literature, exposures should generally be managed conservatively. Contact a regional poison control center (see Table I–42, p 55) or medical toxicologist for expert assistance in managing specific emergency exposures.

REFERENCES

Air Contaminants: Permissible Exposure Limits. *Fed Reg* 1989;**54**:2332.
Barlow SM, Sullivan FM (editors): *Reproductive Hazards of Industrial Chemicals.* Academic Press, 1982.
Emergency Response Planning Committee: *Emergency Response Planning Guidelines.* American Industrial Hygiene Association, 1998.
Fire Protection Guide on Hazardous Materials, 11th ed. National Fire Protection Association, 1994.
Hathaway G et al: *Proctor and Hughes' Chemical Hazards of the Workplace,* 3rd ed. Lippincott, 1991.
Hayes WJ Jr: *Pesticides Studied in Man.* Williams & Wilkins, 1982.

IARC Monographs on the Evaluation of the Carcinogenic Risk of Chemicals to Humans. 54 vols. World Health Organization, 1972–1992.

Morgan DP: *Recognition and Management of Pesticide Poisonings,* 4th ed. US Environmental Protection Agency, 1989.

National Toxicology Program: *Sixth Annual Report on Carcinogens.* US Department of Health & Human Services, 1991.

NIOSH: *Occupational Diseases: A Guide to Their Recognition.* US Department of Health & Human Services, 1977.

NIOSH: Recommendations for occupational safety and health standards. *MMWR* 1988;**37** (Suppl 7).

NIOSH/OSHA: *Occupational Health Guidelines for Chemical Hazards.* DHHS (NIOSH) Publication No. 81-123. US Department of Health & Human Services, 1981.

NIOSH/OSHA: *Pocket Guide to Chemical Hazards.* NIOSH Publication No. 78-210. US Department of Health & Human Services, 1985.

NIOSH: *NIOSH Chemical Listing and Documentation of Revised IDLH Values (3-1-95).* http://www.cdc.gov/niosh/intridl4.html

Rumack BH (editor): *TOMES,* vol 16. Micromedex, 1993.

Schardein JL: *Chemically Induced Birth Defects.* Marcel Dekker, 1985.

Schardein JL, Schwetz BA, Kenel MF: Species sensitivities and prediction of teratogenic potential. *Environ Health Perspect* 1985;**61**:55.

Threshold Limit Values and Biological Exposure Indices. American Council of Governmental Industrial Hygienists, 1996.

TABLE IV–4. HEALTH HAZARD SUMMARIES FOR INDUSTRIAL AND OCCUPATIONAL CHEMICALS

Abbreviations and designations used in this table are defined as follows:

IARC	=	International Agency for Research on Cancer overall classification (see p 428): 1 = known human carcinogen; 2A = probable human carcinogen; 2B = possible human carcinogen; 3 = inadequate data available.
TLV	=	American Conference of Governmental Industrial Hygienists (ACGIH) threshold limit value 8-hour time weighted average (TLV-TWA) air concentration (see p 429): A1 = ACGIH-confirmed human carcinogen; A2 = ACGIH-suspected human carcinogen; A3 = ACGIH animal carcinogen.
ppm	=	Parts of chemical per million parts of air.
mg/m³	=	Milligrams of chemical per cubic meter of air.
mppcf	=	Million particles of dust per cubic foot of air.
(C)	=	Ceiling air concentration (TLV-C) that should not be exceeded at any time.
S	=	Skin absorption can be significant route of exposure.
NIOSH CA	=	Judged by National Institute for Occupational Safety and Health to be a known or suspected human carcinogen (see p 430).
OSHA CA	=	Regulated by the Occupational Safety and Health Administration as an occupational carcinogen (see p 430).
IDLH	=	Immediately Dangerous to Life or Health air concentration (see p 430).
LEL	=	Lower explosive limit.
ERPG	=	Emergency Response Planning Guidelines air concentration values for a one-hour period of exposure (see p 430).
NFPA Codes	=	National Fire Protection Association hazard classification codes (see p 413 and p 430): 0 (no hazard) <—> 4 (severe hazard)
	H =	Health hazard
	F =	Fire hazard
	R =	Reactivity hazard
	Ox =	Oxidizing agent
	W =	Water-reactive substance

Health Hazard Summaries	ACGIH TLV	IDLH	NFPA Codes H F R	Comments
Acetaldehyde [CAS: 75-07-0]: Corrosive; severe burns to eyes and skin may occur. Vapors strongly irritating to eyes and respiratory tract; evidence for adverse effects on fetal development in animals. A carcinogen in test animals (IARC 2B).	25 ppm (C), A3	2000 ppm ERPG-1: 10 ppm ERPG-2: 200 ppm ERPG-3: 1000 ppm	3 4 2	Colorless liquid. Fruity odor and irritation are both adequate warning properties. Vapor pressure is 750 mm Hg at 20 °C (68 °F). Highly flammable.
Acetic acid (vinegar acid) [CAS: 64-19-7]: Concentrated solutions are corrosive; severe burns to eyes and skin may occur. Vapors strongly irritating to eyes and respiratory tract.	10 ppm	50 ppm	3 2 0	Colorless liquid. Pungent, vinegarlike odor and irritation both occur near the TLV and are adequate warning properties. Vapor pressure is 11 mm Hg at 20 °C (68 °F). Flammable.

Chemical	TLV		H	F	R	Comments
Acetic anhydride (CAS: 108-24-7): Corrosive; severe burns to eyes and skin may result. Dermal sensitization has been reported. Vapors highly irritating to eyes and respiratory tract.	5 ppm	200 ppm	3	2	1	Colorless liquid. Odor and irritation both occur below the TLV and are good warning properties. Vapor pressure is 4 mm Hg at 20 °C (68 °F). Flammable. Evolves heat upon contact with water.
Acetone (dimethyl ketone, 2-propanone [CAS: 67-64-1]): Vapors mildly irritating to eyes and respiratory tract. A CNS depressant at high levels. Eye irritation and headache are common symptoms of moderate overexposure.	500 ppm	2500 ppm [LEL]	1	3	0	Colorless liquid with a sharp, aromatic odor. Eye irritation is an adequate warning property. Vapor pressure is 266 mm Hg at 25 °C (77 °F). Highly flammable.
Acetonitrile (methyl cyanide, cyanomethane, ethanenitrile [CAS: 75-05-8]): Vapors mildly irritating to eyes and respiratory tract. Inhibits several metabolic enzyme systems. Dermal absorption occurs. Metabolized to cyanide (see p 150); fatalities have resulted. Symptoms include headache, nausea, vomiting, weakness, and stupor. Limited evidence for adverse effects on fetal development in test animals given large doses.	40 ppm	500 ppm	2	3	0	Colorless liquid. Etherlike odor, detectable at the TLV, is an adequate warning property. Vapor pressure is 73 mm Hg at 20 °C (68 °F). Flammable. Thermal breakdown products include oxides of nitrogen and cyanide. May be found in products for removing sculptured nails.
Acetophenone (phenyl methyl ketone [CAS: 98-86-2]): Direct contact mildly irritating to eyes and skin. A CNS depressant at high levels.	10 ppm		1	2	0	
Acetylene tetrabromide (tetrabromoethane [CAS: 79-27-6]): Direct contact is irritating to eyes and skin. Vapors irritating to eyes and respiratory tract. Dermal absorption occurs. Highly hepatotoxic; liver injury can result from low-level exposures.	1 ppm	8 ppm	3	0	1	Viscous, pale yellow liquid. Pungent, chloroformlike odor. Vapor pressure is less than 0.1 mm Hg at 20 °C (68 °F). Not combustible. Thermal breakdown products include hydrogen bromide and carbonyl bromide.

(C) = ceiling air concentration (TLV-C); S = skin absorption can be significant; A1 = ACGIH-confirmed human carcinogen; A2 = ACGIH-suspected human carcinogen; NFPA Hazard Codes: H = health, F = fire, R = reactivity, Ox = oxidizer, W = water-reactive, 0 (none) <—> 4 (severe). ERPG = Emergency Response Planning Guideline. See p 434 for explanation of definitions.

(continued)

TABLE IV–4. HEALTH HAZARD SUMMARIES FOR INDUSTRIAL AND OCCUPATIONAL CHEMICALS (CONTINUED)

Health Hazard Summaries	ACGIH TLV	IDLH	NFPA Codes H	F	R	Comments
Acrolein (acraldehyde, 2-propenal [CAS: 107-02-8]): Highly corrosive; severe burns to eyes or skin may result. Vapors extremely irritating to eyes, skin, and respiratory tract; pulmonary edema has been reported. Permanent pulmonary function changes may result.	0.1 ppm (C), S	2 ppm ERPG-1: 0.1 ppm ERPG-2: 0.5 ppm ERPG-3: 3 ppm	4	3	3	Colorless to yellow liquid. An unpleasant odor. Eye irritation occurs at low levels and provides a good warning property. Formed in the pyrolysis of many substances. Vapor pressure is 214 mm Hg at 20 °C (68 °F). Highly flammable.
Acrylamide (propenamide, acrylic amide [CAS: 79-06-1]): Concentrated solutions are slightly irritating. Well absorbed by all routes. A potent neurotoxin causing peripheral neuropathy. Contact dermatitis also reported. Testicular toxicity in test animals. A carcinogen in test animals (IARC 2B).	0.03 mg/m³, S, A3	60 mg/m³	2	2	2	Colorless solid. Vapor pressure is 0.007 mm Hg at 20 °C (68 °F). Not flammable. Decomposes around 80 °C (176 °F). Breakdown products include oxides of nitrogen. Monomer used in the synthesis of polyacrylamide plastics.
Acrylic acid (propenoic acid [CAS: 79-10-7]): Corrosive; severe burns may result. Vapors highly irritating to eyes, skin, and respiratory tract. Limited evidence of adverse effects on fetal development at high doses in test animals. Based on structural analogies, compounds containing the acrylate moiety may be carcinogens.	2 ppm, S	ERPG-1: 2 ppm ERPG-2: 50 ppm ERPG-3: 750 ppm	3	2	2	Colorless liquid with characteristic acrid odor. Vapor pressure is 31 mm Hg at 25 °C (77 °F). Flammable. Inhibitor added to prevent explosive self-polymerization.
Acrylonitrile (cyanoethylene, vinyl cyanide, propenenitrile the ([CAS: 107-13-1]): Direct contact can be strongly irritating to eyes and skin. Well absorbed by all routes. A CNS depressant at high levels. Metabolized to cyanide (see p 150). Moderate acute overexposure will produce headache, weakness, nausea, and vomiting. Evidence of adverse effects on fetal development at high doses in animals. A carcinogen in test animals with limited epidemiologic evidence for carcinogenicity in humans (IARC 2A).	2 ppm, S, A2 OSHA CA NIOSH CA	85 ppm ERPG-1: 10 ppm ERPG-2: 35 ppm ERPG-3: 75 ppm	4	3	2	Colorless liquid with a mild odor. Vapor pressure is 83 mm Hg at 20 °C (68 °F). Flammable. Polymerizes rapidly. Thermal decomposition products include hydrogen cyanide and oxides of nitrogen. Used in the manufacture of ABS and SAN resins.
Aldicarb (CAS: 116-06-3): A potent, carbamate-type cholinesterase inhibitor (see p 244). Well absorbed dermally.						Absorption by fruits has caused human poisonings.

Substance	TLV	Other	NFPA (H R F)
Aldrin (CAS: 309-00-2): Chlorinated insecticide (see p 133). Minor skin irritant. Convulsant. Hepatotoxin. Well absorbed dermally. Limited evidence for carcinogenicity in test animals. (IARC 3).	0.25 mg/m³, S, A3 NIOSH CA	25 mg/m³	Tan to dark brown solid. A mild chemical odor. Vapor pressure is 0.000006 mm Hg at 20°C (68 °F). Not flammable but breaks down, yielding hydrogen chloride gas. Most uses have been banned in US.
Allyl alcohol (2-propen-1-ol) [CAS: 107-18-6]: Strongly irritating to eyes and skin; severe burns may result. Vapors highly irritating to eyes and respiratory tract. Systemic poisoning can result from dermal exposures. May cause liver and kidney injury.	2 ppm, S [proposed: 0.5 ppm]	20 ppm	4 3 1 — Colorless liquid. Mustardlike odor and irritation occur near the TLV and serve as good warning properties. Vapor pressure is 17 mm Hg at 20 °C (68 °F). Flammable. Used in chemical synthesis and as a pesticide.
Allyl chloride (3-chloro-1-propene) [CAS: 107-05-1]: Highly irritating to eyes and skin. Vapors highly irritating to eyes and respiratory tract. Well absorbed by the skin, producing both superficial and penetrating irritation and pain. Causes liver and kidney injury in test animals. Chronic exposures have been associated with reports of mild neuropathy.	1 ppm, A3	250 ppm ERPG-1: 3 ppm ERPG-2: 40 ppm ERPG-3: 300 ppm	3 3 1 — Colorless, yellow, or purple liquid. Pungent. Pungent, disagreeable odor and irritation occur only at levels far above the TLV, so exposure is accompanied by poor warning. Vapor pressure is 295 mm Hg at 20 °C (68 °F). Highly flammable. Breakdown products include hydrogen chloride and phosgene.
Allyl glycidyl ether (AGE) [CAS: 106-92-3]: Highly irritating to eyes and skin; severe burns may result. Vapors irritating to eyes and respiratory tract. Sensitization dermatitis has been reported. Hematopoietic and testicular toxicity occurs in test animals at modest doses. Well absorbed through the skin.	1 ppm	50 ppm	Colorless liquid. Unpleasant odor. Vapor pressure is 2 mm Hg at 20 °C (68 °F). Flammable.
Allyl propyl disulfide (onion oil) [CAS: 2179-59-1]: Mucous membrane irritant and lacrimator.	2 ppm		Liquid with a pungent, irritating odor. A synthetic flavorant and food additive. Thermal breakdown products include sulfur oxide fumes.
α-Alumina (aluminum oxide) [CAS: 1344-28-1]: Nuisance dust and physical irritant.	10 mg/m³		

(C) = ceiling air concentration (TLV-C); S = skin absorption can be significant; A1 = ACGIH-confirmed human carcinogen; A2 = ACGIH-suspected human carcinogen; NFPA Hazard Codes: H = health, F = fire, R = reactivity, Ox = oxidizer, W = water-reactive, 0 (none) <—> 4 (severe). ERPG = Emergency Response Planning Guideline. See p 434 for explanation of definitions.

(continued)

TABLE IV–4. HEALTH HAZARD SUMMARIES FOR INDUSTRIAL AND OCCUPATIONAL CHEMICALS (CONTINUED)

Health Hazard Summaries	ACGIH TLV	IDLH	NFPA Codes H F R	Comments
Aluminum metal (CAS: 7429-90-5): Dusts can cause mild eye and respiratory tract irritation. Long-term inhalation of large amounts of fine aluminum powders or fumes from aluminum ore (bauxite) has been associated with reports of pulmonary fibrosis (Shaver's disease). Acute exposures in aluminum refining ("pot room") has been associated with asthmalike responses. Industrial processes used to produce aluminum have been associated with an increased incidence of cancer in workers.	10 mg/m^3 (metal and oxide) 5 mg/m^3 (pyrophoric powders, welding fumes) 2 mg/m^3 (soluble salts, alkyls NOC)		0 3 1 (powder)	Oxidizes readily. Fine powders and flakes are flammable and explosive when mixed with air. Reacts with acids and caustic solutions to produce flammable hydrogen gas.
Aluminum phosphide (CAS: 20859-73-8): Effects caused by phosphine gas that is produced on contact with moisture. Severe respiratory tract irritant.			4 4 2 W	
4-Aminodiphenyl (p-aminobiphenyl, p-phenylaniline [CAS: 92-67-1]): Potent bladder carcinogen in humans (IARC 1). Causes methemoglobinemia (see p 220).	A1 OSHA CA NIOSH CA			Colorless crystals.
2-Aminopyridine (CAS: 504-29-0): Mild irritant. Potent CNS convulsant. Very well absorbed by inhalation and skin contact. Signs and symptoms include headache, dizziness, nausea, elevated blood pressure, and convulsions.	0.5 ppm	5 ppm		Colorless solid with a distinctive odor and a very low vapor pressure at 20 °C (68 °F). Combustible.
Amitrole (3-amino-1,2,4-triazole [CAS: 61-82-5]): Mild irritant. Well absorbed by inhalation and skin contact. Shows antithyroid activity in test animals. Evidence of adverse effects on fetal development in test animals at high doses. A carcinogen in test animals (IARC 2B).	0.2 mg/m^3, A3			Crystalline solid. Appearance and some hazardous properties vary with the formulation.

Substance	TLV	Other	H	F	R	Comments
Ammonia (CAS: 7664-41-7): Corrosive; severe burns to eyes and skin result. Vapors highly irritating to eyes and respiratory tract; pulmonary edema has been reported. Severe responses are associated with anhydrous ammonia or with concentrated ammonia solutions (see p 67).	25 ppm	300 ppm; ERPG-1: 25 ppm; ERPG-2: 200 ppm; ERPG-3: 1000 ppm	3	1	0	Colorless gas or aqueous solution. Pungent odor and irritation are good warning properties. Flammable. Breakdown products include oxides of nitrogen. Although widely used in industry, concentrated forms are most frequently encountered in agriculture and from its use as a refrigerant.
***n*-Amyl acetate (CAS: 628-63-7):** Defats the skin, producing a dermatitis. Vapors mildly irritating to eyes and respiratory tract. A CNS depressant at very high levels. Reversible liver and kidney injury may occur at very high exposures.	100 ppm	1000 ppm	1	3	0	Colorless liquid. Its bananalike odor detectable below the TLV is a good warning property. Vapor pressure is 4 mm Hg at 20 °C (68 °F). Flammable.
***sec*-Amyl acetate (α-methylbutyl acetate [CAS: 628-38-0]):** Defats the skin, producing a dermatitis. Vapors irritating to eyes and respiratory tract. A CNS depressant at very high levels. Reversible liver and kidney injury may occur at high-level exposures.	125 ppm	1000 ppm	1	3	0	Colorless liquid. A fruity odor occurs below the TLV and is a good warning property. Vapor pressure is 7 mm Hg at 20 °C (68 °F). Flammable.
Aniline (aminobenzene, phenylamine [CAS: 62-53-3]): Mildly irritating to eyes upon direct contact, with corneal injury possible. Potent inducer of methemoglobinemia (see p 220). Well absorbed via inhalation and dermal routes. Limited evidence of carcinogenicity in test animals (IARC 3).	2 ppm, S, A3	100 ppm	3	2	0	Colorless to brown viscous liquid. Distinctive amine odor and mild eye irritation occur well below the TLV and are good warning properties. Vapor pressure is 0.6 mm Hg at 20 °C (68 °F). Combustible. Breakdown products include oxides of nitrogen.
***o*-Anisidine (*o*-methoxyaniline [CAS: 29191-52-4]):** Mild skin sensitizer causing dermatitis. Causes methemoglobinemia (see p 220). Well absorbed through skin. Headaches and vertigo are signs of exposure. Possible liver and kidney injury. A carcinogen in test animals (IARC 2B).	0.1 ppm, S, A3	50 mg/m³	2	1	0	Colorless, red, or yellow liquid with the fishy odor of amines. Vapor pressure is less than 0.1 mm Hg at 20 °C (68 °F). Combustible. Primarily used in the dye-stuffs industry.

(C) = ceiling air concentration (TLV-C); S = skin absorption can be significant; A1 = ACGIH-confirmed human carcinogen; A2 = ACGIH-suspected human carcinogen; NFPA Hazard Codes: H = health, F = fire, R = reactivity; Ox = oxidizer, 0 (none) <—> 4 (severe). ERPG = Emergency Response Planning Guideline. See p 434 for explanation of definitions.

(continued)

TABLE IV-4. HEALTH HAZARD SUMMARIES FOR INDUSTRIAL AND OCCUPATIONAL CHEMICALS (CONTINUED)

Health Hazard Summaries	ACGIH TLV	IDLH	NFPA Codes H F R	Comments
Antimony and salts (antimony trichloride, antimony trioxide, antimony pentachloride [CAS: 7440-36-0]): Dusts and fumes irritating to eyes, skin, and respiratory tract. Toxicity through contamination with silica or arsenic may occur. Antimony trioxide is carcinogenic in test animals with limited evidence for carcinogenicity among antimony trioxide production in workers (IARC 2B). See also p 86.	0.5 mg/m³ (as Sb)	50 mg/m³ (as Sb)	3 0 1 (SbCl$_5$) 4 0 1 (SbF$_5$)	The metal is silver-white and has a very low vapor pressure. Some chloride salts release HCl upon contact with air.
ANTU (α-naphthylthiourea [CAS: 86-88-4]): Well absorbed by skin contact and inhalation. Pulmonary edema and liver injury may result from ingestion. Repeated exposures can injure the thyroid and adrenals, producing hypothyroidism. Possible slight contamination with a 2-naphthylamine, a human bladder carcinogen.	0.3 mg/m³	100 mg/m³		Colorless to gray solid powder. Odorless. A rodenticide. Breakdown products include oxides of nitrogen and sulfur dioxide.
Arsenic (CAS: 7440-38-2): Irritating to eyes and skin; hyperpigmentation, hyperkeratoses, and skin cancers have been described. A general cellular poison. May cause bone marrow suppression, peripheral neuropathy, and gastrointestinal, liver, and cardiac injury. Some arsenic compounds have adverse effects on fetal development in test animals. Exposure linked to skin, respiratory tract, and liver cancer in workers (IARC 1). See also p 95.	0.01 mg/m³ (as As) A1 OSHA CA NIOSH CA	5 mg/m³ (as As)		Elemental forms vary in appearance. Crystals are gray. Amorphous forms may be yellow or black. Vapor pressure is very low—about 1 mm Hg at 372 °C (701 °F).
Arsine (CAS: 7784-42-1): Extremely toxic hemolytic agent. Symptoms include abdominal pain, jaundice, hemoglobinuria, and renal failure. Low-level chronic exposures reported to cause anemia. See also p 97.	0.05 ppm NIOSH CA	3 ppm	4 4 2	Colorless gas with an unpleasant garliclike odor. Flammable. Breakdown products include arsenic trioxide and arsenic fumes. Used in the semiconductor industry.
Asbestos (chrysotile, amosite, crocidolite, tremolite, anthophyllite): Effects of exposure include asbestosis (fibrosis of the lung), lung cancer, mesothelioma, and possible digestive tract cancer (IARC 1). Signs of toxicity are usually delayed at least 15–30 years. See also p 98.	0.1 fibers/cm³, A1 OSHA CA NIOSH CA			Fibrous materials. Not combustible. TLVs vary with type: amosite, 0.5 fibers/cm³; A1; chrysotile, 2 fibers/cm³, A1; crocidolite, 0.2 fibers/cm³, A1; other forms, 2 fibers/cm³, A1.

Substance	TLV	IDLH	NFPA (H R F)	Comments
Asphalt fumes (CAS: 8052-42-4): Vapors and fumes irritating to eyes, skin, and respiratory tract. Skin contact can produce hyperpigmentation, dermatitis, or photosensitization. Some constituents are carcinogenic in test animals.	5 mg/m³ [proposed: 0.5 mg/m³]			Smoke with an acrid odor. Asphalt is a complex mixture of parrafinic, aromatic, and heterocyclic hydrocarbons formed by the evaporation of lighter hydrocarbons from petroleum and the partial oxidation of the residue.
Atrazine (CAS: 1912-24-9): A triazine herbicide. Minor skin and eye irritant.	5 mg/m³			
Azinphos-methyl (Guthion [CAS: 86-50-0]: Low-potency organophosphate anticholinesterase insecticide (see p 244). Requires metabolic activation.	0.2 mg/m³, S	10 mg/m³		Brown waxy solid with a negligible vapor pressure. Not combustible. Breakdown products include sulfur dioxide, oxides of nitrogen, and phosphoric acid.
Barium and soluble compounds (CAS: 7440-39-3): Powders irritating to eyes, skin, and respiratory tract. Although not typical of workplace exposures, ingestion of soluble barium salts (as opposed to the insoluble medical compounds used in radiography) are associated with muscle paralysis. See also p 103.	0.5 mg/m³ (as Ba)	50 mg/m³ (as Ba)		Most soluble barium compounds (eg, barium chloride, barium carbonate) are odorless white solids. Elemental barium spontaneously ignites on contact with air and reacts with water to form flammable hydrogen gas.
Benomyl (methyl1-[butylcarbamoyl]-2-benzimidazolecarbamate, Benlate [CAS: 17804-35-2]): A carbamate cholinesterase inhibitor (see p 244). Mildly irritating to eyes and skin. Of low systemic toxicity in test animals by all routes. Evidence of adverse effects on fetal development in test animals.	10 mg/m³			White crystalline solid with a negligible vapor pressure at 20 °C (68 °F). Fungicide and miticide. Appearance and some hazardous properties vary with the formulation.
Benzene (CAS: 71-43-2): Vapors mildly irritating to eyes and respiratory tract. Well absorbed by all routes. A CNS depressant at high levels Symptoms include headache, nausea, tremors, cardiac arrhythmias, and coma. Chronic exposure may result in hematopoietic system depression, aplastic anemia, and leukemia (IARC 1). See also p 104.	0.5 ppm, A1, S, OSHA CA, NIOSH CA	500 ppm, ERPG-1: 50 ppm, ERPG-2: 150 ppm, ERPG-3: 1000 ppm	2 3 0	Colorless liquid. Aromatic hydrocarbon odor. Vapor pressure is 75 mm Hg at 20 °C (68 °F). Flammable.

(C) = ceiling air concentration (TLV-C); S = skin absorption can be significant; A1 = ACGIH-confirmed human carcinogen; A2 = ACGIH-suspected human carcinogen; NFPA Hazard Codes: H = health, F = fire, R = reactivity, Ox = oxidizer, W = water-reactive, 0 (none) <—> 4 (severe). ERPG = Emergency Response Planning Guideline. See p 434 for explanation of definitions.

(continued)

TABLE IV–4. HEALTH HAZARD SUMMARIES FOR INDUSTRIAL AND OCCUPATIONAL CHEMICALS (CONTINUED)

Health Hazard Summaries	ACGIH TLV	IDLH	NFPA Codes H F R	Comments
Benzidine (*p*-diaminodiphenyl [CAS: 92-87-5]): Extremely well absorbed by inhalation and through skin. Caused bladder cancer in exposed workers (IARC 1)	S, A1 OSHA CA NIOSH CA			White or reddish solid crystals. Breakdown products include oxides of nitrogen. Found in dye-stuffs, rubber industry, and analytical laboratories.
Benzoyl peroxide (CAS: 94-36-0): Dusts cause skin, eye, and respiratory tract irritation. A skin sensitizer.	5 mg/m³	1500 mg/m³		White granules or crystalline solids with a very faint odor. Vapor pressure is negligible at 20 °C (68 °F). Strong oxidizer, reacting with combustible materials. Decomposes at 75 °C (167 °F). Unstable and explosive at high temperatures.
Benzyl chloride (α-chlorotoluene, [chloro-methyl]benzene [CAS: 100-44-7]): Highly irritating to skin and eyes. A potent lacrimator. Vapors highly irritating to respiratory tract. Symptoms include weakness, headache, and irritability. May injure liver. Limited evidence for carcinogenicity and adverse effects on fetal development in test animals.	1 ppm, A3	10 ppm ERPG-1: 1 ppm ERPG-2: 10 ppm ERPG-3: 25 ppm	3 2 1	Colorless liquid with a pungent odor. Vapor pressure is 0.9 mm Hg at 20 °C (68 °F). Combustible. Breakdown products include phosgene and hydrogen chloride.
Beryllium (CAS: 7440-41-7): Very high acute exposure to dusts and fumes cause eye, skin, and respiratory tract irritation. However, more importantly, chronic low-level exposures to beryllium oxide dusts can produce interstitial lung disease called berylliosis, which is a sarcoid-like condition that can have extrapulmonary manifestations. A carcinogen in test animals. There is limited evidence of carcinogenicity in humans (IARC 1).	0.002 mg/m³, A1 NIOSH CA	4 mg/m³ (as Be) ERPG-2: 25 µg/m³ ERPG-3: 100 µg/m³	3 1 0	Silver-white metal or dusts. Reacts with some acids to produce flammable hydrogen gas.
Biphenyl (diphenyl [CAS: 92-52-4]): Fumes mildly irritating to eyes. Chronic overexposures can cause bronchitis and liver injury. Peripheral neuropathy and CNS injury have also been reported.	0.2 ppm	100 mg/m³	2 1 0	White crystals. Unusual but pleasant odor. Combustible.

Borates (anhydrous sodium tetraborate, borax [CAS: 1303-96-4]): Contact with dusts is highly irritating to eyes, skin, and respiratory tract. Contact with tissue moisture may cause thermal burns because hydration of borates generates heat. See also p 111.

- TLV: 1 mg/m³ (anhydrous and pentahydrate); 5 mg/m³ (decahydrate)
- White or light gray solid crystals. Odorless.

Boron oxide (boric anhydride, boric oxide [CAS: 1303-86-2]): Contact with moisture generates boric acid (see p 111). Direct eye or skin contact with dusts is irritating. Occupational inhalation exposure has caused sore throat and cough. Evidence for adverse effects on the testes in test animals.

- TLV: 10 mg/m³
- IDLH: 2000 mg/m³
- Colorless glassy granules, flakes, or powder. Odorless. Not combustible.

Boron tribromide (CAS: 10294-33-4): Corrosive; decomposed by tissue moisture to hydrogen bromide (see p 115) and boric acid (see p 111). Severe skin and eye burns may result from direct contact. Vapors highly irritating to eyes and respiratory tract.

- TLV: 1 ppm (C)
- NFPA: 3 0 2 W
- Colorless fuming liquid. Reacts with water, forming hydrogen bromide and boric acid. Vapor pressure is 40 mm Hg at 14 °C (57 °F).

Boron trifluoride (CAS: 7637-07-2): Corrosive; decomposed by tissue moisture to hydrogen fluoride (see p 186) and boric acid (see p 111). Severe skin and eye burns may result. Vapors highly irritating to eyes, skin, and respiratory tract.

- TLV: 1 ppm (C)
- IDLH: 25 ppm
- NFPA: 4 0 1
- Colorless gas. Dense white irritating fumes produced on contact with moist air. These fumes contain boric acid and hydrogen fluoride.

Brodifacoum (CAS: 56073-10-1): Long-acting anticoagulant causing hemorrhage. Blocks vitamin K_1-2, 3 epoxide reductase to inhibit vitamin K-dependent clotting factor synthesis. See also p 148.

Bromine (CAS: 7726-95-6): Corrosive; severe skin and eye burns may result. Vapors highly irritating to eyes and respiratory tract; pulmonary edema may result. Measleslike eruptions may appear on the skin several hours after a severe exposure.

- TLV: 0.1 ppm
- IDLH: 3 ppm; ERPG-1: 0.2 ppm; ERPG-2: 1 ppm; ERPG 3: 5 ppm
- NFPA: 3 0 0 Ox
- Heavy red-brown fuming liquid. Odor and irritation thresholds are below the TLV and are adequate warning properties. Vapor pressure is 175 mm Hg at 20 °C (68 °F). Not combustible.

(C) = ceiling air concentration (TLV-C); S = skin absorption can be significant; A1 = ACGIH-confirmed human carcinogen; A2 = ACGIH-suspected human carcinogen; NFPA Hazard Codes: H = health, F = fire, R = reactivity, Ox = oxidizer, W = water-reactive, 0 (none) <—> 4 (severe). ERPG = Emergency Response Planning Guideline. See p 434 for explanation of definitions.

(continued)

TABLE IV–4. HEALTH HAZARD SUMMARIES FOR INDUSTRIAL AND OCCUPATIONAL CHEMICALS (CONTINUED)

Health Hazard Summaries	ACGIH TLV	IDLH	NFPA Codes H F R	Comments
Bromine pentafluoride (CAS: 7789-30-2): Corrosive; severe skin and eye burns may result. Vapors extremely irritating to eyes and respiratory tract. Chronic overexposures caused severe liver and kidney injury in test animals. See also p 129.	0.1 ppm		4 0 3 W, Ox	Pale yellow liquid. Pungent odor. Not combustible. Highly reactive, igniting most organic materials and corroding many metals. Highly reactive with acids. Breakdown products include bromine and fluorine.
Bromoform (tribromomethane [CAS: 75-25-2]): Vapors highly irritating to eyes and respiratory tract. Well absorbed by inhalation and skin contact. CNS depressant. Liver and kidney injury may occur. Two preliminary tests indicate that it may be an animal carcinogen.	0.5 ppm, S, A3	850 ppm		Colorless to yellow liquid. Chloroformlike odor and irritation are adequate warning properties. Vapor pressure is 5 mm Hg at 20 °C (68°F). Not combustible. Thermal breakdown products include hydrogen bromide and bromine.
1,3-Butadiene (CAS: 106-99-0): Vapors mildly irritating. A CNS depressant at very high levels. Evidence of adverse effects on reproductive organs and fetal development in test animals. A very potent carcinogen in test animals; evidence of carcinogenicity in exposed workers (IARC 2A).	2 ppm, A2 NIOSH CA	2000 ppm [LEL] ERPG-1: 10 ppm ERPG-2: 200 ppm ERPG-3: 5000 ppm	2 4 2	Colorless gas. Mild aromatic odor is a good warning property. Readily polymerizes. Inhibitor added to prevent peroxide formation. Used in the formation of styrene-butadiene and ABS plastics.
2-Butoxyethanol (ethylene glycol monobutyl ether, butyl Cellosolve [CAS: 111-76-2]): Liquid very irritating to eyes and slightly irritating to skin. Vapors irritating to eyes and respiratory tract. Mild CNS depressant. A hemolytic agent in test animals. Well absorbed dermally. Liver and kidney toxicity in test animals. Reproductive toxicity much less than certain other glycol ethers such as ethylene glycol monomethyl ether. See also p 166.	25 ppm, S [proposed: 20 ppm]	700 ppm		Colorless liquid with a mild etherlike odor. Irritation occurs below the TLV and is a good warning property. Vapor pressure is 0.6 mm Hg at 20 °C (68 °F). Flammable.
n-Butyl acetate (CAS: 123-86-4): Vapors irritating to eyes and respiratory tract. A CNS depressant at high levels. Limited evidence for adverse effects on fetal development in test animals.	150 ppm	1700 ppm [LEL]	1 3 0	Colorless liquid. Fruity odor is a good warning property. Vapor pressure is 10 mm Hg at 20 °C (68 °F). Flammable.

Substance	TLV	Other limit	H	F	R	Comments
sec-Butyl acetate (2-butanol acetate) [CAS: 105-46-4]: Vapors irritating to eyes and respiratory tract. A CNS depressant at high levels.	200 ppm	1700 ppm [LEL]	1	3	0	
tert-Butyl acetate (tert-butyl ester of acetic acid [CAS: 540-88-5]): Vapors irritating to eyes and respiratory tract. A CNS depressant at high levels.	200 ppm	1500 ppm [LEL]				
n-Butyl acrylate (CAS: 141-32-2): Highly irritating to skin and eyes; corneal necrosis may result. Vapors highly irritating to eyes and respiratory tract. Based on structural analogies, compounds containing the acrylate moiety may be carcinogens (IARC 3).	10 ppm [proposed: 5 ppm]	ERPG-1: 0.05 ppm / ERPG-2: 25 ppm / ERPG-3: 250 ppm	2	2	2	Colorless liquid. Vapor pressure is 3.2 mm Hg at 20 °C (68 °F). Flammable. Contains inhibitor to prevent polymerization.
n-Butyl alcohol (CAS: 71-36-3): Irritating upon direct contact. Vapors mildly irritating to eyes and respiratory tract. A CNS depressant at very high levels. Chronic occupational overexposures associated with hearing loss and vestibular impairment.	50 ppm (C), S [proposed: 25 ppm (C)]	1400 ppm [LEL]	1	3	0	Colorless liquid. Strong odor and irritation occur below the TLV and are both good warning properties. Flammable.
sec-Butyl alcohol (CAS: 78-92-2): Vapors mildly irritating to eyes and respiratory tract. A CNS depressant at high levels.	100 ppm	2000 ppm	1	3	0	Colorless liquid. Pleasant odor occurs well below the TLV and is an adequate warning property. Vapor pressure is 13 mm Hg at 20 °C (68 °F). Flammable.
tert-Butyl alcohol (CAS: 75-65-0): Vapors mildly irritating to eyes and respiratory tract. A CNS depressant at high levels.	100 ppm	1600 ppm	1	3	0	Colorless liquid. Camphorlike odor and irritation occur slightly below the TLV and are good warning properties. Vapor pressure is 31 mm Hg at 20 °C (68 °F). Flammable.
Butylamine (CAS: 109-73-9): Caustic alkali. Liquid highly irritating to eyes and skin upon direct contact; severe burns may result. Vapors highly irritating to eyes and respiratory tract. May cause histamine release.	5 ppm (C), S	300 ppm	3	3	0	Colorless liquid. Ammonia or fishlike odor occurs below the TLV and is an adequate warning property. Vapor pressure is about 82 mm Hg at 20 °C (68 °F). Flammable.

(C) = ceiling air concentration (TLV-C); S = skin absorption can be significant; A1 = ACGIH-confirmed human carcinogen; A2 = ACGIH-suspected human carcinogen; NFPA Hazard Codes: H = health, F = fire, R = reactivity, Ox = oxidizer, W = water-reactive, 0 (none) <—> 4 (severe). ERPG = Emergency Response Planning Guideline. See p 434 for explanation of definitions.

(continued)

TABLE IV-4. HEALTH HAZARD SUMMARIES FOR INDUSTRIAL AND OCCUPATIONAL CHEMICALS (CONTINUED)

Health Hazard Summaries	ACGIH TLV	IDLH	NFPA Codes H F R	Comments
***tert*-Butyl chromate (CAS: 1189-85-1):** Liquid highly irritating to eyes and skin; severe burns may result. Vapors or mists irritating to eyes and respiratory tract. A liver and kidney toxin. By analogy to other Cr(VI) compounds, a possible carcinogen. See also p 139.	0.1 mg/m³ (C) (as CrO₃) NIOSH CA S	15 mg/m³ (as Cr VI)		Liquid. Reacts with moisture.
***n*-Butyl glycidyl ether (BGE, glycidylbutylether, 1,2-epoxy-3-butoxy propane [CAS: 2426-08-6]):** Liquid irritating to eyes and skin. Vapors irritating to the respiratory tract. A CNS depressant. Causes sensitization dermatitis upon repeated exposures. Testicular atrophy and hematopoietic injury at modest doses in test animals.	25 ppm	250 ppm		Colorless liquid. Vapor pressure is 3 mm Hg at 20 °C (68 °F).
***n*-Butyl lactate (CAS: 138-22-7):** Vapors irritating to eyes and respiratory tract. Workers have complained of sleepiness, headache, coughing, nausea, and vomiting.	5 ppm		1 2 0	Colorless liquid. Vapor pressure is 0.4 mm Hg at 20 °C (68 °F). Combustible.
***n*-Butyl mercaptan (butanethiol [CAS: 109-79-5]):** Vapors mildly irritating to eyes and respiratory tract. Pulmonary edema occurred at high exposure levels in test animals. A CNS depressant at very high levels. Limited evidence for adverse effects on fetal development in test animals at high doses.	0.5 ppm [proposed: 5 ppm]	500 ppm	2 3 0	Colorless liquid. Strong, offensive garliclike odor. Vapor pressure is 35 mm Hg at 20 °C (68 °F). Flammable.
***o*-sec-Butylphenol (CAS: 89-72-5):** Irritating to skin upon direct, prolonged contact; burns have resulted. Vapors mildly irritating to eyes and respiratory tract.	5 ppm, S			A liquid.
***p*-tert-Butyltoluene (CAS: 98-51-1):** Mild skin irritant upon direct contact. Defatting agent causing dermatitis. Vapors irritating to eyes and respiratory tract. A CNS depressant. Limited evidence of adverse effects on fetal development in test animals at high doses.	1 ppm	100 ppm		Colorless liquid. Gasolinelike odor and irritation occur below the TLV and are both good warning properties. Vapor pressure is less than 1 mm Hg at 20 °C (68 °F). Combustible.

Substance	Exposure limits	NFPA codes	Comments / Properties
Cadmium and compounds: Acute fumes and dust exposures can injure the respiratory tract; pulmonary edema can occur. Chronic exposures associated primarily with kidney injury and lung injury. Adverse effects on the testes and on fetal development in test animals. Cadmium and some of its compounds are carcinogenic in test animals. Limited direct evidence for carcinogenicity in humans (IARC 2A). See also p 117.	0.01 mg/m³ (total dust, as Cd) 0.002 mg/m³ (respirable dust, as Cd) 9 mg/m³ (dust and fumes, as Cd) A2 NIOSH CA		Compounds vary in color. Give off fumes when heated or burned. Generally poor warning properties. Metal has a vapor pressure of about 1 mm Hg at 394 °C (741 °F) and reacts with acids to produce flammable hydrogen gas.
Calcium cyanamide (calcium carbimide, lime nitrogen [CAS: 156-62-7]): Dusts highly irritating to eyes, skin, and respiratory tract. Causes sensitization dermatitis. Systemic symptoms include nausea, fatigue, headache, chest pain, and shivering. A disulfiramlike interaction with alcohol (see p 158), "cyanamide flush," may occur in exposed workers.	0.5 mg/m³		Gray crystalline material. Reacts with water, generating ammonia and flammable acetylene.
Calcium hydroxide (hydrated lime, caustic lime [CAS: 1305-62-0]): Corrosive (see p 129); severe eye and skin burns may result. Dusts moderately irritating to eyes and respiratory tract.	5 mg/m³		White, deliquescent crystalline powder. Odorless.
Calcium oxide (lime, quicklime, burnt lime [CAS: 1305-78-8]): Corrosive (see p 129). Exothermic reactions with moisture. Highly irritating to eyes and skin upon direct contact. Dusts highly irritating to skin, eyes, and respiratory tract.	2 mg/m³	3 0 1	White or gray solid powder. Odorless. Hydration generates heat.
Camphor, synthetic (CAS: 76-22-2): Irritating to eyes and skin upon direct contact. Vapors irritating to eyes and nose; may cause loss of sense of smell. A convulsant at doses typical of overdose ingestion, rather than industrial exposure. See also p 122.	2 ppm	0 2 0	Colorless glassy solid. Sharp, obnoxious, aromatic odor near the TLV is an adequate warning property. Vapor pressure is 0.18 mm Hg at 20 °C (68 °F). Combustible.
Caprolactam (CAS: 105-60-2): Highly irritating to eyes and skin upon direct contact. Vapors, dusts, and fumes highly irritating to eyes and respiratory tract. Convulsant activity in test animals.	1 mg/m³ (dust) 5 ppm (vapor) [proposed: 5 mg/m³ (aerosol and vapor)]		White solid crystals. Unpleasant odor. Vapor pressure is 6 mm Hg at 120 °C (248 °F). Thermal breakdown products include oxides of nitrogen.

(C) = ceiling air concentration (TLV-C); S = skin absorption can be significant; A1 = ACGIH-confirmed human carcinogen; A2 = ACGIH-suspected human carcinogen; NFPA Hazard Codes: H = health, F = fire, R = reactivity, Ox = oxidizer, W = water-reactive, 0 (none) <—> 4 (severe); ERPG = Emergency Response Planning Guideline. See p 434 for explanation of definitions.

(continued)

TABLE IV–4. HEALTH HAZARD SUMMARIES FOR INDUSTRIAL AND OCCUPATIONAL CHEMICALS (CONTINUED)

Health Hazard Summaries	ACGIH TLV	IDLH	NFPA Codes H F R	Comments
Captafol (Difolatan [CAS: 2425-06-1]): Dusts irritating to eyes, skin, and respiratory tract. A skin and respiratory tract sensitizer. May cause photoallergic dermatitis. Evidence for carcinogenicity in animal tests (IARC 2A).	0.1 mg/m³, S			White solid crystals. Distinctive, pungent odor. Fungicide. Thermal breakdown products include hydrogen chloride and oxides of nitrogen or sulfur.
Carbaryl (1-naphthyl N-methylcarbamate, Sevin [CAS: 63-25-2]): A carbamate-type cholinesterase inhibitor (see p 244). Evidence of adverse effects on fetal development in test animals at high doses.	5 mg/m³	100 mg/m³		Colorless, white or gray solid. Odorless. Vapor pressure is 0.005 mm Hg at 20 °C (68 °F). Breakdown products include oxides of nitrogen and methylamine.
Carbofuran (2,3-dihydro-2,2′-dimethyl-7-benzofuranylmethylcarbamate, Furadan [CAS: 1563-66-2]): A carbamate-type cholinesterase inhibitor (see p 244). Not well absorbed by skin contact.	0.1 mg/m³			White solid crystals. Odorless. Vapor pressure is 0.00005 mm Hg at 33 °C (91 °F). Thermal breakdown products include oxides of nitrogen.
Carbon black [CAS: 1333-86-4]: Causes eye and respiratory irritation. A lung carcinogen in test animals (IARC 2B).	3.5 mg/m³ NIOSH CA			Extremely fine powdery forms of elemental carbon; may have adsorbed polycyclic organic hydrocarbons.
Carbon disulfide [CAS: 75-15-0]: Vapors mildly irritating to eyes and respiratory tract. A CNS depressant causing coma at high concentrations. Well absorbed by all routes. Acute symptoms include headache, dizziness, nervousness, and fatigue. Neuropathies, parkinsonianlike syndromes, and psychosis may occur. A liver and kidney toxin. An atherogenic agent causing stroke and heart disease. Adversely affects male and female reproductive systems in test animals and humans. Evidence for adverse effects on fetal development in test animals.	10 ppm, S	500 ppm ERPG-1: 1 ppm ERPG-2: 50 ppm ERPG-3: 500 ppm	3 3 0	Colorless to pale yellow liquid. Disagreeable odor occurs below the TLV and is a good warning property. Vapor pressure is 300 mm Hg at 20 °C (68 °F). Highly flammable. Major use in viscose rayon manufacture but its also used in chemical synthesis and as an industrial solvent.

Substance	TLV / exposure	ERPG / other	NFPA (H F R)	Physical properties / comments
Carbon monoxide (CAS: 630-08-0): Binds to hemoglobin, forming carboxyhemoglobin and causing cellular hypoxia. Persons with heart disease are more susceptible. Signs and symptoms include headache, dizziness, coma, and convulsions. Permanent CNS impairment and adverse effects on fetal development may occur after severe poisoning. See also p 125.	25 ppm	1200 ppm	3 4 0	Colorless, odorless gas. No warning properties. Important sources of exposure include indoor use of internal combustion engines, structural fires, and faulty space heaters.
Carbon tetrabromide (CAS: 558-13-4): Highly irritating to eyes upon direct contact. Vapors highly irritating to eyes and respiratory tract. The liver and kidneys are also likely target organs.	0.1 ppm			White to yellow-brown solid. Vapor pressure is 40 mm Hg at 96 °C (204 °F). Nonflammable; thermal breakdown products may include hydrogen bromide and bromine.
Carbon tetrachloride (tetrachloromethane [CAS 56-23-5]): Mildly irritating upon direct contact. A CNS depressant. May cause cardiac arrhythmias. Highly toxic to kidney and liver. Alcohol abuse increases risk of liver toxicity. A carcinogen in test animals (IARC 2B). See also p 127.	5 ppm, S, A2 NIOSH CA	200 ppm ERPG-1: 20 ppm ERPG-2: 100 ppm ERPG-3: 750 ppm	3 0 0	Colorless. Etherlike odor is a poor warning property. Vapor pressure is 91 mm Hg at 20 °C (68 °F). Not combustible. Breakdown products include hydrogen chloride, chlorine gas, and phosgene.
Carbonyl fluoride (COF$_2$ [CAS: 353-50-4]): Extremely irritating to eyes and respiratory tract; pulmonary edema may result. Toxicity results from its hydrolysis to hydrofluoric acid (see p 186).	2 ppm			Colorless, odorless gas. Decomposes upon contact with water to produce hydrofluoric acid.
Catechol (1,2-benzenediol [CAS: 120-80-9]): Highly irritating upon direct contact; severe eye and deep skin burns result. Well absorbed by skin. Systemic toxicity similar to that of phenol (see p 255); however, catechol may be more likely to cause convulsions and hypertension. At high doses, renal and liver injury may occur.	5 ppm, S, A3			Colorless solid crystals.
Cesium hydroxide (cesium hydrate [CAS: 21351-79-1]): Corrosive (see p 129). Highly irritating upon direct contact; severe burns may result. Dusts are irritating to eyes and respiratory tract.	2 mg/m^3			Colorless or yellow crystals that absorb moisture. Negligible vapor pressure.

(C) = ceiling air concentration (TLV-C); S = skin absorption can be significant; A1 = ACGIH-confirmed human carcinogen; A2 = ACGIH-suspected human carcinogen; NFPA Hazard Codes: H = health, F = fire, R = reactivity, Ox = oxidizer, W = water-reactive, 0 (none) <——> 4 (severe), ERPG = Emergency Response Planning Guideline. See p 434 for explanation of definitions.

(continued)

TABLE IV–4. HEALTH HAZARD SUMMARIES FOR INDUSTRIAL AND OCCUPATIONAL CHEMICALS (CONTINUED)

Health Hazard Summaries	ACGIH TLV	IDLH	NFPA Codes H F R	Comments
Chlordane (CAS: 57-74-9): Irritating to skin. A CNS convulsant. Skin absorption is rapid and has caused convulsions and death. Hepatotoxic. Evidence of carcinogenicity in test animals (IARC 2B). See also p 133.	0.5 mg/m³, S, A3	100 mg/m³		Viscous amber liquid. Formulations vary in appearance. A chlorinelike odor. Vapor pressure is 0.00001 mm Hg at 20 °C (68 °F). Not combustible. Thermal breakdown products include hydrogen chloride, phosgene, and chlorine gas. EPA banned this insecticide in 1976.
Chlorinated camphene (toxaphene [CAS: 8001-35-2]): Moderately irritating upon direct contact. A CNS convulsant. Acute symptoms include nausea, confusion, tremors, and convulsions. Well absorbed by skin. Potential liver and kidney injury. See also p 133.	0.5 mg/m³, S, A3	200 mg/m³		Waxy amber-colored solid. Formulations vary in appearance. Turpentinelike odor. Vapor pressure is about 0.3 mm Hg at 20 °C (68 °F).
Chlorinated diphenyl oxide (CAS: 55720-99-5): Chloracne may result from even small exposures. A hepatotoxin in chronically exposed test animals. Signs and symptoms include gastrointestinal upset, jaundice, and fatigue.	0.5 mg/m³	5 mg/m³		Waxy solid or liquid. Vapor pressure is 0.00006 mm Hg at 20 °C (68 °F).
Chlorine (CAS: 7782-50-5): Extremely irritating to eyes, skin, and respiratory tract; severe burns and pulmonary edema may occur. Symptoms include lacrimation, sore throat, headache, coughing, and wheezing. High concentrations may cause rapid tissue swelling and airway obstruction through laryngeal edema. See also p 134.	0.5 ppm	10 ppm ERPG-1: 1 ppm ERPG-2: 3 ppm ERPG-3: 20 ppm	4 0 0 Ox	Amber liquid or greenish-yellow gas. Irritating odor and irritation occur near the TLV and are both good warning properties. Can be formed when acid cleaners are mixed with hypochlorite bleach cleaners.
Chlorine dioxide (chlorine peroxide [CAS: 10049-04-4]): Extremely irritating to eyes and respiratory tract. Symptoms and signs are those of chlorine gas above (see p 134).	0.1 ppm	5 ppm		Yellow-green or orange gas or liquid. Sharp odor at the TLV is a good warning property. Reacts with water to produce perchloric acid. Decomposes explosively in sunlight, with heat, or with shock to produce chlorine gas. Bleaching agent widely used in paper industry.

Substance	Exposure limit	ERPG	NFPA Codes	Comments
Chlorine trifluoride (chlorine fluoride [CAS: 7790-91-2]): Upon contact with moist tissues, hydrolyzes to chlorine (see p 134), hydrogen fluoride (see p 186), and chlorine dioxide. Extremely irritating to eyes, skin, and respiratory tract; severe burns or delayed pulmonary edema could result.	0.1 ppm (C)	20 ppm ERPG-1: 0.1 ppm ERPG-2: 1 ppm ERPG-3: 10 ppm	4 0 3 W, Ox	Greenish-yellow or colorless liquid or gas, or white solid. Possesses a suffocating, sweet odor. Not combustible. Water-reactive, yielding hydrogen fluoride and chlorine gas. Used as incendiary and rocket fuel additive.
Chloroacetaldehyde (CAS: 107-20-0): Extremely corrosive upon direct contact; severe burns will result. Vapors extremely irritating to eyes, skin, and respiratory tract.	1 ppm (C)	45 ppm ERPG-1: 0.1 ppm ERPG-2: 1.0 ppm ERPG-3: 10 ppm		Colorless liquid with a pungent, irritating odor. Vapor pressure is 100 mm Hg at 20 °C (68 °F). Combustible. Readily polymerizes. Thermal breakdown products include phosgene and hydrogen chloride.
α-Chloroacetophenone (tear gas, chemical Mace [CAS: 532-27-4]): Extremely irritating to mucous membranes and respiratory tract. With extremely high inhalational exposures, lower respiratory injury is possible. A potent skin sensitizer. See also p 181.	0.05 ppm	15 mg/m³	2 1 0	Sharp, irritating odor and irritation occur near the TLV and are adequate warning properties. Vapor pressure is 0.012 mm Hg at 20 °C (68 °F). Mace is a common crowd control agent.
Chlorobenzene (monochlorobenzene [CAS: 108-90-7]): Irritating; skin burns may result from prolonged contact. Vapors irritating to eyes and respiratory tract. A CNS depressant. May cause methemoglobinemia (see p 220). Prolonged exposure to high levels has caused lung, liver, and kidney injury in test animals.	10 ppm, A3	1000 ppm	2 3 0	Colorless liquid. Aromatic odor occurs below the TLV and is a good warning property. Vapor pressure is 8.8 mm Hg at 20 °C (68 °F). Flammable. Thermal breakdown products include hydrogen chloride and and phosgene.
o-Chlorobenzylidene malononitrile (tear gas, OCBM, CS [CAS: 2698-41-11]): Highly irritating on direct contact; severe burns may result. Aerosols and vapors very irritating to mucous membranes and upper respiratory tract. With extremely high inhalational exposures, lower respiratory injury is possible. Potent skin sensitizer. Symptoms include headache, nausea and vomiting, severe eye and nose irritation, excess salivation, and coughing. See also p 181.	0.05 ppm (C), S	2 mg/m³		White solid crystals. Pepperlike odor. Vapor pressure is much less than 1 mm Hg at 20 °C (68 °F). CS is a common crowd control agent.

(C) = ceiling air concentration (TLV-C); S = skin absorption can be significant; A1 = ACGIH-confirmed human carcinogen; A2 = ACGIH-suspected human carcinogen; NFPA Hazard Codes: H = health, F = fire, R = reactivity, Ox = oxidizer, W = water-reactive, 0 (none) <—> 4 (severe); ERPG = Emergency Response Planning Guideline. See p 434 for explanation of definitions.

(continued)

TABLE IV–4. HEALTH HAZARD SUMMARIES FOR INDUSTRIAL AND OCCUPATIONAL CHEMICALS (CONTINUED)

Health Hazard Summaries	ACGIH TLV	IDLH	NFPA Codes H F R	Comments
Chlorobromomethane (bromochloromethane, Halon 1011 [CAS: 74-97-5]): Irritating upon direct contact. Vapors mildly irritating to eyes and respiratory tract. A CNS depressant. Disorientation, nausea, headache, seizures, and coma have been reported at high exposure. Chronic high doses caused liver and kidney injury in test animals.	200 ppm	2000 ppm		Colorless to pale yellow liquid. Sweet, pleasant odor detectable far below the TLV. Vapor pressure is 117 mm Hg at 20 °C (68 °F). Thermal breakdown products include hydrogen chloride, hydrogen bromide, and phosgene.
Chlorodifluoromethane (Freon 22 [CAS: 75-45-6]): Irritating upon direct contact. Vapors mildly irritating to eyes and respiratory tract. A CNS depressant. Vapors may cause arrhythmias. There is evidence at high doses for adverse effects on fetal development in test animals. See also p 178.	1000 ppm			Colorless, almost odorless gas. Nonflammable. Thermal breakdown products may include hydrogen fluoride.
Chloroform (trichloromethane [CAS: 67-66-3]): Mildly irritating upon direct contact; dermatitis may result from prolonged exposure. Vapors slightly irritating to eyes and respiratory tract. A CNS depressant. High levels (15,000–20,000 ppm) can cause coma and cardiac arrhythmias. Can produce liver and kidney damage. Limited evidence of adverse effects on fetal development in test animals. A carcinogen in test animals (IARC 2B). See also p 136.	10 ppm, A3 NIOSH CA	500 ppm	2 0 0	Colorless liquid. Pleasant, sweet odor. Not combustible. Vapor pressure is 160 mm Hg at 20 °C (68 °F). Breakdown products include hydrogen chloride, phosgene, and chlorine gas.
bis(Chloromethyl) ether (BCME [CAS: 542-88-1]): A human and animal carcinogen (IARC 1).	0.001 ppm, A1 OSHA CA NIOSH CA			Colorless liquid with a suffocating odor. Vapor pressure is 100 mm Hg at 20 °C (68 °F). Used in the manufacture of ion-exchange resins.
Chloromethyl methyl ether (CMME, methyl chloromethyl ether [CAS: 107-30-2]): Vapors irritating to eyes and respiratory tract. Workers show increased risk of lung cancer, possibly owing to contamination of CMME with 1–7% BCME. (See above)	A2 OSHA CA NIOSH CA		3 3 2	Combustible. Breakdown products include oxides of nitrogen and hydrogen chloride. Used in the manufacture of ion-exchange resins.
1-Chloro-1-nitropropane (CAS: 600-25-9): Based on animal studies, vapors highly irritating to eyes and respiratory tract and may cause pulmonary edema. High levels may cause injury to cardiac muscle, liver, and kidney.	2 ppm	100 ppm	– 2 3	Colorless liquid. Unpleasant odor and tearing occur near the TLV and are good warning properties. Vapor pressure is 5.8 mm Hg at 20 °C (68 °F).

Chloropentafluoroethane (fluorocarbon 115 [CAS: 76-15-3]): Irritating upon direct contact. Vapors mildly irritating to eyes and respiratory tract. Produces coma and cardiac arrhythmias, but only at very high levels in test animals. See also p 178.

1000 ppm

Colorless, odorless gas. Thermal breakdown products include hydrogen fluoride and hydrogen chloride.

Chloropicrin (trichloronitromethane [CAS: 76-06-2]): Extremely irritating upon direct contact; severe burns may result. Vapors extremely irritating to eyes, skin, and respiratory tract; delayed pulmonary edema has been reported. Kidney and liver injuries have been observed in test animals.

0.1 ppm
ERPG-2: 0.2 ppm
ERPG-3: 3 ppm

4   0   3

Colorless, oily liquid. Sharp, penetrating odor and tearing occur near the TLV and are good warning properties. Vapor pressure is 20 mm Hg at 20 °C (68 °F). Breakdown products include oxides of nitrogen, phosgene, nitrosyl chloride, and chlorine gas. Used in fumigants.

β-Chloroprene (2-chloro-1,3-butadiene [CAS: 126-99-8]): Irritating upon direct contact. Vapors irritating to eyes and respiratory tract. A CNS depressant at high levels. Liver and kidneys are major target organs. Limited evidence for adverse effects on fetal development and male reproduction in test animals. Equivocal evidence of carcinogenicity in test animals (IARC 3).

10 ppm,
S
NIOSH CA

300 ppm

2   3   0

Colorless liquid with an etherlike odor. Vapor pressure is 179 mm Hg at 20 °C (68 °F). Highly flammable. Breakdown products include hydrogen chloride. Used in making neoprene.

---

o-Chlorotoluene (2-chloro-1-methylbenzene [CAS: 95-49-8]): In test animals, direct contact produced skin and eye irritation; high vapor exposures resulted in tremors, convulsions, and coma. By analogy to toluene and chlorinated compounds, may cause cardiac arrhythmias.

50 ppm

2   2   0

Colorless liquid. Vapor pressure is 10 mm Hg at 43 °C (109 °F). Flammable.

Chlorpyrifos (Dursban, O,O-diethyl-O-(3,5,6-trichloro-2-pyridinyl [CAS: 2921-88-2]): An organophosphate-type cholinesterase inhibitor (see p 244).

0.2 mg/m³,
S

White solid crystals. Vapor pressure is 0.00002 mm Hg at 25 °C (77 °F).

(continued)

(C) = ceiling air concentration (TLV-C); S = skin absorption can be significant; A1 = ACGIH-confirmed human carcinogen; A2 = ACGIH-suspected human carcinogen; NFPA Hazard Codes: H = health, F = fire, R = reactivity, Ox = oxidizer, W = water-reactive, 0 (none) <—> 4 (severe). ERPG = Emergency Response Planning Guideline. See p 434 for explanation of definitions.

TABLE IV–4. HEALTH HAZARD SUMMARIES FOR INDUSTRIAL AND OCCUPATIONAL CHEMICALS (CONTINUED)

Health Hazard Summaries	ACGIH TLV	IDLH	NFPA Codes H F R	Comments
Chromic acid and chromates (chromium trioxide, sodium dichromate, potassium chromate): Highly irritating upon direct contact; severe eye and skin ulceration (chrome ulcers) may result. Dusts and mists highly irritating to eyes and respiratory tract. Skin and respiratory sensitization (asthma) may occur. Chromium trioxide is a teratogen in test animals. Certain hexavalent chromium compounds are carcinogenic in test animals and humans (IARC 1). See also p 139.	0.5 mg/m³ (Cr III compounds) 0.05 mg/m³, A1 (water-soluble Cr VI, compounds) 0.01 mg/m³, A1 (insoluble Cr IV compounds)	15 mg/m³ (Cr VI)		Soluble chromate compounds are water-reactive.
Chromium metal and insoluble chromium salts: Irritating upon direct contact with skin and eyes; dermatitis may result. Ferrochrome alloys possibly associated with pneumoconiotic changes. See also p 139.	0.5 mg/m³ (metal, as Cr) 0.01 mg/m³, A1 (Cr VI compounds, as Cr)	250 mg/m³ (Cr II compounds) 25 mg/m³ (Cr III compounds) 250 mg/m³ (Cr metal)		Chromium metal, silver luster; copper chromite, greenish-blue solid. Odorless.
Chromyl chloride (CAS: 14977-61-8): Hydrolyzes upon contact with moisture to produce chromic trioxide, HCl, chromic trichloride, and chlorine. Highly irritating upon direct contact; severe burns may result. Mists and vapors highly irritating to eyes and respiratory tract. Certain hexavalent chromium VI compounds are carcinogenic in test animals and humans. See also p 139.	0.025 ppm NIOSH CA			Dark red fuming liquid. Water-reactive, yielding hydrogen chloride, chlorine gas, chromic acid, and chromic chloride.
Coal tar pitch volatiles (particulate polycyclic aromatic hydrocarbons [CAS: 65996-93-2]): Irritating upon direct contact. Contact dermatitis, acne, hypermelanosis, and photosensitization may occur. Fumes irritating to eyes and respiratory tract. A carcinogen in test animals and humans.	0.2 mg/m³, A1 NIOSH CA	80 mg/m³		A complex mixture composed of a high percentage of polycyclic aromatic hydrocarbons. A smoky odor. Combustible. Creosote is an important source of exposure.

	TLV	IDLH	Comments
Cobalt and compounds: Irritating upon direct contact; dermatitis and skin sensitization may occur. Fumes and dusts irritate the respiratory tract; chronic interstitial pneumonitis and respiratory tract sensitization reported. Cardiotoxicity associated with occupational exposures. Evidence of carcinogenicity in test animals (IARC 2B).	0.02 mg/m³ (elemental and inorganic compounds, as Co), A3	20 mg/m³ (as Co)	Elemental cobalt is a black or gray, odorless solid with a negligible vapor pressure. "Hard metal" used in specialty grinding and cutting is a tungsten carbide-cobalt amalgam.
Cobalt hydrocarbonyl (CAS: 16842-03-8): In animal testing, overexposure produces symptoms similar to those of nickel carbonyl and iron pentacarbonyl. Effects include headache, nausea, vomiting, dizziness, fever, and pulmonary edema.	0.1 mg/m3 (as Co)		Flammable gas.
Copper fumes, dusts, and salts: Irritation upon direct contact varies with the compound. The salts are more irritating and can cause corneal ulceration. Allergic contact dermatitis is rare. Dusts and mists irritating to the respiratory tract; nasal ulceration has been described. A syndrome like metal fume fever (see p 146) can result from over-exposure to fumes or fine dusts.	0.2 mg/m³ (fume) 1 mg/m³ (dust & mists) [proposed: 0.05 mg/m³ (fume & respirable particulate); 1 mg/m³ (inhalable particulate, dust & mists)]	100 mg/m³ (as Cu)	Salts vary in color. Generally odorless.
Cotton dust: Chronic exposure causes a respiratory syndrome called byssinosis. Symptoms include cough and wheezing, typically appearing on the first day of the workweek and continuing for a few days or all week, although they may subside within an hour after leaving work. Can lead to irreversible obstructive airway disease.	0.2 mg/m³	100 mg/m³	Cotton textile manufacture is the principal source of exposure.

(C) = ceiling air concentration (TLV-C); S = skin absorption can be significant; A1 = ACGIH-confirmed human carcinogen; A2 = ACGIH-suspected human carcinogen; NFPA Hazard Codes: H = health, F = fire, R = reactivity, Ox = oxidizer, W = water-reactive, 0 (none) <—> 4 (severe). ERPG = Emergency Response Planning Guideline. See p 434 for explanation of definitions.

(continued)

TABLE IV–4. HEALTH HAZARD SUMMARIES FOR INDUSTRIAL AND OCCUPATIONAL CHEMICALS (CONTINUED)

Health Hazard Summaries	ACGIH TLV	IDLH	NFPA Codes H F R	Comments
Creosote (coal tar creosote [CAS: 8001-58-9]): A primary irritant, photosensitizer, and corrosive. Direct eye contact can cause severe keratitis and corneal scarring. Prolonged skin contact can cause chemical acne, pigmentation changes, and severe penetrating burns. Exposure to the fumes or vapors causes irritation of mucous membranes and the respiratory tract. Systemic toxicity results from phenolic and cresolic constituents. Liver and kidney injury may occur with heavy exposure. A carcinogen in test animals. Some evidence for carcinogenicity in humans (IARC 2A). See also phenol, p 255.	NIOSH CA		2 2 0	Oily, dark liquid. Appearance and some hazardous properties vary with the formulation. Sharp, penetrating smoky odor. Combustible. Creosote is produced by the fractional distillation of coal tar. See entry on coal tar pitch volatiles.
Cresol (methylphenol, cresylic acid, hydroxymethylbenzene [CAS: 1319-77-3]): Corrosive. Skin and eye contact can cause severe burns. Exposure may be prolonged owing to local anesthetic action on skin. Well absorbed by all routes. Dermal absorption is a major route of systemic poisoning. Induces methemoglobinemia (see p 220). CNS depressant. Symptoms include headache, nausea and vomiting, tinnitus, dizziness, weakness, and confusion. Severe lung, liver and kidney injury may occur. See also phenol, p 255.	5 ppm, S	250 ppm	3 2 0 (*ortho*) 3 2 0 (*meta, para*)	Colorless, yellow, or pink liquid with a phenolic odor. Vapor pressure is 0.2 mm Hg at 20 °C (68 °F). Combustible.
Crotonaldehyde (2-butenal [CAS: 4170-30-3]): Highly irritating upon direct contact; severe burns may result. Vapors highly irritating to eyes and respiratory tract; delayed pulmonary edema may occur. Evidence for carcinogenicity in test animals.	0.3 ppm (C) S, A3	50 ppm ERPG-1: 2 ppm ERPG-2: 10 ppm ERPG-3: 50 ppm	4 3 2	Colorless to straw-colored liquid. Pungent, irritating odor occurs below the TLV and is an adequate warning property. A warning agent added to fuel gases. Vapor pressure is 30 mm Hg at 20 °C (68 °F). Flammable. Polymerizes when heated.
Crufomate (4-*tert*-butyl-2-chlorophenyl *N*-methyl *O*-methylphosphoramidate [CAS: 299-86-5]): An organophosphate cholinesterase inhibitor (see p 244).	5 mg/m³			Crystals or yellow oil. Pungent odor. Flammable.

Compound		NFPA Codes	Comments
Cumene (isopropylbenzene) [CAS: 98-82-8]: Mildly irritating upon direct contact. A CNS depressant at moderate levels. Well absorbed through skin. Adverse effects in fetal development in rats at high doses.	50 ppm, S — 900 ppm [LEL]	2 3 1	Colorless liquid. Sharp, aromatic odor below the TLV is a good warning property. Vapor pressure is 8 mm Hg at 20 °C (68 °F). Flammable.
Cyanamide (carbodiimide) [CAS: 420-04-2]: Causes transient vasomotor flushing. Highly irritating and caustic to eyes and skin. Has a disulfiramlike interaction with alcohol, producing flushing, headache, and dyspnea (see p 158).	2 mg/m^3	4 1 3	Combustible. Thermal breakdown products include oxides of nitrogen.
Cyanide salts (sodium cyanide, potassium cyanide): Potent and rapidly fatal metabolic asphyxiants that inhibit cytochrome oxidase and stop cellular respiration. Well absorbed through skin; caustic action can promote dermal absorption. See also p 150.	5 mg/m^3 (C) (as cyanide), S — 25 mg/m^3 (as cyanide)		Solids. Mild, almondlike odor. In presence of moisture or acids, hydrogen cyanide may be released. Odor is a poor indicator of exposure to hydrogen cyanide. May be generated in fires from the pyrolysis of such products as polyurethane and polyacrylonitrile.
Cyanogen (dicyan, oxalonitrile [CAS: 460-19-5]): Hydrolyzes to release hydrogen cyanide and cyanic acid. Toxicity similar to that of hydrogen cyanide (see p 150). Vapors irritating to eyes and respiratory tract.	10 ppm	4 4 2	Colorless gas. Pungent, almondlike odor. Breaks down on contact with water to yield hydrogen cyanide and cyanate. Flammable.
Cyanogen chloride (CAS: 506-77-4): Vapors extremely irritating to eyes and respiratory tract; pulmonary edema may result. Cyanide interferes with cellular respiration (see p 150).	0.3 ppm (C)		Colorless liquid or gas with a pungent odor. Thermal breakdown products include hydrogen cyanide and hydrogen chloride. Formed by a reaction with hypochlorite in the treatment of cyanide-containing waste water.
Cyclohexane (CAS: 110-82-7): Mildly irritating upon direct contact. Vapors irritating to eyes and respiratory tract. A CNS depressant at high levels. Chronically exposed test animals developed liver and kidney injury.	300 ppm [proposed: 200 ppm] — 1300 ppm [LEL]	1 3 0	Colorless liquid with a sweet, chloroformlike odor. Vapor pressure is 95 mm Hg at 20 °C (68 °F). Highly flammable.

(C) = ceiling air concentration (TLV-C); S = skin absorption can be significant; A1 = ACGIH-confirmed human carcinogen; A2 = ACGIH-suspected human carcinogen; NFPA Hazard Codes: H = health, F = fire, R = reactivity, Ox = oxidizer, W = water-reactive, 0 (none) <——> 4 (severe). ERPG = Emergency Response Planning Guideline. See p 434 for explanation of definitions.

(continued)

TABLE IV-4. HEALTH HAZARD SUMMARIES FOR INDUSTRIAL AND OCCUPATIONAL CHEMICALS (CONTINUED)

Health Hazard Summaries	ACGIH TLV	IDLH	NFPA Codes H F R	Comments
Cyclohexanol (CAS: 108-93-0): Irritating to eyes and respiratory tract. Vapors irritating at high levels. Based on animal tests, it may injure the liver and kidneys at high doses.	50 ppm, S	400 ppm	1 2 0	Colorless viscous liquid. Mild camphorlike odor. Irritation occurs near the TLV and is a good warning property. Vapor pressure is 1 mm Hg at 20 °C (68 °F). Combustible.
Cyclohexanone (CAS: 108-94-1): Irritating upon direct contact. Vapors irritate the eyes and respiratory tract. A CNS depressant at very high levels. Chronic, moderate doses caused slight liver injury in test animals.	25 ppm, S	700 ppm	1 2 0	Clear to pale yellow liquid with peppermintlike odor. Vapor pressure is 2 mm Hg at 20 °C (68 °F). Flammable.
Cyclohexene (1,2,3,4-tetrahydrobenzene [CAS: 110-83-8]): By structural analogy to cyclohexane, may cause respiratory tract irritation. A CNS depressant.	300 ppm	2000 ppm	1 3 0	Colorless liquid with a sweet odor. Vapor pressure is 67 mm Hg at 20 °C (68 °F). Flammable. Readily forms peroxides and polymerizes.
Cyclohexylamine (aminocyclohexane [CAS: 108-91-8]): Corrosive and highly irritating upon direct contact. Vapors highly irritating to eyes and respiratory tract. Pharmacologically active, possessing sympathomimetic activity. Weak methemoglobin-forming activity (see p 220). Very limited evidence for adverse effects on reproduction in test animals. Animal studies suggest brain, liver, and kidneys are target organs.	10 ppm		3 3 0	Liquid with an obnoxious, fishy odor. Flammable.
Cyclonite (RDX, trinitrotrimethylenetriamine [CAS: 121-82-4]): Dermal and inhalation exposures affect the CNS with symptoms of confusion, headache, nausea, vomiting, convulsions, and coma. Does not have nitratelike toxicity.	0.5 mg/m³, S			Crystalline solid. Vapor pressure is negligible at 20 °C (68 °F). Thermal breakdown products include oxides of nitrogen. Explosive.
Cyclopentadiene [CAS: 542-92-7]): Mildly irritating upon direct contact. Vapors irritating to eyes and respiratory tract. A CNS depressant at high levels. Animal studies suggest some potential for kidney and liver injury at high doses.	75 ppm	750 ppm		Colorless liquid. Sweet, turpentinelike odor. Irritation occurs near the TLV and is a good warning property. Vapor pressure is high at 20 °C (68 °F). Flammable.

Chemical	TLV	ERPG	NFPA (H F R)	Comments
Cyclopentane [CAS: 287-92-3]: Mildly irritating upon direct contact. Vapors irritating to eyes and respiratory tract. A CNS depressant at very high levels. Solvent mixtures containing cyclopentane have caused peripheral neuropathy although this may have been related to n-hexane in combination.	600 ppm		1 3 0	Colorless liquid with a faint hydrocarbon odor. Vapor pressure is about 400 mm Hg at 31 °C (88°F). Flammable.
DDT (dichlorodiphenyltrichloroethane) [CAS: 50-29-3]: Dusts irritating to eyes. Ingestion may cause tremor and convulsions. Chronic low-level exposure results in bioaccumulation. A carcinogen in test animals (IARC 2B). See also p 133.	1 mg/m³, A3 NIOSH CA	500 mg/m³		Colorless, white, or yellow solid crystals with a faint aromatic odor. Vapor pressure is 0.0000002 mm Hg at 20 °C (68 °F). Combustible. Banned for use in US in 1973.
Decaborane [CAS: 17702-41-9]: A potent CNS toxin. Symptoms include headache, dizziness, nausea, loss of coordination, and fatigue. Symptoms may be delayed in onset for 1–2 days; convulsions occur in more severe poisonings. Systemic poisonings can result from dermal absorption. Animal studies suggest a potential for liver and kidney injury.	0.05 ppm, S	15 mg/m³	3 2 1	Colorless solid crystals with a pungent odor. Vapor pressure is 0.05 mm Hg at 25 °C (77 °F). Combustible. Reacts with water to produce flammable hydrogen gas. Used as a rocket fuel additive and as a rubber vulcanization agent.
Demeton (Systox, mercaptophos [CAS: 8065-48-3]: An organophosphate-type cholinesterase inhibitor (see p 244).	0.01 ppm, S	10 mg/m³		A sulfurlike odor. A very low vapor pressure at 20 °C (68 °F). Thermal breakdown products include oxides of sulfur.
Diacetone alcohol (4-hydroxy-4-methyl-2 pentanone [CAS: 123-42-2]: Irritating upon direct contact. Vapors very irritating to eyes and respiratory tract. A CNS depressant at high levels. Possibly some hemolytic activity.	50 ppm	1800 ppm [LEL]	1 2 0	Colorless liquid with an agreeable odor. Vapor pressure is 0.8 mm Hg at 20 °C (68 °F). Flammable.
Diazinon (0,0-diethyl 0-2-isopropyl-4-methyl-6-pyrimidinylthiophosphate [CAS: 333-41-5]: An organophosphate-type cholinesterase inhibitor (see p 244). Well absorbed dermally. Limited evidence for adverse effects on male reproduction and fetal development in test animals at high doses.	0.1 mg/m³, S			Commercial grades are yellow to brown liquids with a faint odor. Vapor pressure is 0.00014 mm Hg at 20 °C (68 °F). Thermal breakdown products include oxides of nitrogen and sulfur.

(C) = ceiling air concentration (TLV-C); S = skin absorption can be significant; A1 = ACGIH–confirmed human carcinogen; A2 = ACGIH–suspected human carcinogen; A3 = ACGIH-suspected human carcinogen; NFPA Hazard Codes: H = health, F = fire, R = reactivity, Ox = oxidizer, W = water-reactive, 0 (none) <—> 4 (severe). ERPG = Emergency Response Planning Guideline. See p 434 for explanation of definitions.

(continued)

TABLE IV–4. HEALTH HAZARD SUMMARIES FOR INDUSTRIAL AND OCCUPATIONAL CHEMICALS (CONTINUED)

Health Hazard Summaries	ACGIH TLV	IDLH	NFPA Codes H F R	Comments
Diazomethane (azimethylene, diazirine [CAS: 334-88-3]): Extremely irritating to eyes and respiratory tract; pulmonary edema has been reported. Immediate symptoms include cough, chest pain, and respiratory distress. A potent methylating agent and respiratory sensitizer.	0.2 ppm, A2	2 ppm		Yellow gas with a musty odor. Air mixtures and compressed liquids can be explosive when heated or shocked.
Diborane (boron hydride [CAS: 19287-45-7]): Extremely irritating to the respiratory tract; pulmonary edema may result. Repeated exposures have been associated with headache, fatigue, and dizziness; muscle weakness or tremors; and chills or fever. Animal studies suggest the liver and kidney are also target organs.	0.1 ppm	15 ppm ERPG-2: 1 ppm ERPG-3: 3 ppm	4 4 3 W	Colorless gas. Obnoxious, nauseatingly sweet odor. Highly flammable. Water-reactive; ignites spontaneously with moist air at room temperatures. A strong reducing agent. Breakdown products include boron oxide fumes. Used in microelectronic industry. Reacts violently with halogenated extinguishing agents.
1,2-Dibromo-3-chloropropane (DBCP [CAS: 96-12-8]): Irritant of eyes and respiratory tract. Has caused sterility (aspermia, oligospermia) in overexposed men. Well absorbed by skin contact and inhalation. A carcinogen in test animals (IARC 2B).	OSHA CA NIOSH CA			Brown liquid with a pungent odor. Combustible. Thermal breakdown products include hydrogen bromide and hydrogen chloride.
1,2-Dibromo-2,2-dichloroethyl dimethyl phosphate (Naled, Dibrom [CAS: 300-76-5]): An organophosphate anticholinesterase agent (see p 244). Highly irritating upon contact; eye injury is likely. Dermal sensitization can occur. Well absorbed dermally; localized muscular twitching results within minutes of contact.	3 mg/m³, S			Has a pungent odor. Vapor pressure is 0.002 mm Hg at 20 °C (68 °F). Not combustible. Thermal breakdown products include hydrogen bromide, hydrogen chloride, and phosphoric acid.
Dibutyl phosphate (di-*n*-butyl phosphate [CAS: 107-66-4]): A moderately strong acid likely to be irritating upon direct contact. Vapors and mists are irritating to the respiratory tract and have been associated with headache at low levels.	1 ppm	30 ppm		Colorless to brown liquid. Odorless. Vapor pressure is much less than 1 mm Hg at 20 °C (68 °F). Decomposes at 100 °C (212 °F) to produce phosphoric acid fumes.

Chemical (CAS)	TLV	Air conc.	NFPA (H F R)	Comments
Dibutyl phthalate (CAS: 84-74-2): Mildly irritating upon direct contact. Ingestion has produced nausea, dizziness, photophobia, and lacrimation but no permanent effects. Adverse effects on fetal development and male reproduction in test animals at very high doses.	5 mg/m³	4000 mg/m³	0 1 0	Colorless, oily liquid with a faint aromatic odor. Vapor pressure is less than 0.01 mm Hg at 20 °C (68 °F). Combustible.
1, 2-Dichloroacetylene (CAS: 7572-29-4): Vapors extremely irritating to eyes and respiratory tract; pulmonary edema may result. CNS toxicity includes nausea and vomiting, headache, involvement of trigeminal nerve and facial muscles, and outbreaks of facial herpes. Limited evidence for carcinogenicity in test animals.	0.1 ppm (C), A3			Colorless liquid.
o-Dichlorobenzene (1,2-dichlorobenzene [CAS: 95-50-1]): Irritating upon direct contact; skin blisters and hyperpigmentation may result from prolonged contact. Vapor also irritating to eyes and respiratory tract. Highly hepatotoxic in test animals. Evidence for adverse effects on male reproduction in test animals.	25 ppm	200 ppm	2 2 0	Colorless to pale yellow liquid. Aromatic odor and eye irritation occur well below the TLV and are adequate warning properties. Thermal breakdown products include hydrogen chloride and chlorine gas.
p-Dichlorobenzene (1,4-dichlorobenzene [CAS: 106-46-7]): Irritating upon direct contact with the solid. Vapors irritating to eyes and respiratory tract. Systemic effects include headache, nausea, vomiting, and liver injury. The *ortho* isomer is more toxic to the liver. A carcinogen in test animals (IARC 2B).	10 ppm, A3	150 ppm	2 2 0	Colorless or white solid. Mothball odor and irritation occur near the TLV and are adequate warning properties. Vapor pressure is 0.4 mm Hg at 20 °C (68 °F). Combustible. Thermal breakdown products include hydrogen chloride. Used as a moth repellant.
3,3´-Dichlorobenzidine (CAS: 91-94-1): Well absorbed by the dermal route. Animal studies suggest that severe eye injury and respiratory tract irritation may occur. A potent carcinogen in test animals (IARC 2B).	S, A3 OSHA CA NIOSH CA			Crystalline needles with a faint odor.
Dichlorodifluoromethane (Freon 12, Fluorocarbon 12 [CAS: 75-71-8]): Mild eye and respiratory tract irritant. Extremely high exposures (eg, 100,000 ppm) can cause coma and cardiac arrhythmias. See also p 178.	1000 ppm	15,000 ppm		Colorless gas. Etherlike odor is a poor warning property. Vapor pressure is 5.7 mm Hg at 20 °C (68 °F). Not combustible. Decomposes slowly on contact with water or heat to produce hydrogen chloride, hydrogen fluoride, and phosgene.

(C) = ceiling air concentration (TLV-C); S = skin absorption can be significant; A1 = ACGIH-confirmed human carcinogen; A2 = ACGIH-suspected human carcinogen; A3 = ACGIH-suspected human carcinogen; NFPA Hazard Codes: H = health, F = fire, R = reactivity, Ox = oxidizer, W = water-reactive, 0 (none) <—> 4 (severe). ERPG = Emergency Response Planning Guideline. See p 434 for explanation of definitions.

(continued)

TABLE IV–4. HEALTH HAZARD SUMMARIES FOR INDUSTRIAL AND OCCUPATIONAL CHEMICALS (CONTINUED)

Health Hazard Summaries	ACGIH TLV	IDLH	NFPA Codes H F R	Comments
1,3-Dichloro-5,5-dimethylhydantoin (Halane, Dactin [CAS: 118-52-5]): Releases hypochlorous acid and chlorine gas (see p 134) on contact with moisture. Direct contact with the dust or concentrated solutions irritating to eyes, skin, and respiratory tract.	0.2 mg/m³	5 mg/m³		White solid with a chlorinelike odor. Odor and eye irritation occur below the TLV and are adequate warning properties. Not combustible. Thermal breakdown products include hydrogen chloride, phosgene, oxides of nitrogen, and chlorine gas.
1,1-Dichloroethane (ethylidene chloride [CAS: 75-34-3]): Mild eye and skin irritant. Vapors irritating to the respiratory tract. A CNS depressant at high levels. By analogy with its 1,2-isomer, may cause arrhythmias. Animal studies suggest some potential for kidney and liver injury.	100 ppm	3000 ppm	2 3 0	Colorless, oily liquid. Chloroformlike odor occurs at the TLV. Vapor pressure is 182 mm Hg at 20 °C (68 °F). Flammable. Thermal breakdown products include vinyl chloride, hydrogen chloride, and phosgene.
1,2-Dichloroethane (ethylene dichloride [CAS: 107-06-2]): Irritating upon prolonged contact; burns may occur. Well absorbed dermally. Vapors irritating to eyes and respiratory tract. A CNS depressant at high levels. May cause cardiac arrhythmias. Severe liver and kidney injury in test animals. A carcinogen in test animals (IARC 2B).	10 ppm NIOSH CA	50 ppm	2 3 0	Flammable. Thermal breakdown products include hydrogen chloride and phosgene.
1,1-Dichloroethylene (vinylidine chloride [CAS: 75-35-4]): Irritating upon direct contact. Vapors very irritating to eyes and respiratory tract. A CNS depressant. May cause cardiac arrhythmias. In test animals, damages the liver and kidneys. Limited evidence of carcinogenicity in test animals (IARC 3).	5 ppm, A3 NIOSH CA [proposed: A4]		4 4 2	Colorless liquid. Sweet, etherlike or chloroformlike odor occurs below the TLV and is a good warning property. Polymerizes readily.
1,2-Dichloroethylene (1,2-dichloroethene, acetylene dichloride [CAS: 540-59-0]): Vapors mildly irritating to respiratory tract. A CNS depressant at high levels; once used as an anesthetic agent. May cause cardiac arrhythmias. Low hepatotoxicity.	200 ppm	1000 ppm	2 3 2	Colorless liquid with a slightly acrid, etherlike or chloroformlike odor. Vapor pressure is about 220 mm Hg at 20 °C (68 °F). Thermal breakdown products include hydrogen chloride and phosgene.

Chemical	Ceiling air concentration	ERPG	NFPA (H F R)	Comments
Dichloroethyl ether (bis[2-chloroethyl] ether, dichloroethyl oxide [CAS: 111-44-4]): Irritating upon direct contact; corneal injury may result. Vapors highly irritating to respiratory tract. A CNS depressant at high levels. Dermal absorption occurs. Animal studies suggest the liver and kidneys are also target organs at high exposures. Limited evidence for carcinogenicity in test animals.	5 ppm, S	100 ppm	3 2 1	Colorless liquid. Obnoxious, chlorinated solvent odor occurs at the TLV and is a good warning property. Flammable. Breaks down on contact with water. Thermal breakdown products include hydrogen chloride.
Dichlorofluoromethane (fluorocarbon 21, Freon 21, Halon 112 [CAS: 75-43-4]): Animal studies suggest much greater hepatotoxicity than most common chlorofluorocarbons. Causes CNS depression, respiratory irritation, and cardiac arrhythmias at very high air levels (eg, 100,000 ppm). Evidence for adverse effects on fetal development (preimplantation losses) in test animals at high levels. See also p 178.	10 ppm	5000 ppm		Colorless liquid or gas with a faint etherlike odor. Thermal breakdown products include hydrogen chloride, hydrogen fluoride, and phosgene.
1,1-Dichloro-1-nitroethane [CAS: 594-72-9]): Based on animal studies, highly irritating upon direct contact. Vapors highly irritating to eyes, skin, and respiratory tract; pulmonary edema may result. In test animals, lethal doses also injured the liver, heart, and kidneys.	2 ppm	25 ppm	2 2 3	Colorless liquid. Obnoxious odor and tearing occur only at dangerous levels and are poor warning properties. Vapor pressure is 15 mm Hg at 20 °C (68 °F).
2,4-Dichlorophenoxyacetic acid (2,4-D [CAS: 94-75-9]): Direct skin contact can produce a rash. Overexposed workers have rarely experienced peripheral neuropathy. Severe rhabdomyolysis and minor liver and kidney injury may occur. Adverse effects on fetal development at high doses in test animals. There are weak epidemiologic associations of phenoxy herbicides with soft tissue sarcomas. See also p 137.	10 mg/m³	100 mg/m³	2 2 3	White to yellow crystals. Appearance and some hazardous properties vary with the formulation. Odorless. Vapor pressure is negligible at 20 °C (68 °F). Thermal breakdown products include hydrogen chloride and phosgene.
1,3-Dichloropropene (1,3-dichloropropylene, Telone [CAS: 542-75-6]): Based on animal studies, irritating upon direct contact. Well absorbed dermally. Vapors irritating to eyes and respiratory tract. In test animals, moderate doses caused severe injuries to the liver, pancreas, and kidneys. A carcinogen in test animals (IARC 2B).	1 ppm, S		2 3 0	Colorless or straw-colored liquid. Sharp, chloroformlike odor. Polymerizes readily. Vapor pressure is 28 mm Hg at 25 °C (77 °F). Thermal breakdown products include hydrogen chloride and phosgene.

(C) = ceiling air concentration (TLV-C); S = skin absorption can be significant; A1 = ACGIH-confirmed human carcinogen; A2 = ACGIH-suspected human carcinogen; NFPA Hazard Codes: H = health, F = fire, R = reactivity, Ox = oxidizer, W = water-reactive, 0 (none) <—> 4 (severe). ERPG = Emergency Response Planning Guideline. See p 434 for explanation of definitions.

(continued)

TABLE IV–4. HEALTH HAZARD SUMMARIES FOR INDUSTRIAL AND OCCUPATIONAL CHEMICALS (CONTINUED)

Health Hazard Summaries	ACGIH TLV	IDLH	NFPA Codes H F R	Comments
2,2-Dichloropropionic acid (CAS: 75-99-0): Corrosive upon direct contact with concentrate; severe burns may result. Vapors mildly irritating to eyes and respiratory tract.	1 ppm			Colorless liquid. The sodium salt is a solid.
Dichlorotetrafluoroethane (fluorocarbon 114, Freon 114 [CAS: 76-14-2]): Vapors may sensitize the myocardium to arrhythmogenic effects of epinephrine at modestly high air levels (25,000 ppm). Other effects at higher levels (100,000–200,000 ppm) include respiratory irritation and CNS depression. See also p 178.	1000 ppm	15,000 ppm		Colorless gas with a mild etherlike odor. Thermal breakdown products include hydrogen chloride, hydrogen fluoride, and phosgene.
Dichlorvos (DDVP, 2,2-dichlorovinyl dimethyl phosphate [CAS: 62-73-7]): An organophosphate-type cholinesterase inhibitor (see p 244). Extremely well absorbed through skin. Evidence of carcinogenicity in test animals (IARC 2B).	0.9 ppm, S	100 mg/m^3		Colorless to amber liquid with a slight chemical odor. Vapor pressure is 0.032 mm Hg at 32 °C (90 °F).
Dicrotophos (dimethyl cis-2-dimethylcarbamoyl-1-methylvinyl phosphate, Bidrin [CAS: 141-66-2]): An organophosphate cholinesterase inhibitor (see p 244). Dermal absorption occurs.	0.25 mg/m^3, S			Brown liquid with a mild ester odor.
Dieldrin (CAS: 60-57-1): Minor skin irritant. Potent convulsant and hepatotoxin. Dermal absorption is a major route of systemic poisoning. Overexposures produce headache, dizziness, twitching, and convulsions. Limited evidence for adverse effects on fetal development and carcinogenicity in test animals (IARC 3). See also p 133.	0.25 mg/m^3, S NIOSH CA	50 mg/m^3		Light brown solid flakes with a mild chemical odor. Appearance and some hazardous properties vary with the formulation. Vapor pressure is 0.0000002 mm Hg at 32 °C (90 °F). Not combustible.
Diesel exhaust: A respiratory irritant. Animal and epidemiological studies provide evidence of pulmonary carcinogenicity.	[proposed: 0.15 mg/m^3, A2 (particulate < 1μm)]			Diesel engines emit a complex mixture of gases, vapors, and respirable particles, including many polycyclic aromatic and nitroaromatic hydrocarbons and oxides of nitrogen, sulfur, and carbon including carbon monoxide.

Diethylamine (CAS: 109-89-7): Corrosive. Highly irritating upon direct contact; severe burns may result. Vapors highly irritating to eyes and respiratory tract; pulmonary edema may occur. Subacute animal studies suggest liver and heart may be target organs.

5 ppm, S | 200 ppm | 3 3 0 | Colorless liquid. Fishy, ammonialike odor occurs below the TLV and is a good warning property. Vapor pressure is 195 mm Hg at 20 °C (68 °F). Highly flammable. Thermal breakdown products include oxides of nitrogen.

2-Diethylaminoethanol (N,N-diethylthanolamine, DEAE [CAS: 100-37-8]): Based on animal studies, highly irritating upon direct contact and a skin sensitizer. Vapors likely irritating to eyes, skin, and respiratory tract. Reports of nausea and vomiting after a momentary exposure to 100 ppm.

2 ppm, S | 100 ppm | 3 2 0 | Colorless liquid. Weak to nauseating ammonia odor. Flammable. Thermal breakdown products include oxides of nitrogen.

Diethylenetriamine (DETA [CAS: 111-40-0]): Corrosive; highly irritating upon direct contact; severe burns may result. Vapors highly irritating to eyes and respiratory tract. Dermal and respiratory sensitization can occur.

1 ppm, S | | 3 1 0 | Viscous yellow liquid with an ammonialike odor. Vapor pressure is 0.37 mm Hg at 20 °C (68 °F). Combustible. Thermal breakdown products include oxides of nitrogen.

Diethyl ketone (3-pentanone [CAS: 96-22-0]): Mildly irritating upon direct contact. Vapors mildly irritating to eyes and respiratory tract.

200 ppm | | 1 3 0 | Colorless liquid with an acetonelike odor. Flammable.

Diethyl sulfate (CAS: 64-67-5): Strong eye and respiratory tract irritant. Sufficient evidence of carcinogenicity in test animals. Limited evidence (laryngeal cancers) in humans (IARC 2A).

| | 3 1 1 | An alkylating agent. Colorless oily liquid with a peppermint odor.

Difluorodibromomethane (dibromodifluoromethane, Freon 12B2 [CAS: 75-61-6]): Based on animal tests, vapors irritate the respiratory tract. A CNS depressant. By analogy to other freons, may cause cardiac arrhythmias. In test animals, high-level chronic exposures caused lung, liver, and CNS injury. See also p 178.

100 ppm | 2000 ppm | | Heavy, volatile, colorless liquid with an obnoxious, distinctive odor. Vapor pressure is 620 mm Hg at 20 °C (68 °F). Not combustible. Thermal breakdown products include hydrogen bromide and hydrogen fluoride.

Diglycidyl ether (di[2,3-epoxypropyl]-ether, DGE [CAS: 2238-07-5]): Extremely irritating upon direct contact; severe burns result. Vapors highly irritating to eyes and respiratory tract; pulmonary edema may result. Testicular atrophy and adverse effects on the hematopoietic system at low doses in test animals. CNS depression also noted. An alkylating agent and a carcinogen in test animals.

0.1 ppm NIOSH CA | 10 ppm | | Colorless liquid with a very irritating odor. Vapor pressure is 0.09 mm Hg at 25 °C (77 °F).

(continued)

(C) = ceiling air concentration (TLV-C); S = skin absorption can be significant; A1 = ACGIH-confirmed human carcinogen; A2 = ACGIH-suspected human carcinogen; NFPA Hazard Codes: H = health, F = fire, R = reactivity, Ox = oxidizer, W = water-reactive, 0 (none) <—> 4 (severe). ERPG = Emergency Response Planning Guideline. See p 434 for explanation of definitions.

TABLE IV–4. HEALTH HAZARD SUMMARIES FOR INDUSTRIAL AND OCCUPATIONAL CHEMICALS (CONTINUED)

Health Hazard Summaries	ACGIH TLV	IDLH	NFPA Codes H F R	Comments
Diisobutyl ketone (2,6-dimethyl-4-heptanone [CAS: 108-83-8]): Mildly irritating upon direct contact. Vapors mildly irritate eyes and respiratory tract. A CNS depressant at high levels.	25 ppm	500 ppm	1 2 0	Colorless liquid with a weak, etherlike odor. Vapor pressure is 1.7 mm Hg at 20 °C (68 °F).
Diisopropylamine (CAS: 108-18-9): Corrosive. Highly irritating upon direct contact; severe burns may result. Vapors very irritating to eyes and respiratory tract. Workers exposed to levels of 25–50 ppm have complained of hazy vision, nausea, and headache.	5 ppm, S	200 ppm	3 3 0	Colorless liquid with an ammonialike odor. Vapor pressure is 60 mm Hg at 20 °C (68 °F). Flammable. Thermal breakdown products include oxides of nitrogen.
Dimethyl acetamide (DMAC [CAS: 127-19-5]): Potent hepatotoxin. Inhalation and skin contact are major routes of absorption. Limited evidence for adverse effects on fetal development in test animals at high doses.	10 ppm, S	300 ppm	2 2 0	Colorless liquid with a weak ammonialike odor. Vapor pressure is 1.5 mm Hg at 20 °C (68 °F). Combustible. Thermal breakdown products include oxides of nitrogen.
Dimethylamine (DMA [CAS: 124-40-3]): Corrosive upon direct contact; severe burns may result. Vapors extremely irritating to eyes and respiratory tract. Animal studies suggest liver is a target organ.	5 ppm	500 ppm ERPG-1: 1 ppm ERPG-2: 100 ppm ERPG-3: 500 ppm	3 4 0	Colorless liquid or gas. Fishy or ammonialike odor far below TLV is a good warning property. Flammable. Thermal breakdown products include oxides of nitrogen.
N,N-Dimethylaniline (CAS: 121-69-7): Causes methemoglobinemia (see p 220). A CNS depressant. Well absorbed dermally. Limited evidence for carcinogenicity in test animals.	5 ppm, S	100 ppm	3 2 0	Straw- to brown-colored liquid with an aminelike odor. Vapor pressure is less than 1 mm Hg at 20 °C (68 °F). Combustible. Thermal breakdown products include oxides of nitrogen.
Dimethylcarbamoyl chloride (CAS: 79-44-7): Rapidly hydrolyzed by moisture to dimethylamine, carbon dioxide, and hydrochloric acid. Expected to be extremely irritating upon direct contact or by inhalation. A carcinogen in test animals (IARC 2A).	A2			Liquid. Rapidly reacts with moisture to yield dimethylamine and hydrogen chloride.

Chemical	TLV	Other	H	F	R	Properties
***N,N*-Dimethylformamide (DMF [CAS: 68-12-2]):** Dermally well absorbed. Symptoms of overexposure include abdominal pain, nausea, and vomiting. This chemical is a potent hepatotoxin in humans. Interferes with ethanol to cause disulfiramlike reactions (see p 158). Limited epidemiologic association with an increased risk of testicular cancer (IARC 2B). Limited evidence for adverse effects on fetal development in animals.	10 ppm, S	500 ppm ERPG-1: 2 ppm ERPG-2: 100 ppm ERPG-3: 200 ppm	1	2	0	Colorless to pale yellow liquid. Faint ammonialike odor is a poor warning property. Vapor pressure is 2.7 mm Hg at 20 °C (68 °F). Flammable. Thermal breakdown products include oxides of nitrogen.
1,1-Dimethylhydrazine (DMH, UDMH [CAS: 57-14-7]): Corrosive upon direct contact; severe burns may result. Vapors extremely irritating to eyes and respiratory tract; pulmonary edema may occur. Well absorbed through the skin. May cause methemoglobinemia (see p 220); may cause hemolysis. A potent hepatotoxin and carcinogen in test animals (IARC 2B).	0.01 ppm, S, NIOSH CA	15 ppm	4	3	1	Colorless liquid with yellow fumes. Amine odor. Vapor pressure is 1.3 mm Hg at 20 °C (68 °F). Thermal breakdown products include oxides of nitrogen.
Dimethyl sulfate (CAS: 77-78-1): Powerful vesicant action; hydrolyzes to sulfuric acid and methanol. Extremely irritating upon direct contact; severe burns have resulted. Vapors irritating to eyes and respiratory tract; delayed pulmonary edema may result. Skin absorption is rapid. A carcinogen in test animals (IARC 2A).	0.1 ppm, S, A3	7 ppm	4	2	0	Colorless, oily liquid. Very mild onion odor is barely perceptible and is a poor warning property. Vapor pressure is 0.5 mm Hg at 20 °C (68 °F). Combustible. Thermal breakdown products include sulfur oxides.
Dinitrobenzene: May stain tissues yellow upon direct contact. Vapors are irritating to respiratory tract. Potent inducer of methemoglobinemia (see p 220). Chronic exposures may result in anemia and liver damage. Injuries testes in test animals. Very well absorbed through the skin.	0.15 ppm, S	50 mg/m^3	3	1	4	Pale yellow crystals. Explosive; detonated by heat or shock. Vapor pressure is much less than 1 mm Hg at 20 °C (68 °F). Thermal breakdown products include oxides of nitrogen.
Dinitro-o-cresol (2-methyl-4,6-dinitrophenol [CAS: 534-52-1]): Highly toxic; uncouples oxidative phosphorylation in mitochondria, increasing metabolic rate and leading to fatigue, sweating, rapid breathing, tachycardia, and fever. Liver and kidney injury may occur. Symptoms may last for days, as it is very slowly excreted. May induce methemoglobinemia (see p 220). Poisonings may result from dermal exposure. Yellow-stained skin may mark exposure. See also p 255.	0.2 mg/m^3, S	5 mg/m^3				Yellow solid crystals. Odorless. Dust is explosive. Vapor pressure is 0.00005 mm Hg at 20 °C (68 °F). Thermal breakdown products include oxides of nitrogen.

(C) = ceiling air concentration (TLV-C); S = skin absorption can be significant; A1 = ACGIH-confirmed human carcinogen; A2 = ACGIH-suspected human carcinogen; NFPA Hazard Codes: H = health, F = fire, R = reactivity, Ox = oxidizer, W = water-reactive, 0 (none) <—> 4 (severe). ERPG = Emergency Response Planning Guideline. See p 434 for explanation of definitions.

(continued)

TABLE IV-4. HEALTH HAZARD SUMMARIES FOR INDUSTRIAL AND OCCUPATIONAL CHEMICALS (CONTINUED)

Health Hazard Summaries	ACGIH TLV	IDLH	NFPA Codes H F R	Comments
2,4-Dinitrophenol (CAS: 25550-58-7): Potent uncoupler of oxidative phosphorylation. Initial findings include hypertension, fever, dyspnea, and tachypnea. May cause methemoglobinemia and harm liver and kidneys. May stain skin at point of contact. Limited evidence for adverse effects on fetal development. See also p 252.				
2,4-Dinitrotoluene (DNT [CAS: 25321-14-6]): May cause methemoglobinemia (see p 220). Uncouples oxidative phosphorylation, leading to increased metabolic rate and hyperthermia, tachycardia, and fatigue. A hepatotoxin. May cause vasodilation; headache and drop in blood pressure are common. Cessation of exposure may precipitate angina pectoris in pharmacologically dependent workers. Well absorbed by all routes. May stain skin yellow. Injures testes in test animals and possibly, exposed workers. A carcinogen in test animals.	0.2 mg/m³, A3, S NIOSH CA	50 mg/m³	3 1 3	Orange-yellow solid (pure) or oily liquid with a characteristic odor. Explosive. Thermal breakdown products include oxides of nitrogen. Vapor pressure is 1 mm Hg at 20 °C (68 °F).
1,4-Dioxane (1,4-diethylene dioxide [CAS: 123-91-1]): Vapors irritating to eyes and respiratory tract. Inhalation or dermal exposures may cause gastrointestinal upset and liver and kidney injury. A carcinogen in test animals (IARC 2B).	25 ppm, S, A3 NIOSH CA [proposed: 20 ppm, S, A3]	500 ppm	2 3 1	Colorless liquid. Mild etherlike odor occurs only at dangerous levels and is a poor warning property. Vapor pressure is 29 mm Hg at 20 °C (68 °F). Flammable.
Dioxathion (2,3-*p*-dioxanedithiol *S,S*-bis [*O,O*-diethyl phosphorodithioate] [CAS: 78-34-2]): An organophosphate-type cholinesterase inhibitor (see p 244). Well absorbed dermally.	0.2 mg/m³, S			Amber liquid. Vapor pressure is negligible at 20 °C (68 °F). Thermal breakdown products include oxides of sulfur.
Dipropylene glycol methyl ether (DPGME [CAS: 34590-94-8]): Mildly irritating to eyes upon direct contact. A CNS depressant at very high levels.	100 ppm, S	600 ppm	0 2 0	Colorless liquid with a mild etherlike odor. Nasal irritation is a good warning property. Vapor pressure is 0.3 mm Hg at 20 °C (68 °F). Combustible.

Compound	TLV	NFPA (H F R)	Comments
Diquat (1,1'-ethylene-2,2'-dipyridinium dibromide, Reglone, Dextrone [CAS: 85-00-7]): Corrosive in high concentrations. Acute renal failure and reversible liver injury may occur. Chronic feeding studies caused cataracts in test animals. Although pulmonary edema might occur, unlike paraquat, pulmonary fibrosis has not been shown with human diquat exposures. See also p 250.	0.5 mg/m³ (total dust) 0.1 mg/m³ (respirable dust), S		Yellow solid crystals. Appearance and some hazardous properties vary with the formulation.
Disulfiram (tetraethylthiuram disulfide, Antabuse [CAS: 97-77-8]): Inhibits aldehyde dehydrogenase, an enzyme involved in ethanol metabolism. Exposure to disulfiram and alcohol will produce flushing, headache, and hypotension. Disulfiram may also interact with other industrial solvents that share metabolic pathways with ethanol. Limited evidence for adverse effects on fetal development in test animals. See also p 158.	2 mg/m³		Crystalline solid. Thermal breakdown products include oxides of sulfur.
Disulfoton (O,O-diethyl-S-ethylmercapto-ethyl dithiophosphate [CAS: 298-04-4]): An organophosphate-type cholinesterase inhibitor (see p 244). Dermally well absorbed.	0.1 mg/m³, S		Vapor pressure is 0.00018 mm Hg at 20 °C (68 °F). Thermal breakdown products include oxides of sulfur.
Divinylbenzene (DVB, vinylstyrene [CAS: 1321-74-0]): Mildly irritating upon direct contact. Vapors mildly irritating to eyes and respiratory tract.	10 ppm	1 2 2	Pale yellow liquid. Combustible. Must contain inhibitor to prevent explosive polymerization.
Emery (corundum, impure aluminum oxide [CAS: 112-62-9]): An abrasive, nuisance dust causing physical irritation to eyes, skin, and respiratory tract.	10 mg/m³		Solid crystals of aluminum oxide. Often used for its abrasive properties (eg, emery cloth, emery wheel).
Endosulfan (CAS: 115-29-7): Inhalation and skin absorption are major routes of exposure. Symptoms include nausea, confusion, excitement, twitching, and convulsions. Animal studies suggest liver and kidney injury from very high exposures. Limited evidence for adverse effects on male reproduction and fetal development in animal studies. See also p 133.	0.1 mg/m³, S		Chlorinated hydrocarbon insecticide. Tan, waxy solid with a mild sulfur dioxide odor. Thermal breakdown products include oxides of sulfur and hydrogen chloride.

(C) = ceiling air concentration (TLV-C); S = skin absorption can be significant; A1 = ACGIH-confirmed human carcinogen; A2 = ACGIH-suspected human carcinogen; NFPA Hazard Codes: H = health, F = fire, R = reactivity, Ox = oxidizer, W = water-reactive, 0 (none) <—> 4 (severe). ERPG = Emergency Response Planning Guideline. See p 434 for explanation of definitions.

(continued)

TABLE IV–4. HEALTH HAZARD SUMMARIES FOR INDUSTRIAL AND OCCUPATIONAL CHEMICALS (CONTINUED)

Health Hazard Summaries	ACGIH TLV	IDLH	NFPA Codes H F R	Comments
Endrin (CAS: 72-20-8): Endrin is the stereoisomer of dieldrin, and its toxicity is very similar. Well absorbed through skin. Overexposure may produce headache, dizziness, nausea, confusion, twitching, and convulsions. Adverse effects on fetal development in test animals. See also p 133.	0.1 mg/m^3, S	2 mg/m^3		Colorless, white, or tan solid. A stereoisomer of dieldrin. A mild chemical odor and negligible vapor pressure of 0.0000002 mm Hg at 20 °C (68 °F). Not combustible. Thermal breakdown products include hydrogen chloride.
Environmental tobacco smoke: Passive smoking causes respiratory irritation and small reductions in lung function. It increases severity and frequency of asthmatic attacks in children. May cause coughing, phlegm production, chest discomfort, and reduced lung function in adults. Causes developmental toxicity in infants and children and reproductive toxicity in adult females. Epidemiological studies show passive smoking causes lung cancer (IARC 1).				
Epichlorohydrin (chloropropylene oxide [CAS: 106-89-8]): Extremely irritating upon direct contact; severe burns may result. Vapors highly irritating to eyes and respiratory tract; pulmonary edema has been reported. Other effects include nausea, vomiting, and abdominal pain. Sensitization has been occasionally reported. Animal studies suggest a potential for liver and kidney injury. High doses reduce fertility in test animals (IARC 2A).	0.5 ppm, S, A3 NIOSH CA	75 ppm ERPG-1: 2 ppm ERPG-2: 20 ppm ERPG-3: 100 ppm	3 3 2	Colorless liquid. The irritating, chloroformlike odor is detectable only at extremely high exposures and is a poor warning property. Vapor pressure is 13 mm Hg at 20 °C (68 °F). Flammable. Thermal breakdown products include hydrogen chloride and phosgene.
EPN (O-ethyl O-p-nitrophenyl phenylphosphonothioate [CAS: 2104-64-5]): An organophosphate-type cholinesterase inhibitor (see p 244).	0.1 mg/m^3, S	5 mg/m^3		Yellow solid or brown liquid. Vapor pressure is 0.0003 mm Hg at 100 °C (212 °F).
Ethanolamine (2-aminoethanol [CAS: 141-43-5]): Highly irritating upon direct contact; severe burns may result. Prolonged contact with skin is irritating. Animal studies suggest that, at high levels, vapors are irritating to eyes and respiratory tract and liver and kidney injury may occur. Limited evidence for adverse effects on fetal development in animal studies.	3 ppm	30 ppm	3 2 0	Colorless liquid. A mild ammonialike odor occurs at the TLV and is an adequate warning property. Vapor pressure is less than 1 mm Hg at 20 °C (68 °F). Combustible. Thermal breakdown products include oxides of nitrogen.

Substance	TLV	Other limit	NFPA (H F R)	Comments
Ethion (phosphorodithioic acid [CAS: 563-12-2]): An organophosphate-type cholinesterase inhibitor (see p 244). Well absorbed dermally.	0.4 mg/m³, S			Colorless, odorless liquid when pure. Technical products have an objectionable odor. Vapor pressure is 0.000002 mm Hg at 20 °C (68 °F). Thermal breakdown products include oxides of sulfur.
2-Ethoxyethanol (ethylene glycol monoethyl ether, EGEE, Cellosolve [CAS: 110-80-5]): Mildly irritating on direct contact. Skin contact is a major route of absorption. Overexposures may reduce sperm counts in men. A potent teratogen in both rats and rabbits. Large doses cause lung, liver, testes, kidney, and spleen injury in test animals. See also p 166.	5 ppm, S	500 ppm	2 2 0	OSHA is in the process of greatly lowering its permissible exposure limit (proposed value 0.1 ppm) to provide some protection against the reproductive toxicity of this agent. Colorless liquid. Very mild, sweet odor occurs only at very high levels and is a poor warning property. Vapor pressure is 4 mm Hg at 20 °C (68 °F).
2-Ethoxyethyl acetate (ethylene glycol monoethyl ether acetate, Cellosolve acetate): Mildly irritating upon direct contact. May produce CNS depression and kidney injury. Skin contact is a major route of absorption. Metabolized to 2-ethoxyethanol. Adverse effects on fertility and fetal development in animals. See also p 166.	5 ppm, S	500 ppm	2 2 0	OSHA is in the process of greatly lowering its permissible exposure limit (proposed value 0.1 ppm) to provide some protection against the reproductive toxicity of this agent. Colorless liquid. Mild ether-like odor occurs at the TLV and is a good warning property. Flammable.
Ethyl acetate (CAS: 141-78-6): Slightly irritating to eyes and skin. Vapors irritating to eyes and respiratory tract. A CNS depressant at very high levels. Metabolized to ethanol and acetic acid, so may have some of the fetotoxic potential of ethanol.	400 ppm	2000 ppm [LEL]	1 3 0	Colorless liquid. Fruity odor occurs at the TLV and is a good warning property. Vapor pressure is 76 mm Hg at 20 °C (68 °F). Flammable.
Ethyl acrylate (CAS: 140-88-5): Extremely irritating upon direct contact; severe burns may result. A skin sensitizer. Vapors highly irritating to eyes and respiratory tract. In animal tests, heart, liver, and kidney damage was observed at high doses. A carcinogen in test animals (IARC 2B).	5 ppm	300 ppm	2 3 2	Colorless liquid. Acrid odor occurs below the TLV and is a good warning property. Vapor pressure is 29.5 mm Hg at 20 °C (68 °F). Flammable. Contains an inhibitor to prevent dangerous self-polymerization.

(C) = ceiling air concentration (TLV-C); S = skin absorption can be significant; A1 = ACGIH-confirmed human carcinogen; A2 = ACGIH-suspected human carcinogen; NFPA Hazard Codes: H = health, F = fire, R = reactivity, Ox = oxidizer, W = water-reactive, 0 (none) <—> 4 (severe). ERPG = Emergency Response Planning Guideline. See p 434 for explanation of definitions.

(continued)

TABLE IV–4. HEALTH HAZARD SUMMARIES FOR INDUSTRIAL AND OCCUPATIONAL CHEMICALS (CONTINUED)

Health Hazard Summaries	ACGIH TLV	IDLH	NFPA Codes H F R	Comments
Ethyl alcohol (alcohol, grain alcohol, ethanol, EtOH [CAS: 64-17-5]): At high levels, vapors irritating to eyes and respiratory tract. A CNS depressant at high levels of exposure. Strong evidence for adverse effects on fetal development in test animals and humans with chronic ingestion (fetal alcohol syndrome). See also p 162.	1000 ppm	3300 ppm [LEL]	0 3 0	Colorless liquid with a mild, sweet odor. Vapor pressure is 43 mm Hg at 20 °C (68 °F). Flammable.
Ethylamine (CAS: 75-04-7): Corrosive upon direct contact; severe burns may result. Vapors highly irritating to eyes, skin, and respiratory tract; delayed pulmonary edema may result. Animal studies suggest potential for liver and kidney injury at moderate doses.	5 ppm, S	600 ppm	3 4 0	Colorless liquid or gas with an ammonialike odor. Highly flammable. Thermal breakdown products include oxides of nitrogen.
Ethyl amyl ketone (5-methyl-3-heptanone [CAS: 541-85-5]): Irritating to eyes upon direct contact. Vapors irritating to eyes and respiratory tract. A CNS depressant at high levels.	25 ppm			Colorless liquid with a strong, distinctive odor. Flammable.
Ethylbenzene (CAS: 100-41-4): Mildly irritating to eyes upon direct contact. May cause skin burns upon prolonged contact. Dermally well absorbed. Vapors irritating to eyes and respiratory tract. A CNS depressant at high levels of exposure.	100 ppm [proposed: 100 ppm, A3]	800 ppm [LEL]	2 3 0	Colorless liquid. Aromatic odor and irritation occur at levels close to the TLV and are adequate warning properties. Vapor pressure is 7.1 mm Hg at 20 °C (68 °F). Flammable.
Ethyl bromide (CAS: 74-96-4): Irritating to skin upon direct contact. Irritating to respiratory tract. A CNS depressant at high levels, and may cause cardiac arrhythmias. Former use as an anesthetic agent was discontinued because of fatal liver, kidney, and myocardial injury. Evidence for carcinogenicity in test animals.	5 ppm, S, A3	2000 ppm	2 1 0	Colorless to yellow liquid. Etherlike odor detectable only at high, dangerous levels. Vapor pressure is 375 mm Hg at 20 °C (68 °F). Highly flammable. Thermal breakdown products include hydrogen bromide and bromine gas.
Ethyl butyl ketone (3-heptanone [CAS: 106-35-4]): Mildly irritating to eyes upon direct contact. Vapors irritating to eyes and respiratory tract. A CNS depressant at high levels.	50 ppm	1000 ppm	1 2 0	Colorless liquid. Fruity odor is a good warning property. Vapor pressure is 4 mm Hg at 20 °C (68 °F). Flammable.

Substance	TLV	Other	NFPA (H F R)	Comments
Ethyl chloride (CAS: 75-00-3): Mildly irritating to eyes and respiratory tract. A CNS depressant at high levels; has caused cardiac arrhythmias at anesthetic doses. Animal studies suggest the kidneys and liver are target organs at high doses. Structurally similar to the carcinogenic chloroethanes.	100 ppm, A3, S	3800 ppm [LEL]	1 4 0	Colorless liquid or gas with a pungent, etherlike odor. Highly flammable. Thermal breakdown products include hydrogen chloride and phosgene.
Ethylene chlorohydrin (2-chloroethanol) [CAS: 107-07-3]: Irritating to eyes upon direct contact. Skin contact is extremely hazardous because it is not irritating and absorption is rapid. Vapors irritating to eyes and respiratory tract; pulmonary edema has been reported. Systemic effects include CNS depression, myocardiopathy, shock, and liver and kidney damage.	1 ppm (C), S	7 ppm	4 2 0	Colorless liquid with a weak etherlike odor. Vapor pressure is 5 mm Hg at 20 °C (68 °F). Combustible. Thermal breakdown products include hydrogen chloride and phosgene.
Ethylenediamine (CAS: 107-15-3): Highly irritating upon direct contact; burns may result. Respiratory and dermal sensitization may occur. Vapors irritating to eyes and respiratory tract. Animal studies suggest potential for kidney injury at high doses.	10 ppm, S	1000 ppm	3 2 0	Colorless viscous liquid or solid. Ammonialike odor occurs at the PEL and is an adequate warning property. Vapor pressure is 10 mm Hg at 20 °C (68 °F). Flammable. Thermal breakdown products include oxides of nitrogen.
Ethylene dibromide (1,2-dibromoethane, EDB [CAS: 106-93-4]): Highly irritating upon direct contact; severe burns result. Highly toxic by all routes. Vapors highly irritating to eyes and respiratory tract. Severe liver and kidney injury may occur. A CNS depressant. Adverse effects on the testes in test animals and, possibly, humans. A carcinogen in test animals (IARC 2A). See p 164.	S, A3 NIOSH CA	100 ppm	3 0 0	Colorless liquid or solid. Mild, sweet odor is a poor warning property. Vapor pressure is 11 mm Hg at 20 °C (68 °F). Not combustible. Thermal breakdown products include hydrogen bromide and bromine gas. Fumigant and chemical intermediate used in organic synthesis.
Ethylene glycol (antifreeze [CAS: 107-21-1]): A CNS depressant. Metabolized to oxalic and other acids; severe acidosis may result. Precipitation of calcium oxalate crystals in tissues can cause extensive injury. Adversely affects fetal development in animal studies at very high doses. Not well absorbed dermally. See also p 166.	100 mg/m³ (C)		1 1 0	Colorless viscous liquid. Odorless with a very low vapor pressure.

(C) = ceiling air concentration (TLV-C); S = skin absorption can be significant; A1 = ACGIH-confirmed human carcinogen; A2 = ACGIH-suspected human carcinogen; A3 = ... NFPA Hazard Codes: H = health, F = fire, R = reactivity, Ox = oxidizer, W = water-reactive, 0 (none) <—> 4 (severe). ERPG = Emergency Response Planning Guideline. See p 434 for explanation of definitions.

(continued)

TABLE IV–4. HEALTH HAZARD SUMMARIES FOR INDUSTRIAL AND OCCUPATIONAL CHEMICALS (CONTINUED)

Health Hazard Summaries	ACGIH TLV	IDLH	NFPA Codes H F R	Comments
Ethylene glycol dinitrate (EGDN [CAS: 628-96-6]): Causes vasodilation similar to other nitrite compounds. Headache, hypotension, flushing, palpitation, delirium, and CNS depression may occur. Well absorbed by all routes. Tolerance and dependence may develop to vasodilatory effects; cessation after repeated exposures may cause angina pectoris. Weak inducer of methemoglobinemia (see p 220).	0.05 ppm, S	75 mg/m^3		Yellow oily liquid. Vapor pressure is 0.05 mm Hg at 20 °C (68 °F). Explosive.
Ethyleneimine (CAS: 151-56-4): Strong caustic. Highly irritating upon direct contact; severe burns may result. Vapors irritating to eyes and respiratory tract; delayed-onset pulmonary edema may occur. Overexposures have resulted in nausea, vomiting, headache, and dizziness. Well absorbed dermally. A carcinogen in animals.	0.5 ppm, S, A3 OSHA CA NIOSH CA	100 ppm	4 3 3	Colorless liquid with an aminelike odor. Vapor pressure is 160 mm Hg at 20 °C (68 °F). Flammable. Contains inhibitor to prevent explosive self-polymerization.
Ethylene oxide (CAS: 75-21-8): Highly irritating upon direct contact. Vapors irritating to eyes and respiratory tract; delayed pulmonary edema has been reported. A CNS depressant at very high levels. Chronic overexposures can cause peripheral neuropathy and possible permanent CNS impairment. Adverse effects on fetal development and fertility in test animals and limited evidence in humans. A carcinogen in animal studies. Limited evidence of carcinogenicity in humans (IARC 2A). See also p 169.	1 ppm, A2 OSHA CA NIOSH CA	800 ppm ERPG-2: 50 ppm ERPG-3: 500 ppm	3 4 3	Colorless. Highly flammable. Etherlike odor is a poor warning property. Important source of exposures is sterilization operations in health care industry.
Ethyl ether (diethyl ether [CAS: 60-29-7]): Vapors irritating to eyes and respiratory tract. A CNS depressant and anesthetic agent; tolerance may develop to this effect. Overexposure produces nausea, headache, dizziness, anesthesia, and respiratory arrest. Evidence for adverse effects on fetal development in test animals.	400 ppm	1900 ppm [LEL]	1 4 1	Colorless liquid. Etherlike odor occurs at low levels and is a good warning property. Vapor pressure is 439 mm Hg at 20 °C (68 °F). Highly flammable.

Substance	TLV	ERPG	H	F	R	Comments
Ethyl formate (CAS: 109-94-4): Slightly irritating to the skin upon direct contact. Vapors mildly irritating to eyes and upper respiratory tract. In test animals, very high levels caused rapid narcosis and pulmonary edema.	100 ppm	1500 ppm	2	3	0	Colorless liquid. Fruity odor and irritation occur near the TLV and are good warning properties. Vapor pressure is 194 mm Hg at 20 °C (68 °F). Highly flammable.
Ethyl mercaptan (ethanethiol [CAS: 75-08-1]): Vapors mildly irritating to eyes and respiratory tract. Respiratory paralysis and CNS depression at very high levels. Headache, nausea, and vomiting likely owing to strong odor.	0.5 ppm [proposed: 10 ppm]	500 ppm	2	4	0	Colorless liquid. Penetrating, offensive, mercaptan-like odor. Vapor pressure is 442 mm Hg at 20 °C (68 °F).
N-Ethylmorpholine (CAS: 100-74-3): Irritating to eyes upon direct contact. Vapors irritating to eyes and respiratory tract. Workers exposed to levels near the TLV reported drowsiness and temporary visual distrubances, including corneal edema. Animal testing suggests potential for skin absorption.	5 ppm, S	100 ppm	2	3	0	Colorless liquid with ammonialike odor. Vapor pressure is 5 mm Hg at 20 °C (68 °F). Flammable. Thermal breakdown products include oxides of nitrogen.
Ethyl silicate (tetraethyl orthosilicate, tetraethoxysilane [CAS: 78-10-4]): Irritating upon direct contact. Vapors irritating to eyes and respiratory tract. All human effects noted at vapor exposures above the odor threshold. In subchronic animal testing, high vapor levels produced liver, lung, and kidney damage, and delayed-onset pulmonary edema.	10 ppm	700 ppm	2	2	0	Colorless liquid. Faint alcohollike odor and irritation are good warning properties. Vapor pressure is 2 mm Hg at 20 °C (68 °F). Flammable.
Fenamiphos (ethyl 3-methyl-4-(methylthio)-phenyl(1-methylethyl)phosphoramide [CAS: 22224-92-6]): An organophosphate-type cholinesterase inhibitor (see p 244). Well absorbed dermally.	0.1 mg/m³, S					Tan, waxy solid. Vapor pressure is 0.000001 mm Hg at 30 °C (86 °F).
Fensulfothion (O,O-diethyl O-[4-(methyl-sulfinyl)phenyl]phos-phorothioate [CAS: 115-90-2]): An organophosphate-type cholinesterase inhibitor (see p 244).	0.1 mg/m³					Brown liquid.

(C) = ceiling air concentration (TLV-C); S = skin absorption can be significant; A1 = ACGIH-confirmed human carcinogen; A2 = ACGIH-suspected human carcinogen; NFPA Hazard Codes: H = health, F = fire, R = reactivity, Ox = oxidizer, W = water-reactive, 0 (none) <—> 4 (severe). ERPG = Emergency Response Planning Guideline. See p 434 for explanation of definitions.

(continued)

TABLE IV–4. HEALTH HAZARD SUMMARIES FOR INDUSTRIAL AND OCCUPATIONAL CHEMICALS (CONTINUED)

Health Hazard Summaries	ACGIH TLV	IDLH	NFPA Codes H F R	Comments
Fenthion (O,O-dimethyl O-[3-methyl-4-(methylthio)phenyl]phosphorothioate [CAS: 55-38-9]): An organophosphate-type cholinesterase inhibitor (see p 244). Highly lipid soluble; toxicity may be prolonged. Dermal absorption is rapid.	0.2 mg/m³, S			Yellow to tan viscous liquid with a mild garliclike odor. Vapor pressure is 0.00003 mm Hg at 20 °C (68 °F).
Ferbam (ferric dimethyldithiocarbamate [CAS: 14484-64-1]): Thiocarbamates do not act through cholinesterase inhibition. Dusts irritating upon direct contact; causes dermatitis in persons sensitized to sulfur. Dusts are mild respiratory tract irritants. Limited evidence for adverse effects on fetal development in test animals.	10 mg/m³	800 mg/m³		Odorless, black solid. Vapor pressure is negligible at 20 °C (68 °F). Thermal breakdown products include oxides of nitrogen and sulfur. Used as a fungicide.
Ferrovanadium dust (CAS: 12604-58-9): Mild irritant of eyes and respiratory tract.	1 mg/m³	500 mg/m³		Odorless, dark-colored powders.
Fluoride dust (as fluoride): Irritating to eyes and respiratory tract. Workers exposed to levels 10 mg/m³ suffered nasal irritation and bleeding. Lower level exposures have produced nausea and eye and respiratory tract irritation. Chronic overexposures may result in skin rashes. Fluorosis, a bone disease with chronic high-level fluoride ingestion, is not associated with occupational dust inhalation. See also p 170.	2.5 mg/m³ (as F)	250 mg/m³ (as F)		Appearance varies with the compound. Sodium fluoride is a colorless to blue solid.
Fluorine (CAS: 7782-41-4): Rapidly reacts with moisture to form ozone and hydrofluoric acid. The gas is a severe eye, skin, and respiratory tract irritant; severe penetrating burns and pulmonary edema have resulted. Systemic hypocalcemia can occur with fluorine or hydrogen fluoride exposure. See also p 186.	1 ppm ERPG-1: 0.5 ppm ERPG-2: 5.0 ppm ERPG-3: 20 ppm	25 ppm	4 0 4 W	Pale yellow gas. Sharp odor is a poor warning property. Highly reactive; will ignite many oxidizable materials. Uses include rocket fuel oxidizer.

Chemical	TLV-C / Exposure	ERPG	NFPA (H F R)	Comments
Fonofos (*O*-ethyl *S*-phenyl ethylphosphono-thiolothionate, Dyfonate [CAS: 944-22-9]): An organophosphate-type cholinesterase inhibitor (see p 244). Highly toxic; oral toxicity in test animals ranged from 3 to 13 mg/kg for rats, and rabbits died after eye instillation.	0.1 mg/m³, S			Vapor pressure is 0.00021 mm Hg at 20 °C (68 °F). Thermal breakdown products include oxides of sulfur.
Formaldehyde (formic aldehyde, methanal, HCHO, formalin [CAS: 50-00-0]): Highly irritating to eyes upon direct contact; severe burns result. Irritating to skin; may cause a sensitization dermatitis. Vapors highly irritating to eyes and respiratory tract. Sensitization may occur. A carcinogen in test animals (IARC 2A). See also p 177.	0.3 ppm (C), A2 OSHA CA NIOSH CA	20 ppm ERPG-1: 1 ppm ERPG-2: 10 ppm ERPG-3: 25 ppm	3 4 0 (gas) 3 2 0 (formalin)	Colorless gas with a suffocating odor. Combustible. Formalin (15% methanol) solutions are flammable.
Formamide (methanamide [CAS: 75-12-7]): In animal tests, mildly irritating upon direct contact. Adverse effects on fetal development in test animals at very high doses.	10 ppm, S		2 1 –	Clear, viscous liquid. Odorless. Vapor pressure is 2 mm Hg at 70 °C (158 °F). Combustible. Thermal breakdown products include oxides of nitrogen.
Formic acid (CAS: 64-18-6): Acid is corrosive; severe burns may result from contact of eyes and skin with concentrated acid. Vapors highly irritating to eyes and respiratory tract. Ingestion may produce severe metabolic acidosis and blindness (see methanol, p 218).	5 ppm	30 ppm	3 2 0	Colorless liquid. Pungent odor and irritation occur near the TLV and are adequate warning properties. Vapor pressure is 30 mm Hg at 20 °C (68 °F). Combustible.
Furfural (bran oil [CAS: 98-01-1]): Highly irritating upon direct contact; burns may result. Vapors highly irritating to eyes and respiratory tract; pulmonary edema may result. Animal studies indicate the liver is a target organ. Hyperreflexia and convulsions occur at large doses in test animals.	2 ppm, S, A3	100 ppm ERPG-1: 2 ppm ERPG-2: 10 ppm ERPG-3: 100 ppm	3 2 0	Colorless to light brown liquid. Almondlike odor occurs below the TLV and is a good warning property. Vapor pressure is 2 mm Hg at 20 °C (68 °F). Combustible. Thermal breakdown products include oxides of nitrogen.
Furfuryl alcohol (CAS: 98-00-0): Dermal absorption occurs. Vapors irritating to eyes and respiratory tract. A CNS depressant at high air levels.	10 ppm, S	75 ppm	1 2 1	Clear, colorless liquid. Upon exposure to light and air, changes color to red or brown. Vapor pressure is 0.53 mm Hg at 20 °C (68 °F). Combustible.

(C) = ceiling air concentration (TLV-C); S = skin absorption can be significant; A1 = ACGIH-confirmed human carcinogen; A2 = ACGIH-suspected human carcinogen; OSHA CA = OSHA carcinogen; NIOSH CA = NIOSH carcinogen; NFPA Hazard Codes: H = health, F = fire, R = reactivity, Ox = oxidizer, W = water-reactive, 0 (none) <—> 4 (severe); ERPG = Emergency Response Planning Guideline. See p 434 for explanation of definitions.

(continued)

TABLE IV-4. HEALTH HAZARD SUMMARIES FOR INDUSTRIAL AND OCCUPATIONAL CHEMICALS (CONTINUED)

Health Hazard Summaries	ACGIH TLV	IDLH	NFPA Codes H F R	Comments
Gasoline (CAS: 8006-61-9): Although exact composition varies, the acute toxicity of all gasolines is similar. Vapors irritating to eyes and respiratory tract at high levels. A CNS depressant; symptoms include incoordination, dizziness, headaches, and nausea. Benzene (generally < 1%) is one significant chronic health hazard. Other additives such as ethylene dibromide and tetraethyl and tetramethyl lead are present in low amounts and may be absorbed through the skin. Very limited evidence for carcinogenicity in test animals. See also p 183.	300 ppm, A3		1 3 0	Clear to amber liquid with a characteristic odor. Highly flammable. Gasoline is sometimes inappropriately used as a solvent. Substance abuse via inhalation has been reported.
Germanium tetrahydride (CAS: 7782-65-2): A hemolytic agent with effects similar to but less potent than arsine in animals. Symptoms include abdominal pain, hematuria, anemia, and jaundice.	0.2 ppm			Colorless gas. Highly flammable.
Glutaraldehyde (1,5-pentandial (CAS: 111-30-8)): The purity and therefore the toxicity of glutaraldehyde varies widely. Allergic dermatitis may occur. Highly irritating on contact; severe burns may result. Vapors highly irritating to eyes and respiratory tract; respiratory sensitization may occur. In animal studies, the liver is a target organ at high doses.	0.05 ppm (C)			Colorless solid crystals. Vapor pressure is 0.0152 mm Hg at 20 °C (68 °F). Can undergo hazardous self-polymerization. Commonly used as a sterilizing agent in medical settings.
Glycidol (2,3-epoxy-1-propanol (CAS: 556-52-5)): Highly irritating to eyes on contact; burns may result. Moderately irritating to skin and respiratory tract. Evidence for carcinogenicity and testicular toxicity in test animals.	2 ppm, A3	150 ppm		Colorless liquid. Vapor pressure is 0.9 mm Hg at 25 °C (77 °F). Combustible.
Hafnium (CAS: 7440-58-6): Based on animal studies, dusts are mildly irritating to eyes and skin. Liver injury may occur at very high doses.	0.5 mg/m^3	50 mg/m^3		The metal is a gray solid. Other compounds vary in appearance.

Substance	Exposure	H	R	F	Comments
Heptachlor (CAS: 76-44-8): CNS convulsant. Skin absorption is rapid and has caused convulsions and death. Hepatotoxic. Stored in fatty tissues. Limited evidence for adverse effects on fetal development in test animals at high doses. A carcinogen in test animals. See also p 133.	0.05 mg/m³, S, A3				White or light tan, waxy solid with a camphorlike odor. Vapor pressure is 0.0003 mm Hg at 20 °C (68 °F). Thermal breakdown products include hydrogen chloride. Not combustible.
n-Heptane (CAS: 142-82-5): Vapors only slightly irritating to eyes and respiratory tract. May cause euphoria, vertigo, CNS depression, and cardiac arrhythmias at high levels.	400 ppm	1	3	0	Colorless clear liquid. Mild gasolinelike odor occurs below the TLV and is a good warning property. Vapor pressure is 40 mm Hg at 20 °C (68 °F). Flammable.
Hexachlorobutadiene (CAS: 87-68-3): Based on animal studies, rapid dermal absorption is expected. The kidney is the major target organ. A carcinogen in test animals (IARC 3).	0.02 ppm, S, A3				Heavy, colorless liquid. Thermal breakdown products include hydrogen chloride and phosgene.
Hexachlorocyclopentadiene (CAS: 77-47-4): Vapors extremely irritating to eyes and respiratory tract; lacrimation, salivation. In animal studies, a potent kidney and liver toxin. At higher levels the brain, heart, and adrenal glands were affected. Tremors occurred at high doses.	0.01 ppm				Yellow to amber liquid with a pungent odor. Vapor pressure is 0.08 mm Hg at 20 °C (68 °F). Not combustible.
Hexachloroethane (perchloroethane) [CAS: 67-72-1]: Hot fumes irritating to eyes, skin, and mucous membranes. Based on animal studies, causes CNS depression and kidney and liver injury at high doses. Limited evidence of carcinogenicity in test animals. (IARC 3).	1 ppm, S, A3 NIOSH CA				White solid with a camphorlike odor. Vapor pressure is 0.22 mm Hg at 20 °C (68 °F). Not combustible. Thermal breakdown products include phosgene, chlorine gas, and hydrogen chloride.
Hexachloronaphthalene (Halowax 1014 [CAS: 1335-87-1]: Based on workplace experience, a potent toxin causing severe chloracne and severe, occasionally fatal, liver injury. Skin absorption can occur.	0.2 mg/m³, S				Light yellow solid with an aromatic odor. Vapor pressure is less than 1 mm Hg at 20 °C (68 °F). Not combustible.
Hexamethylphosphoramide (CAS: 680-31-9): Low-level exposures produced nasal cavity cancer in rats (IARC 2B). Adverse effects on the testes in test animals.	S, A3				Colorless liquid with an aromatic odor. Vapor pressure is 0.07 mm Hg at 20 °C (68 °F). Thermal breakdown products include oxides of nitrogen.

ERPG-1: 3 ppm
ERPG-2: 10 ppm
ERPG-3: 30 ppm

2 1 1

300 ppm

35 mg/m³

2 mg/m³, S

750 ppm

(C) = ceiling air concentration (TLV-C); S = skin absorption can be significant; A1 = ACGIH-confirmed human carcinogen; A2 = ACGIH-suspected human carcinogen; NFPA Hazard Codes: H = health, F = fire, R = reactivity, Ox = oxidizer, W = water-reactive, 0 (none) <—> 4 (severe). ERPG = Emergency Response Planning Guideline. See p 434 for explanation of definitions.

(continued)

TABLE IV–4. HEALTH HAZARD SUMMARIES FOR INDUSTRIAL AND OCCUPATIONAL CHEMICALS (CONTINUED)

Health Hazard Summaries	ACGIH TLV	IDLH	NFPA Codes H F R			Comments
n-Hexane (normal hexane [CAS: 110-54-3]): Vapors mildly irritating to eyes and respiratory tract. A CNS depressant at high levels, producing headache, dizziness, and gastrointestinal upset. Occupational overexposures have resulted in peripheral neuropathies. Methyl ethyl ketone potentiates this toxicity. Testicular toxicity in animal studies.	50 ppm, S	1100 ppm [LEL]	1	3	0	Colorless, clear liquid with a mild gasoline odor. Vapor pressure is 124 mm Hg at 20 °C (68 °F). Highly flammable.
Hexane isomers (other than *n*-hexane, isohexane, 2,3-demethyl-butane): Vapors mildly irritating to eyes and respiratory tract. A CNS depressant at high levels, producing headache, dizziness, and gastrointestinal upset.	500 ppm					Colorless liquids with a mild petroleum odor. Vapor pressures are high at 20 °C (68 °F). Highly flammable.
sec-Hexyl acetate (1,3-dimethylbutyl acetate [CAS: 108-84-9]): At low levels, vapors irritating to eyes and respiratory tract. Based on animal studies, a CNS depressant at high levels.	50 ppm	500 ppm	1	2	0	Colorless liquid. Unpleasant fruity odor and irritation are both good warning properties. Vapor pressure is 4 mm Hg at 20 °C (68 °F). Flammable.
Hexylene glycol (2-methyl-2,4-pentanediol [CAS: 107-41-5]): Irritating upon direct contact; vapors irritating to eyes and respiratory tract. A CNS depressant at very high doses in animal studies.	25 ppm (C)		1	1	0	Liquid with a faint sweet odor. Vapor pressure is 0.05 mm Hg at 20 °C (68 °F). Combustible.
Hydrazine (diamine [CAS: 302-01-2]): Corrosive upon direct contact; severe burns result. Vapors extremely irritating to eyes and respiratory tract; pulmonary edema may occur. Highly hepatotoxic. A convulsant and hemolytic agent. Kidneys are also target organs. Well absorbed by all routes. A carcinogen in test animals (IARC 2B).	0.01 ppm, S, A3 NIOSH CA	50 ppm	3	3	3 (vapors explosive)	Colorless, fuming, viscous liquid with an amine odor. Vapor pressure is 10 mm Hg at 20 °C (68 °F). Flammable. Thermal breakdown products include oxides of nitrogen. Used as rocket fuel.
Hydrogen bromide (HBr [CAS: 10035-10-6]): Direct contact with concentrated solutions may cause corrosive acid burns. Vapors highly irritating to eyes and respiratory tract; pulmonary edema may result.	3 ppm (C)	30 ppm	3	0	0	Colorless gas or pressurized liquid. Acrid odor and irritation occur near the TLV and are adequate warning properties. Not combustible.

Chemical	TLV	ERPG	NFPA	Comments
Hydrogen chloride (muriatic acid, HCl [CAS: 7647-01-0]): Direct contact with concentrated solutions may cause corrosive acid burns. Vapors highly irritating to eyes and respiratory tract; pulmonary edema has resulted.	5 ppm (C)	50 ppm ERPG-1: 3 ppm ERPG-2: 20 ppm ERPG-3: 100 ppm	3 0 1	Colorless gas with a pungent, choking odor. Irritation occurs near the TLV and is a good warning property. Not combustible.
Hydrogen cyanide (hydrocyanic acid, prussic acid, HCN [CAS: 74-90-8]): A rapidly acting, potent metabolic asphyxiant that inhibits cytochrome oxidase and stops cellular respiration. See also p 150.	4.7 ppm (C), S	50 ppm ERPG-2: 10 ppm ERPG-3: 25 ppm	4 4 2 (vapors extremely toxic)	Colorless to pale blue liquid or colorless gas with a sweet, bitter almond smell that is an inadequate warning property even for those sensitive to it. Vapor pressure is 620 mm Hg at 20 °C (68 °F). Cyanide salts will release HCN gas with exposure to acids or heat.
Hydrogen fluoride (hydrofluoric acid, HF [CAS: 7664-39-3]): Produces severe, penetrating burns to eyes, skin, and deeper tissues upon direct contact with solutions. Onset of pain and erythema may be delayed as much as 12–16 hours. As a gas, highly irritating to the eyes and respiratory tract; pulmonary edema has resulted. Severe hypocalcemia may occur with overexposure. See p 186.	3 ppm (C) (as F)	30 ppm ERPG-1: 2 ppm ERPG-2: 20 ppm ERPG-3: 50 ppm	4 0 1	Colorless fuming liquid or gas. Irritation occurs at levels below the TLV and is an adequate warning property. Vapor pressure is 760 mm Hg at 20 °C (68 °F). Not combustible. Commercial rust-removing products may contain HF, but generally at lower concentrations (< 10%).
Hydrogen peroxide (CAS: 7722-84-1): A strong oxidizing agent. Direct contact with concentrated solutions can produce severe eye damage and skin irritation, including erythema and vesicle formation. Vapors irritating to eyes, skin, mucous membranes, and respiratory tract.	1 ppm	75 ppm ERPG-1: 10 ppm ERPG-2: 50 ppm ERPG-3: 100 ppm	2 0 3 Ox (60% or greater) 2 0 1 Ox (40–60%)	Colorless liquid with a slightly sharp, distinctive odor. Vapor pressure is 5 mm Hg at 30 °C (86 °F). Because of instability, usually found in aqueous solutions. Not combustible but a very powerful oxidizing agent.
Hydrogen selenide (CAS: 7783-07-5): Vapors extremely irritating to eyes and respiratory tract. Systemic symptoms from low-level exposure include nausea and vomiting, fatigue, metallic taste in mouth, and a garlicky breath odor. Animal studies indicate hepatotoxicity.	0.05 ppm	1 ppm		Colorless gas. The strongly offensive odor and irritation occur only at levels far above the TLV and are poor warning properties. Flammable. Water-reactive.

(C) = ceiling air concentration (TLV-C); S = skin absorption can be significant; A1 = ACGIH-confirmed human carcinogen; A2 = ACGIH-suspected human carcinogen; NFPA Hazard Codes: H = health, F = fire, R = reactivity, Ox = oxidizer, W = water-reactive, 0 (none) <—> 4 (severe); ERPG = Emergency Response Planning Guideline. See p 434 for explanation of definitions.

(continued)

TABLE IV-4. HEALTH HAZARD SUMMARIES FOR INDUSTRIAL AND OCCUPATIONAL CHEMICALS (CONTINUED)

Health Hazard Summaries	ACGIH TLV	IDLH	NFPA Codes H F R	Comments
Hydrogen sulfide (sewer gas [CAS: 7783-06-4]): Vapors irritating to eyes and respiratory tract. At higher levels, a potent, rapid systemic toxin causing cellular asphyxia and death. Systemic effects of low-level exposure include headache, cough, nausea, and vomiting. See also p 188.	10 ppm [proposed: 5 ppm]	100 ppm ERPG-1: 0.1 ppm ERPG-2: 30 ppm ERPG-3: 100 ppm	4 4 0	Colorless gas. Although the strong rotten egg odor can be detected at very low levels, olfactory fatigue occurs. Odor is therefore a poor warning property. Flammable. Produced by the decay of organic material as may occur in sewers, manure pits, and fish processing. Fossil fuel production also may generate the gas.
Hydroquinone (1,4-dihydroxybenzene [CAS: 123-31-9]): Highly irritating to eyes upon direct contact. Chronic occupational exposures may cause partial discoloration and opacification of the cornea. Systemic effects reported result from ingestion and include tinnitus, headache, dizziness, gastrointestinal upset, CNS excitation, and skin depigmentation. May cause methemoglobinemia (see p 220). Limited evidence of carcinogenicity in test animals.	2 mg/m³, A3	50 mg/m³	2 1 0	White solid crystals. Vapor pressure is less than 0.001 mm Hg at 20 °C (68 °F). Combustible.
2-Hydroxypropyl acrylate (HPA [CAS: 999-61-1]): Highly irritating upon direct contact; severe burns may result. Vapors highly irritating to eyes and respiratory tract. Based on structural analogies, compounds containing the acrylate moiety may be carcinogens.	0.5 ppm, S		3 1 2	Combustible liquid.
Indene [CAS: 95-13-6]: Repeated direct contact with the skin produced a dry dermatitis but no systemic effects. Vapors likely irritating to eyes and respiratory tract. Based on animal studies, high air levels may cause liver and kidney damage.	10 ppm			Colorless liquid.
Indium [CAS: 7440-74-6]: Based on animal studies, the soluble salts are extremely irritating to eyes upon direct contact. Dusts irritating to eyes and respiratory tract. In animal studies, indium compounds are highly toxic parenterally but much less toxic orally.	0.1mg/m³			Appearance varies with the compound. The elemental metal is a silver-white lustrous solid.

Name and description	TLV	Other	H	F	R	Comments
Iodine [CAS: 7553-56-2]: Extremely irritating upon direct contact; severe burns result. Vapors extremely irritating and corrosive to eyes and respiratory tract. Rarely, a skin sensitizer. Medicinal use of iodine-containing drugs has been associated with fetal goiter, a potentially life-threatening condition for the fetus or infant. Iodine causes adverse effects on fetal development in test animals. See also p 190.	0.1 ppm (C)	2 ppm ERPG-1: 0.1 ppm ERPG-2: 0.5 ppm ERPG-3: 5 ppm				Violet-colored solid crystals. Sharp, characteristic odor is a poor warning property. Vapor pressure is 0.3 mm Hg at 20 °C (68 °F). Not combustible.
Iron oxide fume [CAS: 1309-37-1]: Fumes and dusts can produce a benign pneumoconiosis (siderosis) with shadows on chest radiographs.	5 mg/m³ (as Fe)	2500 mg/m³ (as Fe)				Red-brown fume with a metallic taste. Vapor pressure is negligible at 20 °C (68 °F).
Iron pentacarbonyl (Iron carbonyl) [CAS: 13463-40-6]): Acute toxicity resembles that of nickel carbonyl. Inhalation of vapors can cause lung and systemic injury without warning signs. Symptoms of overexposure include headache, nausea and vomiting, and dizziness. Symptoms of severe poisoning are fever, extreme weakness, and pulmonary edema; effects may be delayed for up to 36 hours.	0.1 ppm					Colorless to yellow viscous liquid. Vapor pressure is 40 mm Hg at 30.3 °C (86.5 °F). Highly flammable.
Isoamyl acetate (banana oil, 3-methyl butyl acetate [CAS: 123-92-21]: May be irritating to skin upon prolonged contact. Vapors mildly irritating to eyes and respiratory tract. Symptoms in men exposed to 950 ppm for 0.5 hour included headache, weakness, dyspnea, and irritation of the nose and throat. A CNS depressant at high doses in test animals.	100 ppm	1000 ppm	1	3	0	Colorless liquid. Bananalike odor and irritation occur at low levels and are good warning properties. Vapor pressure is 4 mm Hg at 20 °C (68 °F). Flammable.
Isoamyl alcohol (3-methyl-1-butanol [CAS: 123-51-3]: Vapors irritating to eyes and respiratory tract. A CNS depressant at high levels.	100 ppm	500 ppm	1	2	0	Colorless liquid. Irritating alcohollike odor and irritation are good warning properties. Vapor pressure is 2 mm Hg at 20 °C (68 °F). Flammable.
Isobutyl acetate (2-methylpropyl acetate [CAS: 110-19-0]: Vapors mildly irritating to eyes and respiratory tract. A CNS depressant at high levels.	150 ppm	1300 ppm [LEL]	1	3	0	Colorless liquid. Pleasant fruity odor is a good warning property. Vapor pressure is 13 mm Hg at 20 °C (68 °F). Flammable.

(C) = ceiling air concentration (TLV-C); S = skin absorption can be significant; A1 = ACGIH-confirmed human carcinogen; A2 = ACGIH-suspected human carcinogen; NFPA Hazard Codes: H = health, F = fire, R = reactivity, Ox = oxidizer, W = water-reactive, 0 (none) <—> 4 (severe). ERPG = Emergency Response Planning Guideline. See p 434 for explanation of definitions.

(continued)

TABLE IV–4. HEALTH HAZARD SUMMARIES FOR INDUSTRIAL AND OCCUPATIONAL CHEMICALS (CONTINUED)

Health Hazard Summaries	ACGIH TLV	IDLH	NFPA Codes H F R	Comments
Isobutyl alcohol (2-methyl-1 propanol [CAS: 78-83-1]): A CNS depressant at high levels.	50 ppm	1600 ppm	1 3 0	Colorless liquid. Mild characteristic odor is a good warning property. Vapor pressure is 9 mm Hg at 20 °C (68 °F). Flammable.
Isophorone (trimethylcyclohexenone [CAS: 78-59-1]): Vapors irritating to eyes and respiratory tract. Workers exposed to 5–8 ppm complained of fatigue and malaise after 1 month. Higher exposures result in nausea, headache, dizziness, and a feeling of suffocation at 200–400 ppm. Limited evidence for adverse effects on fetal development in test animals.	5 ppm (C), A3	200 ppm	2 2 0 W	Colorless liquid with a camphorlike odor. Vapor pressure is 0.2 mm Hg at 20 °C (68 °F). Flammable.
Isophorone diisocyanate (CAS: 4098-71-9]): Based on animal studies, extremely irritating upon direct contact; severe burns may result. By analogy with other isocyanates, vapors or mists likely to be potent respiratory sensitizers, causing asthma. See also p 194.	0.005 ppm		2 2 1 W	Colorless to pale yellow liquid. Vapor pressure is 0.0003 mm Hg at 20 °C (68 °F). Possible thermal breakdown products include oxides of nitrogen and hydrogen cyanide.
2-Isopropoxyethanol (isopropyl Cellosolve, ethylene glycol mono-isopropyl ether [CAS: 109-59-1]): Defatting agent causing dermatitis. May cause hemolysis.	25 ppm, S			Clear colorless liquid with a characteristic odor.
Isopropyl acetate (CAS: 108-21-4): Vapors irritating to the eyes and respiratory tract. A weak CNS depressant.	250 ppm	1800 ppm	1 3 0	Colorless liquid. Fruity odor and irritation are good warning properties. Vapor pressure is 43 mm Hg at 20 °C (68 °F). Flammable.
Isopropyl alcohol (isopropanol, 2-propanol [CAS: 67-63-0]): Vapors produce mild eye and respiratory tract irritation. High exposures can produce CNS depression. See also p 197.	400 pm [proposed: 200 ppm]	2000 ppm [LEL]	1 3 0	Rubbing alcohol. Sharp odor and irritation are adequate warning properties. Vapor pressure is 33 mm Hg at 20 °C (68 °F). Flammable.

Compound	TLV-C		NFPA Codes (H R F)	Comments
Isopropylamine (2-aminopropane [CAS: 75-31-0]): Corrosive upon direct contact; severe burns may result. Vapors highly irritating to the eyes and respiratory tract. Exposure to vapors can cause transient corneal edema.	5 ppm	750 ppm	3 4 0	Colorless liquid. Strong ammonia oror and irritation are good warning properties. Vapor pressure is 478 mm Hg at 20 °C (68 °F). Highly flammable. Thermal breakdown products include oxides of nitrogen.
Isopropyl ether (diisopropyl ether [CAS: 108-20-3]): A skin irritant upon prolonged contact with liquid. Vapors mildly irritating to the eyes and respiratory tract. A CNS depressant.	250 ppm	1400 ppm [LEL]	1 3 1	Colorless liquid. Offensive and sharp etherlike odor and irritation are good warning properties. Vapor pressure is 119 mm Hg at 20 °C (68 °F). Highly flammable. Contact with air causes formation of explosive peroxides.
Isopropyl glycidyl ether [CAS: 4016-14-2]: Irritating upon direct contact. Allergic dermatitis may occur. Vapors irritating to eyes and respiratory tract. In animals. A CNS depressant at high oral doses; chronic exposures produced liver injury. Some glycidyl ethers possess hematopoietic and testicular toxicity.	50 ppm	400 ppm		Flammable. Vapor pressure is 9.4 mm Hg at 25 °C (77 °F).
Kepone (chlordecone [CAS: 143-50-0]): Neurotoxin; overexposure causes slurred speech, memory impairment, incoordination, weakness, tremor, and convulsions. Causes infertility in males. Hepatotoxic. Well absorbed by all routes. A carcinogen in test animals. See also p 133.	NIOSH CA			A solid.
Ketene (ethenone [CAS: 463-51-4]): Vapors extremely irritating to the eyes and respiratory tract; pulmonary edema may result and can be delayed for up to 72 hours. Toxicity similar to that of phosgene (see p 262), of which it is the nonchlorinated analog, in both magnitude and time course.	0.5 ppm	5 ppm		Colorless gas with a sharp odor. Polymerizes readily. Acetylating agent. Water-reactive.

(C) = ceiling air concentration (TLV-C); S = skin absorption can be significant; A1 = ACGIH-confirmed human carcinogen; A2 = ACGIH-suspected human carcinogen; NFPA Hazard Codes: H = health, F = fire, R = reactivity, Ox = oxidizer, W = water-reactive, 0 (none) <—> 4 (severe); ERPG = Emergency Response Planning Guideline. See p 434 for explanation of definitions.

(continued)

TABLE IV–4. HEALTH HAZARD SUMMARIES FOR INDUSTRIAL AND OCCUPATIONAL CHEMICALS (CONTINUED)

Health Hazard Summaries	ACGIH TLV	IDLH	NFPA Codes H F R	Comments
Lead (inorganic compounds, dusts, and fumes): Toxic to CNS and peripheral nerves, kidneys, and hematopoietic system. Toxicity may result from acute or chronic exposures. Inhalation and ingestion are the major routes of absorption. Symptoms and signs include abdominal pain, anemia, mood or personality changes, and peripheral neuropathy. Encephalopathy may develop with high blood levels. Adversely affects reproductive functions in men and women. Adverse effects on fetal development in test animals. Such inorganic lead compounds are carcinogenic in animal studies (IARC 2B). See also p 199.	0.05 mg/m³, A3	100 mg/m³ (as Pb)		The elemental metal is dark gray. Vapor pressure is low, about 2 mm Hg at 1000 °C (1832 °F). Major industrial sources include smelting, battery manufacture, radiator repair, and glass and ceramic processing.
Lead arsenate (CAS: 10102-48-4): Most common acute poisoning symptoms are caused by arsenic, with lead being responsible for chronic toxicity. Symptoms include abdominal pain, headache, vomiting, diarrhea, nausea, itching, and lethargy. Liver and kidney damage may also occur. See both lead and arsenic, pp 199 and 95.	0.15 mg/m³			White powder often dyed pink. Not combustible.
Lead chromate (chrome yellow [CAS: 7758-97-6]): Toxicity may result from both the chromium and the lead components. Lead chromate is a suspect human carcinogen owing to the carcinogenicity of hexavalent chromium and inorganic lead compounds. See both lead and hexavalent chromium, pp 199 and 139.	0.05 mg/m³ (as Pb) 0.012 mg/m³ (as Cr), A2			Yellow pigment in powder or crystal form.
Lindane (gamma-hexachlorocyclohexane [CAS: 58-89-9]): A CNS stimulant and convulsant. Vapors irritating to the eyes and mucous membranes and produce severe headaches and nausea. Well absorbed by all routes. Animal feeding studies have resulted in lung, liver, and kidney damage. May injure bone marrow. Equivocal evidence of carcinogenicity in test animals. See also p 133.	0.5 mg/m³, S, A3	50 mg/m³		White crystalline substance with a musty odor if impure. Not combustible. Vapor is 0.0000094 mm Hg at 20 °C (68 °F). Although an agricultural chemical, lindane is more commonly found as a pediculocide in dilute solution (Kwell ®).

Substance	Ceiling air concentration (TLV-C)	Value	NFPA (H R F)	Comments
Lithium hydride (CAS: 7580-67-8): Strong vesicant and alkaline corrosive. Extremely irritating upon direct contact; severe burns result. Dusts extremely irritating to eyes and respiratory tract; pulmonary edema may develop. Symptoms of systemic toxicity include nausea, tremors, confusion, blurring of vision, and coma.	0.025 mg/m³	0.5 mg/m³ ERPG-1: 25µg1m³ ERPG-2: 100µg1m³ ERPG-3: 500 µg1m³	3 2 2 W	Off-white, translucent solid powder that darkens on exposure. Odorless. Very water-reactive, yielding highly flammable hydrogen gas and caustic lithium hydroxide. Finely dispersed powder may ignite spontaneously.
LPG (liquified petroleum gas [CAS: 68476-85-7]): A simple asphyxiant and possible CNS depressant. Flammability dangers greatly outweigh toxicity concerns. See also hydrocarbons, p 183.	1000 ppm	2000 ppm [LEL]		Colorless gas. An odorant is usually added as the pure product is odorless. Highly flammable.
Magnesium oxide fume (CAS: 1309-48-4): Slightly irritating to eyes and upper respiratory tract. May cause syndrome like metal fume fever (see p 217).	10 mg/m³	750 mg/m³		White fume.
Malathion (O,O-dimethyl dithiophosphate of diethyl mercaptosuccinate [CAS: 121-75-5]): An organophosphate-type cholinesterase inhibitor (see p 244). May cause skin sensitization. Absorbed dermally.	10 mg/m³, S	250 mg/m³		Colorless to brown liquid with mild skunklike odor. Vapor pressure is 0.00004 mm Hg at 20 °C (68 °F). Thermal breakdown products include oxides of sulfur and phosphorus.
Maleic anhydride (2,5-furandione [CAS: 108-31-6]): Extremely irritating upon direct contact; severe burns may result. Vapors and mists extremely irritating to eyes, skin, and respiratory tract. A skin and respiratory tract sensitizer (asthma).	0.25 ppm	10 mg/m³	3 1 1	Colorless to white solid. Strong, penetrating odor. Eye irritation occurs at the TLV and is an adequate warning property. Vapor pressure is 0.16 mm Hg at 20 °C (68 °F). Combustible.
Manganese (CAS: 7439-96-5): Chronic overexposure results in a CNS toxicity manifested as psychosis which may be followed by a progressive toxicity similar to parkinsonism (Manganism). See also p 211.	0.2 mg/m³ (elemental and inorganic compounds, as Mn)	500 mg/m³ (Mn compounds, as Mn)		Elemental metal is a gray, hard, brittle solid. Other compounds vary in appearance. Exposure occurs in mining and milling of the metal, in ferromanganese steel production, and through electric arc welding.

(C) = ceiling air concentration (TLV-C); S = skin absorption can be significant; A1 = ACGIH-confirmed human carcinogen; A2 = ACGIH-suspected human carcinogen; NFPA Hazard Codes: H = health, F = fire, R = reactivity, Ox = oxidizer, W = water-reactive, 0 (none) <——> 4 (severe). ERPG = Emergency Response Planning Guideline. See p 434 for explanation of definitions.

(continued)

TABLE IV–4. HEALTH HAZARD SUMMARIES FOR INDUSTRIAL AND OCCUPATIONAL CHEMICALS (CONTINUED)

Health Hazard Summaries	ACGIH TLV	IDLH	NFPA Codes H F R	Comments
Mercury (quicksilver [CAS: 7439-97-6]): Acute exposures to high vapor levels reported to cause toxic pneumonitis and pulmonary edema. Well absorbed by inhalation. Skin contact can produce irritation and sensitization dermatitis. Mercury salts but not metallic mercury are primarily toxic to the kidneys by acute ingestion. High acute or chronic overexposures can result in CNS toxicity (erythrism), chronic renal disease, brain injury, and peripheral neuropathies. Some inorganic mercury compounds have adverse effects on fetal development in test animals. See also p 213.	0.025 mg/m^3 (inorganic and elemental), S	10 mg/m^3		Elemental metal is a dense, silvery liquid. Odorless. Vapor pressure is 0.0012 mm Hg at 20 °C (68 °F). Sources of exposure include small-scale gold refining operations by hobbyists and mercury-containing instruments.
Mercury, alkyl compounds (dimethylmercury, diethyl mercury, ethylmercuric chloride, phenylmercuric acetate): Irritating upon direct contact; some compounds may cause burns. Well absorbed by all routes. Slow excretion may allow accumulation to occur. Readily crosses blood-brain barrier and placenta. High acute or chronic overexposures can cause kidney damage, organic brain disease, and peripheral neuropathy. Methylmercury is teratogenic in humans. See also p 213.	0.01 mg/m^3 (alkyl compounds, as Hg), S	2 mg/m^3 (as Hg)		Colorless liquids or solids. Many alkyl compounds have a disagreeable odor. Inorganic mercury can be converted to alkyl mercury compounds in the environment. Phenylmercuric acetate until recently was used as a fungicide in paints.
Mesityl oxide (4-methyl-3-penten-2-one [CAS: 141-79-7]): Causes dermatitis upon prolonged contact. Vapors very irritating to eyes and respiratory tract. Based on animal tests, a CNS depressant and injures kidney and liver at high levels.	15 ppm	1400 ppm [LEL]	2 3 1	Colorless viscous liquid with a peppermintlike odor. Irritation is an adequate warning property. Vapor pressure is 8 mm Hg at 20 °C (68 °F). Flammable. Readily forms peroxides.
Methacrylic acid (2-methylpropenoic acid [CAS: 79-41-4]): Corrosive upon direct contact; severe burns result. Vapors highly irritating to eyes and, possibly, respiratory tract. Based on structural analogies, compounds containing the acrylate moiety may be carcinogens.	20 ppm		3 2 2	Liquid with an acrid, disagreeable odor. Vapor pressure is less than 0.1 mm Hg at 20 °C (68 °F). Combustible. Polymerizes above 15 °C (59 °F), emitting toxic gases.

Compound	TLV		H	F	R	Comments
Methomyl (S-methyl N ((methylcarbamoyl)oxy) thioacetimidate, Lannate, Nudrin [CAS: 16752-77-5]): A carbamate-type cholinesterase inhibitor (see p 244).	2.5 mg/m³					A slight sulfur odor. Vapor pressure is 0.00005 mm Hg at 20 °C (68 °F). Thermal breakdown products include oxides of nitrogen and sulfur.
Methoxychlor (dimethoxy-DDT, 2,2-bis(p-methoxyphenol)-1,1,1-trichloroethane [CAS: 72-43-5]): A convulsant at very high doses in test animals. Limited evidence for adverse effects on male reproduction and fetal development in test animals at high doses. See also p 133.	10 mg/m³	5000 mg/m³				Colorless to tan solid with a mild fruity odor. Appearance and some hazardous properties vary with the formulation. Vapor pressure is very low at 20 °C (68 °F).
2-Methoxyethanol (ethylene glycol monomethyl ether, methyl Cellosolve [CAS: 109-86-4]): Workplace overexposures have resulted in depression of the hematopoietic system and encephalopathy. Symptoms include disorientation, lethargy, and anorexia. Well absorbed dermally. Animal testing revealed testicular atrophy and teratogenicity at low doses. Overexposure associated with reduced sperm counts in workers. See also p 166.	5 ppm, S	200 ppm	2	2	0	Clear, colorless liquid with a faint odor. Vapor pressure is 6 mm Hg at 20 °C (68 °F). Flammable.
2-Methoxyethyl acetate (ethylene glycol monomethyl ether acetate, methyl Cellosolve acetate [CAS: 110-49-6]): Mildly irritating to eyes upon direct contact. Dermally well absorbed. Vapors slightly irritating to the respiratory tract. A CNS depressant at high levels. Based on animal studies, may cause kidney damage, leukopenia, testicular atrophy, and birth defects. See also p 166.	5 ppm, S	200 ppm	1	2	–	Colorless liquid with a mild, pleasant odor. Flammable.
Methyl acetate [CAS: 79-20-9]: Vapors moderately irritating to the eyes and respiratory tract. A CNS depressant at high levels. Hydrolyzed to methanol in the body with possible consequent toxicity similar to that of methanol (see p 218).	200 ppm	3100 ppm [LEL]	1	3	0	Colorless liquid with a pleasant, fruity odor that is a good warning property. Vapor pressure is 173 mm Hg at 20 °C (68 °F). Flammable.
Methyl acetylene (propyne [CAS: 74-99-7]): A CNS depressant and respiratory irritant at very high air concentrations in test animals.	1000 ppm	1700 ppm [LEL]	2	4	2	Colorless gas with sweet odor. Flammable.

(C) = ceiling air concentration (TLV-C); S = skin absorption can be significant; A1 = ACGIH-confirmed human carcinogen; A2 = ACGIH-suspected human carcinogen; NFPA Hazard Codes: H = health, F = fire, R = reactivity, Ox = oxidizer, W = water-reactive, 0 (none) <—> 4 (severe); ERPG = Emergency Response Planning Guideline. See p 434 for explanation of definitions.

(continued)

TABLE IV–4. HEALTH HAZARD SUMMARIES FOR INDUSTRIAL AND OCCUPATIONAL CHEMICALS (CONTINUED)

Health Hazard Summaries	ACGIH TLV	IDLH	NFPA Codes H F R	Comments
Methyl acrylate (2-propenoic acid methyl ester [CAS: 96-33-3]): Highly irritating upon direct contact; severe burns may result. A possible skin sensitizer. Vapors highly irritating to the eyes and respiratory tract. Based on structural analogies, compounds containing the acrylate moiety may be carcinogens.	2 ppm, S	250 ppm	3 3 2	Colorless liquid with a sharp, fruity odor. Vapor pressure is 68.2 mm Hg at 20 °C (68 °F). Inhibitor included to prevent violent polymerization.
Methylal (dimethoxymethane [CAS: 109-87-5]): Mildly irritating to eyes and respiratory tract. A CNS depressant at very high levels. Animal studies suggest a potential to injure heart, liver, kidneys, and lungs at very high air levels.	1000 ppm	2200 ppm [LEL]	2 3 2	Colorless liquid with pungent, chloroformlike odor. Highly flammable.
Methylacrylonitrile (2-methyl-2-pro-penenitrile, methacrylonitrile [CAS: 126-98-7]): Mildly irritating upon direct contact. Well absorbed dermally. Metabolized to cyanide (see p 150). In animal tests, acute inhalation at high levels caused death without signs of irritation, probably by a mechanism similar to that of acrylonitrile. Lower levels produced convulsions and loss of motor control in hind limbs.	1 ppm, S			Liquid. Vapor pressure is 40 mm Hg at 13 °C (55 °F).
Methyl alcohol (methanol, wood alcohol [CAS: 67-56-1]): Mildly irritating to eyes and skin. Systemic toxicity may result from absorption by all routes. Toxic metabolites are formate and formaldehyde. A CNS depressant. Signs and symptoms include headache, nausea, abdominal pain, dizziness, shortness of breath, metabolic acidosis, and coma. Visual disturbances (optic neuropathy) range from blurred vision to blindness. See also p 218.	200 ppm, S	6000 ppm ERPG-1: 200 ppm ERPG-2: 1000 ppm ERPG-3: 5000 ppm	1 3 0	Colorless liquid with a distinctive, sharp odor that is a poor warning property. Flammable. Found in windshield fluids and antifreezes.
Methylamine (CAS: 74-89-5): Corrosive. Vapors highly irritating to eyes, skin, and respiratory tract; severe burns and pulmonary edema may result.	5 ppm	100 ppm ERPG-1: 10 ppm ERPG-2: 100 ppm ERPG-3: 500 ppm	3 4 0	Colorless gas with a fishy or ammonialike odor. Odor is a poor warning property owing to olfactory fatigue. Flammable.
Methyl-*n*-amyl ketone (2-heptanone [CAS: 110-43-0]): Vapors are irritating to eyes and respiratory tract. A CNS depressant.	50 ppm	800 ppm	1 2 0	Colorless or white liquid with a fruity odor. Vapor pressure is 2.6 mm Hg at 20 °C (68 °F). Flammable.

Chemical	TLV	H	R	F	Comments
***N*-methylaniline (CAS: 100-61-8):** A potent inducer of methemoglobinemia (see p 220). Well absorbed by all routes. Animal studies suggest potential for liver and kidney injury.	0.5 ppm, S				Yellow to light brown liquid with a weak ammonia-like odor. Vapor pressure is less than 1 mm Hg at 20 °C (68 °F). Thermal breakdown products include oxides of nitrogen
Methyl bromide (bromomethane [CAS: 74-83-9]): Causes severe irritation and burns upon direct contact. Vapors irritating to the lung; pulmonary edema may result. The CNS, liver, and kidneys are major target organs; acute poisoning causes nausea, vomiting, delirium, and convulsions. Both inhalation and skin exposure may cause systemic toxicity. Chronic exposures associated with peripheral neuropathy in humans. Evidence for adverse effects on fetal development in test animals. Limited evidence of carcinogenicity in test animals (IARC 3). See also p 222, and chloropicrin in this table.	1 ppm, S NIOSH CA	250 ppm ERPG-2: 50 ppm ERPG-3: 200 ppm	3	1	0	Colorless liquid or gas with a mild chloroformlike odor that is a poor warning property. Chloropicrin, a lacrimator, is often added as a warning agent. Methyl bromide is a widely used fumigant in agriculture and in structural pesticide control.
Methyl *n*-butyl ketone (MBK, 2-hexanone [CAS: 591-78-6]): Vapors irritating to eyes and respiratory tract at high levels. A CNS depressant at high doses. Causes peripheral neuropathy by a mechanism thought to be the same as that of *n*-hexane. Well absorbed by all routes. Causes testicular toxicity in animal studies.	5 ppm, S	1600 ppm	2	3	0	Colorless liquid with an acetonelike odor. Vapor pressure is 3.8 mm Hg at 20 °C (68 °F). Flammable. NIOSH recommended exposure limit is 1.0 ppm.
Methyl chloride (CAS: 74-87-3): Once used as an anesthetic. Symptoms include headache, confusion, ataxia, convulsions, and coma. Liver, kidney, and bone marrow are other target organs. Evidence for adverse effects on both the testes and fetal development in test animals at high doses.	50 ppm, S NIOSH CA	2000 ppm ERPG-2: 400 ppm ERPG-3: 1000 ppm	1	4	0	Colorless gas with a mild, sweet odor that is a poor warning property. Highly flammable.
Methyl-2-cyanoacrylate (CAS: 137-05-3): Vapors irritating to the eyes and upper respiratory tract. May act as a sensitizer. A strong and fast-acting glue that can fasten body parts to each other or surfaces. Direct contact with the eye may result in mechanical injury if the immediate bonding of the eyelids is followed by forced separation.	0.2 ppm				Colorless viscous liquid. Commonly, this compound and related ones are known as "super glues."

(C) = ceiling air concentration (TLV-C); S = skin absorption can be significant; A1 = ACGIH-confirmed human carcinogen; A2 = ACGIH-suspected human carcinogen; NFPA Hazard Codes: H = health, F = fire, R = reactivity, Ox = oxidizer, 0 (none) <—> 4 (severe). ERPG = Emergency Response Planning Guideline. See p 434 for explanation of definitions.

(continued)

TABLE IV–4. HEALTH HAZARD SUMMARIES FOR INDUSTRIAL AND OCCUPATIONAL CHEMICALS (CONTINUED)

Health Hazard Summaries	ACGIH TLV	IDLH	NFPA Codes H F R	Comments
Methylcyclohexane (CAS: 108-87-2): Irritating upon direct contact. Vapors irritating to eyes and respiratory tract. A CNS depressant at high levels. Based on animal studies, some liver and kidney injury may occur at chronic high doses.	400 ppm	1200 ppm [LEL]	2 3 0	Colorless liquid with a faint benzenelike odor. Vapor pressure is 37 mm Hg at 20 °C (68 °F). Highly flammable.
o-Methylcyclohexanone (CAS: 583-60-8): Based on animal studies, irritating upon direct contact. Dermal absorption occurs. Vapors irritating to eyes and respiratory tract. A CNS depressant at high levels.	50 ppm, S	600 ppm	– 2 0	Colorless liquid with mild peppermint odor. Irritation is a good warning property. Vapor pressure is about 1 mm Hg at 20 °C (68 °F). Flammable.
Methyl demeton (O,O-dimethyl 2-ethylmercaptoethyl thiophosphate [CAS: 8022-00-2]): An organophosphate-type cholinesterase inhibitor (see p 244).	0.5 mg/m³, S			Colorless to pale yellow liquid with an unpleasant odor. Vapor pressure is 0.00036 mm Hg at 20 °C (68 °F). Thermal breakdown products include oxides of sulfur and phosphorus.
4,4´-Methylene-bis(2-chloroaniline) (MOCA [CAS: 101-14-4]): A carcinogen in test animals (IARC 2A). Dermal absorption occurs.	0.01 ppm, S, A2 NIOSH CA			Tan solid. Thermal breakdown products include oxides of nitrogen and hydrogen chloride.
Methylene bis(4-cyclohexylisocyanate [CAS: 5124-30-1]): A strong irritant and skin sensitizer. Based on analogy to other isocyanates, vapors are likely to be potent respiratory tract irritants and sensitizers. See also p 194.	0.005 ppm			White to pale yellow solid flakes. Odorless Possible thermal breakdown products include oxides of nitrogen and hydrogen cyanide.
Methylene bisphenyl isocyanate (4,4-di-phenylmethane diisocyanate, MDI [CAS: 101-68-81]): Irritating upon direct contact. Vapors and dusts highly irritating to eyes and respiratory tract. Potent respiratory tract sensitizer (asthma). See also p 194.	0.005 ppm	75 mg/m³		White to pale yellow flakes. Odorless. Vapor pressure is 0.05 mm Hg at 20 °C (68 °F). Possible thermal breakdown products include oxides of nitrogen and hydrogen cyanide. Component of urethanes.

Chemical / Toxicology	Exposure limits	NFPA (H F R)	Comments / Physical properties
Methylene chloride (methylene dichloride, dichloromethane [CAS: 75-09-2]): Irritating upon prolonged direct contact. Dermal absorption occurs. Vapors irritating to eyes and respiratory tract. A CNS depressant. May cause cardiac arrhythmias. Liver and kidney injury at high concentrations. Converted to carbon monoxide in the body with resultant carboxyhemoglobin formation. A carcinogen in test animals (IARC 2B). See also p 224.	50 ppm, A3, OSHA CA, NIOSH CA / 2300 ppm, ERPG-1: 200 ppm, ERPG-2: 750 ppm, ERPG-3: 4000 ppm	2 1 0	Heavy colorless liquid with a chloroformlike odor that is a poor warning property. Vapor pressure is 350 mm Hg at 20 °C (68 °F). Possible thermal breakdown products include phosgene and hydrogen chloride. Methylene chloride is a solvent with many industrial and commercial uses (eg, furniture strippers, carburetor cleaners).
4,4′-Methylene dianiline (4,4′-diaminodiphenylmethane [CAS: 101-77-9]): Vapors highly irritating to eyes and respiratory tract. Hepatotoxicity (cholestatic jaundice) observed in overexposed workers. Systemic toxicity may result from inhalation, ingestion, or skin contact. Methemoglobinemia (see p 220), kidney injury, retinal injury, and evidence of carcinogenicity in animals (IARC 2B).	0.1 ppm, S, A3, NIOSH CA	3 1 0	Light brown solid crystals with a faint amine odor. Combustible. Thermal breakdown products include oxides of nitrogen.
Methyl ethyl ketone (2-butanone, MEK [CAS: 78-93-3]): Vapors irritating to eyes and respiratory tract. A CNS depressant at high levels. Limited evidence for adverse effects on fetal development in test animals. Potentiates neurotoxicity of methyl butyl ketone and n-hexane.	200 ppm / 3000 ppm	1 3 0	Colorless liquid with a mild acetone odor. Vapor pressure is 77 mm Hg at 20 °C (68 °F). Flammable.
Methyl ethyl ketone peroxide (CAS: 1338-23-4): Based on chemical reactivity, highly irritating upon direct contact; severe burns may result. Vapors or mists likely to be highly irritating to the eyes and respiratory tract. In animal tests, overexposure resulted in liver, kidney, and lung damage.	0.2 ppm (C)		Colorless liquid with a characteristic odor. Shock sensitive. Breaks down above 50 °C (122 °F). Explodes upon rapid heating. May contain additives such as dimethyl phthalate, cyclohexanone peroxide, or diallylphthalate to add stability.
Methyl formate (CAS: 107-31-3): Vapors highly irritating to eyes and respiratory tract. A CNS depressant at high levels. Exposure has been associated with visual disturbances, including temporary blindness.	100 ppm / 4500 ppm	2 4 0	Colorless liquid with a pleasant odor at high levels. Odor is a poor warning property. Vapor pressure is 476 mm Hg at 20 °C (68 °F). Highly flammable.

(C) = ceiling air concentration (TLV-C); S = skin absorption can be significant; A1 = ACGIH-confirmed human carcinogen; A2 = ACGIH-suspected human carcinogen; NFPA Hazard Codes: H = health, F = fire, R = reactivity, Ox = oxidizer, W = water-reactive, 0 (none) <—> 4 (severe). ERPG = Emergency Response Planning Guideline. See p 434 for explanation of definitions.

(continued)

TABLE IV–4. HEALTH HAZARD SUMMARIES FOR INDUSTRIAL AND OCCUPATIONAL CHEMICALS (CONTINUED)

Health Hazard Summaries	ACGIH TLV	IDLH	NFPA Codes H F R	Comments
Methylhydrazine (monomethylhydrazine [CAS: 60-34-4]): Similar to hydrazine in toxic actions. Vapors likely to be highly irritating to the eyes and respiratory tract. Causes methemoglobinemia (see p 220). Potent hemolysin. Highly hepatotoxic. Causes kidney injury. A convulsant. A carcinogen in test animals.	0.01 ppm, S, A3 NIOSH CA	20 ppm	4 3 2	Colorless clear liquid. Vapor pressure is 36 mm Hg at 20 °C (68 °F). Flammable. In addition to potential industrial uses, exposure to methylhydrazine can occur from ingestion of false morel mushrooms.
Methyl iodide: (iodomethane [CAS: 74-88-4]): An alkylating agent. Based on chemical properties, likely to be highly irritating upon direct contact; severe burns may result. Dermal absorption is likely. Vapors highly irritating to respiratory tract; pulmonary edema has resulted. Neurotoxic; signs and symptoms include nausea, vomiting, dizziness, slurred speech, visual disturbances, ataxia, tremor, irritability, convulsions, and coma. Delusions and hallucinations may last for weeks during recovery. Severe hepatic injury may also occur. Limited evidence of carcinogenicity in test animals (IARC 3).	2 ppm, S, NIOSH CA	100 ppm ERPG-1: 25 ppm ERPG-2: 50 ppm ERPG-3: 125 ppm		Colorless, yellow, red, or brown liquid. Not combustible. Vapor pressure is 375 mm Hg at 20 °C (68 °F). Thermal breakdown products include iodine and hydrogen iodide.
Methyl isoamyl ketone (5-methyl-2-hexanone [CAS: 110-12-3]): By analogy to other aliphatic-ketones, vapors are likely to be irritating to eyes and respiratory tract. Likely to be a CNS depressant.	50 ppm		1 2 0	Colorless liquid with a pleasant odor. Vapor pressure is 4.5 mm Hg at 20 °C (68 °F). Flammable.
Methyl isobutyl ketone (4-methyl-2-pentanone, hexone [CAS: 108-10-1]): Irritating to eyes upon direct contact. Vapors irritating to eyes and respiratory tract. Reported systemic symptoms in humans are weakness, dizziness, ataxia, nausea, vomiting, and headache. High-dose studies in animals suggest a potential for liver and kidney injury.	50 ppm	500 ppm	2 3 1	Colorless liquid with a mild odor. Vapor pressure is 7.5 mm Hg at 25 °C (77 °F). Flammable.

Chemical	Air concentration	ERPG	NFPA Codes	Comments

Methyl isocyanate (MIC [CAS: 624-83-9]): Highly reactive; highly corrosive upon direct contact. Vapors extremely irritating to eyes, skin, and respiratory tract; severe burns and pulmonary edema have resulted. A sensitizing agent. Toxicity is not related to cyanide. Evidence that severe poisonings have adverse effects on fetal development. See also p 194.

0.02 ppm, S

3 ppm
ERPG-1: 0.025 ppm
ERPG-2: 0.5 ppm
ERPG-3: 5 ppm

4 3 2
W

Colorless liquid with a sharp, disagreeable odor that is a poor warning property. Vapor pressure is 348 mm Hg at 20 °C (68 °F). Flammable. Reacts with water to release methylamine. Polymerizes upon heating. Thermal breakdown products include hydrogen cyanide and oxides of nitrogen. Used as a chemical intermediate in pesticide synthesis. MIC is not in urethanes.

Methyl mercaptan (CAS: 74-93-1): Causes delayed-onset pulmonary edema. CNS effects include narcosis and convulsions. Reported to have caused methemoglobinemia and hemolysis in a patient with G6PD deficiency (see p 220).

0.5 ppm
[proposed:
5 ppm]

150 ppm
ERPG-1: 0.005 ppm
ERPG-2: 25 ppm
ERPG-3: 100 ppm

4 4 0

Colorless liquid with an offensive rotten egg odor. Odor and irritation are good warning properties.

Methyl methacrylate (CAS: 80-62-6): Irritating upon direct contact. Vapors irritating to the eyes, skin, and respiratory tract. A sensitizer (asthma). At very high levels may produce headache, nausea, vomiting, dizziness. Limited evidence for adverse effects on fetal development in animal tests at very high doses.

100 ppm

1000 ppm

2 3 2

Colorless liquid with a pungent, acrid, fruity odor. Vapor pressure is 35 mm Hg at 20 °C (68 °F). Flammable. Contains inhibitors to prevent self-polymerization. Used in resin polymers, including medical applications.

Methyl parathion (O,O-dimethyl O-p-nitro-phenylphosphorothioate [CAS: 298-00-0]): A highly potent organophosphate cholinesterase inhibitor (see p 244).

0.2 mg/m³, S

Tan liquid with a strong garliclike odor. Vapor pressure is 0.5 mm Hg at 20 °C (68 °F). Appearance may vary with formulation.

Methyl propyl ketone (2-pentanone [CAS: 107-87-9]): Vapors irritating to eyes and respiratory tract. Based on animal studies, a CNS depressant at high levels.

200 ppm

1500 ppm

2 3 0

Colorless liquid with a characteristic odor. Vapor pressure is 27 mm Hg at 20 °C (68 °F). Flammable.

Methyl silicate (tetramethoxy silane [CAS: 681-84-5]): Highly reactive; corrosive upon direct contact; severe burns and loss of vision may result. Vapors extremely irritating to eyes and respiratory tract; severe eye burns and pulmonary edema may result.

1 ppm

Colorless crystals. Reacts with water, forming silicic acid and methanol.

(C) = ceiling air concentration (TLV-C); S = skin absorption can be significant; A1 = ACGIH-confirmed human carcinogen; A2 = ACGIH-suspected human carcinogen; NFPA Hazard Codes: H = health, F = fire, R = reactivity, Ox = oxidizer; W = water-reactive, 0 (none) <—> 4 (severe). ERPG = Emergency Response Planning Guideline. See p 434 for explanation of definitions.

(continued)

TABLE IV–4. HEALTH HAZARD SUMMARIES FOR INDUSTRIAL AND OCCUPATIONAL CHEMICALS (CONTINUED)

Health Hazard Summaries	ACGIH TLV	IDLH	NFPA Codes H F R	Comments
α-Methylstyrene (CAS: 98-83-9): Slightly irritating upon direct contact. Vapors irritating to eyes and respiratory tract. A CNS depressant at high levels.	50 ppm	700 ppm	1 2 1	Colorless liquid with a characteristic odor. Irritation is an adequate warning property. Vapor pressure is 1.9 mm Hg at 20 °C (68 °F). Flammable.
Methyl tert butyl ether (MTBE [CAS: 1634-04-4]): Vapors mildly irritating to eyes and respiratory tract. A CNS depressant. Acute exposure at high levels can cause nausea, vomiting, dizziness, and sleepiness. Adverse effects on liver and kidney in test animals at high levels. Evidence for adverse effects on reproduction and carcinogenicity in test animals exposed to very high concentrations.				A volatile colorless liquid at room temperature. Gasoline additive. Vapor pressure is 248 mm Hg at 25 °C.
Metribuzin (4-amino-6-[1,1-dimethylethyl]-3-[methylthio]-1,2,4-triazin-5 [4H]-one [CAS: 21087-64-9]): Human data available reveal no irritation or sensitization after dermal exposure. In animal testing, was poorly absorbed through the skin and produced no direct skin or eye irritation. Repeated high doses caused CNS depression and liver and thryoid effects.	5 mg/m³			Vapor pressure is 0.00001 mm Hg at 20 °C (68 °F). Thermal breakdown products include oxides of sulfur and nitrogen.
Mevinphos (2-carbomethoxy-1-methylvinyl dimethyl phosphate, phosdrin [CAS: 7786-34-7]): An organophosphate cholinesterase inhibitor (see p 244). Well absorbed by all routes. Repeated exposures to low levels can accumulate to produce symptoms.	0.09 mg/m³, S	4 ppm		Colorless or yellow liquid with a faint odor. Vapor pressure is 0.0022 mm Hg at 20 °C (68 °F). Combustible. Thermal breakdown products include phosphoric acid mist.
Mica (CAS: 12001-25-2): Dusts may cause pneumoconiosis upon chronic inhalation.	3 mg/m³ (respirable dust)	1500 mg/m³		Colorless solid flakes or sheets. Odorless. Vapor pressure is negligible at 20 °C (68 °F). Noncombustible.

Chemical	Exposure limit	NFPA (H F R)	Comments
Monocrotophos (dimethyl 2-methylcarbamoyl-1-methylvinyl phosphate [CAS: 6923-22-4]): An organophosphate-type cholinesterase inhibitor (see p 244). Limited human data indicate it is well absorbed through the skin but is rapidly metabolized and excreted.	0.25 mg/m³, S		Reddish-brown solid with a mild odor.
Morpholine (tetrahydro-1,4-oxazine [CAS: 110-91-8]): Corrosive; extremely irritating upon direct contact; severe burns may result. Well absorbed dermally. Vapors irritating to eyes and respiratory tract. Exposure to vapors has caused transient corneal edema. May cause severe liver and kidney injury.	20 ppm, S; 1400 ppm [LEL]	3 3 0	Colorless liquid with mild ammonialike odor. Vapor pressure is 7 mm Hg at 20 °C (68 °F). Flammable. Thermal breakdown products include oxides of nitrogen. Found in some consumer polish and wax products.
Naphthalene (CAS: 91-20-3): Highly irritating to eyes upon direct contact. Vapors are irritating to eyes and may cause cataracts upon chronic exposure. Dermally well absorbed. May induce methemoglobinemia (see p 220). Symptoms of overexposure include headache and nausea. See also p 230.	10 ppm	2 2 0	White to brown solid. The mothball odor and respiratory tract irritation are good warning properties. Current mothball formulations in the US do not contain naphthalene. Vapor pressure is 0.05 mm Hg at 20 °C (68 °F). Combustible.
β-Naphthylamine (2-aminonaphthalene [CAS: 91-59-8]): Acute overexposures can cause methemoglobinemia (see p 000) or acute hemorrhagic cystitis. Well absorbed through skin. Known human bladder carcinogen.	A1 OSHA CA NIOSH CA		White to reddish crystals. Vapor pressure is 1 mm Hg at 108°C (226 °F). Combustible.
Nickel carbonyl (nickel tetracarbonyl [CAS: 13463-39-3]): Inhalation of vapors can cause severe lung and systemic injury without irritant warning signs. Symptoms include headache, nausea, vomiting, fever, and extreme weakness. Based on animal studies, liver and brain damage may occur. Adverse effects on fetal development in test animals. A carcinogen in test animals.	0.05 ppm (as Ni) NIOSH CA; 2 ppm (as Ni)	4 3 3	Colorless liquid or gas. The musty odor is a poor warning property. Vapor pressure is 321 mm Hg at 20 °C (68 °F). Highly flammable. Exposures largely limited to nickel refining.

(C) = ceiling air concentration (TLV-C); S = skin absorption can be significant; A1 = ACGIH-confirmed human carcinogen; A2 = ACGIH-suspected human carcinogen; NFPA Hazard Codes: H = health, F = fire, R = reactivity, Ox = oxidizer, W = water-reactive, 0 (none) <—> 4 (severe). ERPG = Emergency Response Planning Guideline. See p 434 for explanation of definitions.

(continued)

TABLE IV–4. HEALTH HAZARD SUMMARIES FOR INDUSTRIAL AND OCCUPATIONAL CHEMICALS (CONTINUED)

Health Hazard Summaries	ACGIH TLV	IDLH	NFPA Codes H F R	Comments
Nickel metal and soluble inorganic salts (nickel chloride, nickel sulfate, nickel nitrate, nickel oxide): May cause a severe sensitization dermatitis, "nickel itch," upon repeated contact. Fumes highly irritating to the respiratory tract. Some compounds have adverse effects on fetal development in test animals. Some compounds are human nasal and lung carcinogens (IARC 1).	1.5 mg/m^3 (elemental) 0.1 mg/m^3 (soluble compounds), as Ni 0.2 mg/m^3, A1 (insoluble compounds), as Ni	10 mg/m^3 (as Ni)		Gray metallic powder or green solids. All forms are odorless.
Nicotine (CAS: 54-11-5): A potent nicotinic cholinergic receptor agonist. Well absorbed by all routes of exposure. Symptoms include dizziness, confusion, weakness, nausea and vomiting, tachycardia and hypertension, tremors, convulsions, and muscle paralysis. Death from respiratory paralysis can be very rapid. Adverse effects on fetal development in animal studies. See also p 231.	0.5 mg/m^3, S	5 mg/m^3	4 1 0	Pale yellow to dark brown viscous liquid with a fishy or aminelike odor. Vapor pressure is 0.0425 mm Hg at 20 °C (68 °F). Combustible. Thermal breakdown products include oxides of nitrogen. Although generally thought of in context of tobacco use and abstinence products, nicotine is a widely used pesticide.
Nitric acid (aqua fortis, engraver's acid [CAS: 7697-37-2]): Concentrated solutions corrosive to eyes and skin; very severe penetrating burns result. Vapors highly irritating to eyes and respiratory tract; pulmonary edema has resulted. Chronic inhalation exposure can produce bronchitis and erosion of the teeth.	2 ppm	25 ppm	3 0 0 Ox (≤ 40%) 4 0 1 Ox (fuming)	Colorless, yellow, or red fuming liquid with an acrid, suffocating odor. Vapor pressure is approximately 62 mm Hg at 25 °C (77 °F). Not combustible.
Nitric oxide (NO, nitrogen monoxide [CAS: 10102-43-9]): Nitric oxide slowly converts to nitrogen dioxide in air; eye and mucous membrane irritation and pulmonary edema are likely from nitrogen dioxide. Overexposures have been reported to result in acute and chronic obstructive airway disease. Based on animal studies, may cause methemoglobinemia (see p 220). Binds to hemoglobin at the same site as oxygen and this may contribute to the toxicity. See also p 234.	25 ppm	100 ppm		Colorless or brown gas. The sharp, sweet odor occurs below the TLV and is a good warning property.

Chemical / Toxicology	TLV	ERPG	NFPA (H R F)	Comments
p-Nitroaniline (CAS: 100-01-6): Irritating to eyes upon direct contact; may injure cornea. Well absorbed by all routes. Overexposure results in headache, weakness, respiratory distress, and methemoglobinemia (see p 220). Liver damage may also occur.	3 mg/m³, S	300 mg/m³	3 1 2	Yellow solid with an ammonialike odor that is a poor warning property. Vapor pressure is much less than 1 mm Hg at 20 °C (68 °F). Combustible. Thermal breakdown products include oxides of nitrogen.
Nitrobenzene (CAS: 98-95-3): Irritating upon direct contact; sensitization dermatitis may occur. Well absorbed by all routes. Causes methemoglobinemia (see p 220). Symptoms include headache, cyanosis, weakness, and gastrointestinal upset. May injure liver. Injures testes in animals. Limited evidence for adverse effects on fetal development in animals.	1 ppm, S, A3	200 ppm	3 2 1	Pale yellow to dark brown viscous liquid. Shoe polish-like odor is a good warning property. Vapor pressure is much less than 1 mm Hg at 20 °C (68 °F). Combustible. Thermal breakdown products include oxides of nitrogen.
p-Nitrochlorobenzene (CAS: 100-00-5): Irritating upon direct contact; sensitization dermatitis may occur upon repeated exposures. Well absorbed by all routes. Causes methemoglobinemia (see p 220). Symptoms include headache, cyanosis, weakness, and gastrointestinal upset. May cause liver and kidney injury.	0.1 ppm, S, A3	100 mg/m³	3 1 1	Yellow solid with a sweet odor. Vapor pressure is 0.009 mm Hg at 25 °C (77 °F). Combustible. Thermal breakdown products include oxides of nitrogen and hydrogen chloride.
4-Nitrodiphenyl (4-nitrobiphenyl) [CAS: 92-93-3]: Extremely well absorbed through skin. Produces bladder cancer in dogs and rabbits. Metabolized to 4-aminodiphenyl which is a potent carcinogen in humans.	S, A2 OSHA CA NIOSH CA			White solid with a sweet odor. Thermal breakdown products include oxides of nitrogen.
Nitroethane (CAS: 79-24-3): Based on high-exposure studies in animals, vapors are irritating to the respiratory tract. A CNS depressant. Causes liver injury at high levels of exposure in test animals. A structurally similar compound, 2-nitropropane, is a carcinogen.	100 ppm	1000 ppm	1 3 3 (explodes on heating)	Colorless viscous liquid with a fruity odor that is a poor warning property. Vapor pressure is 15.6 mm Hg at 20 °C (68 °F). Flammable. Thermal breakdown products include oxides of nitrogen.
Nitrogen dioxide (CAS: 10102-44-0): Gases and vapors irritating to eyes and respiratory tract; fatal pulmonary edema has resulted. Initial symptoms include cough and dyspnea. Pulmonary edema may appear after a delay of several hours. The acute phase may be followed by a fatal secondary stage, with fever and chills, dyspnea, cyanosis, and delayed-onset pulmonary edema. See p 234.	3 ppm	20 ppm	3 0 0 Ox	Dark brown fuming liquid or gas. Pungent odor and irritation occur only slightly above the TLV and are adequate warning properties. Vapor pressure is 720 mm Hg at 20 °C (68 °F). Important exposures include structural fires, sillage (silo-filling), and gas-shielded (MIG or TIG) welding.

(C) = ceiling air concentration (TLV-C); S = skin absorption can be significant; A1 = ACGIH-confirmed human carcinogen; A2 = ACGIH-suspected human carcinogen; NFPA Hazard Codes: H = health, F = fire, R = reactivity, Ox = oxidizer, W = water-reactive, 0 (none) <—> 4 (severe). ERPG = Emergency Response Planning Guideline. See p 434 for explanation of definitions.

(continued)

TABLE IV-4. HEALTH HAZARD SUMMARIES FOR INDUSTRIAL AND OCCUPATIONAL CHEMICALS (CONTINUED)

Health Hazard Summaries	ACGIH TLV	IDLH	NFPA Codes H F R	Comments
Nitrogen trifluoride (nitrogen fluoride [CAS: 7783-54-2]): Vapors may cause eye irritation. Based on animal studies, may cause methemoglobinemia (see p 220) and liver and kidney damage.	10 ppm	1000 ppm		Colorless gas with a moldy odor that is a poor warning property. Not combustible. Highly reactive and explosive under a number of conditions.
Nitroglyercin (glycerol trinitrate [CAS: 55-63-0]): Causes vasodilation, including coronary arteries. Headache and drop in blood pressure are common. Well absorbed by all routes. Tolerance to vasodilation can occur; cessation of exposure may precipitate angina pectoris in pharmacologically dependent workers. See also p 233.	0.05 ppm, S	75 mg/m³	2 2 4	Pale yellow viscous liquid. Vapor pressure is 0.00026 mm Hg at 20 °C (68 °F). Highly explosive.
Nitromethane (CAS: 75-52-5): Based on high-dose animal studies, causes respiratory tract irritation, liver and kidney injury, and CNS depression with ataxia, weakness, convulsions, and, possibly, methemoglobinemia (see p 220).	20 ppm	750 ppm	1 3 4	Colorless liquid with a faint fruity odor that is a poor warning property. Vapor pressure is 27.8 mm Hg at 20 °C (68 °F). Thermal breakdown products include oxides of nitrogen.
1-Nitropropane (CAS: 108-03-2): Vapors mildly irritating to eyes and respiratory tract. Liver and kidney injury may occur.	25 ppm	1000 ppm	1 3 2 (may explode on heating)	Colorless liquid with a faint fruity odor that is a poor warning property. Vapor pressure is 7.5 mm Hg at 20 °C (68 °F). Flammable. Thermal breakdown products include oxides of nitrogen.
2-Nitropropane (CAS: 79-46-9): Mildly irritating, CNS depressant at high exposures. Highly hepatotoxic; fatalities have resulted. Renal toxicity also occurs. Well absorbed by all routes. Limited evidence for adverse effects on fetal development in test animals. A carcinogen in test animals (IARC 2B).	10 ppm, A3 NIOSH CA	100 ppm	1 3 2 (may explode on heating)	Colorless liquid. Vapor pressure is 12.9 mm Hg at 20 °C (68 °F). Flammable. Thermal breakdown products include oxides of nitrogen.
N-Nitrosodimethylamine (dimethylnitrosamine [CAS: 62-75-9]): Overexposed workers suffered severe liver damage. Based on animal studies, well absorbed by all routes. A potent animal carcinogen producing liver, kidney, and lung cancers (IARC 2A).	A3, S OSHA CA NIOSH CA			Yellow viscous liquid. Combustible.

Substance	TLV	(second value)	H	F	R	Comments
Nitrotoluene (*o*-, *m*-, *p*-nitrotoluene [CAS: 99-08-1]): Weak inducer of methemoglobinemia (see p 220). By analogy to structurally similar compounds, dermal absorption is likely.	2 ppm, S	200 ppm	3	1	1	*Ortho* and *meta*, yellow liquid or solid. *Para*, yellow solid. All isomers have a weak, aromatic odor. Vapor pressure is approximately 0.15 mm Hg at 20 °C (68 °F). Thermal breakdown products include oxides of nitrogen. Intermediate in synthesis of dye-stuffs and explosives.
Nitrous oxide [CAS: 10024-97-2]: A CNS depressant. Hematopoietic effects from chronic exposure include megaloblastic anemia. Substance abuse has resulted in neuropathies. May have an adverse effect on human fertility and fetal development. See also p 236.	50 ppm					Colorless gas. Sweet odor. Not combustible. Widely used in dentistry.
Octachloronaphthalene (Halowax 1051 [CAS: 2234-13-1]): By analogy to other chlorinated naphthalenes, workers overexposed by inhalation or skin contact may experience chloracne and liver damage.	0.1 mg/m³, S					Pale yellow solid with an aromatic odor. Vapor pressure is less than 1 mm Hg at 20 °C (68 °F). Not combustible. Thermal breakdown products include hydrogen chloride.
Octane [CAS: 111-65-9]: Vapors mildly irritating to eyes and respiratory tract. A CNS depressant at very high concentrations.	300 ppm	1000 ppm [LEL]	0	3	0	Colorless liquid. Gasolinelike odor and irritation are good warning properties. Vapor pressure is 11 mm Hg at 20 °C (68 °F). Flammable.
Osmium tetroxide (osmic acid [CAS: 20816-12-0]): Corrosive upon direct contact; severe burns may result. Fumes are highly irritating to eyes and respiratory tract. Based on high-dose animal studies, bone marrow and kidney damage may occur.	0.0002 ppm (as Os)	1 mg/m³ (as Os)				Colorless to pale yellow solid with a sharp and irritating odor like chlorine. Vapor pressure is 7 mm Hg at 20 °C (68 °F). Not combustible. Catalyst and laboratory reagent.
Oxalic acid (ethanedioic acid [CAS: 144-62-7]): A strong acid; corrosive to eyes and to skin upon direct contact (see p 129). Fumes irritating to respiratory tract. Highly toxic upon ingestion; precipitation of calcium oxalate crystals can cause hypocalcemia and renal damage. See also p 248.	1 mg/m³	500 mg/m³	3	1	0	Colorless or white solid. Odorless. Vapor pressure is less than 0.001 mm Hg at 20 °C (68 °F).

(C) = ceiling air concentration (TLV-C); S = skin absorption can be significant; A1 = ACGIH-confirmed human carcinogen; A2 = ACGIH-suspected human carcinogen; NFPA Hazard Codes: H = health, F = fire, R = reactivity, Ox = oxidizer, W = water-reactive, 0 (none) <—> 4 (severe), ERPG = Emergency Response Planning Guideline. See p 434 for explanation of definitions.

(continued)

TABLE IV-4. HEALTH HAZARD SUMMARIES FOR INDUSTRIAL AND OCCUPATIONAL CHEMICALS (CONTINUED)

Health Hazard Summaries	ACGIH TLV	IDLH	NFPA Codes H F R	Comments
Oxygen difluoride (oxygen fluoride, fluorine monoxide [CAS: 7783-41-7]): Extremely irritating to the eyes, skin, and respiratory tract. Effects similar to hydrofluoric acid (see p 186.) Based on animal studies, may also injure kidney, internal genitalia, and other organs. Workers have complained of severe headaches after low-level exposures.	0.05 ppm (C)	0.5 ppm		Colorless gas with a strong and foul odor. Olfactory fatigue is common, so odor is a poor warning property. A strong oxidizing agent.
Ozone (triatomic oxygen [CAS: 10028-15-6]): Irritating to eyes and respiratory tract. Pulmonary edema has been reported. See also p 181.	0.05 ppm (heavy work); 0.08 ppm (moderate work); 0.1 ppm (light work); [proposed: 0.2 ppm (≤2 hours)]	5 ppm		Colorless or bluish gas. Sharp, distinctive odor is an adequate warning property. A strong oxidizing agent. Gas-shielded and specialty welding are potential sources of exposure.
Paraquat (1,1'-dimethyl-4,4'-bipyridinium dichloride [CAS: 4687-14-7]): Extremely irritating upon direct contact; severe corrosive burns may result. Well absorbed through skin. A potent toxin causing acute multiorgan failure as well as progressive fatal pulmonary fibrosis after ingestion. See also p 250.	0.5 mg/m^3 (total dust) 0.1 mg/m^3 (respirable fraction)	1 mg/m^3		Odorless white to yellow solid. Vapor pressure is negligible at 20 °C (68 °F). Not combustible. Thermal breakdown products include oxides of nitrogen and sulfur and hydrogen chloride. While widely used as a herbicide, most deaths occur as a result of ingestion.
Parathion (O,O-diethyl O-p-nitrophenyl phosphorothioate [CAS: 56-38-2]): Highly potent organophosphate cholinesterase inhibitor (see p 244). Systemic toxicity has resulted from inhalation, ingestion, and dermal exposures. Evidence for adverse effects on fetal development in test animals at high doses.	0.1 mg/m^3, S	10 mg/m^3		Yellow to dark brown liquid with garliclike odor. Odor threshold of 0.04 ppm suggests it has good warning properties. Vapor pressure is 0.0004 mm Hg at 20 °C (68 °F). Thermal breakdown products include oxides of sulfur, nitrogen, and phosphorus. In the field, weathering/oxidation can convert parathion to the even more toxic organophosphate, paraoxon.

Compound [CAS]			NFPA Codes (H F R)	Comments
Pentaborane [CAS: 19624-22-7]: Highly irritating upon direct contact; severe burns may result. Vapors irritating to the respiratory tract. A potent CNS toxin; symptoms include headache, nausea, weakness, confusion, hyperexcitability, tremors, seizures, and coma. CNS effects may persist. Liver and kidney injury may also occur.	0.005 ppm	1 ppm	4 4 2	Colorless liquid. Vapor pressure is 171 mm Hg at 20 °C (68 °F). The pungent sour-milk odor occurring only at air levels well above the TLV is a poor warning property. May ignite spontaneously. Reacts violently with halogenated extinguishing media. Thermal breakdown products include boron acids.
Pentachloronaphthalene (Halowax 1013) [CAS: 1321-64-8]: Chloracne results from prolonged skin contact or inhalation. May cause severe, potentially fatal liver injury or necrosis by all routes of exposure.	0.5 mg/m³, S			Pale yellow waxy solid with a pleasant aromatic odor. Odor threshold not known. Vapor pressure is less than 1 mm Hg at 20 °C (68 °F). Not combustible. Thermal breakdown products include hydrogen chloride fumes.
Pentachlorophenol (Penta, PCP) [CAS: 87-86-5]: Irritating upon direct contact; burns may result. Vapors irritating to eyes and respiratory tract. A potent metabolic poison; uncouples oxidative phosphorylation. Well absorbed by all routes. Evidence for adverse effects on fetal development and carcinogenicity in test animals (IARC 2B). See also p 252.	0.5 mg/m³, S, A3	2.5 mg/m³	3 0 0	Eye and nose irritation occur slightly above the TLV and are good warning properties. Vapor pressure is 0.0002 mm Hg at 20 °C (68 °F). Not combustible. Thermal breakdown products include hydrogen chloride, chlorinated phenols, and octachlorodibenzodioxin. Widely used as a wood preservative.
Pentane (n-pentane) [CAS: 109-66-0]: Vapors mildly irritating to eyes and respiratory tract. A CNS depressant at high levels.	600 ppm	1500 ppm [LEL]	1 4 0	Colorless liquid with a gasolinelike odor that is an adequate warning property. Vapor pressure is 426 mm Hg at 20 °C (68 °F). Flammable.
Petroleum distillates (petroleum naphtha, petroleum ether): Vapors irritating to eyes and respiratory tract. A CNS depressant. If n-hexane, benzene, or other toxic contaminants are present, those hazards should be addressed. See also p 183.		1100 ppm [LEL]	1 4 0 (petroleum ether)	Colorless liquid. Kerosenelike odor at levels below the TLV serves as a warning property. Highly flammable. Vapor pressure is about 40 mm Hg at 20 °C (68 °F).

(C) = ceiling air concentration (TLV-C); S = skin absorption can be significant; A1 = ACGIH-confirmed human carcinogen; A2 = ACGIH-suspected human carcinogen; NFPA Hazard Codes: H = health, F = fire, R = reactivity, Ox = oxidizer, W = water-reactive, 0 (none) <——> 4 (severe). ERPG = Emergency Response Planning Guideline. See p 434 for explanation of definitions.

(continued)

TABLE IV–4. HEALTH HAZARD SUMMARIES FOR INDUSTRIAL AND OCCUPATIONAL CHEMICALS (CONTINUED)

Health Hazard Summaries	ACGIH TLV	IDLH	NFPA Codes H F R	Comments
Phenol (carbolic acid, hydroxybenzene [CAS: 108-95-2]): Corrosive acid and protein denaturant. Direct eye or skin contact causes severe tissue damage or blindness. Deep skin burns can occur without warning pain. Systemic toxicity by all routes; percutaneous absorption of vapor occurs. Vapors highly irritating to eyes and respiratory tract. Symptoms include nausea, vomiting, cardiac arrhythmias, circulatory collapse, convulsions, and coma. Toxic to liver and kidney. A tumor promoter. See also p 255.	5 ppm, S	250 ppm ERPG-1: 10 ppm ERPG-2: 50 ppm ERPG-3: 200 ppm	4 2 0	Colorless to pink crystalline solid, or viscous liquid. Its odor has been described as being distinct, acrid, and aromatic or as being sweet and tarry. As the odor is detected at or below the TLV, it is a good warning property. Vapor pressure is 0.36 mm Hg at 20 °C (68 °F). Combustible.
Phenylenediamine (p-diaminobenzene, p-aminoaniline [CAS: 106-50-3]): Irritating upon direct contact. May cause skin and respiratory tract sensitization (asthma). Inflammatory reactions of larynx and pharynx have often been noted in exposed workers.	0.1 mg/m³	25 mg/m³	– 1 0	White to light purple or brown solid, depending on degree of oxidation. Combustible. Thermal breakdown products include oxides of nitrogen.
Phenyl ether (diphenyl ether [CAS: 101-84-8]): Mildly irritating upon prolonged direct contact. Vapors irritating to eyes and respiratory tract. Based on high-dose experiments in animals, liver and kidney damage may occur after ingestion.	1 ppm	100 ppm		Colorless liquid or solid. Mildly disagreeable odor detected below the TLV serves as a good warning property. Vapor pressure is 0.02 mm Hg at 25 °C (77 °F). Combustible.
Phenyl glycidyl ether (PGE, 1,2-epoxy-3-phenoxypropane [CAS: 122-60-1]): Irritating upon direct contact. A skin sensitizer. Based on animal studies, vapors are very irritating to eyes and respiratory tract. In high-dose animal studies, a CNS depressant producing liver, kidney, spleen, testes, thymus, and hematopoietic system injury. A carcinogen in test animals (IARC 2B).	0.1 ppm, S	100 ppm		Colorless liquid with an unpleasant, sweet odor. Vapor pressure is 0.01 mm Hg at 20 °C (68 °F). Combustible. Readily forms peroxides.
Phenylhydrazine [CAS: 100-63-0]: A strong base and corrosive upon direct contact. A potent skin sensitizer. Dermal absorption occurs. Vapors very irritating to eyes and respiratory tract. May cause hemolytic anemia with secondary kidney damage. Limited evidence of carcinogenicity in test animals.	0.1 ppm, S, A3 NIOSH CA	15 ppm	3 2 0	Pale yellow crystals or oily liquid with a weakly aromatic odor. Darkens upon exposure to air and light. Vapor pressure is less than 0.1 mm Hg at 20 °C (68 °F). Combustible. Thermal breakdown products include oxides of nitrogen.

Compound	TLV	Other limits	NFPA (H F R)	Comments
Phenylphosphine (CAS: 638-21-1): In animals, subchronic inhalation at 2 ppm caused loss of appetite, diarrhea, tremor, hemolytic anemia, dermatitis, and irreversible testicular degeneration.	0.05 ppm (C)			Crystalline solid. Spontaneously combustible at high air concentrations.
Phorate (*O,O*-diethyl S-(ethylthio)methyl phosphorodithioate, Thimet, Timet(CAS: 298-02-2)): An organophosphate-type cholinesterase inhibitor (see p 244). Well absorbed by all routes.	0.05 mg/m³, S			Clear liquid. Vapor pressure is 0.002 mm Hg at 20 °C (68 °F).
Phosgene (carbonyl chloride, COCl₂ [CAS: 75-44-5]): Extremely irritating to the lower respiratory tract. Exposure can be insidious because irritation and smell are inadequate as warning properties for pulmonary injury. Higher levels cause irritation of the eyes, skin, and mucous membranes. See also p 262.	0.1 ppm	2 ppm ERPG-2: 0.2 ppm ERPG-3: 1 ppm	4 0 1	Colorless gas. Sweet haylike odor at low concentrations; sharp and pungent odor at high concentrations. Dangerous concentrations may not be detected by odor.
Phosphine (hydrogen phosphide [CAS: 7803-51-2]): Extremely irritating to the respiratory tract; fatal pulmonary edema has resulted. A multisystem poison. Symptoms in moderately overexposed workers included diarrhea, nausea, vomiting, cough, headache, and dizziness. See also p 263.	0.3 ppm	50 ppm	4 4 2	Colorless gas. A fishy or garliclike odor detected well below the TLV is considered to be a good warning property. May ignite spontaneously on contact with air. A common fumigant, generated on-site by aluminum phosphide and moisture.
Phosphoric acid (CAS: 7664-38-2): A strong corrosive acid; severe burns may result from direct contact. Mist or vapors irritating to eyes and respiratory tract.	1 mg/m³	1000 mg/m³	3 0 0	Colorless, syrupy, odorless liquid. Solidifies at temperatures below 20 °C (68 °F). Vapor pressure is 0.03 mm Hg at 20 °C (68 °F). Not combustible.
Phosphorus (yellow phosphorus, white phosphorus, P [CAS: 7723-14-0]): Severe, penetrating burns may result upon direct contact. Material may ignite upon contact with skin. Fumes irritating to eyes and respiratory tract; pulmonary edema may occur. Potent hepatotoxin. Systemic symptoms include abdominal pain, jaundice, and garlic odor on the breath. Historically, chronic poisoning caused jaw bone necrosis (phossy jaw). See also p 264.	0.02 ppm (yellow phosphorus)	5 mg/m³	4 4 2	White to yellow, waxy or crystalline solid with acrid fumes. Flammable. Vapor pressure is 0.026 mm Hg at 20 °C (68 °F). Ignites spontaneously on contact with air. Thermal breakdown products include phosphoric acid fume. Historical exposures involved the match industry which has long since substituted other forms of phosphorus. Current uses include munitions and pesticides.

(C) = ceiling air concentration (TLV-C); S = skin absorption can be significant; A1 = ACGIH-confirmed human carcinogen; A2 = ACGIH-suspected human carcinogen; NFPA Hazard Codes: H = health, F = fire, R = reactivity, Ox = oxidizer, W = water-reactive, 0 (none) <—> 4 (severe). ERPG = Emergency Response Planning Guideline. See p 434 for explanation of definitions.

(continued)

TABLE IV–4. HEALTH HAZARD SUMMARIES FOR INDUSTRIAL AND OCCUPATIONAL CHEMICALS (CONTINUED)

Health Hazard Summaries	ACGIH TLV	IDLH	NFPA Codes H F R	Comments
Phosphorus oxychloride (CAS: 10025-87-3): Reacts with moisture to release phosphoric and hydrochloric acids; highly corrosive upon direct contact. Fumes extremely irritating to eyes and respiratory tract. Systemic effects include headache, dizziness, and dyspnea. Kidney toxicity may occur.	0.1 ppm		4 0 2 W	Clear colorless to pale yellow, fuming liquid possessing a pungent odor. Vapor pressure is 40 mm Hg at 27.3 °C (81 °F). Not combustible.
Phosphorus pentachloride (CAS: 10026-13-8): Reacts with moisture to release phosphoric and hydrochloric acids; highly corrosive upon direct contact. Fumes extremely irritating to eyes and respiratory tract.	0.1 ppm	70 mg/m³	3 0 2 W	Pale yellow solid with a hydrochloric acidlike odor. Not combustible.
Phosphorus pentasulfide (CAS: 1314-80-3): Rapidly reacts with moisture and moist tissues to form hydrogen sulfide (see p 188) and phosphoric acid. Severe burns may result from prolonged contact with tissues. Dusts or fumes extremely irritating to eyes and respiratory tract. Systemic toxicology is predominantly caused by hydrogen sulfide.	1 mg/m³	250 mg/m³	2 1 2 W	Greenish-yellow solid with odor of rotten eggs. Olfactory fatigue reduces value of smell as a warning property. Thermal breakdown products include sulfur dioxide, hydrogen sulfide, phosphorus pentoxide, and phosphoric acid fumes. Ignites spontaneously in the presence of moisture.
Phosphorus trichloride (CAS: 7719-12-2): Reacts with moisture to release phosphoric and hydrochloric acids; highly corrosive upon direct contact. Fumes extremely irritating to eyes and respiratory tract.	0.2 ppm	25 ppm	4 0 2 W	Fuming colorless to yellow liquid. Irritation provides a good warning property. Vapor pressure is 100 mm Hg at 20 °C (68 °F). Not combustible.
Phthalic anhydride (phthalic acid anhydride [CAS: 85-44-9]): Extremely irritating upon direct contact; chemical burns occur after prolonged contact. Dusts and vapors extremely irritating to respiratory tract. A potent skin and respiratory tract sensitizer (asthma).	1 ppm	60 mg/m³	3 1 0	White crystalline solid with choking odor at very high air concentrations. Vapor pressure is 0.05 mm Hg at 20 °C (68 °F). Combustible. Thermal breakdown products include phthalic acid fumes.

Chemical / Comments	Exposure limit	IDLH	H	F	R	Physical description
Picloram (4-amino-3,5,6-trichloropicolinic acid [CAS: 1918-02-1]): Dusts mildly irritating to skin, eyes, and respiratory tract. Has low oral toxicity in test animals. Limited evidence of carcinogenicity in animals.	10 mg/m³					White powder possessing a bleachlike odor. Vapor pressure is 0.0000006 mm Hg at 35 °C (95 °F). Thermal breakdown products include oxides of nitrogen and hydrogen chloride.
Picric acid (2,4,6-trinitrophenol [CAS: 88-89-1]): Irritating upon direct contact. Dust stains skin yellow and can cause a sensitization dermatitis. Symptoms of low-level exposure are headache, dizziness, and gastrointestinal upset. May induce methemoglobinemia (see p 220). Ingestion of large amounts causes hemolysis, nephritis, and hepatitis. Staining of the conjunctiva and aqueous humor can give vision a yellow hue. A weak uncoupler of oxidative phosphorylation.	0.1 mg/m³	75 mg/m³	3	4	4	Pale yellow crystalline solid or paste. Odorless. Vapor pressure is much less than 1 mm Hg at 20 °C (68 °F). Decomposes explosively above 120 °C (248 °F). May detonate when shocked. Contact with metals, ammonia, or calcium compounds can form salts that are much more sensitive to shock detonation.
Pindone (Pival, 2-pivaloyl-1,3-indanedione [CAS: 83-26-1]): A vitamin K antagonist anticoagulant (see p 148).	0.1 mg/m³	100 mg/m³				Bright yellow crystalline substance.
Piperazine dihydrochloride (CAS: 142-64-3): Irritating upon direct contact; burns may result. A moderate skin and respiratory sensitizer. Nausea, vomiting, and diarrhea are side effects of medicinal use. Overdosage has caused confusion, lethargy, coma, and seizures.	5 mg/m³					White crystalline solid with a mild fishy odor.
Piperidine (CAS: 110-89-4): Highly irritating upon direct contact; severe burns may result. Vapors irritating to eyes and respiratory tract. Small doses initially stimulate autonomic ganglia; larger doses depress them. A 30–60 mg/kg dose may produce symptoms in humans.			3	3	0	Flammable.
Platinum—soluble salts (sodium chloroplatinate; ammonium chloroplatinate, platinum tetrachloride): Sensitizers causing asthma and dermatitis. Metallic platinum does not share these effects. Soluble platinum compounds are also highly irritating to eyes, mucous membranes, and respiratory tract.	0.002 mg/m³ (as Pt)	4 mg/m³ (as Pt)				Appearance varies with the compound. Thermal breakdown products of some chloride salts include chlorine gas. Used as industrial catalysts and in specialized photographic applications.

(C) = ceiling air concentration (TLV-C); S = skin absorption can be significant; A1 = ACGIH-confirmed human carcinogen; A2 = ACGIH-suspected human carcinogen; NFPA Hazard Codes: H = health, F = fire, R = reactivity, W = water-reactive, Ox = oxidizer, 0 (none) <—> 4 (severe). ERPG = Emergency Response Planning Guideline. See p 434 for explanation of definitions.

(continued)

TABLE IV–4. HEALTH HAZARD SUMMARIES FOR INDUSTRIAL AND OCCUPATIONAL CHEMICALS (CONTINUED)

Health Hazard Summaries	ACGIH TLV	IDLH	NFPA Codes H F R	Comments
Polychlorinated biphenyls (chlorodiphenyls, Aroclor 1242, PCBs): Exposure to high concentrations is irritating to eyes, nose, and throat. Chronically overexposed workers suffer from chloracne and liver injury. Reported symptoms are anorexia, gastrointestinal upset, and peripheral neuropathies. Some health effects may be caused by contaminants or thermal decomposition products. Adverse effects on fetal development and fertility in test animals. A carcinogen in test animals (IARC 2A). See also p 274.	1 mg/m³ (42%chlorine), S, NIOSH CA 0.5 mg/m³ (54% chlorine), S, A3 NIOSH CA		2 1 0	42% chlorinated: a colorless to dark brown liquid with a slight hydrocarbon odor and a vapor pressure of 0.001 mm Hg at 20 °C (68 °F). 54% chlorinated: light yellow oily liquid with a slight hydrocarbon odor and a vapor pressure of 0.00006 mm Hg at 20 °C (68 °F). Thermal breakdown products include chlorinated dibenzofurans and chlorodibenzodioxins. Although no longer used, old transformers may still contain PCBs.
Polytetrafluoroethylene decomposition products: Overexposures result in polymer fume fever, a disease with flulike symptoms including chills, fever, and cough. See also p 217.				Produced by pyrolysis of Teflon and related materials. Perisofluorobutylene and carbonyl fluoride are among the pyrolysis products.
Polyvinyl chloride decomposition products: Fumes are irritating to the respiratory tract and may cause "meat wrapper's" asthma.				Produced by the high-temperature partial breakdown of polyvinyl chloride plastics.
Portland cement (a mixture of mostly tricalcium silicate and dicalcium silicate with some alumina, calcium aluminate, and iron oxide): Irritant of the eyes, nose, and skin; corrosive burns may occur. Long-term heavy exposure has been associated with dermatitis and bronchitis.	10 mg/m³ (< 1% quartz)	5000 mg/m³		Gray powder. Odorless. Portland cement manufacture is typically associated with sulfur dioxide exposure.
Potassium hydroxide (KOH [CAS: 1310-58-3]): A caustic alkali causing severe burns to tissues upon direct contact. Exposure to dust or mist causes eye, nose, and respiratory tract irritation.	2 mg/m³ (C)		3 0 1	White solid that absorbs moisture. Vapor pressure is negligible at 20 °C (68 °F). Gives off heat and a corrosive mist when in contact with water.
Propane (CAS: 74-98-6): Simple asphyxiant. See also hydrocarbons, p 183.	2500 ppm	2100 ppm [LEL]	1 4 0	

Chemical	(C)	ERPG	H F R	Comments
Propargyl alcohol (2-propyn-1-ol [CAS: 107-19-7]): Irritating to skin upon direct contact. Dermally well absorbed. A CNS depressant. Causes liver and kidney injury in test animals.	1 ppm, S		4 3 3	Light to straw-colored liquid with a geraniumlike odor. Vapor pressure is 11.6 mm Hg at 20 °C (68 °F). Flammable.
Propionic acid [CAS: 79-09-4]: Irritating to eyes and skin upon direct contact with concentrated solutions; burns may result. Vapors irritating to eyes, skin, and respiratory tract. A food additive of low systemic toxicity.	10 ppm		3 2 0	Colorless oily liquid with a pungent, somewhat rancid odor. Vapor pressure is 10 mm Hg at 39.7 °C (103.5 °F). Flammable.
Propoxur (o-isopropoxyphenyl N-methylcarbamate, DDVP, Baygon [CAS: 114-26-1]): A carbamate anticholinesterase insecticide (see p 244). Limited evidence for adverse effects on fetal development in test animals.	0.5 mg/m^3, A3			White crystalline solid with a faint characteristic odor. Vapor pressure is 0.01 mm Hg at 120 °C (248 °F). Common insecticide found in many OTC formulations.
n-Propyl acetate [CAS: 109-60-4]: Vapors irritating to eyes and respiratory tract. Excessive inhalation may cause weakness, nausea, and chest tightness. Based on high-exposure studies in test animals, a CNS depressant.	200 ppm	1700 ppm	1 3 0	Colorless liquid. Mild fruity odor and irritant properties provide good warning properties. Vapor pressure is 25 mm Hg at 20 °C (68 °F). Flammable.
Propyl alcohol (1-propanol [CAS: 71-23-8]): Vapors mildly irritating to eyes and respiratory tract. A CNS depressant. See also isopropyl alcohol, p 197.	200 ppm, S	800 ppm	1 3 0	Colorless volatile liquid. Vapor pressure is 15 mm Hg at 20 °C (68 °F). Mild alcohollike odor is an adequate warning property.
Propylene dichloride (1,2-dichloropropane [CAS: 78-87-5]): Vapors very irritating to eyes and respiratory tract. Causes CNS depression and severe liver and kidney damage in animal studies. Testicular toxicity at high doses in test animals.	75 ppm	400 ppm	2 3 0	Colorless liquid. Chloroformlike odor is considered to be an adequate warning property. Vapor pressure is 40 mm Hg at 20 °C (68 °F). Flammable. Thermal breakdown products include hydrogen chloride. An agricultural nematocide.

(C) = ceiling air concentration (TLV-C); S = skin absorption can be significant; A1 = ACGIH-confirmed human carcinogen; A2 = ACGIH-suspected human carcinogen; NFPA Hazard Codes: H = health, F = fire, R = reactivity, Ox = oxidizer, W = water-reactive, 0 (none) <---> 4 (severe), ERPG = Emergency Response Planning Guideline. See p 434 for explanation of definitions.

(continued)

TABLE IV–4. HEALTH HAZARD SUMMARIES FOR INDUSTRIAL AND OCCUPATIONAL CHEMICALS (CONTINUED)

Health Hazard Summaries	ACGIH TLV	IDLH	NFPA Codes H F R	Comments
Propylene glycol dinitrate (1,2-propylene glycol dinitrate, PGDN [CAS: 6423-43-4]): Mildly irritating upon direct contact. Dermal absorption occurs. May cause methemoglobinemia (see p 220). Causes vasodilation, including coronary arteries. Headache and drop in blood pressure are common. Well absorbed by all routes. Tolerance to vasodilation can occur; cessation of exposure may precipitate angina pectoris in pharmacologically dependent workers. See also nitrates, p 233.	0.05 ppm, S			Colorless liquid with an unpleasant odor. Thermal breakdown products include oxides of nitrogen.
Propylene glycol monomethyl ether (1-methoxy-2-propanol [CAS: 107-98-2]): Vapors very irritating to the eyes and possibly the respiratory tract. A mild CNS depressant.	100 ppm		0 3 0	Colorless, flammable liquid.
Propylene imine (2-methylaziridine [CAS: 75-55-8]): Very irritating upon direct contact; severe burns may result. Vapors highly irritating to eyes and respiratory tract. May also injure liver and kidneys. Well absorbed dermally. A carcinogen in test animals.	2 ppm, S, A3	100 ppm		A fuming colorless liquid with a strong ammonialike odor. Flammable. Thermal breakdown products include oxides of nitrogen.
Propylene oxide (2-epoxypropane [CAS: 75-56-9]): Highly irritating upon direct contact; severe burns result. Vapors highly irritating to eyes and respiratory tract. Based on high-dose animal studies, may cause CNS depression and peripheral neuropathy. A carcinogen in test animals (IARC 2A).	20 ppm, A3	400 ppm	3 4 2	Colorless liquid. Its sweet, etherlike odor is considered to be an adequate warning property. Vapor pressure is 442 mm Hg at 20 °C (68 °F). Highly flammable. Polymerizes violently.
n-Propyl nitrate (nitric acid n-propyl ester [CAS: 627-13-4]): Vasodilator causing headaches and hypotension. Causes methemoglobinemia (see p 220). See also nitrates, p 233.	25 ppm	500 ppm	2 3 3 Ox (may explode on heating)	Pale yellow liquid with an unpleasant sweet odor. Vapor pressure is 18 mm Hg at 20 °C (68 °F). Flammable. Thermal breakdown products include oxides of nitrogen.

Substance	TLV		NFPA (H R F)	Comments
Pyrethrum (pyrethrin I or II; cinerin I or II; jasmolin I or II): Dusts can cause primary contact dermatitis and skin and respiratory tract sensitization (asthma). Of very low systemic toxicity. See also p 276.	5 mg/m³	5000 mg/m³		Vapor pressure is negligible at 20 °C (68 °F). Combustible. Widely used insecticide.
Pyridine (CAS: 110-86-1): Irritating upon prolonged direct contact; occasional reports of skin sensitization. Vapors irritating to eyes and respiratory tract. A CNS depressant. Induces methemoglobinemia. Chronic ingestion of small amounts has caused fatal liver and kidney injury. Workers exposed to 6–12 ppm have complained of headache, dizziness, and gastrointestinal upset. Dermally well absorbed.	5 ppm	1000 ppm	3 3 0	Colorless or yellow liquid with a nauseating odor and a definite "taste" that serves as a good warning property. Vapor pressure is 18 mm Hg at 20 °C (68 °F). Flammable. Thermal breakdown products include oxides of nitrogen and cyanide.
Pyrogallol (1,2,3-trihydroxybenzene; pyrogallic acid [CAS: 87-66-1]): Highly irritating upon direct contact; severe burns may result. Potent reducing agent and general cellular poison. Causes methemoglobinemia (see p 220). Attacks heart, lungs, liver, kidneys, red blood cells, bone marrow, and muscle. Causes sensitization dermatitis. Deaths have resulted from the topical application of salves containing pyrogallol.				White to gray odorless solid.
Quinone (1,4-cyclohexadienedione, p-benzoquinone [CAS: 106-51-4]): A severe irritant of the eyes and respiratory tract. May induce methemoglobinemia (see p 220). Acute overexposure to dust or vapors can cause conjunctival irritation and discoloration, corneal edema, ulceration, and scarring. Chronic exposures can permanently reduce visual acuity. Skin contact can cause irritation, ulceration, and pigmentation changes.	0.1 ppm	100 mg/m³		Pale yellow crystalline solid. The acrid odor is not a reliable warning property. Vapor pressure is 0.1 mm Hg at 20 °C (68 °F). Sublimes when heated.
Resorcinol (1,3-dihydroxybenzene [CAS: 108-46-3]): Corrosive acid and protein denaturant; extremely irritating upon direct contact; severe burns result. May cause methemoglobinemia (see p 220). A sensitizer. Dermally well absorbed. See also phenol, p 255.	10 ppm		— 1 0	White crystalline solid with a faint odor. May turn pink on contact with air. Vapor pressure is 1 mm Hg at 108 °C (226 °F). Combustible.

(C) = ceiling air concentration (TLV-C); S = skin absorption can be significant; A1 = ACGIH-confirmed human carcinogen; A2 = ACGIH-suspected human carcinogen; NFPA Hazard Codes: H = health, F = fire, R = reactivity, Ox = oxidizer, W = water-reactive, 0 (none) <—> 4 (severe). ERPG = Emergency Response Planning Guideline. See p 434 for explanation of definitions.

(continued)

TABLE IV–4. HEALTH HAZARD SUMMARIES FOR INDUSTRIAL AND OCCUPATIONAL CHEMICALS (CONTINUED)

Health Hazard Summaries	ACGIH TLV	IDLH	NFPA Codes H F R	Comments
Ronnel (O,O-dimethyl-O-(2,4,5-trichlorophenyl)phosphorothioate, Fenchlorphos [CAS: 299-84-3]): One of the least toxic organophosphate anticholinesterase insecticides (see p 244).	10 mg/m³	300 mg/m³		Vapor pressure is 0.0008 mm Hg at 20 °C (68 °F). Not combustible. Unstable above 149 °C (300 °F); harmful gases such as sulfur dioxide, dimethyl sulfide, and trichlorophenol may be released.
Rotenone (tubatoxin, cube root, derris root, derrin [CAS: 83-79-4]): Irritating upon direct contact. Dusts irritate the respiratory tract. A metabolic poison; depresses cellular respiration and inhibits mitotic spindle formation. Ingestion of large doses numbs oral mucosa and causes nausea and vomiting, muscle tremors, and convulsions. Chronic exposure caused liver and kidney damage in animal studies. Limited evidence for adverse effects on fetal development in animals at high doses.	5 mg/m³	2500 mg/m³		White to red crystalline solid. Vapor pressure is negligible at 20 °C (68 °F). A natural pesticide extracted from such plants as cube, derris, and timbo. Odorless. Decomposes upon contact with air or light. Unstable to alkali.
Selenium and inorganic compounds (as selenium): Fumes, dusts, and vapors irritating to eyes, skin, and respiratory tract; pulmonary edema may occur. Many compounds are well absorbed dermally. A general cellular poison. Chronic intoxication causes depression, nervousness, dermatitis, gastrointestinal upset, metallic taste in mouth and garlicky odor of breath, excess caries, and loss of fingernails or hair. The liver and kidneys are also target organs. Some selenium compounds have been found to cause birth defects and cancers in test animals. See also p 289.	0. 2 mg/m³ (as Se)	1 mg/m³ (as Se)		Elemental selenium is a black, gray, or red crystalline or amorphous solid and is odorless.
Selenium dioxide (selenium oxide [CAS: 7446-08-4]): Strong vesicant; severe burns result from direct contact. Converted to selenious acid in the presence of moisture. Well absorbed dermally. Fumes and dusts very irritating to eyes and respiratory tract. See also p 289.				White solid. Reacts with water to form selenious acid.

Agent	TLV	Comments
Selenium hexafluoride (CAS: 7783-79-1): Vesicant. Reacts with moisture to form selenium acids and hydrofluoric acid; severe HF burns may result from direct contact (see p 186). Fumes highly irritating to eyes and respiratory tract; pulmonary edema may result.	0.05 ppm	Colorless gas. Not combustible.
Selenium oxychloride (CAS: 7791-23-3): Strong vesicant. Direct contact can cause severe burns. Dermally well absorbed. Fumes extremely irritating to eyes and respiratory tract; delayed pulmonary edema may result.	2 ppm	Colorless to yellow liquid. Hydrogen chloride and selenious acid fumes produced on contact with moisture.
Silica, amorphous (diatomaceous earth, precipitated and gel silica): Possesses little or no potential to cause silicosis. Most sources of amorphous silica contain quartz (see crystalline silica, below). If greater than 1% quartz is present, the quartz hazard must be addressed. When strongly heated (calcined) with limestone, diatomaceous earth becomes crystalline and can cause silicosis. Amorphous silica has been associated with lung fibrosis but the role of crystalline silica contamination remains controversial.	10 mg/m³ (precipitated silica, diatomaceous earth, silica gel) 3 mg/m³ (respirable dust) 2 mg/m³ (silica fume)	3000 mg/m³	White to gray powders. Odorless with a negligible vapor pressure. The TLV for dusts is 10 mg/m³ if no asbestos and less than 1% quartz are present.
Silica, crystalline (quartz; fused amorphous silica; cristobolite; tridymite; tripoli [CAS: 14464-46-1]): Inhalation of dusts causes silicosis, a progressive, fibrotic scarring of the lung. Individuals with silicosis are much more susceptible to tuberculosis. Some forms of crystalline silica are carcinogenic (IARC 2A).	0.1 mg/m³ (respirable dust; quartz, fused silica, tripoli) 0.05 mg/m³ (respirable dust; cristobolite, tridymite)	25 mg/m³ (cristobolite, tridymite) 50 mg/m³ (quartz, tripoli)	Colorless, odorless solid with a negligible vapor pressure. A component of many mineral dusts.
Silicon (CAS: 7440-21-3): A nuisance dust that does not cause pulmonary fibrosis. Parenteral exposure has been associated with systemic toxicity.	10 mg/m³	Gray to black, lustrous needlelike crystals. Vapor pressure is negligible at 20 °C (68 °F).

(C) = ceiling air concentration (TLV-C); S = skin absorption can be significant; A1 = ACGIH-confirmed human carcinogen; A2 = ACGIH-suspected human carcinogen; NFPA Hazard Codes: H = health, F = fire, R = reactivity, Ox = oxidizer, W = water-reactive, 0 (none) <—> 4 (severe); ERPG = Emergency Response Planning Guideline. See p 434 for explanation of definitions.

(continued)

TABLE IV–4. HEALTH HAZARD SUMMARIES FOR INDUSTRIAL AND OCCUPATIONAL CHEMICALS (CONTINUED)

Health Hazard Summaries	ACGIH TLV	IDLH	NFPA Codes H F R	Comments
Silicon tetrachloride (CAS: 10026-04-7): Generates hydrochloric acid vapor upon contact with moisture; severe burns may result. Extremely irritating to eyes and respiratory tract; pulmonary edema may result.			3 0 2 W	Not combustible.
Silver (CAS: 7440-22-4): Silver compounds cause argyria, a blue-gray discoloration of tissues, which may be generalized throughout the viscera or localized to the conjunctiva, nasal septum, and gums. Some silver salts are corrosive upon direct contact with tissues.	0.01 mg/m³ (soluble compounds, as Ag) 0.1 mg/m³ (metal)	10 mg/m³ (Ag compounds, as Ag)		Compounds vary in appearance. Silver nitrate is a strong oxidizer.
Sodium azide (hydrazoic acid, sodium salt; NaN₃ [CAS: 26628-22-8]): Potent cellular toxin; inhibits cytochrome oxidase. Eye irritation, bronchitis, headache, hypotension, and collapse have been reported in overexposed workers. See also p 99.	0.11 ppm (C) (as hydrazoic acid vapor)			White, odorless, crystalline solid.
Sodium bisulfide (NaSH [CAS: 16721-80-5]): Decomposes in the presence of water to form hydrogen sulfide (see p 188) and sodium hydroxide (see p 129). Highly corrosive and irritating to eyes, skin, and respiratory tract.				White crystalline substance with a slight odor of sulfur dioxide.
Sodium bisulfite (sodium hydrogen sulfite, NaHSO₃ [CAS: 7631-90-5]): Irritating to eyes, skin, and respiratory tract. Hypersensitivity reactions (angioedema, bronchospasm, or anaphylaxis) may occur.	5 mg/m³			White crystalline solid with a slight sulfur dioxide odor and disagreeable taste. Widely used as a food additive.
Sodium fluoroacetate (compound 1080 [CAS: 62-74-8]): A highly toxic metabolic poison. Metabolized to fluorocitrate, which prevents the oxidation of acetate in the Krebs cycle. Human lethal oral dose ranges from 2 to 10 mg/kg. See also p 172.	0.05 mg/m³, S	2.5 mg/m³		Fluffy white solid or a fine white powder. Sometimes dyed black. Hygroscopic. Odorless. Vapor pressure is negligible at 20 °C (68 °F). Not combustible. Thermal breakdown products include hydrogen fluoride. Used as a rodenticide.

Compound	TLV	Other	NFPA (H F R)	Comments
Sodium hydroxide (NaOH [CAS: 1310-73-2]): A caustic alkali; may cause severe burns. Fumes or mists are highly irritating to eyes, skin, and respiratory tract. See also p 129.	2 mg/m³ (C)	10 mg/m³	3 0 1 W	White solid that absorbs moisture. Odorless. Evolves great heat upon solution in water. Soda lye is an aqueous solution.
Sodium metabisulfite (sodium pyrosulfite [CAS: 7681-57-4]): Very irritating to eyes and skin upon direct contact. Dusts irritating to eyes and respiratory tract; pulmonary edema may result. Hypersensitivity reactions may occur.	5 mg/m³			White powder or crystalline material with a slight odor of sulfur dioxide. Reacts to form sulfur dioxide in the presence of moisture.
Stibine (antimony hydride [CAS: 7803-52-3]): A potent hemolytic agent similar to arsine. Gases irritating to the lung; pulmonary edema may occur. Liver and kidney are secondary target organs. See also p 86.	0.1 ppm	5 ppm	4 4 2	Colorless gas. Odor similar to that of hydrogen sulfide but may not be a reliable warning property. Formed when acid solutions of antimony are treated with zinc or strong reducing agents.
Stoddard solvent (mineral spirits, a mixture of aliphatic and aromatic hydrocarbons [CAS: 8052-41-3]): Dermal absorption can occur. Vapors irritating to eyes and respiratory tract. A CNS depressant. Chronic overexposures associated with headache, fatigue, bone marrow hypoplasia, and jaundice. May contain a small amount of benzene. See also hydrocarbons, p 183.	100 ppm	20,000 mg/m³	0 2 0	Colorless liquid. Kerosenelike odor and irritation are good warning properties. Vapor pressure is approximately 2 mm Hg at 20 °C (68 °F). Flammable.
Strychnine (CAS: 57-24-9): Neurotoxin binds to inhibitory, postsynaptic glycine receptors, which results in excessive motor activity associated with convulsions and muscular hyperrigidity leading to respiratory impairment or paralysis. See also p 298.	0.15 mg/m³	3 mg/m³		White solid. Odorless. Vapor pressure is negligible at 20 °C (68 °F). Thermal breakdown products include oxides of nitrogen. Street drugs may be adulterated with strychnine.
Styrene monomer (vinylbenzene [CAS: 100-42-5]): Irritating upon direct contact. Dermal absorption occurs. Vapors irritating to respiratory tract. A CNS depressant. Symptoms include headache, nausea, dizziness, and fatigue. Cases of peripheral neuropathy have been reported. Limited evidence for adverse effects on fetal development and cancer in test animals (IARC 2B).	20 ppm	700 ppm ERPG-1: 50 ppm ERPG-2: 250 ppm ERPG-3: 1000 ppm	2 3 2	Colorless viscous liquid. Sweet aromatic odor at low concentrations is an adequate warning property. Odor at high levels is acrid. Vapor pressure is 4.5 mm Hg at 20 °C (68 °F). Flammable. Inhibitor must be included to avoid explosive polymerization. Used in SBR, ABS, and SAN polymers.

(C) = ceiling air concentration (TLV-C); S = skin absorption can be significant; A1 = ACGIH-confirmed human carcinogen; A2 = ACGIH-suspected human carcinogen; NFPA Hazard Codes: H = health, F = fire, R = reactivity, Ox = oxidizer, W = water-reactive, 0 (none) <—> 4 (severe); ERPG = Emergency Response Planning Guideline. See p 434 for explanation of definitions.

(continued)

TABLE IV–4. HEALTH HAZARD SUMMARIES FOR INDUSTRIAL AND OCCUPATIONAL CHEMICALS (CONTINUED)

Health Hazard Summaries	ACGIH TLV	IDLH	NFPA Codes H F R	Comments
Subtilisins (proteolytic enzymes of _Bacillus subtilis_ [CAS: 1395-21-7]): Primary skin and respiratory tract irritants. Potent sensitizers causing primary bronchoconstriction and asthma.	0.06 μg/m³ (C)			Light-colored powder. Occupational asthma associated with their introduction into detergent in a powder formulation.
Sulfur dioxide (CAS: 7446-09-5): Forms sulfurous acid upon contact with moisture. Strongly irritating to eyes and skin; burns may result. Extremely irritating to the respiratory tract; irritation of the upper airways has caused obstruction of the upper airways and pulmonary edema. Asthmatics are of documented increased sensitivity to the bronchoconstrictive effects of sulfur dioxide air pollution. See also p 300.	2 ppm	100 ppm ERPG-1: 0.3 ppm ERPG-2: 3 ppm ERPG-3: 15 ppm	3 0 0 (liquified)	Colorless gas. Pungent, suffocating odor with a "taste" and irritative effects that are good warning properties.
Sulfur hexafluoride (CAS: 2551-62-4): Considered to be essentially a nontoxic gas. Asphyxiation by the displacement of air is suggested as the greatest hazard.	1000 ppm			Odorless, colorless dense gas. May be contaminated with other fluorides of sulfur, including the highly toxic sulfur pentafluoride, which release HF or oxyfluorides on contact with moisture.
Sulfuric acid (oil of vitriol, H₂SO₄ [CAS: 7664-93-9]): Highly corrosive upon direct contact; severe burns may result. Breakdown may release sulfur dioxide (see p 300). Exposure to the mist can irritate the eyes, skin, and respiratory tract.	1 mg/m³, A2 (strong acid mists)	15 mg/m³ ERPG-1: 2 mg/m³ ERPG-2: 10 mg/m³ ERPG-3: 30 mg/m³	3 0 2 W	Colorless to dark brown heavy, oily liquid. Odorless. Eye irritation may be an adequate warning property. A strong oxidizer. Addition of water creates strong exothermic reaction. Vapor pressure is less than 0.001 mm Hg at 20 °C (68 °F).
Sulfur monochloride (CAS: 10025-67-9): Forms hydrochloric acid and sulfur dioxide (see p 300) upon contact with water; direct contact can cause burns. Vapors highly irritating to the eyes, skin, and the respiratory tract.	1 ppm (C)	5 ppm	3 1 1	Fuming, amber to red, oily liquid with a pungent, irritating, sickening odor. Eye irritation is a good warning property. Vapor pressure is 6.8 mm Hg at 20 °C (68 °F). Combustible. Breakdown products include hydrogen sulfide, hydrogen chloride, and sulfur dioxide.

Sulfur pentafluoride (disulfur decafluoride [CAS: 5714-22-7]): Vapors are extremely irritating to the lungs; causes pulmonary edema at low levels (0.5 ppm) in test animals.	0.01 ppm (C)	1 ppm	Colorless liquid or vapor with a sulfur dioxidelike odor. Vapor pressure is 561 mm Hg at 20 °C (68 °F). Not combustible. Thermal breakdown products include sulfur dioxide and hydrogen fluoride.
Sulfur tetrafluoride (SF₄ [CAS: 7783-60-0]): Readily hydrolyzed by moisture to form sulfur dioxide (see p 300) and hydrogen fluoride (see p 186). Extremely irritating to the respiratory tract; pulmonary edema may occur. Vapors also highly irritating to eyes and skin.	0.1 ppm (C)		Colorless gas. Reacts with moisture to form sulfur dioxide and hydrogen fluoride.
Sulfuryl fluoride (Vikane, SO₂F₂ [CAS: 2699-79-8]): Irritating to eyes and respiratory tract; fatal pulmonary edema has resulted. Acute high exposure causes tremors and convulsions in test animals. Chronic exposures may cause kidney and liver injury and elevated fluoride. See also p 186.	5 ppm	200 ppm	Colorless, odorless gas with no warning properties. Chloropicrin, a lacrimator, is often added to provide a warning property. Thermal breakdown products include sulfur dioxide and hydrogen fluoride. A widely used fumigant.
Sulprofos (O-ethyl O-[4-(methylthio)phenyl] S-propylphosphorodithioate [CAS: 35400-43-2]): An organophosphate anticholinesterase insecticide (see p 244).	1 mg/m³		Tan-colored liquid with a characteristic sulfide odor.
Talc, containing no asbestos fibers or crystalline silica (CAS: 14807-96-6): A tissue irritant. Pulmonary aspiration may cause serious pneumonitis.	2 mg/m³ (C) (respirable dust; if talc contains asbestos fibers, see asbestos TLV)	1000 mg/m³	
Tantalum compounds (as Ta): Of low acute toxicity. Dusts mildly irritating to the lungs.(metal and oxide)	5 mg/m³	2500 mg/m³ (as Ta)	Metal is a gray-black solid, platinum-white if polished. Odorless. Tantalum pentoxide is a colorless solid. Used in aerospace and other specialty alloys.

(C) = ceiling air concentration (TLV-C); S = skin absorption can be significant; A1 = ACGIH-confirmed human carcinogen; A2 = ACGIH-suspected human carcinogen; NFPA Hazard Codes: H = health, F = fire, R = reactivity, Ox = oxidizer, W = water-reactive, 0 (none) <—> 4 (severe). ERPG = Emergency Response Planning Guideline. See p 434 for explanation of definitions.

(continued)

TABLE IV–4. HEALTH HAZARD SUMMARIES FOR INDUSTRIAL AND OCCUPATIONAL CHEMICALS (CONTINUED)

Health Hazard Summaries	ACGIH TLV	IDLH	NFPA Codes H F R	Comments
Tellurium and compounds (as Te): Complaints of sleepiness, nausea, metallic taste, and garlicky odor on breath and perspiration associated with workplace exposures. Neuropathies have been noted in high-dose studies. Hydrogen telluride causes pulmonary irritation and hemolysis; however, its ready decomposition reduces likelihood of a toxic exposure. Some tellurium compounds are fetotoxic or teratogenic in test animals.	0.1 mg/m³ (as Te)	25 mg/m³ (as Te)		Metallic tellurium is a solid with a silvery-white or grayish luster.
Tellurium hexafluoride (CAS: 7783-80-4): Slowly hydrolyzes to release hydrofluoric acid (see p 186) and telluric acid. Extremely irritating to the eyes and respiratory tract; pulmonary edema may occur. Has caused headaches, dyspnea, and garlicky odor on the breath of overexposed workers.	0.02 ppm	1 ppm		Colorless gas. Offensive odor. Not combustible. Thermal breakdown products include hydrogen fluoride.
Temephos (Abate, O,O,O',O'-tetramethyl O,O-thiodi-p-phenylene phosphorothioate [CAS: 3383-96-8]): Primary irritant of eyes, skin, and respiratory tract; a moderately toxic organophosphate-type cholinesterase inhibitor (see p 244). Well absorbed by all routes.	10 mg/m³			
Terphenyls (diphenyl benzenes, triphenyls [CAS: 26140-60-3]): Irritating upon direct contact. Vapors and mists irritating to respiratory tract; pulmonary edema has occured at very high levels in test animals. Animal studies also suggest a slight potential for liver and kidney injury.	5 mg/m³ (C)	500 mg/m³	0 1 0	White to light yellow crystalline solids. Irritation is a possible warning property. Vapor pressure is very low at 20 °C (68 °F). Combustible. Commercial grades are mixtures of o-, m-, p-isomers.
1,1,1,2-Tetrachloro-2,2-difluoroethane (halocarbon 112a; refrigerant 112a [CAS: 76-11-9]): Of low acute toxicity. Very high air levels irritating to the eyes and respiratory tract. A CNS depressant at high levels. By analogy to other freons, may cause cardiac arrhythmias. High-dose studies in animals suggest possible kidney and liver injury. See also p 178.	500 ppm	2000 ppm		Colorless liquid or solid with a slight etherlike odor. Vapor pressure is 40 mm Hg at 20 °C (68 °F). Not combustible. Thermal breakdown products include hydrogen chloride and hydrogen fluoride.

1,1,2,2-Tetrachloro-1,2-difluoroethane (halocarbon 112; refrigerant 112 [CAS: 76-12-0]): Of low acute toxicity. Once used as an anthelminthic. Very high air levels cause CNS depression. Vapors mildly irritating. By analogy to other freons, may cause cardiac arrhythmias. See also p 178.

500 ppm | 2000 ppm

Colorless liquid or solid with a slight etherlike odor. Odor is of unknown value as a warning property. Vapor pressure is 40 mm Hg at 20 °C (68 °F). Not combustible. Thermal breakdown products include hydrogen chloride and hydrogen fluoride.

1,1,2,2-Tetrachloroethane (acetylene tetrachloride [CAS: 79-34-5]): Dermal absorption may cause systemic toxicity. Vapors irritating to the eyes and respiratory tract. A CNS depressant. By analogy to other chlorinated ethane derivatives, may cause cardiac arrhythmias. May cause hepatic or renal injury. Limited evidence of carcinogenicity in test animals (IARC 3).

1 ppm, S NIOSH CA | 100 ppm

Colorless to light yellow liquid. Sweet, suffocating, chloroform like odor is a good warning property. Vapor pressure is 8 mm Hg at 20 °C (68 °F). Not combustible. Thermal breakdown products include hydrogen chloride and phosgene.

Tetrachloroethylene (perchloroethylene [CAS: 127-18-4]): Irritating upon prolonged contact; mild burns may result. Vapors irritating to eyes and respiratory tract. A CNS depressant. By analogy to other trichloroethylene and other chlorinated solvents, may cause arrhythmias. May cause liver and kidney injury. Chronic overexposure may cause short-term memory loss and personality changes. Limited evidence of adverse effects on reproductive function in males and fetal development in test animals. Evidence for carcinogenicity in test animals (IARC 2B). See also p 308.

25 ppm, A3 NIOSH CA | 150 ppm ERPG-1: 100 ppm ERPG-2: 200 ppm ERPG-3: 1000 ppm | 2 0 0

Colorless liquid. Chloroformlike or etherlike odor and eye irritation are adequate warning properties. Vapor pressure is 14 mm Hg at 20 °C (68 °F). Not combustible. Thermal breakdown products include phosgene and hydrochloric acid. Used in the dry cleaning industry.

Tetrachloronaphthalene (Halowax [CAS: 1335-88-2]): Causes chloracne and jaundice. Stored in body fat. Dermal absorption occurs.

2 mg/m³

White to light yellow solid. Aromatic odor of unknown value as a warning property. Vapor pressure is less than 1 mm Hg at 20 °C (68 °F). Thermal breakdown products include hydrogen chloride and phosgene.

Tetraethyl-di-thionopyrophosphate (TEDP, sulfotepp [CAS: 3689-24-5]): An organophosphate anticholinesterase insecticide (see p 244). Well absorbed dermally.

10 mg/m³

Yellow liquid with garlic odor. Not combustible. Thermal breakdown products include sulfur dioxide and phosphoric acid mist.

(C) = ceiling air concentration (TLV-C); S = skin absorption can be significant; A1 = ACGIH-confirmed human carcinogen; A2 = ACGIH-suspected human carcinogen; A3 = ACGIH-confirmed animal carcinogen; NFPA Hazard Codes: H = health, F = fire, R = reactivity, Ox = oxidizer, W = water-reactive, 0 (none) <—> 4 (severe). ERPG = Emergency Response Planning Guideline. See p 434 for explanation of definitions.

(continued)

TABLE IV–4. HEALTH HAZARD SUMMARIES FOR INDUSTRIAL AND OCCUPATIONAL CHEMICALS (CONTINUED)

Health Hazard Summaries	ACGIH TLV	IDLH	NFPA Codes H F R	Comments
Tetraethyl lead (CAS: 78-00-2): A potent CNS toxin. Dermally well absorbed. Can cause psychosis, mania, convulsions, and coma. Reports of reduced sperm counts and impotence in overexposed workers. See also p 199.	0.1 mg/m^3 (as Pb), S	40 mg/m^3 (as Pb)	3 2 3	Colorless liquid. May be dyed blue, red, or orange. Slight musty odor of unknown value as a warning property. Vapor pressure is 0.2 mm Hg at 20 °C (68 °F). Combustible. Decomposes in light. As a gasoline additive, heavy exposure can occur through inappropriate use of gasoline as a solvent and in substance abuse.
Tetraethyl pyrophosphate (TEPP [CAS: 107-49-3]): A potent organophosphate cholinesterase inhibitor (see p 244). Rapidly absorbed through skin.	0.05 mg/m^3, S	5 mg/m^3		Colorless to amber liquid with a faint fruity odor. Slowly hydrolyzed in water. Vapor pressure is 1 mm Hg at 140 °C (284 °F). Not combustible. Thermal breakdown products include phosphoric acid mist.
Tetrahydrofuran (THF, diethylene oxide [CAS: 109-99-9]): Mildly irritating upon direct contact. Vapors mildly irritating to eyes and respiratory tract. A CNS depressant at high levels. A liver and kidney toxin at high doses in test animals.	200 ppm	2000 ppm [LEL]	2 3 1	Colorless liquid. The etherlike odor is detectable well below the TLV and provides a good warning property. Flammable. Vapor pressure is 145 mm Hg at 20 °C (68 °F).
Tetramethyl lead (CAS: 75-74-1): A potent CNS toxin thought to be similar to tetraethyl lead. See also p 199.	0.15 mg/m^3 (as Pb), S	40 mg/m^3 (as Pb)	3 3 3	Colorless liquid. May be dyed red, orange, or blue. Slight musty odor is of unknown value as a warning property. Vapor pressure is 22 mm Hg at 20 °C (68 °F).
Tetramethyl succinonitrile (TMSN [CAS: 3333-52-6]): A potent neurotoxin. Headaches, nausea, dizziness, convulsions, and coma have occurred in overexposed workers.	0.5 ppm, S	5 ppm		Colorless, odorless solid. Thermal breakdown products include oxides of nitrogen.

Compound	Air concentration	Appearance/Comments
Tetranitromethane (CAS: 509-14-8): Highly irritating upon direct contact; mild burns may result. Vapors extremely irritating to eyes and respiratory tract; pulmonary edema has been reported. May cause methemoglobinemia (see p 220). Liver, kidney, and CNS injury in test animals at high doses. Overexposure associated with headaches, fatigue, dyspnea. See also nitrates, p 233.	0.005 ppm, A3	Colorless to light yellow liquid or solid with a pungent, acrid odor. Irritative effects are a good warning property. Vapor pressure is 8.4 mm Hg at 20 °C (68 °F). Not combustible. A weak explosive and oxidizer. Highly explosive in the presence of impurities.
Tetrasodium pyrophosphate (CAS: 7722-88-5): Alkaline; dusts are mild irritants of eyes, skin, and respiratory tract.	5 mg/m³	White powder. Alkaline in aqueous solution.
Tetryl (nitramine, 2,4,6-trinitrophenylmethylnitramine [CAS: 479-45-8]): Causes severe sensitization dermatitis. Dusts extremely irritating to the eyes and respiratory tract. Stains tissues bright yellow. May injure the liver and kidneys. Overexposures also associated with malaise, headache, nausea, and vomiting.	1.5 mg/m³	White to yellow solid. Odorless. A strong oxidizer. Vapor pressure is much less than 1 mm Hg at 20 °C (68 °F). Explosive used in detonators and primers.
Thallium, soluble compounds (thallium sulfate, thallium acetate, thallium nitrate): A potent toxin causing diverse chronic effects including psychosis, peripheral neuropathy, optic neuritis, alopecia, abdominal pain, irritability, and weight loss. Liver and kidney injury may occur. Ingestion causes severe hemorrhagic gastroenteritis. Absorption possible by all routes. See also p 302.	0.1 mg/m³ (as Tl), S	15 mg/m³ (as Tl) — Appearance varies with the compound. The elemental form is a bluish-white, ductile heavy metal with a negligible vapor pressure. Thallium has been used as a rodenticide.
Thioglycolic acid (mercaptoacetic acid [CAS: 68-11-1]): Skin or eye contact with concentrated acid causes severe burns. Vapors irritating to eyes and respiratory tract.	1 ppm, S	Colorless liquid. Unpleasant mercaptanlike odor. Vapor pressure is 10 mm Hg at 18 °C (64 °F). Found in some coldwave and depilatory formulations.
Thiram (tetramethylthiuram disulfide [CAS: 137-26-8]): Dusts mildly irritating to eyes, skin, and respiratory tract. A moderate allergen and a potent skin sensitizer. Has disulfiramlike effects in exposed persons who consume alcohol (see p 158). Experimentally a goitrogen. Adverse effects on fetal development in test animals at very high doses.	1 mg/m³	100 mg/m³ — White to yellow powder with a characteristic odor. May be dyed blue. Vapor pressure is negligible at 20 °C (68 °F). Thermal breakdown products include sulfur dioxide and carbon disulfide. Used in rubber manufacture and as a fungicide.

(C) = ceiling air concentration (TLV-C); S = skin absorption can be significant; A1 = ACGIH-confirmed human carcinogen; A2 = ACGIH-suspected human carcinogen; A3 = ACGIH-suspected animal carcinogen; NFPA Hazard Codes: H = health, F = fire, R = reactivity, Ox = oxidizer, W = water-reactive, 0 (none) <—> 4 (severe), ERPG = Emergency Response Planning Guideline. See p 434 for explanation of definitions.

(continued)

TABLE IV–4. HEALTH HAZARD SUMMARIES FOR INDUSTRIAL AND OCCUPATIONAL CHEMICALS (CONTINUED)

Health Hazard Summaries	ACGIH TLV	IDLH	NFPA Codes H F R	Comments
Tin, metal, and inorganic compounds: Dusts irritating to the eyes, nose, throat, and skin. Prolonged inhalation may cause chest x-ray abnormalities. Some compounds react with water to form acids (tin tetrachloride, stannous chloride, and stannous sulfate) or bases (sodium and potassium stannate).	2 mg/m^3 (as Sn)	100 mg/m^3 (as Sn)		Metallic tin is odorless with a dull, silvery color.
Tin, organic compounds: Highly irritating upon direct contact; burns may result. Dusts, fumes, or vapors highly irritating to the eyes and respiratory tract. Triethyltin is a potent neurotoxin; triphenyltin acetate is highly hepatotoxic. Trialkyltins are the most toxic, followed in order by the dialkyltins and monoalkyltins. Within each of these classes, the ethyltin compounds are the most toxic. All are well absorbed dermally.	0.1 mg/m^3 (as Sn)	25 mg/m^3 (as Sn)		There are many kinds of organotin compounds: mono-, di-, tri-, and tetra-alkyltin and -aryltin compounds exist. Combustible. Organic tin compounds are used in some polymers and paints.
Titanium dioxide (CAS: 13463-67-7): A mild pulmonary irritant.	10 mg/m^3	5000 mg/m^3		White odorless powder. Rutile is a common crystalline form. Vapor pressure is negligible.
Tolidine (o-tolidine, 3,3'-dimethylbenzidine [CAS: 119-93-7]): A carcinogen in test animals (IARC 2B).	S, A3 NIOSH CA			White to reddish solid. Oxides of nitrogen are among thermal breakdown products.
Toluene (toluol, methylbenzene [CAS: 108-88-3]): Vapors mildly irritating to eyes and respiratory tract. A CNS depressant; may cause brain, kidney and muscle damage with frequent intentional abuse. May cause cardiac arrhythmias. Liver and kidney injury with heavy exposures. Abusive sniffing during pregnancy associated with birth defects. See also p 307.	50 ppm, S	500 ppm ERPG-1: 50 ppm ERPG-2: 300 ppm ERPG-3: 1000 ppm	2 3 0	Colorless liquid. Aromatic, benzenelike odor detectable at very low levels. Irritation serves as a good warning property. Vapor pressure is 22 mm Hg at 20 °C (68 °F). Flammable.

Chemical	TLV-C (ppm)	H F R	Physical description
Toluene 2,4-diisocyanate (CAS: 584-84-9): A potent respiratory tract sensitizer (asthma) and potent irritant of the eyes, skin, and respiratory tract. Pulmonary edema has resulted with higher exposures. A carcinogen in test animals (IARC 2B). See also p 194.	0.005 ppm	3 1 3 W	Colorless needles or a liquid with a sharp, pungent odor. Vapor pressure is approximately 0.04 mm Hg at 20 °C (68 °F). Combustible.
o-Toluidine (2-methylaniline) [CAS: 95-53-4]: A corrosive alkali; can cause severe burns. May cause methemoglobinemia (see p 220). Dermal absorption occurs. A carcinogen in test animals. (IARC 2A).	2 ppm, S, A3	3 2 0	Colorless to pale yellow liquid. The weak aromatic odor is thought to be a good warning property. Vapor pressure is less than 1 mm Hg at 20 °C (68 °F).
m-Toluidine (3-methylaniline) [CAS: 108-44-1]: A corrosive alkali; can cause severe burns. May cause methemoglobinemia (see p 220). Dermal absorption occurs.	2 ppm, S		Pale yellow liquid. Vapor pressure is less than 1 mm Hg at 20 °C (68 °F).
p-Toluidine (4-methylaniline) [CAS: 106-49-0]: A corrosive alkali; can cause severe burns. May cause methemoglobinemia (see p 220). Dermal absorption occurs. A carcinogen in test animals.	2 ppm, S, A3	3 2 0	White solid. Vapor pressure is 1 mm Hg at 20 °C (68 °F).
Tributyl phosphate (CAS: 126-73-8): Highly irritating upon direct contact; causes severe eye injury and skin irritation. Vapors or mists irritating to the eyes and respiratory tract; high exposure in test animals caused pulmonary edema. Weak anticholinesterase activity. Headache and nausea are reported.	0.2 ppm	2 1 0	Colorless to pale yellow liquid. Odorless. Vapor pressure is very low at 20 °C (68 °F). Combustible. Thermal breakdown products include phosphoric acid fume.
Trichloroacetic acid (CAS: 76-03-9): A strong acid. A protein denaturant. Corrosive to eyes and skin upon direct contact.	1 ppm		Deliquescent crystalline solid. Vapor pressure is 1 mm Hg at 51 °C (128.3 °F). Thermal breakdown products include hydrochloric acid and phosgene.
1,2,4-Trichlorobenzene (CAS: 120-82-1): Prolonged or repeated contact can cause skin and eye irritation. Vapors irritating to the eyes, skin, and respiratory tract. High-dose animal exposures injure the liver, kidneys, lungs, and CNS. Does not cause chloracne.	5 ppm (C)	2 1 0	A colorless liquid with an unpleasant, mothball-like odor. Vapor pressure is 1 mm Hg at 38.4 °C (101.1 °F). Combustible. Thermal breakdown products include hydrogen chloride and phosgene.

(C) = ceiling air concentration (TLV-C); S = skin absorption can be significant; A1 = ACGIH-confirmed human carcinogen; A2 = ACGIH-suspected human carcinogen; A3 = ACGIH-confirmed animal carcinogen; NFPA Hazard Codes: H = health, F = fire, R = reactivity, Ox = oxidizer, W = water-reactive, 0 (none) <—> 4 (severe). ERPG = Emergency Response Planning Guideline. See p 434 for explanation of definitions.

(continued)

TABLE IV–4. HEALTH HAZARD SUMMARIES FOR INDUSTRIAL AND OCCUPATIONAL CHEMICALS (CONTINUED)

Health Hazard Summaries	ACGIH TLV	IDLH	NFPA Codes H F R	Comments
1,1,1-Trichloroethane (methyl chloroform, TCA [CAS: 71-55-6]): Vapors mildly irritating to eyes and respiratory tract. A CNS depressant. May cause cardiac arrhythmias. Some dermal absorption occurs. Liver and kidney injury may occur. See also p 308.	350 ppm	700 ppm ERPG-1: 350 ppm ERPG-2: 700 ppm ERPG-3: 3500 ppm	2 1 0	Colorless liquid. Vapor pressure is 100 mm Hg at 20 °C (68 °F). Not combustible. Thermal breakdown products include hydrogen chloride and phosgene. Widely used chlorinated solvent.
1,1,2-Trichloroethane [CAS: 79-00-5]: Dermal absorption may occur. Vapors mildly irritating to eyes and respiratory tract. A CNS depressant. May cause cardiac arrhythmias. Causes liver and kidney injury in test animals. Limited evidence for carcinogenicity in test animals (IARC 3). See also p 308.	10 ppm, S NIOSH CA	100 ppm	2 1 0	Colorless liquid. Sweet, chloroformlike odor is of unknown value as a warning property. Vapor pressure is 19 mm Hg at 20 °C (68 °F). Not combustible. Thermal breakdown products include phosgene and hydrochloric acid.
Trichloroethylene (trichloroethene, TCE [CAS: 79-01-6]): Dermal absorption may occur. Vapors mildly irritating to eyes and respiratory tract. A CNS depressant. May cause cardiac arrhythmias. May cause cranial and peripheral neuropathies and liver damage. Has a disulfiramlike effect, "degreasers' flush" (see p 158). Reported to cause liver and lung cancers in mice (IARC 3). See also p 308.	50 ppm NIOSH CA	1000 ppm ERPG-1: 100 ppm ERPG-2: 500 ppm ERPG-3: 5000 ppm	2 1 0	Colorless liquid. Sweet chloroformlike odor. Vapor pressure is 58 mm Hg at 20 °C (68 °F). Not combustible at room temperatures. Decomposition products include hydrogen chloride and phosgene.
Trichlorofluoromethane (Freon 11 [CAS: 75-69-4]): Vapors mildly irritating to eyes and respiratory tract. A CNS depressant. May cause cardiac arrhythmias. See also p 178.	1000 ppm (C)			Colorless liquid or gas at room temperature. Vapor pressure is 690 mm Hg at 20 °C (68 °F). Not combustible. Thermal breakdown products include hydrogen chloride and hydrogen fluoride.
Trichloronaphthalene (Halowax [CAS: 1321-65-9]): Causes chloracne. A hepatotoxin a low doses, causing jaundice. Stored in body fat. Systemic toxicity may occur following dermal exposure.	5 mg/m³, S			Colorless to pale yellow solid with an aromatic odor of uncertain value as a warning property. Vapor pressure is less than 1 mm Hg at 20 °C (68 °F). Flammable. Decomposition products include phosgene and hydrogen chloride.

Chemical			NFPA	Comments
2,4,5-Trichlorophenoxyacetic acid (2,4,5-T) [CAS: 93-76-5]: Moderately irritating to eyes, skin, and respiratory tract. Ingestion can cause gastroenteritis and injury to the CNS, muscle, kidney, and liver. A weak uncoupler of oxidative phosphorylation. Polychlorinated dibenzodioxin compounds are contaminants (see p 156). There are reports of sarcomas occurring in applicators. Adverse effects on fetal development in test animals.	10 mg/m³	250 mg/m³		Colorless to tan solid. Appearance and some hazardous properties vary with the formulation. Odorless. Vapor pressure is negligible at 20 °C (68 °F). Not combustible. Thermal breakdown products include hydrogen chloride and dioxins. A herbicide once widely used as a defoliant and in Vietnam, "Agent Orange."
1,1,2-Trichloro-1,2,2-trifluoroethane (Freon 113): Vapors mildly irritating to eyes and mucous membranes. Very high air levels cause CNS depression and may injure the liver. May cause cardiac arrhythmias at air concentrations as low as 2000 ppm in test animals. See also p 178.	1000 ppm	2000 ppm		Colorless liquid. Sweetish, chloroformlike odor occurs only at very high concentrations and is a poor warning property. Vapor pressure is 284 mm Hg at 20 °C (68 °F). Not combustible. Thermal breakdown products include hydrogen chloride, hydrogen fluoride, and phosgene.
Triethylamine [CAS: 121-44-8]: An alkaline corrosive; highly irritating to eyes and skin; severe burns may occur. Vapors very irritating to eyes and respiratory tract; pulmonary edema may occur. High doses in animals cause heart, liver, and kidney injury. CNS stimulation possibly resulting from inhibition of monoamine oxidase.	1 ppm, S	200 ppm	3 3 0	Colorless liquid with a fishy, ammonialike odor of unknown value as a warning property. Vapor pressure is 54 mm Hg at 20 °C (68 °F). Flammable.
Trifluorobromomethane (Halon 1301; Freon 13B1) [CAS: 75-63-8]: Extremely high air levels (150,000–200,000) can cause CNS depression and cardiac arrhythmias. See also p 178.	1000 ppm	40,000 ppm		Colorless gas with a weak etherlike odor at high levels and poor warning properties. Not combustible.
Trifluoromethane (Freon 23) [CAS: 75-46-7]: Vapors mildly irritating to the eyes and mucous membranes. Very high air levels cause CNS depression and cardiac arrhythmias. See also p 178.				Not combustible.
Trimellitic anhydride (TMAN) [CAS: 552-30-7]: Dusts and vapors extremely irritating to eyes, nose, throat, skin, and respiratory tract. Potent respiratory sensitizer (asthma). Can also cause diffuse lung hemorrhage.	0.04 mg/m³ (C)			Colorless solid. Hydrolyzes to trimellitic acid in aqueous solutions. Vapor pressure is 0.000004 mm Hg at 25 °C (77 °F). TMAN is an important component of certain epoxy coatings.

(C) = ceiling air concentration (TLV-C); S = skin absorption can be significant; A1 = ACGIH-confirmed human carcinogen; A2 = ACGIH-suspected human carcinogen; NFPA Hazard Codes: H = health, F = fire, R = reactivity, Ox = oxidizer, W = water-reactive, 0 (none) <—> 4 (severe). ERPG = Emergency Response Planning Guideline. See p 434 for explanation of definitions.

(continued)

TABLE IV–4. HEALTH HAZARD SUMMARIES FOR INDUSTRIAL AND OCCUPATIONAL CHEMICALS (CONTINUED)

Health Hazard Summaries	ACGIH TLV	IDLH	NFPA Codes H F R			Comments
Trimethylamine (CAS: 75-50-3): An alkaline corrosive; highly irritating upon direct contact; severe burns may occur. Vapors very irritating to respiratory tract.	5 ppm	ERPG-1: 0.1 ppm ERPG-2: 100 ppm ERPG-3: 500 ppm	3	4	0	Highly flammable gas with a pungent, fishy, ammonialike odor. May be used as a warning agent in natural gas.
Trimethyl phosphite (phosphorous acid trimethylester [CAS: 121-45-9]): Very irritating upon direct contact; severe burns may result. Vapors highly irritating to respiratory tract. Cataracts have developed in test animals exposed to high air levels. Evidence for adverse effects on fetal development in test animals.	2 ppm		0	2	0	Colorless liquid with a characteristic, strong, fishy, or ammonialike odor. Hydrolyzed in water. Vapor pressure is 24 mm Hg at 25 °C (77 °F). Combustible.
Trinitrotoluene (2,4,6-trinitrotoluene, TNT [CAS: 118-96-7]): Irritating upon direct contact. Stains tissues yellow. Causes sensitization dermatitis. Vapors irritating to the respiratory tract. May cause liver injury, methemoglobinemia (see p 220). Occupational overexposure associated with cataracts. Causes vasodilation, including coronary arteries. Headache and drop in blood pressure are common. Well absorbed by all routes. Tolerance to vasodilation can occur; cessation of exposure may precipitate angina pectoris in pharmacologically dependent workers. See also nitrates, p 233.	0.1 mg/m^3, S	500 mg/m^3				White to light yellow crystalline solid. Odorless. Vapor pressure is 0.05 mm Hg at 85 °C (185 °F). Explosive upon heating or shock.
Triorthocresyl phosphate (TOCP [CAS: 78-30-8]): Inhibits acetylcholinesterase (see p 244). Potent neurotoxin causing delayed, partially reversible peripheral neuropathy by all routes.	0.1 mg/m^3, S	40 mg/m^3				Colorless viscous liquid. Odorless. Not combustible. Although an anticholinesterase inhibitor, it is widely used as a chemical additive and in chemical synthesis.
Triphenyl phosphate (CAS: 115-86-6): Weak anticholinesterase activity in humans (see p 244). Delayed neuropathy reported in test animals.	3 mg/m^3	1000 mg/m^3	2	1	0	Colorless solid. Faint phenolic odor. Not combustible. Thermal breakdown products include phosphoric acid fumes.

Substance and comments	TLV	IDLH/ERPG	H	F	R	Physical description
Tungsten and compounds: Few reports of human toxicity. Some salts may release acid upon contact with moisture. Chronic exposure to tungsten carbide cobalt amalgams in the hard-metals industry may be associated with fibrotic lung disease. See cobalt.	5 mg/m³ (insoluble compounds) 1 mg/m³ (soluble compounds)					Elemental tungsten is a gray, hard, brittle metal. Finely divided powders are flammable.
Turpentine (CAS: 8006-64-2): Irritating to eyes upon direct contact. Dermal sensitizer. Dermal absorption occurs. Vapors irritating to respiratory tract. A CNS depressant at high air levels. See also hydrocarbons, p 183.	100 ppm	800 ppm	1	3	0	Colorless to pale yellow liquid with a characteristic paintlike odor that serves as a good warning property. Vapor pressure is 5 mm Hg at 20 °C (68 °F). Flammable.
Uranium compounds: Many salts are irritating to the respiratory tract; soluble salts are potent kidney toxins. Uranium is a weakly radioactive element (alpha emitter); decays to the radionuclide, thorium 230. Uranium has the potential to cause radiation injury to the lungs, tracheobronchial lymph nodes, bone marrow, and skin.	0.2 mg/m³ (soluble and insoluble compounds, as U), A1	10 mg/m³				Dense, silvery-white, lustrous metal. Finely divided powders are pyrophoric. Radioactive.
Valeraldehyde (pentanal) [CAS: 110-62-3]: Very irritating to eyes and skin; severe burns may result. Vapors highly irritating to the eyes and respiratory tract.	50 ppm		1	3	0	Colorless liquid with a fruity odor. Flammable.
Vanadium pentoxide (CAS: 1314-62-1): Dusts or fumes highly irritating to eyes, skin, and respiratory tract. Acute overexposures have been associated with a persistent bronchitis and asthmalike responses, "boilermakers' asthma." Sensitization dermatitis reported. Low-level exposure may cause a greenish discoloration of the tongue, metallic taste, and cough.	0.05 mg/m³	35 mg/m³ (as V)				Yellow-orange to rust-brown crystalline powder or dark gray flakes. Odorless. Not combustible.
Vinyl acetate (CAS: 108-05-4): Highly irritating upon direct contact; severe skin and eye burns may result. Vapors irritating to the eyes and respiratory tract. Mild CNS depressant at high levels. Limited evidence for adverse effects on male reproduction in test animals at high doses.	10 ppm, A3	ERPG-1: 5 ppm ERPG-2: 75 ppm ERPG-3: 500 ppm	2	3	2	Volatile liquid with a pleasant fruity odor at low levels. Vapor pressure is 115 mm Hg at 25 °C (77 °F). Flammable. Polymerizes readily. Must contain inhibitor to prevent polymerization.

(C) = ceiling air concentration (TLV-C); S = skin absorption can be significant; A1 = ACGIH-confirmed human carcinogen; A2 = ACGIH-suspected human carcinogen; A3 = ACGIH-suspected human carcinogen; NFPA Hazard Codes: H = health, F = fire, R = reactivity, Ox = oxidizer, W = water-reactive, 0 (none), <―> 4 (severe). ERPG = Emergency Response Planning Guideline. See p 434 for explanation of definitions.

(continued)

TABLE IV-4. HEALTH HAZARD SUMMARIES FOR INDUSTRIAL AND OCCUPATIONAL CHEMICALS (CONTINUED)

Health Hazard Summaries	ACGIH TLV	IDLH	NFPA Codes H F R	Comments
Vinyl bromide (CAS: 593-60-2): At high air levels, an eye and respiratory tract irritant and CNS depressant; a kidney and liver toxin. Animal carcinogen (IARC 2A).	5 ppm, A2 NIOSH CA [proposed: 0.5 ppm]		2 0 1	Colorless, highly flammable gas with a distinctive odor.
Vinyl chloride (CAS: 75-01-4): An eye and respiratory tract irritant at high air levels. Degeneration of distal phalanges with "acroosteolysis," Raynaud's disease, and scleroderma have been associated with heavy workplace overexposures. A CNS depressant at high levels, formerly used as an anesthetic. May cause cardiac arrhythmias. Causes angiosarcoma of the liver in humans (IARC 1).	5 ppm, A1 NIOSH CA [proposed: 1 ppm]		2 4 2	Colorless, highly flammable gas with a sweet ether-like odor. Polymerizes readily. Current potential exposure is limited to vinyl chloride synthesis and polymerization to PVC.
Vinyl cyclohexene dioxide (vinylhexane dioxide [CAS: 106-87-6]): Moderately irritating upon direct contact; severe burns may result. Vapors highly irritating to eyes and respiratory tract. Testicular atrophy, leukemia, and necrosis of the thymus in test animals. Topical application causes skin cancer in animal studies.	0.1 ppm, S, A3			Colorless liquid. Vapor pressure is 0.1 mm Hg at 20 °C (68 °F).
Vinyl toluene (methylstyrene [CAS: 25013-15-4]): Vapors irritating to eyes and respiratory tract. A CNS depressant at high levels. Hepatic, renal, and hematologic toxicities observed at high doses in test animals. Limited evidence for adverse effects on the developing fetus at high doses.	50 ppm	400 ppm	2 2 2	Colorless liquid. Strong, unpleasant odor is considered to be an adequate warning property. Vapor pressure is 1.1 mm Hg at 20 °C (68 °F). Flammable. Inhibitor added to prevent explosive polymerization.
VM&P naphtha (varnish makers' and printers' naphtha; ligroin [CAS: 8032-32-4]): Vapors irritating to eyes and respiratory tract. A CNS depressant at high levels. May contain a small amount of benzene. See also hydrocarbons, p 183.	300 ppm, A3			Colorless volatile liquid.

Substance	TLV	ERPG	NFPA (H F R)	Comments
Warfarin (CAS: 81-81-2): An anticoagulant by ingestion. Medicinal dosages associated with adverse effects on fetal development in test animals and humans. See also p 148.	0.1 mg/m³	100 mg/m³		Colorless crystalline substance. Odorless. Used as a rodenticide. Exposure is typically from inadvertent or deliberate ingestion, rather than through workplace contamination.
Xylene (mixture of o-, m-, p-dimethylbenzenes [CAS: 1330-20-7]): Vapors irritating to eyes and respiratory tract. By analogy to toluene and benzene, may cause cardiac arrhythmias. May injure kidneys. Limited evidence for adverse effects on fetal development at very high doses. See also p 307.	100 ppm	900 ppm	2 3 0	Colorless liquid or solid. Weak, somewhat sweet, aromatic odor. Irritant effects are adequate warning properties. Vapor pressure is approximately 8 mm Hg at 20 °C (68 °F). Flammable.
Xylidine (dimethylaniline [CAS: 1300-73-8]): May cause methemoglobinemia (see p 220). Dermal absorption may occur. Liver and kidney damage seen in test animals.	0.5 ppm, S, A3	50 ppm	3 1 0	Pale yellow to brown liquid. Weak, aromatic amine odor is an adequate warning property. Vapor pressure is less than 1 mm Hg at 20 °C (68 °F). Combustible. Thermal breakdown products include oxides of nitrogen.
Yttrium and compounds (yttrium metal; yttrium nitrate hexahydrate; yttrium chloride; yttrium oxide): Dusts may be irritating to the eyes and respiratory tract.	1 mg/m³ (as Y)	500 mg/m³		Appearance varies with compound.
Zinc chloride (CAS: 7646-85-7): Caustic and highly irritating upon direct contact; severe burns may result. Ulceration of exposed skin from exposure to fumes has been reported. Fumes extremely irritating to respiratory tract; pulmonary edema has resulted.	1 mg/m³ (fume)	50 mg/m³		White powder or colorless crystals that absorb moisture. The fume is white and has an acrid odor. Exposure is principally through smoke bombs.
Zinc chromates (basic zinc chromate, $ZnCrO_4$; zinc potassium chromate, $KZn_2(CrO_4)_2(OH)$; zinc yellow): Contains hexavalent chromium which is associated with lung cancer in workers. See also p 139.	0.01 mg/m³ (as Cr), A1			Basic zinc chromate is a yellow pigment; dichromates are orange.

(C) = ceiling air concentration (TLV-C); S = skin absorption can be significant; A1 = ACGIH-confirmed human carcinogen; A2 = ACGIH-suspected human carcinogen; NFPA Hazard Codes: H = health, F = fire, R = reactivity, Ox = oxidizer, W = water-reactive, 0 (none) <—> 4 (severe). ERPG = Emergency Response Planning Guideline. See p 434 for explanation of definitions.

(continued)

TABLE IV-4. HEALTH HAZARD SUMMARIES FOR INDUSTRIAL AND OCCUPATIONAL CHEMICALS (CONTINUED)

Health Hazard Summaries	ACGIH TLV	IDLH	NFPA Codes H F R	Comments
Zinc oxide (CAS: 1314-13-2): Fumes irritating to the respiratory tract. Causes metal fume fever (see p 217). Symptoms include headache, fever, chills, muscle aches, and vomiting.	5 mg/m^3 (fume) 10 mg/m^3 (dusts)	500 mg/m^3		A white or yellowish-white powder. Fumes of zinc oxide are formed when elemental zinc is heated. Principal exposure is through brass foundries or welding on galvanized steel.
Zirconium compounds (zirconium oxide, ZrO$_2$; zirconium oxychloride, ZrOCl; zirconium tetrachloride, ZrCl$_4$): Zirconium compounds are generally of low toxicity. Some compounds are irritating; zirconium tetrachloride releases HCl upon contact with moisture. Granulomata caused by the use of deodorants containing zirconium have been observed. Dermal sensitization has not been reported.	5 mg/m^3 (as Zr)	50 mg/m^3 (as Zr)		The elemental form is a bluish-black powder or a grayish-white, lustrous metal. The finely divided powder can be flammable.

(C) = ceiling air concentration (TLV-C); S = skin absorption can be significant; A1 = ACGIH-confirmed human carcinogen; A2 = ACGIH-suspected human carcinogen; NFPA Hazard Codes: H = health, F = fire, R = reactivity, Ox = oxidizer, W = water-reactive, 0 (none) <—> 4 (severe). ERPG = Emergency Response Planning Guideline. See p 434 for explanation of definitions.

Subject Index

A-200 Pyrinate. *See* **pyrethrins/pyrethroids, 276–277**
A & D ointment, 240*t*. *See also* low-toxicity products, **238–241**
Abate (temephos). *See also* organophosphates and carbamates, **244–248**
  hazard summary for, 518*t*
  toxicity of, 246*t*
Abdomen
  examination of, in diagnosis of poisoning, 28–29
  x-ray studies of
    in caustic and corrosive agent injuries, 131
    cocaine packets visualized by, 144
    in diagnosis of poisoning, **42–43**, 43*t*
Abelcet. *See* amphotericin, 320*t*
Abrus precatorius, 269*t*, 270*t*. *See also* plants and herbal medicines, **265–274**
Abuse
  child, 56, 58–59
  sexual, 59
AC (hydrogen cyanide gas). *See also* cyanide, **150–152**
  as chemical warfare agent, 245*t*
Acarbose. *See also* antidiabetic agents, **81–84**
  toxicity of, 81, 82*t*, 83
Accupril. *See* quinapril, 330*t*
ACE (angiotensin converting enzyme) inhibitors, **62**
  hyperkalemia caused by, 36*t*
  toxicity of, **62**
Acebutolol. *See also* beta-adrenergic blockers, **107–109**
  pharmacokinetics of, 319*t*
  toxicity of, 108*t*
Acephate. *See also* organophosphates and carbamates, **244–248**
  toxicity of, 246*t*
Acetaldehyde, hazard summary for, 434*t*
Acetaminophen, **62–65**
  acetylcysteine for overdose of, 65, 334–335
  anion gap acidosis caused by, 32*t*
  combination products containing, 63
  elimination of, 53*t*
  hepatic failure/hepatotoxicity caused by, 38, 38*t*, 63, 64–65, 64*f*
  metoclopramide for vomiting caused by, 64, 382–383
  ondansetron for vomiting caused by, 64, 395–396
  pharmacokinetics of, 63, 319*t*
  quantitative levels/potential interventions and, 43*t*
  renal failure caused by, 37*t*, 63
  toxicity of, **62–65**
  in toxicology screens, 39*t*, 40*t*
    interferences and, 41*t*
Acetazolamide. *See also* diuretics, **159–160**
  abdominal x-ray showing, 43*t*
  pharmacokinetics of, 319*t*
  toxicity of, 159*t*

Acetic acid (vinegar)
  for cnidarian envenomation, 199
  hazard summary for, 434*t*
  tert-butyl ester of (*tert*-butyl acetate), hazard summary for, 445*t*
Acetic anhydride, hazard summary for, 436*t*
Acetohexamide. *See also* antidiabetic agents, **81–84**
  pharmacokinetics of, 82*t*, 319*t*
  toxicity of, 82, 82*t*
Acetone
  drugs or toxins causing odor of, 30*t*
  estimation of level of from osmolar gap, 31*t*
  hazard summary for, 436*t*
  isopropyl alcohol causing odor of, 197
  osmolar gap elevation caused by, 31*t*
  in toxicology screens, 39*t*, 40*t*
Acetonitrile. *See also* cyanide, **150–152**
  hazard summary for, 436*t*
  job processes associated with exposure to, 422*t*
  toxicity of, 150
Acetophenone, hazard summary for, 436*t*
Acetylcysteine, **334–335**
  for acetaminophen overdose, 65, 334–335
  anaphylactoid reaction caused by, 26*t*, 334
  for carbon tetrachloride poisoning, 127, 334–335
  for chromium poisoning, 140
  for methyl bromide poisoning, 223
  for pennyroyal oil ingestion, 123, 334–335
  pharmacology/use of, **334–335**
Acetylene dichloride (1,2-dichloroethylene), hazard summary for, 462*t*
Acetylene tetrabromide, hazard summary for, 436*t*
Acetylene tetrachloride (1,1,2,2-tetrachloroethane), hazard summary for, 519*t*
Acetylsalicylic acid. *See also* salicylates, **284–286**
  toxicity of, 284
ACGIH (American Conference of Governmental Industrial Hygienists), Threshold Limit Values set by, 429
Achillea millefolium, 271*t*. *See also* plants and herbal medicines, **265–274**
Acid mists, job processes associated with exposure to, 422*t*
"Acid" (slang). *See* lysergic acid diethylamide (LSD), **207–209**
Acidemia, metabolic, bicarbonate for, 346–347
Acidification, urinary, for phencyclidine overdose, 255
Acidosis, metabolic
  anion gap, 31–33
    drugs and toxins causing, 32, 32*t*
    osmolar gap with, 30, 31, 32
    treatment of, 32–33
  antidiabetic agents causing, 81, 83
  bicarbonate for, 345–346
  osmolar gap elevation caused by, 31*t*

NOTE: A *t* following a page number indicates tabular material and an *f* following a page number indicates an illustration. Both proprietary and generic product names are listed in the index. When a proprietary name is used, the reader is encouraged to review the full reference under the generic name for complete information on the product.

Barium chlorate. *See also* barium, **103–104**
toxicity of, 132–133
Barium sulfate, for radiation poisoning, 283*t*
Bark scorpion envenomation, 286–287
Barometric pressure, increased, occupational exposure to, 425
Baroreceptor reflex, bradycardia and atrioventricular
block and, 10
Barthrin. *See also* pyrethrins/pyrethroids,
276–277
toxicity of, 276*t*
Bath oil beads, 240*t*. *See also* low-toxicity products,
238–241
Batteries, button, toxicity of, 129–131
Battery recycling, toxic exposures and, 422*t*
Baygon (propoxur). *See also* organophosphates and
carbamates, **244–248**
hazard summary for, 509*t*
toxicity of, 247*t*
BCG (intravesical). *See also* antineoplastic agents,
88–93
toxicity of, 91*t*
BCME (bis[chloromethyl] ether), hazard summary
for, 452*t*
BCNU (carmustine). *See also* antineoplastic agents,
88–93
toxicity of, 89*t*
1,4-BD (1,4-butanediol), as GHB precursor, 180
Be-still tree, 266*t*. *See also* plants and herbal medicines, **265–274**
Beech, 266*t*. *See also* plants and herbal medicines,
265–274
Beer, monoamine oxidase inhibitor interaction and,
225*t*
Beer potomania, hyponatremia caused by,
34*t*, 35
Beesix. *See* pyridoxine (vitamin B₆), 317–318,
407–408
Begonia *(Begonia rex)*, 266*t*. *See also* plants and
herbal medicines, **265–274**
Belladonna, 266*t*. *See also* plants and herbal medicines, **265–274**
Bellyache bush, 266*t*. *See also* plants and herbal
medicines, **265–274**
Benadryl. *See* diphenhydramine, 84*t*, 85, 86,
359–360
Benadryl Elixir. *See* diphenhydramine, 84*t*, 85, 86,
359–360
Benazepril, pharmacokinetics of, 320*t*
Bendiocarb. *See also* organophosphates and carbamates, **244–248**
toxicity of, 247*t*
Bendroflumethiazide. *See also* diuretics,
159–160
pharmacokinetics of, 320*t*
toxicity of, 159*t*
Benfuracarb. *See also* organophosphates and car-
bamates, **244–248**
toxicity of, 247*t*
Ben Gay Greaseless Stainless Cream. *See*
menthol, 122*t*
salicylates (methyl salicylate), **284–286**
Benlate (benomyl), hazard summary for, 441*t*
Bennies. *See* amphetamines, **68–70**
Benomyl, hazard summary for, 441*t*
Bensulide. *See also* organophosphates and carbamates, **244–248**
toxicity of, 246*t*
Bentonite, as binding agent, 50*t*
Bentyl. *See* dicyclomine, 78*t*
Benylin Cough Syrup. *See* diphenhydramine, 84*t*,
85, 86, **359–360**
Benzalkonium chloride. *See also* detergents,
154–155
toxicity of, 154*t*

Benzene, **104–105**. *See also* hydrocarbons,
183–185
exposure limits for, 104–105, 441*t*
hazard summary for, 441*t*
hematologic disorders caused by, 425
toxicity of, **104–105**
(chloro-methyl)Benzene (benzyl chloride), hazard
summary for, 442*t*
1,2-Benzenediol (catechol), hazard summary for,
449*t*
Benzethonium chloride. *See also* detergents,
154–155
toxicity of, 154*t*
Benzidine, hazard summary for, 442*t*
Benzocaine. *See also* anesthetics, local, **70–72**
toxicity of, 71*t*
in children, 58*t*
Benzodiazepines, **106–107**, **342–344**
coma caused by, 18*t*, 106, 107
treatment of, 19, 107, 369–370
for drug/alcohol withdrawal, 164, 342–344
flumazenil for overdose of, 19, 107, 369–370
pharmacokinetics of, 106, 342–343
pharmacology/use of, **342–344**
for seizures, 342–344
stupor caused by, 18*t*, 106, 107
treatment of, 19, 107
toxicity of, **106–107**
in toxicology screens, 39*t*, 107
Benzonatate. *See also* anesthetics, local, **70–72**
toxicity of, 71*t*
p-Benzoquinone (quinone), hazard summary for,
511*t*
Benzoylecgonine, in toxicology screens, 39*t*
Benzoyl peroxide, hazard summary for, 442*t*
Benzphetamine. *See also* amphetamines, **68–70**
pharmacokinetics of, 320*t*
toxicity of, 68, 69*t*
Benzthiazide, pharmacokinetics of, 320*t*
Benztropine, 78*t*, 258, **344–345**. *See also* anticholinergic agents, **78–79**
for dystonia, 25, 344–345
pharmacokinetics of, 320*t*
pharmacology/use of, **344–345**
toxicity of, 78*t*, 258
in toxicology screens, 39*t*
Benzyl alcohol, anion gap acidosis caused by, 32*t*
Benzyl chloride, hazard summary for, 442*t*
Bepridil. *See also* calcium antagonists, **119–121**
pharmacokinetics of, 320*t*
toxicity of, 120, 120*t*
Berberis spp, 266*t*. *See also* plants and herbal medicines, **265–274**
Beryllium
fibrotic lung disease caused by, 423
hazard summary for, 442*t*
job processes associated with exposure to, 422*t*
Beta-adrenergic agents, **109–111**
for bronchospasm, 9
esmolol for overdose of, 111, 366–367
hyperglycemia caused by, 33*t*, 110
for hyperkalemia, 36
hypokalemia caused by, 36*t*, 37, 110
hypotension caused by, 15*t*, 110, 111
lactic acidosis caused by, 32*t*, 110
pharmacokinetics of, 110
propranolol for overdose of, 111, 405–406
toxicity of, **109–111**
Beta-adrenergic blockers, **107–109**
amrinone for overdose of, 335–336
atrioventricular block caused by, 9*t*, 108
bradycardia caused by, 9*t*
bronchospasm caused by, 8*t*, 109
epinephrine for overdose of, 109, 365–366
glucagon for overdose of, 109, 371–372

Cleocin. *See* clindamycin, 76*t*
Cleopatra's asp envenomation, 294*t*. *See also* snakebites, **293–296**
Clidinium. *See also* anticholinergic agents, **78–79**
  pharmacokinetics of, 322*t*
  toxicity of, 78*t*
Clindamycin. *See also* antibiotics, **75–78**
  toxicity of, 76*t*
Clinoril. *See* sulindac, 238*t*
Clitocybe mushrooms. *See also* mushroom poisoning, **227–230**
  cerusata, muscarine toxicity and, 227*t*
  clavipes, coprine toxicity and, 227*t*
  dealbata, muscarine toxicity and, 227*t*
Clofibrate
  rhabdomyolysis associated with, 25*t*
  syndrome of inappropriate ADH secretion caused by, 34*t*
Clomipramine. *See also* tricyclic antidepressants, **310–312**
  monoamine oxidase inhibitor interaction and, 225*t*
  pharmacokinetics of, 322*t*
  toxicity of, 310*t*
Clonazepam. *See also* benzodiazepines, **106–107**
  pharmacokinetics of, 322*t*
  toxicity of, 106*t*
Clonidine, **141–142**
  atrioventricular block caused by, 9*t*
  bradycardia caused by, 9*t*
  coma caused by, 18*t*
  hypertension caused by, 17*t*
  hypotension caused by, 15*t*
  miosis caused by, 29*t*
  naloxone for overdose of, 142, 384–386
  pharmacokinetics of, 322*t*
  stupor caused by, 18*t*
  toxicity of, **141–142**
  ventilatory failure caused by, 6*t*
Clorazepate. *See also* benzodiazepines, **106–107**
  pharmacokinetics of, 322*t*
  toxicity of, 106*t*
Clorox Liquid Bleach. *See* hypochlorite, 134–136, 240*t*
Clorox 2 Powdered Laundry Bleach. *See* detergents (sodium carbonate), **154–155**
Clostridium
  botulinum, 112. *See also* botulism, **112–114**
  perfringens, food poisoning caused by, 173*t*. *See also* food poisoning, bacterial, **173–174**
  tetani, 301. *See also* tetanus, **301–302**
Clothing, protective, for response in hazardous materials incident, 416
Clotrimazole cream, 240*t*. *See also* low-toxicity products, **238–241**
Clove oil. *See also* essential oils, **122–123**
  toxicity of, 122*t*
Clover, sweet, 148, 271*t*. *See also* coumarin, **148–150**
Clozapine. *See also* antipsychotic drugs, **257–259**
  pharmacokinetics of, 322*t*
  rhabdomyolysis associated with, 25*t*
  seizures caused by, 22*t*
  toxicity of, 257*t*, 258
Clozaril. *See* clozapine, 257*t*, 258
CMME (chloromethyl methyl ether), hazard summary for, 452*t*
Cnidaria envenomation, **198–199**
CO. *See* carbon monoxide, **125–126**
Coal tar creosote. *See also* phenols, **255–257**
  hazard summary for, 456*t*
  toxicity of, 255–257
Coal tar pitch volatiles, hazard summary for, 454*t*
Coal workers' pneumoconiosis, 423
Cobalt/cobalt compounds, hazard summary for, 455*t*

Cobalt hydrocarbonyl, hazard summary for, 455*t*
Cobalt-tungsten carbide, fibrotic lung disease caused by, 423
Cobra envenomation, 294*t*. *See also* snakebites, **293–296**
Cocaethylene. *See also* cocaine, **142–145**
  toxicity of, 143
Cocaine, **142–145**
  agitation caused by, 23*t*, 143
  bromocriptine to reduce craving for, 349
  dyskinesias caused by, 24*t*
  with heroin ("speedball"), 142
  hypertension caused by, 17*t*, 143
  hyperthermia associated with, 20*t*, 143, 144
  hypoxia caused by, 7*t*
  monoamine oxidase inhibitor interaction and, 225*t*
  mydriasis caused by, 29*t*
  for nasotracheal intubation, 5
  pharmacokinetics of, 143, 322*t*
  phentolamine for overdose of, 145, 400–401
  propranolol for overdose of, 145, 405–406
  psychosis caused by, 23*t*
  renal failure caused by, 37*t*
  rhabdomyolysis associated with, 25*t*, 37*t*, 144
  seizures caused by, 22*t*, 143
  tachycardia caused by, 12*t*, 143, 144
  toxicity of, 71*t*, **142–145**
  in toxicology screens, 39*t*
  ventricular arrhythmias caused by, 13*t*, 143, 144
Cockroach Wipeout Chalk. *See* Chinese chalk, 276
COCl₂ (phosgene), **262–263**. *See also* gases, irritant, **181–183**
  as chemical warfare agent, 245*t*
  exposure limits for, 262–263, 505*t*
  hazard summary for, 505*t*
  job processes associated with exposure to, 422*t*
  toxicity of, 182*t*, 245*t*, **262–263**
Codeine. *See also* opiates/opioids, **242–244**
  pharmacokinetics of, 322*t*
  toxicity of, 242*t*
    in children, 58*t*
  in toxicology screens, 39*t*
  interferences and, 42*t*
Coffeeberry, 267*t*. *See also* plants and herbal medicines, **265–274**
Coffee tree, Kentucky, 269*t*. *See also* plants and herbal medicines, **265–274**
Cogentin. *See* benztropine, 78*t*, 258, **344–345**
Cohosh. *See also* plants and herbal medicines, **265–274**
  black, 266*t*
  blue, 266*t*
"Coke burns," 144. *See also* cocaine, **142–145**
Cola nut, 267*t*. *See also* plants and herbal medicines, **265–274**
ColBENEMID. *See* colchicine, **145–146**
Colchicine, **145–146**
  pharmacokinetics of, 322*t*
  rhabdomyolysis associated with, 25*t*, 145, 146
  toxicity of, 15*t*, **145–146**
Colchicine-specific antibodies, Fab fragments of, for colchicine overdose, 146
Colchicum autumnale, 145, 266*t*, 269*t*. *See also* colchicine, **145–146**; plants and herbal medicines, **265–274**
Cold packs. *See also* nitrites, **233–234**; nontoxic products, **238–241**
  accidental exposure to, 240*t*
Cold remedies, decongestants in, **259–261**
Cold zone (Support Zone), at hazardous materials incident site, 411, 412*f*
  victim management in, 417
Colic, lead, 200, 201
Colocasia spp, 268*t*. *See also* plants and herbal medicines, **265–274**

Cyclophosphamide. *See also* antineoplastic agents, **88–93**
  as teratogen, 57*t*
  toxicity of, 89*t*
Cycloserine
  agitation caused by, 23*t*
  psychosis caused by, 23*t*
  pyridoxine for overdose of, 407–408
Cyclospora, food-borne diarrhea caused by, 173
Cyclosporin, renal failure caused by, 37*t*
Cyclothiazide. *See also* diuretics, **159–160**
  toxicity of, 159*t*
Cycrin. *See* medroxyprogesterone, 91*t*
Cylert. *See* pemoline, 69*t*
Cymethrin. *See also* pyrethrins/pyrethroids, **276–277**
  toxicity of, 276*t*
Cypermethrin. *See also* pyrethrins/pyrethroids, **276–277**
  toxicity of, 276, 276*t*
Cyperus alternifolius, 271*t*. *See also* plants and herbal medicines, **265–274**
Cyproheptadine. *See also* antihistamines, **84–86**
  pharmacokinetics of, 322*t*
  for serotonin syndrome, 21, 81, 227
  toxicity of, 85*t*
Cystospaz. *See* hyoscyamine, 78*t*
Cytarabine. *See also* antineoplastic agents, **88–93**
  as teratogen, 57*t*
  toxicity of, 90*t*
Cythioate. *See also* organophosphates and carbamates, **244–248**
  toxicity of, 246*t*
Cytisus spp, 267*t*, 270*t*. *See also* plants and herbal medicines, **265–274**
Cytosar-U. *See* cytarabine, 90*t*
Cytoxan. *See* cyclophosphamide, 89*t*

2,4-D (dichlorophenoxyacetic acid)
  in Agent Orange, 137
  hazard summary for, 463*t*
  toxicity of, 137
D-con Mouse Prufe. *See* warfarin, 148–150
D-con Mouse Prufe II. *See* brodifacoum, 148
Dacarbazine. *See also* antineoplastic agents, **88–93**
  extravasation of, 93
  toxicity of, 91*t*, 93
Dactin (1,3-dichloro 5,5-dimethylhydantoin), hazard summary for, 462*t*
Dactinomyin. *See also* antineoplastic agents, **88–93**
  extravasation of, 93
  toxicity of, 89*t*, 93
Daffodil (bulb), 267*t*. *See also* plants and herbal medicines, **265–274**
Dalgan. *See* dezocine, 322*t*
Dalmane. *See* flurazepam, 106*t*
"DANs" (slang). *See* carisoprodol, 292, 292*t*
Dantrium. *See* dantrolene, **354–355**
Dantrolene, **354–355**
  for malignant hyperthermia, 21, 354–355
  pharmacology/use of, **354–355**
Daphne, 267*t*. *See also* plants and herbal medicines, **265–274**
Dapsone
  for *Loxosceles* spider envenomation, 298
  pharmacokinetics of, 322*t*
  toxicity of, 76*t*, 77, 78, **152–154**
Daranide. *See* dichlorphenamide, 159*t*
Darvocet N-50/N-100. *See*
  acetaminophen, **62–65**
  propoxyphene, 242*t*, 243
Darvon. *See* propoxyphene, 242*t*, 243
Darvon Compound. *See*
  aspirin, **284–286**

caffeine, **118–119**
  propoxyphene, 242*t*, 243
"Date rape" drug, GHB as, 180
Datura stramonium, 269*t*. *See also* plants and herbal medicines, **265–274**
Daubentonia spp, 270*t*. *See also* plants and herbal medicines, **265–274**
Daunorubicin. *See also* antineoplastic agents, **88–93**
  extravasation of, 93
  toxicity of, 89*t*, 93
DaunoXome. *See* daunorubicin, 89*t*, 93
Day jessamine, 269*t*. *See also* plants and herbal medicines, **265–274**
Daypro. *See* oxaprozin, 238*t*
DBCP (1,2-dibromo-3-chloropropane), hazard summary for, 460*t*
DDT. *See also* chlorinated hydrocarbons, **133–134**
  hazard summary for, 459*t*
  toxicity of, 133, 133*t*
DDVP (dichlorvos). *See also* organophosphates and carbamates, **244–248**
  hazard summary for, 464*t*
  toxicity of, 246*t*
DDVP (propoxur). *See also* organophosphates and carbamates, **244–248**
  hazard summary for, 509*t*
  toxicity of, 247*t*
Deadline for Slugs and Snails. *See* metaldehyde, **216–217**
Deadly nightshade, 267*t*, 270*t*. *See also* plants and herbal medicines, **265–274**
DEAE (2-diethylaminoethanol), hazard summary for, 465*t*
Deapril-ST. *See* ergoloid derivatives, 160–162
Death camas, 267*t*. *See also* plants and herbal medicines, **265–274**
Decaborane, hazard summary for, 459*t*
Decamethrin. *See also* pyrethrins/pyrethroids, **276–277**
  toxicity of, 276*t*
Declomycin. *See* demeclocycline, 77*t*
Decongestants, **259–261**
  pharmacokinetics of, 259
  phentolamine for overdose of, 260, 400–401
  toxicity of, **259–261**
Decontamination
  in emergency evaluation and treatment, 3*f*, **43–50**
  eyes, 44, 45*f*
  gastrointestinal, **45–50**
  for hazardous materials exposure
    at hospital, 418
    at incident site, 416–417
  inhalation, 44–45
  skin, 43–44, 44*t*
  surface, **43–45**
DEET (diethyltoluamide), seizures caused by, 22*t*
DEF. *See also* organophosphates and carbamates, **244–248**
  toxicity of, 246*t*
Deferoxamine, **355–356**
  for iron poisoning, 193–194, 355–356
  pharmacology/use of, **355–356**
Defibrillation (direct-current countershock), for ventricular fibrillation, 14
Degreasers, occupational exposure to, 421, 422*t*
Degreaser's flush, 308, 309
Dehydration, hypernatremia caused by, 34
Delirium, **23–24**
  drugs and toxins causing, 23*t*
  treatment of, 23–24
    haloperidol for, 24, 373–374
Delirium tremens (DTs), 163
Delphinium, 269*t*. *See also* plants and herbal medicines, **265–274**

Fool's parsley, 268t. *See also* plants and herbal medicines, **265–274**
Forced diuresis, for enhanced elimination, 52
Foreign bodies, metallic, abdominal x-ray showing, 43t
Fork lift/compressor operation, indoor, toxic exposures and, 422t
Formaldehyde, **177–178**. *See also* caustic and corrosive agents, **129–131**; gases, irritant, **181–183**
  anion gap acidosis caused by, 32t, 130t, 177
  exposure limits for, 177, 182t, 477t
  hazard summary for, 477t
  methanol metabolized to, 218
  toxicity of, 130t, **177–178**, 182t
Formalin (formaldehyde aqueous solution)
  hazard summary for, 477t
  methanol in, 177, 178
  toxicity of, 177–178
Formamide, hazard summary for, 477t
Formate (formic acid) poisoning, 130t, 177–178
  methanol intoxication and, 218, 219
Formetanate. *See also* organophosphates and carbamates, **244–248**
  toxicity of, 247t
Formic acid, hazard summary for, 477t
Formic aldehyde (formaldehyde), **177–178**. *See also* caustic and corrosive agents, **129–131**; gases, irritant, **181–183**
  anion gap acidosis caused by, 32t, 130t, 177
  exposure limits for, 177, 182t, 477t
  hazard summary for, 477t
  methanol metabolized to, 218
  toxicity of, 130t, **177–178**, 182t
Formicidae (ant) bites, 189–190
Formothion. *See also* organophosphates and carbamates, **244–248**
  toxicity of, 246t
Fosinopril, pharmacokinetics of, 324t
Fosphenytoin, **401–402**. *See also* phenytoin, **261–262**
  pharmacokinetics of, 324t, 401
  pharmacology/use of, **401–402**
Four o'clock, 268t. *See also* plants and herbal medicines, **265–274**
Foxglove, 128, 268t. *See also* cardiac (digitalis) glycosides, **128–129**; plants and herbal medicines, **265–274**
"Free base" cocaine. *See also* cocaine, **142–145**
  toxicity of, 143
Free erythrocyte protoporphyrin (FEP), in lead poisoning, 201
Freon 11 (trichlorofluoromethane)
  hazard summary for, 524t
  toxicity of, 178–179
Freon 12 (dichlorodifluoromethane)
  hazard summary for, 461t
  toxicity of, 178–179
Freon 12B2 (difluorodibromoethane), hazard summary for, 465t
Freon 13B1 (trifluorobromomethane), hazard summary for, 525t
Freon 21 (dichlorofluoromethane)
  hazard summary for, 463t
  toxicity of, 178–179
Freon 22 (chlorodifluoromethane)
  hazard summary for, 452t
  toxicity of, 178–179
Freon 23 (trifluoromethane), hazard summary for, 525t
Freon 113 (1,1,2-trichloro-1,2,2-trifluoroethane)
  hazard summary for, 525t
  toxicity of, 178–179
Freon 114 (dichlorotetrafluoroethane)
  hazard summary for, 464t
  toxicity of, 178–179

Freons (fluorinated hydrocarbons), **178–179**
  exposure limits for, 178–179
  propranolol for poisoning caused by, 405–406
  toxicity of, **178–179**
  ventricular arrhythmias caused by, 13t, 178, 179, 428
Frostbite, liquid sulfur dioxide causing, 300
Fuller's earth, as binding agent, 50t
Fumes, combustion, occupational exposure to, 421
Fumigation, toxic exposures and, 422t
Fungizone. *See* amphotericin, 320t
Furadan (carbofuran). *See also* organophosphates and carbamates, **244–248**
  hazard summary for, 448t
  toxicity of, 247t
Furamethrin. *See also* pyrethrins/pyrethroids, **276–277**
  toxicity of, 276t
2,5-Furandione (maleic anhydride), hazard summary for, 487t
Furazolidone. *See also* monoamine oxidase inhibitors, **225–227**
  toxicity of, 225–227
Furfural, hazard summary for, 477t
Furfuryl alcohol, hazard summary for, 477t
Furniture polish, toxicity of, 184
Furniture refinishing, toxic exposures and, 422t
Furosemide. *See also* diuretics, **159–160**
  for bromide poisoning, 117
  pharmacokinetics of, 324t
  toxicity of, 159t
Furoxone. *See* furazolidone, 225–227

"G caps" (slang). *See* **gamma hydroxybutyrate (GHB), 179–181**
G-CSF (granulocyte colony-stimulating factor), for colchicine overdose, 146
GA (tabun). *See also* organophosphates and carbamates, **244–248**
  as chemical warfare agent, 245t
Gaboon viper envenomation, 294t. *See also* snakebites, **293–296**
Gag reflex, airway assessment and, 1
Galerina mushrooms. *See also* mushroom poisoning, **227–230**
  autumnalis, toxicity of, 228–230
  marginata, toxicity of, 228–230
  toxicity of, 227t, 228–230
Galium odoratum, 271t. *See also* plants and herbal medicines, **265–274**
Gamma butyrolactone, as GHB precursor, 180
Gamma-hexachlorocyclohexane (lindane). *See also* chlorinated hydrocarbons, **133–134**
  hazard summary for, 486t
  toxicity of, 133t
    in children, 58t
  volume of distribution of, 51t
Gamma Hydrate. *See* gamma hydroxybutyrate (GHB), **179–181**
Gamma hydroxybutyrate (GHB), **179–181**
  coma caused by, 18t, 180
  dyskinesias caused by, 24t
  pharmacokinetics of, 324t
  seizures caused by, 22t, 181
  stupor caused by, 18t, 180
  toxicity of, **179–181**
Gamma OH. *See* gamma hydroxybutyrate (GHB), **179–181**
Garamycin. *See* gentamicin, 76t
Garlic. *See also* plants and herbal medicines, **265–274**
  drugs or toxins causing odor of, 30t
  toxicity of, 272t
Gas-shielded welding, toxic exposures and, 422t

food poisoning caused by, 175–176, 176*t*
  cimetidine/H₂ blockers for, 176, 353–354
  diphenhydramine for, 176, 359–360
"Scoop" (slang). *See* gamma hydroxybutyrate (GHB), **179–181**
Scope Mouthwash. *See* ethanol, **162–164**
Scopolamine. *See also* anticholinergic agents, **78–79**
  pharmacokinetics of, 330*t*
  toxicity of, 78*t*
Scorpaenidae envenomation, **203–204**
Scorpion envenomation, **286–287**
Scotch broom, 267*t*, 270*t*. *See also* plants and herbal medicines, **265–274**
Scrub Free Heavy Duty Bathroom Cleaner
  non-phosphate formula (hydroxyacetic acid, sulfamic acid). *See* caustic and corrosive agents, **129–131**
  phosphate formula (hydroxyacetic acid, phosphoric acid). *See* caustic and corrosive agents, **129–131**
Sea nettle envenomation, 198–199
  American (*Chrysaora quinquecirrha*), treatment of, 199
Sea snake envenomation, 294*t*. *See also* snakebites, **293–296**
Sea wasp envenomation, 198–199
Seafood,
  anaphylactic reaction caused by, 26*t*
  arsenobetaine and arsenocholine in, 95, 96
  food poisoning caused by, **175–176**
Secobarbital. *See also* barbiturates, **101–103**
  pharmacokinetics of, 331*t*
  toxicity of, 102*t*
Seconal. *See* secobarbital, 102*t*
Sectral. *See* acebutolol, 108*t*
Sedation, conscious, midazolam for, 342–344
Sedative-hypnotics, **287–289**. *See also* barbiturates, **101–103**; benzodiazepines, **106–107**
  coma caused by, 18*t*
  for dyskinesia, 25
  hypotension caused by, 15*t*
  hypothermia associated with, 19*t*
  hypoxia caused by, 7*t*
  rhabdomyolysis associated with, 25*t*
  for rigidity, 25
  stupor caused by, 18*t*
  toxicity of, **287–289**
  in toxicology screens, 39*t*, 40*t*
  ventilatory failure caused by, 6*t*
  withdrawal from
    confusion caused by, 23*t*
    diazepam and lorazepam for, 342–344
    hypertension caused by, 17*t*
    hyperthermia associated with, 20*t*
    seizures caused by, 22*t*
    tachycardia caused by, 12*t*
Seizures, **21–23**
  anion gap acidosis and, 32*t*
  drugs and toxins causing, 22*t*
  rhabdomyolysis associated with, 25*t*
  treatment of, 22–23
    benzodiazepines for, 342–344
    fosphenytoin for, 401–402
    pentobarbital for, 23, 398–399
    phenobarbital for, 22, 399–400
    phenytoin for, 22–23, 261, 401–402
Seldane. *See* terfenadine, 85*t*, 86
Selegiline. *See also* monoamine oxidase inhibitors, **225–227**
  toxicity of, 225–227
Selenious acid (gun bluing). *See also* selenium, **289–291**
  toxicity of, 289, 290
  in children, 58*t*
Selenium, **289–291**
  hazard summary for, 512*t*

odor caused by, 30*t*, 290
toxicity of, **289–291**
Selenium dioxide (selenium oxide), hazard summary for, 512*t*
Selenium hexafluoride. *See also* selenium, **289–291**
  hazard summary for, 513*t*
  toxicity of, 290*t*
Selenium hydride (hydrogen selenide). *See also* selenium, **289–291**
  hazard summary for, 481*t*
  toxicity of, 290, 290*t*
Selenium oxide (selenium dioxide), hazard summary for, 512*t*
Selenium oxychloride, hazard summary for, 513*t*
Selenomethionine. *See also* selenium, **289–291**
  toxicity of, 289–290
Self-contained breathing apparatus (SCBA), for personal protection during response in hazardous materials incidents, 416
Semprex-D. *See*
  acrivastine, 85*t*
  pseudoephedrine, 259–261
Senecio spp, 267*t*, 268*t*, 270*t*, 271*t*. *See also* plants and herbal medicines, **265–274**
Senna. *See also* plants and herbal medicines, **265–274**
  toxicity of, 273*t*
Sensorcaine. *See* bupivacaine, 71*t*
Septra. *See*
  sulfonamides (sulfamethoxazole), 77*t*
  trimethoprim, 77, 77*t*
Serax. *See* oxazepam, 106*t*
Serentil. *See* mesoridazine, 257*t*
Serotonin reuptake inhibitors (SSRIs), 80
  agitation caused by, 24*t*
  dyskinesias caused by, 24*t*
  psychosis caused by, 23*t*
  seizures caused by, 22*t*
  toxicity of, 80
Serotonin syndrome, 21, 80
  dextromethorphan causing, 155, 156
  in monoamine oxidase inhibitor overdose, 227
  treatment of, 21, 81
Serotonin uptake inhibitors. *See* serotonin reuptake inhibitors (SSRIs), 80
Sertraline. *See also* antidepressants, noncyclic, **79–81**
  monoamine oxidase inhibitor interaction and, 225*t*, 226
  pharmacokinetics of, 331*t*
  toxicity of, 79, 80*t*
Serum osmolality, in diagnosis of poisoning, 30–31, 31*t*
Serzone. *See* nefazodone, 79, 80*t*
Sesbania spp, 268*t*, 270*t*. *See also* plants and herbal medicines, **265–274**
Sevin (carbaryl). *See also* organophosphates and carbamates, **244–248**
  hazard summary for, 448*t*
  pralidoxime in poisoning caused by, 403–404
  toxicity of, 247*t*
Sewage work, toxic exposures and, 422*t*
Sewer gas (hydrogen sulfide), **188**
  anion gap acidosis caused by, 32*t*
  coma caused by, 18*t*, 188
  exposure limits for, 188, 482*t*
  hazard summary for, 482*t*
  hypoxia caused by, 7*t*, 8
  job/occupaional processes associated with exposure to, 422*t*, 425
  nitrites for poisoning caused by, 188, 390–392
  odor caused by, 30*t*, 188
  seizures caused by, 22*t*, 188
  stupor caused by, 18*t*, 188
  tachycardia caused by, 12*t*
  toxicity of, **188**